Nutrition and the Cancer Patient

Nutrition and the Cancer Patient

Edited by

Egidio Del Fabbro

Vickie Baracos

Wendy Demark-Wahnefried

Tim Bowling

Jane Hopkinson

Eduardo Bruera

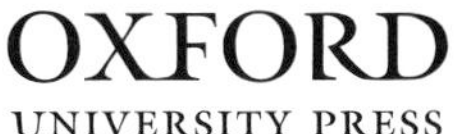

OXFORD
UNIVERSITY PRESS

Great Clarendon Street, Oxford OX2 6DP

Oxford University Press is a department of the University of Oxford.
It furthers the University's objective of excellence in research, scholarship,
and education by publishing worldwide in

Oxford New York

Auckland Cape Town Dar es Salaam Hong Kong Karachi
Kuala Lumpur Madrid Melbourne Mexico City Nairobi
New Delhi Shanghai Taipei Toronto

With offices in

Argentina Austria Brazil Chile Czech Republic France Greece
Guatemala Hungary Italy Japan Poland Portugal Singapore
South Korea Switzerland Thailand Turkey Ukraine Vietnam

Oxford is a registered trade mark of Oxford University Press
in the UK and in certain other countries

Published in the United States
by Oxford University Press Inc., New York

First published 2010

British Library Cataloguing in Publication Data
Data available

Library of Congress Cataloging in Publication Data
Data available

Typeset in Minion by Glyph International, Bangalore, India
Printed in Great Britain
on acid-free paper by
CPI Antony Rowe, Chippenham, Wiltshire

ISBN 978–0–19–955019–7

10 9 8 7 6 5 4 3 2 1

Foreword

Nutrition and its impact on cancer is a topic which captivates public interest. Newspaper articles commonly report on dietary elements which may affect cancer growth. As any family practitioner or oncologist will attest to, our patients and loved ones scour the internet for information, often misleading on nutritional therapies. We must recognize community concerns and benefit from their stimulus to learn more about nutrition, a topic often undertaught and, perhaps, not sufficiently respected within our clinics.

Patients may be concerned about loss of appetite and reduced food intake; but their families are usually more distressed. Their efforts to sustain the nutrition of a loved one must be honored, an enterprise successful when carried out by a health care team, but difficult when left to a busy single practitioner.

Nutrition and the Cancer Patient fully addresses nutritional issues arising in cancer care, with an emphasis on the Cancer Anorexia- Cachexia Syndrome. Indeed, it is the first major textbook to do so. It will certainly be welcomed by oncologists and palliative care physicians and other health professionals concerned with the envelope of care of cancer patients and their families. The book has wider appeal as much of what we know about cancer cachexia informs the all too common wasting syndrome encountered in patients with other chronic disorders such as congestive failure and the frail elderly.

Cachexia, usually linked with anorexia, fatigue and functional loss, is the single biggest symptom complex bedeviling the lives of advanced cancer patients. Symptoms can kill; anorexia-cachexia is estimated to bring about twenty to twenty-five per cent of cancer deaths. Thus, anorexia-cachexia is a source of profound suffering and yet it has received disproportionate attention by researchers and clinicians alike. Few laboratories have studied it and clinical research has lagged. Why the disconnect? There is a Chinese proverb that goes: the start of wisdom is to call things by their right name—well we haven't had a commonly accepted definition of cachexia—not having a clearly defined target makes it difficult to rally around that target. This may lead to despair that such a complex issue can ever be sorted out and coupled with this a lack of intellectual interest; one senses that many oncologists simply regard cachexia as the price of having advanced cancer.

An amazing self-reinforcing system is revealed which can tie together what appear to be disparate effects such as muscle wasting, autonomic dysfunction, mitochondrial changes, anorexia et al into a not as yet quite coherent system. While much remains to be learned, today we know we do have tools to help arrest tumor wasting; we have promising clinical research leads based on our new insights and we know that we must come together to form translational research groups and clinical interdisciplinary teams to contest the nutritional complexities which both enhance tumor progression and induce patient and family suffering.

Nutrition and the Cancer Patient is a comprehensive text. Yes, the basic science of anorexia-cachexia is well covered, as is nutritional assessment and use of dietary aids and drugs, enteral and parenteral therapies. The editors recognize that nutritional success depends on more than food and pharmacy. Thus there are excellent chapters on exercise therapy, the management of depression and other symptoms which impact on energy intake and application. There is a scholarly entry on complimentary and alternative therapies; a very important topic in view of widespread public interest. The spiritual and cultural issues which influence patient and family wishes and the needs of special populations are recognized. All of the above need to be integrated into a therapeutic plan, a task well addressed in Nutrition and Cancer.

Dr Del Fabbro and his associates have published an extremely timely book, bringing us up to date on dietary management today, presaging the advances of the foreseeable future. The chapters by Dr Baracos and her colleagues are the most lucid accounts of the pathophysiology of wasting in our cancer patients that I have read; they translate seamlessly into the subsequent clinical chapters. The chapters on assessment stressing early diagnosis and primary management and emphasizing the role of dietitians in our teams are particularly noted. Indeed, the editors and their selection of authors and the authors' emphasis on teamwork in their texts stress the underlying value of a team approach to cachexia research and care. Of note, patients and families are recognized as team members. In this enterprise they are actively involved and not just passive recipients of care.

Nutrition and the Cancer Patient should be in the library of every health professional sustaining cancer patients with symptom problems. Clinical oncologists are in this coterie. Which oncologists? All of them, as the presence of cachexia colors the decisions equally of the surgeon, the radiotherapist, the hematologist and the medical oncologist. I believe it will also be of interest to the general surgeon and internist, to the dietitian community and rehabilitation experts of all stripes. One fervently hopes that the book may find its way into the hands of students and residents. It will help shed that negative spirit sometimes surrounding the advanced cancer patient and teach them about an exciting field with approaches of great promise.

PROFESSOR NEIL MACDONALD,
Founding Director of McGill Cancer Nutrition and Rehabilitation Programme,
McGill University, Montreal,
Québec, Canada

Contents

Contributors

Inga Andrew MRPharmS BPharm (Hons)
Dip Clin Pharm SP
Senior Clinical Pharmacist,
County Durham and Darlington NHS Foundation Trust,
University Hospital of North Durham,
Durham, UK

Sami Antoun MD
Department of Supportive Care,
Institut Gustave Roussy,
Villejuif, France

Tessa Aston RD MSc BSc (Hons)
Macmillan Specialist Dietitian,
Specialist Palliative Care Team,
North Yorkshire & York NHS Trust
UK

Christopher Bailey RGN PhD MSc BA (Hons)
Lecturer Senior Research Fellow,
School of Health Sciences,
University of Southampton,
Nightingale Building,
Southampton, UK

Casey Balentine Azuero MPH
Holistic Care coordinator,
University of Alabama at Birmingham,
Center for Palliative Care,
and University of Alabama at Birmingham,
Division of Preventive Medicine,
Birmingham, Alabama, USA

Vickie E. Baracos PhD
Professor & Alberta Cancer Foundation Chair in Palliative Medicine,
University of Alberta,
Edmonton, Canada

Rachel A. Barrett
Principal Oncology Dietician
Principal Haematology/Oncology Dietitian,
Guy's and St Thomas' NHS Foundation Trust,
London, UK

Eran Ben-Arye MD
Director,
Integrative Oncology Program,
Oncology Service,
Lin Medical Center,
Clalit Health Services,
Haifa and Western Galilee District, Israel
and Complementary and Traditional Medicine Unit,
Lecturer,
Department of Family Medicine,
Bruce Rappaport Faculty of Medicine,
Technion, Israel Institute of Technology,
Haifa, Israel

Trevelyan Beyer BSc (Hons) PT MCSP
Physiotherapist,
St Cuthbert's Hospice,
Merryoaks
Durham, UK

David Blum MD
Clinical Research Fellow,
Oncological Palliative Medicine,
Division of Oncology/Hematology,
Department of Internal Medicine and Palliative Care Center,
Cantonal Hospital,
St Gallen, Switzerland

Tim E. Bowling MBBS MD FRCP
Consultant in Gastroenterology and
Clinical Nutrition,
Nottingham University Hospitals,
Nottingham, UK

Eduardo Bruera MD
Professor of Medicine,
F.T. McGraw Chair in the treatment of cancer
Department of Palliative Care and
Rehabilitation Medicine,
University of Texas M. D. Anderson Cancer
Center,
Houston, Texas, USA

Jacqueline Cairns BSc (Hons) OT MCOT
Occupational Therapist,
St. Cuthbert's Hospice,
Merryoaks,
Durham,UK

Marina Chiara Garassino MD
Oncology Department,
Fatebenefratelli and Ophthalmic Hospital,
Milan, Italy

Shalini Dalal MD
Assistant Professor,
Department of Palliative Care and
Rehabilitation Medicine,
University of Texas M. D. Anderson Cancer
Center,
Houston, Texas, USA

Mellar P. Davis MD FCCP
Professor of Medicine,
Cleveland Clinic Lerner School of Medicine,
Case Western Reserve University,
Director,Clinical fellowship,
Palliative Medicine and Supportive Oncology
Services,
Division of Solid Tumor,
Taussig Cancer Institute,
The Cleveland Clinic Foundation,
Cleveland, Ohio, USA

Marvin Omar Delgado Guay MD
Assistant Professor,
University of Texas Health Science Center at
Houston,
Department of Internal Medicine,
Division of Geriatrics and Palliative Medicine,
Lyndon B. Johnson General Hospital,
Houston, Texas, USA

Wendy Demark-Wahnefried PhD RD
Professor of Nutrition Science
University of Alaboma at Birmingham
Associate Director of the UAB
Comprehensive Cancer Center, USA

Laura Elliott MPH RD CSO LD
Clinical Dietition,
Mary Greeley Medical Center,
Ames, Iowa, USA,

Egidio del Fabbro MD
Assistant Professor of Palliative Care and
Rehabilitation,
The University of Texas M. D. Anderson
Cancer Center,
Houston, Texas, USA

Nada Fadul MD
Assistant Professor,
Department of Palliative Care and
Rehabilitation Medicine,
University of Texas M. D. Anderson Cancer
Center,
Houston, Texas, USA

Gabriella Farina MD
Oncology Department,
Fatebenefratelli and Ophthalmic Hospital,
Milan, Italy

Moshe Frenkel MD
Associate Professor,
Integrative Medicine Program,
University of Texas M. D. Anderson Cancer
Center, Houston, TX, USA

Jose Garcia MD
Assistant Professor,
Division of Diabetes,
Endocrinology and Metabolism,
Baylor College of Medicine,
Michael DeBakey Veterans
Affairs Medical Center,
Houston, Texas, USA

Ioannis Gioulbasanis MD
Department of Medical Oncology,
University General Hospital of Heraklion,
Heraklion, Crete, Greece

Liz Gwyther MB ChB FCFP MSc Pall Med
Senior Lecturer,
Department of Family Medicine,
University of Cape Town
Cape Town, South Africa,
and Executive Director,
Hospice Palliative Care Association of South Africa

Bob Hansford
Volunteer,
St Benedict's Hospice,
Sunderland, UK

Richard Harding BSc (Joint Hons) MSc DipSW PhD
Senior Lecturer,
King's College London,
Department of Palliative Care,
Policy & Rehabilitation,
London, UK

Colette Hawkins BSc MBBS MRCP
Macmillan Consultant in Palliative Medicine,
University Hospital of North Durham,
County Durham and Darlington NHS Foundation Trust,
Durham, UK

Martin Hewitt BSc BM MD MS FRCP FRCPCH
Consultant in Paediatric Medicine & Paediatric Oncology & Child Health
Department of Child Health,
Queens Medical Centre Campus,
Nottingham University Hospital,
Nottingham, UK

Jane Hopkinson RGN PhD MSc BSc (Hons)
Macmillan Post Doctoral Research Fellow,
School of Health Sciences,
University of Southampton,
Southampton, UK

Richard D. Johnston MSc MRCP
Clinical Research Fellow,
Wolfson Digestive Diseases Centre,
University Hospital Nottingham
Nottingham, UK

Lee W. Jones PhD
Associate Professor,
Scientific Director,
Duke Center for Cancer Survivorship,
Department of Radiation Oncology,
Duke University Medical Center,
Durham, North Carolina, USA

Sian Kirkham BSc (Hons) MBBS MRCPCH
Consultant in Paediatric Gastroenterology,
Hepatology & Nutrition,
Nottingham University Hospitals,
Nottingham, UK

Elizabeth Kvale MD
Assistant Professor,
Birmingham Veterans Administration Medical Center,
and University of Alabama at Birmingham,
Center for Palliative Care,
Birmingham, Alabama, USA

Nicla La Verde MD
Oncology Department,
Fatebenefratelli and Ophthalmic Hospital,
Milan, Italy

Dileep N. Lobo MS DM FRCS
Associate Professor & Reader,
Division of Gastrointestinal Surgery,
Nottingham Digestive Diseases Centre
Biomedical Research Unit,
Nottingham University Hospitals,
Queen's Medical Centre,
Nottingham, UK

Susan E. McClement RN PhD
Associate Professor,
Faculty of Nursing, University of Manitoba,
and Research Associate
Manitoba Palliative Care Research Unit
Winnipeg, Manitoba, Canada

Dena Norton RD
Clinical Dietition,
Integrative Medicine Program,
University of Texas M. D. Anderson Cancer Center, Houston,
Texas, USA

Alejandra Palma MD
Instructor, Program of Palliative Medicine,
Medical School, Pontificia Universidad Católica de Chile,
Santiago, Chile

Barbara Parry MSc RD
Senior Research Dietitian,
Winchester and Andover Breast Unit,
Royal Hampshire County Hospital,
Winchester, UK

Henrique A. Parsons MD
Postdoctorial fellow,
Department of Palliative Care and Rehabilitation Medicine,
University of Texas M. D. Anderson Cancer Center,
Houston, Texas, USA

Carla M. M. Prado PhD
Postdoctorial fellow,
University of Alberta,
Department of Oncology,
Edmonton,
Alberta, Canada

Beatriz Shand MD
Instructor, Center for Bioethics and Department of Neurology,
Pontificia Universidad Católica de Chile,
Santiago, Chile

Florian Strasser MD
Associate Professor,
Head of Oncological Palliative Medicine,
Section Oncology,
Department of Internal Medicine,
Cantonal Hospital,
St Gallen, Switzerland

Carla Ida Ripamonti MD
Head, Day-Hospital and Outpatient Clinic of Pain Therapy and Palliative Care,
Rehabilitation and Palliative Care Operative Unit,
National Cancer Institute,
Milan, Italy

Paulina Taboada MD PhD
Associate Professor,
Director of the Center for Bioethics,
Pontificia Universidad Católica de Chile,
Santiago, Chile

Pradeep F. Thomas FRCS
Specialist Registrar in Surgery,
Nottingham University Hospitals,
Queen's Medical Centre,
Nottingham, UK

Sarah Toule
Cancer & Diet Information Project Lead,
Cancer Equality,
Vauxhall,
London, UK

Eric Walker PA-C, MHS, MSHA
University of Alabama at Birmingham,
Center for Palliative Care,
Birmingham, Alabama, USA

Jeremy Woodward MA PhD FRCP
Consultant Gastroenterologist,
Addenbrooke's Hospital,
Cambridge, UK

Reverend Caroline Worsfold MA BA (Hons)
Chaplain,
Northumberland Tyne & Wear NHS Trust and St Benedict's Hospice,
Sunderland, UK

Part 1

Basic principles

Chapter 1

Introduction and definitions

Vickie E. Baracos

The weight-related behaviour of contemporary populations of cancer patients is in a state of evolution and this is reflected by the various definitions described in this chapter. An increasing prevalence of obesity is noted in virtually all states and nations. The median age of cancer diagnosis (~65 years) occurs at the stage in life where adults reach their highest lifetime body weights. Excess bodyweight, expressed as high body mass index, is associated with the risk of some common adult cancers. These include oesophageal adenocarcinoma, thyroid, colon and renal cancers in men, and endometrial, breast, gallbladder, oesophageal adenocarcinoma and renal cancers in women. These associations were generally similar in studies from North America, Europe and Australia, and the Asia–Pacific region. As a consequence, cancer patients, and even those with metastatic disease, are increasingly presenting as obese. We were surprised to record an average fat mass in excess of 20 kg, in a cohort of metastatic colorectal cancer patients at one month from death, in spite of preceding weight loss and large burden of metastatic disease.

Underneath a mantle of adipose tissue, it appears that muscle wasting goes on unrelentingly. The divergent behaviour of muscle and adipose tissue means that patients may on the one hand rarely present as underweight or severely underweight, but may frequently have an occult condition of lean tissue wasting of significant magnitude. An important inference from this is that a unit of human body weight, or of body weight change, may never be expected to have a constant composition. This is starting to be acknowledged by experts on cachexia, and a recently published consensus definition of cancer cachexia notably makes a distinction between the behaviour of skeletal muscle and adipose tissue: 'cachexia, is a complex metabolic syndrome associated with underlying illness and *characterized by loss of muscle with or without loss of fat mass.*' As the physiognomy of contemporary humans changes over time, it will be an important challenge to adapt both our terminology and our conceptions of malnutrition and nutritional risk.

The terms and definitions, and the contexts in which these are used, are addressed in the following section.

Terms pertaining to nutrition and food intake

Anorexia (deriving from the Greek *an-*, a prefix that denotes absence, + *orexe* = appetite): decreased appetite, lack of desire or interest in food. An important distinction is made between the anorexia of malignant disease and anorexia nervosa, an unrelated psychophysiological disorder characterized by an abnormal fear of becoming obese and distorted self-image, characterized by unwillingness to eat.

Malnutrition: faulty nutrition due to inadequate or unbalanced intake of nutrients or their impaired assimilation or utilization.

Starvation: the most extreme form of malnutrition; a lack of essential nutrients over a prolonged period of time. Starvation is a physiological state characterized by progressive mobilization of body energy and protein reserves, tending to maximize conservation of energy by efficient use of fuels and lowered metabolic energy expenditure.[1]

Nutrition impact symptoms: this is a useful practical term used by several authors to describe symptoms associated with primary disease or treatments which alter normal ingestive behaviour.[2,3] These most often affect the normal function of the digestive tract (constipation, early satiety, diarrhoea, dysphagia, oesophagitis, heartburn, mucositis/stomatitis, nausea, vomiting, taste and smell alterations, xerostomia, thick saliva, dental problems) or more generally act to inhibit feeding (fatigue, pain, dyspnoea).

Nutritional risk: early signs and changes that predict the subsequent development of frank malnutrition. The detection of malnutrition is a different notion than the detection of nutritional risk. Nutritional risk implies a relation between different nutritional criteria (weight, intake, nutritional consequences of treatment) and patient outcomes (weight loss, risk of infection, morbidity, mortality, quality of life). Anthropmetric or biological parameters could be normal at the time of the evaluation, but the overall situation requires a nutritional strategy. For example, a combined treatment of gastric cancer with radiation and chemotherapy can be considered a situation of nutritional risk because the large reduction intake associated with this treatment almost invariably results in the development of malnutrition.

Artificial nutrition: nutrition in any form other than the taking in of food and fluid through the mouth (orally). This can be achieved through a nasogastric tube, gastrostomy or via total parenteral nutrition.

Terms pertaining to weight and weight-related disorders

Cachexia (deriving from the Greek *kakhexiā*: *kako-*, bad, + *hexis*, condition) would seem to be a well-accepted term that most people regard as being equivalent to emaciation. Although the end-stage condition is rather obvious, there has actually been no widely agreed upon operational definition or diagnostic criteria for cachexia. International Classification of Disease Codes for cachexia (ICD-9: 799.4) and unusual weight loss are poorly defined. The lack of a definition accepted by clinicians and researchers has limited identification and treatment of cachectic patients as well as the development and approval of potential therapeutic agents, and several organizations and authors have sought to address this concern. A group of scientists and clinicians met in 2007 in Washington, DC, for the Cachexia Consensus Conference. The definition that emerged is:

> Cachexia, is a complex metabolic syndrome associated with underlying illness and characterized by loss of muscle with or without loss of fat mass. The prominent clinical feature of cachexia is weight loss in adults (corrected for fluid retention) or growth failure in children (excluding endocrine disorders). Anorexia, inflammation, insulin resistance and increased muscle protein breakdown are frequently associated with cachexia. Cachexia is distinct from starvation, age-related loss of muscle mass, primary depression, malabsorption and hyperthyroidism and is associated with increased morbidity.[4]

By this definition, cachexia is distinct from starvation, but in most instances cachexia is associated with anorexia and malnutrition. Others have gone on to suggest several operational definitions specific to cancer cachexia, but these are not yet generally agreed.[5–7]

Anorexia–cachexia: this term is favoured by some authors and is often abbreviated as CACS (cancer cachexia–anorexia syndrome). Since anorexia and impairment to eating by nutrition impact symptoms are agreed by almost everyone to be a part of cachexia,[4–7] this term may be viewed as synonymous with cachexia.

Table 1.1 Total appendicular skeletal muscle index, kg/m² (SD)

	Men	Women
Healthy young adults	9.6 (1.2)	7.3 (0.9)
Healthy adults aged 65 years	7.8 (0.9)	6.1 (0.8)
Sarcopenia	<7.26	<5.45

Sarcopenia is a term denoting a reduced quantity of skeletal muscle and the generally accepted definition is an absolute muscle mass >2 SD below that typical of healthy adults and significantly associated with impaired mobility.[8] Sarcopenia is homologous to a more familiar term, osteopenia (low bone mineral density, a well-known risk factor for fractures). Like osteopenia and osteporosis, our understanding of sarcopenia has been developed with image-based methods for the precise determination of muscle mass, and this is often reported in the units of total appendicular skeletal muscle, determined by dual-energy X-ray absorptiometry (DXA) and adjusted for stature (kg/m²). Some reference values are available from large population-based DXA studies (Table 1.1).[9,10] Sarcopenia was first characterized in the elderly, and is aptly called the 'silent crippler' because of its association with risks of physical disability, falls, fractures and frailty.[11,12]

Sarcopenic obesity is a term denoting the concurrent presence of these two conditions. It seems that muscle loss may be masked by weight stability[13] and that muscle loss with fat gain culminates in sarcopenic obesity. This condition is prevalent all around the world[14–17] and is present in populations with advanced cancer[18] which have conventionally been associated with weight loss.

References

1. Cahill GF Jr (2006) Fuel metabolism in starvation. *Annu Rev Nutr*, **26**, 1–22.
2. Tong H, Isenring E, Yates P (2009) The prevalence of nutrition impact symptoms and their relationship to quality of life and clinical outcomes in medical oncology patients. *Support Care Cancer*, **17**(1), 83–90.
3. Ottery FD (1995) Supportive nutrition to prevent cachexia and improve quality of life. *Semin Oncol*, **22**(2 Suppl 3), 98–111.
4. Evans WJ, Morley JE, Argilés J, *et al.* (2008) Cachexia: a new definition. *Clin Nutr*, **27**(6), 793–9.
5. Bozzetti F, Mariani L (2009) Defining and classifying cancer cachexia: a proposal by the SCRINIO Working Group. *J Parenter Enteral Nutr*, **33**(4), 361–7.
6. Fox KM, Brooks JM, Gandra SR, Markus R, Chiou CF (2009) Estimation of cachexia among cancer patients based on four definitions. *J Oncol*, 693458 [Epub 1 Jul 2009].
7. Fearon KC, Voss AC, Hustead DS (2006) Cancer Cachexia Study Group. Definition of cancer cachexia: effect of weight loss, reduced food intake, and systemic inflammation on functional status and prognosis. *Am J Clin Nutr*, **83**(6), 1345–50.
8. Baumgartner RN, Koehler KM, Gallagher D, *et al.* (1998) Epidemiology of sarcopenia among the elderly in New Mexico. *Am J Epidemiol*, **147**(8), 755–63.
9. Gallagher D, Visser M, De Meersman RE, *et al.* (1997) Appendicular skeletal muscle mass: effects of age, gender, and ethnicity. *J Appl Physiol*, **83**, 229–39.
10. Newman AB, Lee JS, Visser M, *et al.* (2005) Weight change and the conservation of lean mass in old age: the Health, Aging and Body Composition Study. *Am J Clin Nutr*, **82**(4), 872–8.
11. Visser M (2009) Towards a definition of sarcopenia—results from epidemiologic studies. *J Nutr Health Aging*, **13**(8), 713–6.
12. Kinney JM (2004) Nutritional frailty, sarcopenia and falls in the elderly. *Curr Opin Clin Nutr Metab Care*, **7**(1), 15–20.

13. Gallagher D, Ruts E, Visser M, *et al.* (2000) Weight stability masks sarcopenia in elderly men and women. *Am J Physiol Endocrinol Metab*, **279**(2), E366–75.
14. Kim TN, Yang SJ, Yoo HJ, *et al.* (2009) Prevalence of sarcopenia and sarcopenic obesity in Korean adults: the Korean sarcopenic obesity study. *Int J Obes (Lond)*, **33**(8), 885–92.
15. Bouchard DR, Dionne IJ, Brochu M (2009) Sarcopenic/obesity and physical capacity in older men and women: data from the Nutrition as a Determinant of Successful Aging (NuAge) – the Quebec Longitudinal Study. *Obesity (Silver Spring)* [Epub ahead of print] PubMed PMID: 19373219.
16. Rolland Y, Lauwers-Cances V, Cristini C, *et al.* (2009) Difficulties with physical function associated with obesity, sarcopenia, and sarcopenic-obesity in community-dwelling elderly women: the EPIDOS (EPIDemiologie de l'OSteoporose) Study. *Am J Clin Nutr*, **89**(6), 1895–900.
17. Stenholm S, Harris TB, Rantanen T, Visser M, Kritchevsky SB, Ferrucci L (2008) Sarcopenic obesity: definition, cause and consequences. *Curr Opin Clin Nutr Metab Care*, **11**(6), 693–700.
18. Prado CM, Lieffers JR, McCargar LJ, *et al.* (2008) Prevalence and clinical implications of sarcopenic obesity in patients with solid tumours of the respiratory and gastrointestinal tracts: a population-based study. *Lancet Oncol*, **9**(7), 629–35.

Chapter 2

Metabolism and physiology

Vickie E. Baracos and Henrique A. Parsons

Introduction

In this chapter, the adaptive controls of energy balance in health, in starvation and in malignant disease are considered.

Controls of energy balance in healthy individuals

In a healthy adult, body weight is maintained because the number of calories ingested is equal to the amount of energy expended. Under these conditions the size of energy reserve in adipose tissue remains constant. Energy homeostasis has a high priority and specific metabolic changes help to store food energy optimally, or conversely to mobilize reserves under appropriate circumstances. Energy balance is maintained during starvation by a large fall in oxygen consumption. Conversely, during periods of carbohydrate and protein availability, corresponding increases in basal metabolism and energy expenditure are seen.[1] This coupling of intake with energy expenditure is a mechanism to conserve calories when caloric intake is low while disposing of or storing excess ingested calories when caloric intake is excessive. In healthy people, palatable, energy-dense foods retain high incentive value even when immediate physiological energy requirements have been met, and this feature of food intake regulation promotes overeating. This response has adaptive value in developing an energy reserve for potential future food shortages.

The physiological control of energy intake is complex and integrates afferent signals from several organs such as the gastrointestinal tract, and the adipose tissue. Central integration of these signals occurs in the hypothalamus, most specifically in two populations of neurons: one orexigenic pathway (promoting food intake and reducing energy loss) expressing neuropeptide Y (NPY) and the agouti-related protein (AgRP) and one anorexigenic pathway (inhibiting food intake and increasing the use of energy) expressing pro-opiomelanocortin (POMC) and cocaine-amphetamine-related transcript (CART).[2] These neuron populations extend their axons to several parts of the central nervous system in order to deliver their orexigenic/anorexigenic messages. These messages are delivered to at least three effector neuron populations. One, situated in the lateral hypothalamus, contains melanin-concentrating hormone (MCH) neurons,[3] which are associated with orexigenic effects[4] and the orexin/hypocretin neurons[5,6] which are also linked to an increase in food intake.[6] A second effector neuron population expresses thyrotrophin-releasing hormone (TRH), which decreases appetite[7] in addition to its regulatory function via the hypothalamus–hypophysis–thyroid axis.[8] Another second-order neuron population in the paraventricular nucleus secretes γ-aminobutyric acid (GABA), which modulates both orexigenic and anorexigenic effector neurons (Figure 2.1).[9,10]

Corticotrophin-releasing hormone (CRH), CART, TRH are called melanocortins because of their binding to melanocortin receptors and are cleaved from the POMC precursor.[11] Synthetic agonists of the melanocortin-4 receptor are able to suppress food intake, and blockade of its function leads to overfeeding, indicating that these receptors are closely linked to food intake.[12,13]

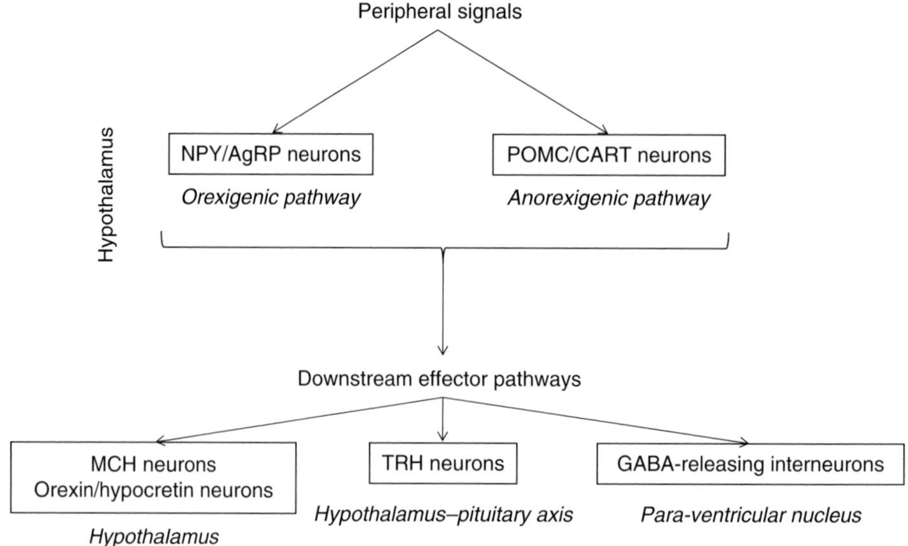

Fig. 2.1 Hypothalamic integration of peripheral signals and second order neuron populations. NPY, neuropeptide Y; AgRP, agouti-related protein; POMC, pro-opiomelanocortin; CART, cocaine- and amphetamine-regulated transcript; MCH, melanin-concentrating hormone; TRH, thyrotrophin-releasing hormone; GABA, gamma-aminobutyric acid.

The peripheral afferent signals come from a variety of organs (mainly gastrointestinal tract and adipose tissue) as seen in Figure 2.2. In response to food, and proportionate to the calories ingested, the L cells in the distal gut release into the circulation a 36-amino-acid hormone, peptide YY,[14,15] which has an inhibitory action on the NPY/AgRP neurons, therefore inhibiting orexigenic signals.

Ghrelin, a 28-amino-acid hormone produced mostly in the stomach, but also in a variety of other tissues, has an interesting effect on the hypothalamus: in addition to directly stimulating the orexigenic effects of the NPY/AgRP neurons, ghrelin is also capable of binding to specific receptors on these neurons and inhibiting the POMC/CART neurons via GABA pathways. This causes

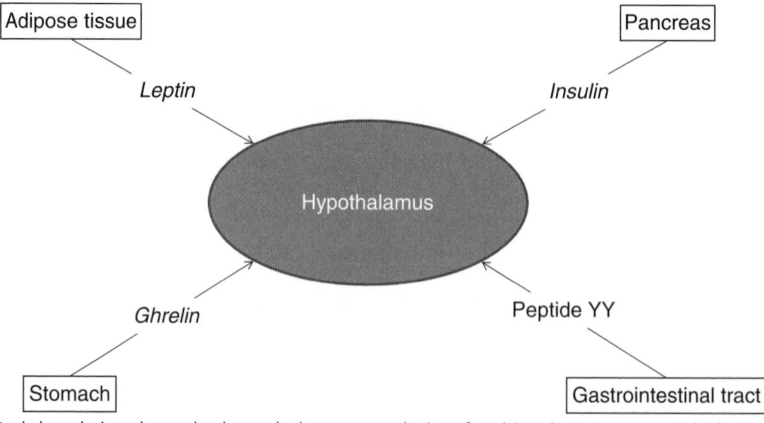

Fig. 2.2 Peripheral signals to the hypothalamus regulating food intake/energy metabolism.

inhibition of the anorexigenic pathway thereby increasing appetite. In addition, ghrelin may also mediate orexigenic effects via the vagus nerve.[16]

Leptin is also an important afferent to the hypothalamus, and produced mostly in adipose tissue but also in smaller amounts by the placenta, the stomach, and breast.[17] Leptin is secreted by the adipose tissue as a response to energy stores: higher energy stores drive an elevation of leptin with subsequent reduction of food intake and increase of the metabolic rate, by a direct inhibitory action on the NPY/AgRP neurons and also an excitatory action on POMC/CART neurons in the hypothalamus.[2,17] Insulin, secreted by the exocrine pancreas, has an anorexigenic effect by an excitatory action on POMC/CART neurons and inhibitory action on NPY/AgRP neurons.[2,18]

Appetite regulation is linked to peripheral metabolism, such that central stimuli for feeding such as NPY also promote energy storage in adipose tissue. Conversely, central inhibition of feeding with the use of melanocortin-4 agonists is associated with raised metabolic rate and lipolysis.[19–21] Central controls serve to orchestrate and unify physiological responses to the availability of food and are fundamental to the coordination of appetite and energy expenditure.

The precision of this regulation is high, so that healthy individuals are particularly resistant to developing a state of negative energy balance that leads to depletion of adipose tissue reserves. Involuntary weight loss, as occurs in many cancer patients, represents an important failure of the normal control of energy balance.

Adaptive response to starvation differs from the tumour-bearing state

While the presence of malignancy is often heralded by loss of appetite and lowered intake of nutrients, important distinctions can be made between the metabolic responses to simple malnutrition or starvation, and the tumour-bearing state. Currently used definitions of cancer cachexia (Chapter 1) underscore the distinctions between starvation and cancer.

Several observations related to food intake help to clarify these differences. Food intake in the cancer patient may not correlate with degree of weight loss or other indices of malnutrition, and attempts to supplement food intake with either consultation by a dietitian or nutrition supplementation may fail to prevent the progressive weight loss. Even when supplementation is conducted with parenteral feeding, weight gain is still often transitory and is associated frequently with gain of water and fat but not protein.[22,23] Unlike starvation, for which the deficits are generally corrected by refeeding, decreased food intake is not the sole actor responsible for the complex array of metabolic alterations present in the tumour-bearing state. Starvation and chronic malnutrition are associated with adaptive decreases in metabolic rate and increased economy of energy fuel utilization, whereas cancer is characterized by hypermetabolism[24,25] and activation of catabolic pathways. The increased energy expenditure results in a rate of depletion of physiological reserves of energy and protein that is greater than would be expected based on the prevailing level of food intake.

Cachexia also differs from starvation in the resulting changes in body tissue composition. During simple starvation, uncomplicated by injury, infection or malignancy, all organs lose mass.[26,27] In the tumour-bearing state, organs such as muscle, skin, and bone are catabolic, while organs such as liver and spleen and many parts of the immune system are anabolic and accumulate protein.[28,29] The anabolic state of the liver exceeds the accumulation of liver protein, because much of its anabolism is not only apparent in the liver itself but is reflected in an increased production of secretory (i.e. acute phase) proteins.[30]

Adipose tissue loses mass because it provides most of the substrate metabolized to meet energy requirements, but the proportions of fat and lean tissues lost during starvation and cancer differ.

During periods of prolonged starvation, fat stores are mobilized preferentially over skeletal muscle protein, and the majority of tissues convert to fat-derived fuels (free fatty acids, ketones) to meet metabolic demands. In starvation, most tissues can preferentially use ketone bodies over glucose production by gluconeogenesis, thereby sparing protein catabolism and lean body mass. By contrast, in the tumour-bearing state, glucose production via gluconeogenesis is maintained, promoting protein catabolism and facilitating muscle wasting and early lean body mass depletion.[31] Increased gluconeogenesis during starvation is transient, as hepatic glucose production is displaced by β-oxidation of lipid; however, gluconeogenesis and hepatic glucose production are not suppressed in the tumour-bearing state.[32] In starvation, fatty acid oxidation is suppressed by glucose administration, but fatty acid oxidation is not as easily suppressed by administered glucose in cancer patients.[33] The displacement of amino acids as fuels by ketone bodies is imperative to a successful preservation of nitrogen balance and lean body mass in starvation, and this critical adaptation is limited or absent in the tumour-bearing state.

Adaptive response to infection, injury and malignancy

The responses of the host organism to infection, trauma or the presence of a malignant tumour appear to be highly organized and conserved. These responses include loss of appetite, sleep and loss of weight, largely consisting of skeletal muscle. There is a functional redistribution of body protein, where somatic protein (muscle) is mobilized for energy needs or serves as the precursors of hepatic and acute-phase response (APR), a universal reaction to infection and trauma.[34–36] Soeters and Grimble[37] suggest the logical and obligatory nature of these events become plain by the simple observation of traumatized wild animals in their natural surroundings. Animals retreat into hiding, sleep and exhibit little mobility. Appetite is minimal and disinterest in food continues even when food is readily available. The animal exhibits a catabolic state, reflected in loss of weight, especially skeletal muscle. When the injury is not life-limiting, the injured area heals, and thereafter the animal resumes normal activity, starts eating and regains muscle mass and function.[34,36] Anorexia is considered an important behavioural adaptation. Limiting the incentive to forage for food reduces exposure to risks of predation and further injury, while in a compromised state. Concurrent mobilization of stored reserves of energy and skeletal muscle protein provides resources to cover basal costs of metabolism, immune responses and wound healing. Mobilization of skeletal muscle via suppression of protein synthesis and activation of proteolysis is a stereotypical event during response to injury.

Tumour burden induces metabolic changes that are dissimilar to those seen in caloric restriction and resemble those found in infection or injury.[38,39] Collectively, these metabolic changes and cellular events are presumed to be adaptive because they contribute to the defeat of invading organisms and supply precursors for immune activation and wound healing. Our intent to reverse some of the features of the adaptive response to injury, infection and cancer must take into account the highly conserved nature of these changes, and the specific mechanisms by which they occur. In the next sections of this chapter, specific controls of appetite and muscle protein turnover are considered.

Cancer-associated dysregulation of controls of appetite

A basic understanding of the control of feeding behaviour and its alteration in the tumour-bearing state is germane to the understanding of cancer-associated malnutrition. Food intake is a primary site of intervention, be it by dietetic counselling, pharmacological agents intended to stimulate appetite, or by artificial nutritional support. Dietary intakes of patients with advanced malignant disease have been reported, with about 40% of patients having energy intake insufficient to support basal metabolism (i.e. 22–24 kcal/kg/day).[24,40,41]

The brain is the primary site where food intake is regulated. Specific hypothalamic nuclei integrate cognitive, visual and sensory inputs, and peripheral signals, indicating the status of body energy reserves, the activity of the gastrointestinal tract and nutrient intake.

The regulation of energy balance in healthy individuals (discussed above) involves a host of mediators that exerts orexigenic or anorexigenic actions in the brain.[2,42–46] NPY, AgRP, MCH, ghrelin and orexins stimulate feeding behaviour, whereas melanocortins [α-melanocyte-stimulating hormone (MSH) and γ-MSH], CART, TRH, and CRH have an inhibitory action. Some of the key systemic hormones modulating energy homeostasis may be dysregulated in cancer, including insulin,[18] leptin,[47,48] corticosteroids,[49,50] ghrelin,[51–53] peptide YY, cholecystokinin and glucagon-like peptide-1. An expanded list of neuropeptides, hormones and paracrine factors that contribute to control of food intake and energy expenditure is given in Table 2.1.

Table 2.1 Signalling molecules in appetite regulation: abbreviations and actions

Abbreviation	Molecule name	Effect on feeding
2AG	2-Arachidonylglycerol (endocannabinoid)	+
AgRP	Agouti-related protein	+
Anandamide	N-Arachidonylethanolamine (endocannabinoid)	+
Cort	Corticosterone, cortisol (species-dependent)	+
DA	Dopamine	+
Ghrelin	Natural ligand of GHS-R	+
GHS-R	Growth hormone secretagogue receptor	+
MCH	Melanin-concentrating hormone	+
NPY	Neuropeptide Y	+
OX	Orexin A and B	+
Y1R, Y5R	NPY-1 and -5 receptors	+
Gal	Galanin	+
Norepinephrine	Noradrenaline	+
Amylin	Gut peptide	–
α-MSH	α-Melanocyte-stimulating hormone	–
5-HT	Serotonin	–
CART	Cocaine- and amphetamine-regulated transcript	–
CCK	Cholecystokinin	–
CRF = CRH	Corticotrophin-releasing factor	–
GIP	Gastrin inhibitory peptide	–
GLP-1, GLP-2	Glucagon-like peptide-1 and -2	–
Insulin	Natural ligand of insulin receptor	–

(Continued)

Table 2.1 (Continued) Signalling molecules in appetite regulation: abbreviations and actions

Abbreviation	Molecule name	Effect on feeding
Il-1β	Interleukin-1 proinflammatory cytokine	–
Leptin	Adipocyte-secreted hormone	–
PYY	Peptide YY–Y2 receptor ligand	–
MC4-R	Melanocortin-4 receptor	–
POMC	Pro-opiomelanocortin	–
TRH	Thyrotrophin-releasing hormone	–
TNFα	Tumour necrosis factor proinflammatory cytokine	–
UCN 1, 2, 3	Urocortins 1, 2 and 3	–
UCP1,2,3	Uncoupling proteins 1,2,3	–
Y2R	NPY-2 receptors	–

Early work on the respective contributions of these regulating signals was based on neuroanatomical lesions of the brain, especially the hypothalamus; current research involves the injection, overexpression or genetic ablation of chemical messengers and/or their receptors.

The neurons of the arcuate nucleus (ARC) of the hypothalamus provide a framework for understanding what may occur in cancer anorexia. The two major groups described earlier in the chapter include: (1) neurons that stimulate appetite through secretion of NPY and AgRP; (2) neurons that depress appetite through secretion of α-MSH; derived from specific proteolytic cleavage of the prohormone, pro-opiomelanocortin (POMC), and CART. A feeling of hunger can be induced through several mechanisms. Activation of the NPY/AgRP-releasing neurons of the ARC will increase appetite, as will inhibition of the αMSH-releasing POMC neurons. Conversely, inhibition of NPY/AgRP neurons will dampen appetite, as will activation of POMC neurons. Research using NPY and Y(1) receptor immunohistochemistry reveals reduced NPY staining in paraventricular (PVN) and ARC of tumour-bearing rats.[54] Y(1) receptor abundance is also reduced in the ARC and PVN of tumour-bearing rats, whereas pair-fed rats exhibit elevated Y(1) R in the PVN. NPY concentrations are decreased in the PVN, ventromedial (VMN), and lateral hypothalamus (LHA) in tumour-bearing rats compared with pair fed controls; these changes are reversed by tumour resection.[55] The results suggest dysfunction of NPY controls and suggest downregulation of Y(1) receptors as well as possible problems in NPY translation.

The central melanocortin system has emerged as a major contributor to body weight regulation. In particular, the melanocortin-4 receptor (MCR-4), its endogenous agonist αMSH, and its endogenous antagonist agouti-related protein (AgRP), have been shown to be vital to the maintenance of body weight. Selective antagonists of MCR-4 can prevent or attenuate the development of cachexia in animal models of acute and chronic disease.[56–59] Stimulation of hypothalamic MCR-4 produces anorexia, increased metabolic rate and activations of lipolysis in white adipose tissue.[19–21] Weight loss induced by endotoxin or IL-1β and by tumour growth is inhibited by MCR-4 blockade.[60–62] A role for MCR signalling is suggested by studies showing that MCR-4 knockout mice, or mice administered AgRP, resist tumour-induced loss of lean body mass.[63,64] The recent advent of non-toxic, orally active, small-molecule MCR-4 antagonists raises the possibility of direct intervention at this level.[64,65]

The level of complexity and comparative lack of knowledge of the regulation of cancer anorexia make it a difficult site for targeted intervention. Regulation of appetite results from a synthesis of the actions of a long list of orexigenic and anorexigenic factors. Cancer anorexia appears multifactorial and appears to involve most of the neuronal signalling pathways modulating energy intake, making it seem unlikely that a single factor may be used to reverse anorexia. The nature of changes in the peripheral metabolic signals that influence appetite regulation in the brain (leptin, insulin, peptide YY, ghrelin, and lipid mediators) is still being evaluated. The status of the hedonic pathway that normally promotes intake of high energy density food in the tumour-bearing state is largely unknown. Also, little is known about whether the metabolic signals of satiety (i.e. cholecystokinin) function normally in cancer patients.

Regulation of muscle protein metabolism

Wasting of lean tissues and especially skeletal muscle is an important component of cancer-associated weight loss. Severe muscle wasting is associated with risks of physical disability, falls, fractures and frailty, extended hospital stays, infectious and non-infectious complications in hospital, mortality, severe toxicity during chemotherapy and mortality. These problems indicate that muscle wasting is an important target for therapeutic interventions.

Muscle mass depends on the balance between the rate of protein synthesis and protein catabolism. There is some debate as to the respective contributions of decreased protein synthesis and increased catabolism in cancer-associated muscle loss;[66] however, most studies have focused on protein catabolism as the key step in muscle wasting. The vast majority of the available evidence on this topic comes from experimental studies in laboratory rodents. Direct measures of protein synthesis and degradation in humans are costly and invasive and thus have been infrequently conducted in cancer patients.[67–71]

A great deal of attention has been paid recently to the identity of proteolytic pathways contributing to muscle catabolism. Skeletal muscle contains lysosomes as well as cytosolic calcium-dependent calpains, which are involved primarily in catabolism of extracellular proteins and cell-surface receptors,[72] and in tissue injury, necrosis, and autolysis,[73] respectively. The ATP ubiquitin-dependent proteolytic pathway appears to be a common proteolytic pathway of cancer-associated muscle catabolism.[74–79] Most intracellular proteins in skeletal muscle are degraded through the ubiquitin proteasome system, in which proteins are marked for proteasomal degradation by the conjugation of ubiquitin molecules. Ubiquitin is the name coined for a highly conserved protein that was found to be ubiquitously present in tissues.

The first step in this pathway is the covalent attachment of polyubiquitin chains to the targeted protein. Ubiquitin conjugation involves a series of enzymatic steps including activation of ubiquitin (E1); transfer of activated Ub to the E2 enzyme that serves as a carrier protein and interacts with a specific E3 enzyme (ubiquitin protein ligase). The ubiquitin ligase binds to the protein substrates to be degraded and catalyses the transfer of ubiquitin to the substrate to generate a ubiquitin chain. Polyubiquitinylated proteins are recognized and degraded by the 26S proteasome complex. The ubiquitin is not degraded but is recycled back into the ubiquitin–proteasome pathway to be used in the breakdown of other proteins.

Further studies are required to better understand the regulation of elements of this system. The importance of the ubiquitin ligase family must be resolved, including identifying the physiological substrates for these enzymes in skeletal muscle, elucidating signalling events that regulate their activity, and analysing the effects of specific inhibition.

Central role of inflammatory mediators in coordination of loss of appetite and coordinated catabolic processes

Inflammation is widely agreed to be a unifying mechanism for the cluster of behaviours associated with injury, infection and cancer that are discussed in the preceding sections. Pro-inflammatory cytokines [specifically, members of the interleukin-6 (IL-6) superfamily, as well as tumour necrosis factor-α (TNFα), interleukin-1 (IL-1β), and interferon-γ (IFNγ], are generated in the brain, by the tumour, by tissues in the locale of the tumour and by a diversity of host cells including skeletal muscle, adipose tissue, and cells of the immune system and liver. Cytokines elicit anorexia, fever, slow wave sleep, lipolysis and muscle proteolysis, in addition to their characteristic immune responses when injected systemically.[80–82] Independent lines of research suggest that these mediators initiate both appetite loss and coordinated mobilization of body energy and protein reserves.[83,84]

A cytokine-inducible ubiquitin ligase has been identified in muscles of tumour-bearing rats.[85] The administration of TNF-α to rats increased skeletal muscle proteolysis associated with an increase in both free and conjugated ubiquitin,[86–88] and to directly induce proteolysis through the ubiquitin–proteasome pathway.[89] IL-1 and IFNγ are also able to upregulate ubiquitin gene expression.[90] There are just a few studies in humans.[91,92] Weight-losing patients with gastric cancer had double the levels of ubiquitin mRNA levels in the rectus abdominus muscle compared with control groups.[91,92]

It is notable that cytokines participate in paracrine amplification of their own responses. In key brain regions, including the arcuate nucleus, microglia and other cells produce cytokines and thereafter respond to them with upregulation of production of cytokine receptors and cytokines.[57] Skeletal muscle shows similar paracrine amplification in response to cytokines, and a variety of authors others have shown a sharp left-shift in the endotoxin dose–response in tumour-bearing animals, with hyper-reactive responses in cytokine production, food intake, muscle protein catabolism and mortality.[93]

Conclusion

The tumour-bearing state is characterized by anorexia and systemic metabolic changes that are distinct from starvation or malnourishment and are similar to the responses to infection and injury. Loss of appetite and muscle protein catabolism reflect adaptive responses intended to enact immune reactions and tissue repair, independent of food supply. These effects are orchestrated by the brain, and by a series of proinflammatory cytokines, which act both centrally and peripherally. The identification of therapeutic pharmacological and nutritional interventions to reverse these alterations will depend on a more complete understanding of the control systems responsible for cancer-associated anorexia and muscle catabolism.

References

1. Chwalibog A, Tauson AH, Thorbek G (2004) Energy metabolism and substrate oxidation in pigs during feeding, starvation and re-feeding. *J Anim Physiol Anim Nutr (Berl)*, **88**(3–4), 101–12.
2. Schwartz MW, Woods SC, Porte D Jr, Seeley RJ, Baskin DG (2000) Central nervous system control of food intake. *Nature*, **404**(6778), 661–71.
3. Qu D, Ludwig DS, Gammeltoft S, *et al.* (1996) A role for melanin-concentrating hormone in the central regulation of feeding behaviour. *Nature*, **380**(6571), 243–7.
4. Shimada M, Tritos NA, Lowell BB, Flier JS, Maratos-Flier E (1998) Mice lacking melanin-concentrating hormone are hypophagic and lean. *Nature*, **396**(6712), 670–4.
5. de Lecea L, Kilduff TS, Peyron C, *et al.* (1998) The hypocretins: hypothalamus-specific peptides with neuroexcitatory activity. *Proc Natl Acad Sci USA*, **95**(1), 322–7.
6. Sakurai T, Amemiya A, Ishii M, *et al.* (1998) Orexins and orexin receptors: a family of hypothalamic neuropeptides and G protein-coupled receptors that regulate feeding behavior. *Cell*, **92**(4), 573–85.
7. Kow LM, Pfaff DW (1991) The effects of the TRH metabolite cyclo(His-Pro) and its analogs on feeding. *Pharmacol Biochem Behav*, **38**(2), 359–64.

8. Flier JS, Harris M, Hollenberg AN (2000) Leptin, nutrition, and the thyroid: the why, the wherefore, and the wiring. *J Clin Invest*, **105**(7), 859–61.
9. Kokare DM, Patole AM, Carta A, Chopde CT, Subhedar NK (2006) GABA(A) receptors mediate orexin-A induced stimulation of food intake. *Neuropharmacology*, **50**(1), 16–24.
10. Tews JK, Repa JJ, Harper AE (1984) Alleviation in the rat of a GABA-induced reduction in food intake and growth. *Physiol Behav*, **33**(1), 55–63.
11. Cone RD, Lu D, Koppula S, *et al.* (1996) The melanocortin receptors: agonists, antagonists, and the hormonal control of pigmentation. *Recent Prog Horm Res*, **51**, 287–317; discussion 18.
12. Fan W, Boston BA, Kesterson RA, Hruby VJ, Cone RD (1997) Role of melanocortinergic neurons in feeding and the agouti obesity syndrome. *Nature*, **385**(6612), 165–8.
13. Vaisse C, Clement K, Guy-Grand B, Froguel P (1998) A frameshift mutation in human MC4R is associated with a dominant form of obesity. *Nat Genet*, **20**(2), 113–4.
14. Vincent RP, le Roux CW (2008) The satiety hormone peptide YY as a regulator of appetite. *J Clin Pathol*, **61**(5), 548–52.
15. Adrian TE, Ferri GL, Bacarese-Hamilton AJ, Fuessl HS, Polak JM, Bloom SR (1985) Human distribution and release of a putative new gut hormone, peptide YY. *Gastroenterology*, **89**(5), 1070–7.
16. De Vriese C, Delporte C (2007) Influence of ghrelin on food intake and energy homeostasis. *Curr Opin Clin Nutr Metab Care*, **10**(5), 615–9.
17. Klok MD, Jakobsdottir S, Drent ML (2007) The role of leptin and ghrelin in the regulation of food intake and body weight in humans: a review. *Obes Rev*, **8**(1), 21–34.
18. Schwartz MW, Figlewicz DP, Baskin DG, Woods SC, Porte D, Jr (1992) Insulin in the brain: a hormonal regulator of energy balance. *Endocr Rev*, **13**(3), 387–414.
19. Song CK, Jackson RM, Harris RB, Richard D, Bartness TJ (2005) Melanocortin-4 receptor mRNA is expressed in sympathetic nervous system outflow neurons to white adipose tissue. *Am J Physiol Regul Integr Comp Physiol*, **289**(5), R1467–76.
20. Song CK, Vaughan CH, Keen-Rhinehart E, Harris RB, Richard D, Bartness TJ (2008) Melanocortin-4 receptor mRNA expressed in sympathetic outflow neurons to brown adipose tissue: neuroanatomical and functional evidence. *Am J Physiol Regul Integr Comp Physiol*, **295**(2), R417–28.
21. Bartness TJ, Kay Song C, Shi H, Bowers RR, Foster MT (2005) Brain-adipose tissue cross talk. *Proc Nutr Soc*, **64**(1), 53–64.
22. Grosvenor M, Bulcavage L, Chlebowski RT (1989) Symptoms potentially influencing weight loss in a cancer population. Correlations with primary site, nutritional status, and chemotherapy administration. *Cancer*, **63**(2), 330–4.
23. Evans WK, Makuch R, Clamon GH, *et al.* (1985) Limited impact of total parenteral nutrition on nutritional status during treatment for small cell lung cancer. *Cancer Res*, **45**(7), 3347–53.
24. Bosaeus I, Daneryd P, Svanberg E, Lundholm K (2001) Dietary intake and resting energy expenditure in relation to weight loss in unselected cancer patients. *Int J Cancer*, **93**(3), 380–3.
25. Jatoi A, Daly BD, Hughes VA, Dallal GE, Kehayias J, Roubenoff R (2001) Do patients with nonmetastatic non-small cell lung cancer demonstrate altered resting energy expenditure? *Ann Thorac Surg*, **72**(2), 348–51.
26. Melchior JC (1998) From malnutrition to refeeding during anorexia nervosa. *Curr Opin Clin Nutr Metab Care*, **1**(6), 481–5.
27. Holecek M, Sprongl L, Tilser I (2001) Metabolism of branched-chain amino acids in starved rats: the role of hepatic tissue. *Physiol Res*, **50**(1), 25–33.
28. Jepson MM, Pell JM, Bates PC, Millward DJ (1986) The effects of endotoxaemia on protein metabolism in skeletal muscle and liver of fed and fasted rats. *Biochem J*, **235**(2), 329–36.
29. Rooyackers OE, Saris WH, Soeters PB, Wagenmakers AJ (1994) Prolonged changes in protein and amino acid metabolism after zymosan treatment in rats. *Clin Sci (Lond)*, **87**(5), 619–26.

30. Gabay C, Kushner I (1999) Acute-phase proteins and other systemic responses to inflammation. *N Engl J Med*, **340**(6), 448–54.
31. Tisdale MJ (1997) Cancer cachexia: metabolic alterations and clinical manifestations. *Nutrition*, **13**(1), 1–7.
32. Tayek JA (1992) A review of cancer cachexia and abnormal glucose metabolism in humans with cancer. *J Am Coll Nutr*, **11**(4), 445–56.
33. Shaw JH, Wolfe RR (1987) Fatty acid and glycerol kinetics in septic patients and in patients with gastrointestinal cancer. The response to glucose infusion and parenteral feeding. *Ann Surg*, **205**(4), 368–76.
34. Ishibashi N, Plank LD, Sando K, Hill GL (1998) Optimal protein requirements during the first 2 weeks after the onset of critical illness. *Crit Care Med*, **26**(9), 1529–35.
35. Plank LD, Hill GL (2000) Sequential metabolic changes following induction of systemic inflammatory response in patients with severe sepsis or major blunt trauma. *World J Surg*, **24**(6), 630–8.
36. Plank LD, Hill GL (2000) Similarity of changes in body composition in intensive care patients following severe sepsis or major blunt injury. *Ann NY Acad Sci*, **904**, 592–602.
37. Soeters PB, Grimble RF (2009) Dangers, and benefits of the cytokine mediated response to injury and infection. *Clin Nutr*, **28**(6), 583–596
38. Argiles JM, Alvarez B, Lopez-Soriano FJ (1997) The metabolic basis of cancer cachexia. *Med Res Rev*, **17**(5), 477–98.
39. Lowry SF (1991) Cancer cachexia revisited: old problems and new perspectives. *Eur J Cancer*, **27**(1), 1–3.
40. Hutton JL, Martin L, Field CJ, *et al.* (2006) Dietary patterns in patients with advanced cancer: implications for anorexia-cachexia therapy. *Am J Clin Nutr*, **84**(5), 1163–70.
41. Fearon KC, Von Meyenfeldt MF, Moses AG, *et al.* (2003) Effect of a protein and energy dense N-3 fatty acid enriched oral supplement on loss of weight and lean tissue in cancer cachexia: a randomised double blind trial. *Gut*, **52**(10), 1479–86.
42. Cone RD (1999) The central melanocortin system and energy homeostasis. *Trends Endocrinol Metab*, **10**(6), 211–16.
43. Elmquist JK (2000) Anatomic basis of leptin action in the hypothalamus. *Front Horm Res*, **26**, 21–41.
44. Sleeman MW, Anderson KD, Lambert PD, Yancopoulos GD, Wiegand SJ (2000) The ciliary neurotrophic factor and its receptor, CNTFR alpha. *Pharm Acta Helv*, **74**(2–3), 265–72.
45. Williams G, Harrold JA, Cutler DJ (2000) The hypothalamus and the regulation of energy homeostasis: lifting the lid on a black box. *Proc Nutr Soc*, **59**(3), 385–96.
46. Woods SC, Schwartz MW, Baskin DG, Seeley RJ (2000) Food intake and the regulation of body weight. *Annu Rev Psychol*, **51**, 255–77.
47. Ahima RS, Flier JS (2000) Leptin. *Annu Rev Physiol*, **62**, 413–37.
48. Friedman JM, Halaas JL (1998) Leptin and the regulation of body weight in mammals. *Nature*, **395**(6704), 763–70.
49. Dallman MF, Akana SF, Strack AM, Hanson ES, Sebastian RJ (1995) The neural network that regulates energy balance is responsive to glucocorticoids and insulin and also regulates HPA axis responsivity at a site proximal to CRF neurons. *Ann NY Acad Sci*, **771**, 730–42.
50. Shih A, Jackson KC, 2nd (2007) Role of corticosteroids in palliative care. *J Pain Palliat Care Pharmacother*, **21**(4), 69–76.
51. Kojima M, Hosoda H, Date Y, Nakazato M, Matsuo H, Kangawa K (1999) Ghrelin is a growth-hormone-releasing acylated peptide from stomach. *Nature*, **402**(6762), 656–60.
52. Nakazato M, Murakami N, Date Y, *et al.* (2001) A role for ghrelin in the central regulation of feeding. *Nature*, **409**(6817), 194–8.
53. Tschop M, Smiley DL, Heiman ML (2000) Ghrelin induces adiposity in rodents. *Nature*, **407**(6806), 908–13.

54. Chance WT, Xiao C, Dayal R, Sheriff S (2007) Alteration of NPY and Y1 receptor in dorsomedial and ventromedial areas of hypothalamus in anorectic tumor-bearing rats. *Peptides*, **28**(2), 295–301.

55. Ramos EJ, Suzuki S, Meguid MM, *et al.* (2004) Changes in hypothalamic neuropeptide Y and monoaminergic system in tumor-bearing rats: pre- and post-tumor resection and at death. *Surgery*, **136**(2), 270–6.

56. Madison LD, Marks DL (2006) Anticatabolic properties of melanocortin-4 receptor antagonists. *Curr Opin Clin Nutr Metab Care*, **9**(3), 196–200.

57. Deboer MD, Marks DL (2006) Cachexia: lessons from melanocortin antagonism. *Trends Endocrinol Metab*, **17**(5), 199–204.

58. DeBoer MD, Marks DL (2006) Therapy insight: Use of melanocortin antagonists in the treatment of cachexia in chronic disease. *Nat Clin Pract Endocrinol Metab*, **2**(8), 459–66.

59. Fletcher AL, Marks DL (2007) Central mechanisms controlling appetite and food intake in a cancer setting: an update. *Curr Opin Support Palliat Care*, **1**(4), 306–11.

60. Marks DL, Butler AA, Turner R, Brookhart G, Cone RD (2003) Differential role of melanocortin receptor subtypes in cachexia. *Endocrinology*, **144**(4), 1513–23.

61. Marks DL, Ling N, Cone RD (2001) Role of the central melanocortin system in cachexia. *Cancer Res*, **61**(4), 1432–8.

62. Whitaker KW, Reyes TM (2008) Central blockade of melanocortin receptors attenuates the metabolic and locomotor responses to peripheral interleukin-1beta administration. *Neuropharmacology*, **54**(3), 509–20.

63. Joppa MA, Gogas KR, Foster AC, Markison S (2007) Central infusion of the melanocortin receptor antagonist agouti-related peptide (AgRP(83-132)) prevents cachexia-related symptoms induced by radiation and colon-26 tumors in mice. *Peptides*, **28**(3), 636–42.

64. Markison S, Foster AC, Chen C, *et al.* (2005) The regulation of feeding and metabolic rate and the prevention of murine cancer cachexia with a small-molecule melanocortin-4 receptor antagonist. *Endocrinology*, **146**(6), 2766–73.

65. Chen C, Jiang W, Tucci F, *et al.* (2007) Discovery of 1-[2-[(1S)-(3-dimethylaminopropionyl)amino-2-methylpropyl]-4-methylphenyl]-4-[(2R)-methyl-3-(4-chlorophenyl)-propionyl]piperazine as an orally active antagonist of the melanocortin-4 receptor for the potential treatment of cachexia. *J Med Chem*, **50**(22), 5249–52.

66. Tisdale MJ (2002) Cachexia in cancer patients. *Nat Rev Cancer*, **2**(11), 862–71.

67. Eden E, Ekman L, Bennegard K, Lindmark L, Lundholm K (1984) Whole-body tyrosine flux in relation to energy expenditure in weight-losing cancer patients. *Metabolism*, **33**(11), 1020–7.

68. Fearon KC, Hansell DT, Preston T, *et al.* (1988) Influence of whole body protein turnover rate on resting energy expenditure in patients with cancer. *Cancer Res*, **48**(9), 2590–5.

69. McMillan DC, Preston T, Fearon KC, Burns HJ, Slater C, Shenkin A (1994) Protein synthesis in cancer patients with inflammatory response: investigations with [15N]glycine. *Nutrition*, **10**(3), 232–40.

70. Melville S, McNurlan MA, Calder AG, Garlick PJ (1990) Increased protein turnover despite normal energy metabolism and responses to feeding in patients with lung cancer. *Cancer Res* **50**(4), 1125–31.

71. Richards EW, Long CL, Nelson KM, *et al.* (1993) Protein turnover in advanced lung cancer patients. *Metabolism*, **42**(3), 291–6.

72. Lecker SH, Solomon V, Mitch WE, Goldberg AL (1999) Muscle protein breakdown and the critical role of the ubiquitin-proteasome pathway in normal and disease states. *J Nutr*, **129**(1S Suppl), 227S–37S.

73. Goll DE, Thompson VF, Taylor RG, Christiansen JA (1992) Role of the calpain system in muscle growth. *Biochimie*, **74**(3), 225–37.

74. Llovera M, Garcia-Martinez C, Agell N, Lopez-Soriano FJ, Argiles JM (1995) Muscle wasting associated with cancer cachexia is linked to an important activation of the ATP-dependent ubiquitin-mediated proteolysis. *Int J Cancer*, **61**(1), 138–41.

75. Llovera M, Garcia-Martinez C, Agell N, Marzabal M, Lopez-Soriano FJ, Argiles JM (1994) Ubiquitin gene expression is increased in skeletal muscle of tumour-bearing rats. *FEBS Lett*, **338**(3), 311–8.
76. Attaix D, Combaret L, Tilignac T, Taillandier D (1999) Adaptation of the ubiquitin-proteasome proteolytic pathway in cancer cachexia. *Mol Biol Rep*, **26**(1–2), 77–82.
77. Khal J, Wyke SM, Russell ST, Hine AV, Tisdale MJ (2005) Expression of the ubiquitin-proteasome pathway and muscle loss in experimental cancer cachexia. *Br J Cancer*, **93**(7), 774–80.
78. Lecker SH, Jagoe RT, Gilbert A, *et al.* (2004) Multiple types of skeletal muscle atrophy involve a common program of changes in gene expression. *FASEB J*, **18**(1), 39–51.
79. Tisdale MJ (2005) The ubiquitin-proteasome pathway as a therapeutic target for muscle wasting. *J Support Oncol*, **3**(3), 209–17.
80. Goshen I, Yirmiya R (2009) Interleukin-1 (IL-1): a central regulator of stress responses. *Front Neuroendocrinol*, **30**(1), 30–45.
81. Dinarello CA (2000) Proinflammatory cytokines. *Chest*, 118(2), 503–8.
82. Argiles JM, Lopez-Soriano FJ (1999) The role of cytokines in cancer cachexia. *Med Res Rev*, **19**(3), 223–48.
83. Turrin NP, Ilyin SE, Gayle DA, *et al.* (2004) Interleukin-1beta system in anorectic catabolic tumor-bearing rats. *Curr Opin Clin Nutr Metab Care*, **7**(4), 419–26.
84. Tracey KJ, Morgello S, Koplin B, et al. (1990) Metabolic effects of cachectin/tumor necrosis factor are modified by site of production. Cachectin/tumor necrosis factor-secreting tumor in skeletal muscle induces chronic cachexia, while implantation in brain induces predominantly acute anorexia. *J Clin Invest*, **86**(6), 2014–24.
85. Kwak KS, Zhou X, Solomon V, *et al.* (2004) Regulation of protein catabolism by muscle-specific and cytokine-inducible ubiquitin ligase E3alpha-II during cancer cachexia. *Cancer Res*, **64**(22), 8193–8.
86. Garcia-Martinez C, Agell N, Llovera M, Lopez-Soriano FJ, Argiles JM (1993) Tumour necrosis factor-alpha increases the ubiquitinization of rat skeletal muscle proteins. *FEBS Lett*, **323**(3), 211–4.
87. Garcia-Martinez C, Lopez-Soriano FJ, Argiles JM (1993) Acute treatment with tumour necrosis factor-alpha induces changes in protein metabolism in rat skeletal muscle. *Mol Cell Biochem*, **125**(1), 11–8.
88. Garcia-Martinez C, Llovera M, Agell N, Lopez-Soriano FJ, Argiles JM (1994) Ubiquitin gene expression in skeletal muscle is increased by tumour necrosis factor-alpha. *Biochem Biophys Res Commun*, **201**(2), 682–6.
89. Llovera M, Garcia-Martinez C, Agell N, Lopez-Soriano FJ, Argiles JM (1997) TNF can directly induce the expression of ubiquitin-dependent proteolytic system in rat soleus muscles. *Biochem Biophys Res Commun*, **230**(2), 238–41.
90. Llovera M, Carbo N, Lopez-Soriano J, *et al.* (1998) Different cytokines modulate ubiquitin gene expression in rat skeletal muscle. *Cancer Lett*, **133**(1), 83–7.
91. Bossola M, Muscaritoli M, Costelli P, *et al.* (2001) Increased muscle ubiquitin mRNA levels in gastric cancer patients. *Am J Physiol Regul Integr Comp Physiol*, **280**(5), R1518–23.
92. Williams A, Sun X, Fischer JE, Hasselgren PO (1999) The expression of genes in the ubiquitin-proteasome proteolytic pathway is increased in skeletal muscle from patients with cancer. *Surgery*, **126**(4), 744–9; discussion 49–50.
93. Mackenzie ML, Bedard N, Wing SS, Baracos VE (2005) A proinflammatory tumor that activates protein degradation sensitizes rats to catabolic effects of endotoxin. *Am J Physiol Endocrinol Metab*, **289**(4), E527–33.

Chapter 3

Assessment of nutritional status

Vickie E. Baracos, Carla M. M. Prado, Sami Antoun, Ioannis Gioulbasanis

Nutritional assessments of oncology patients are necessary in a variety of situations but they do not all require the same personnel or expertise. The essential elements of nutritional assessment are derived from the concepts of malnutrition and of nutritional risk. The primary assessment is screening, which aims to systematically identify individuals who are malnourished or are at risk. The screening assessment must be relevant to the patient population, clinically practical and accessible to front-line health care providers of any category. Nutrition screening tools are a means of grading or scoring nutritional status. Based on this assessment, decisions are made to treat, to continue monitoring, or to refer patients to nutrition professionals with specialized expertise.

In the front lines: screening for nutritional risk and malnutrition

Evaluation of nutritional status and nutritional risk includes several base elements:

- level of energy intake;
- weight and weight loss;
- biological criteria;
- nutritional risk factors associated with the underlying pathology and treatments.

Screening usually includes parameters that are reported by the patient and can be evaluated by any category of health care professional. In addition to the identification of frank malnutrition, an important facet of screening is to identify people at risk for malnutrition before severe changes occur. These individuals are more likely to have a decrease in caloric intake that can be corrected by nutritional intervention.

Screening nutritional assessment

For intake, prospectively collected dietary records are the standard for estimation of total energy and macronutrient intake. Screening tools use surrogate assessments in the form of questions pertaining to the type, number and frequency of meals. Questions related to the patient's ability to purchase, to shop, prepare and eat independently are often included, as are up to a dozen symptoms exerting a negative impact on food intake. These symptoms include nausea, vomiting, constipation, early satiety, taste alteration, pain, difficulty swallowing, mouth sores, and dental problems.

Involuntary weight loss is considered a hallmark of malignant disease. Weight and height may be reported by caregivers or patients. There is evidence to support the reliability of self-reported height, weight and weight history.[1] Height and weight data are used to compute the common anthropometric descriptor, body mass index (BMI; kg/m^2). BMI is used to define patients who are clinically underweight. Low BMI associated with nutritional risk differs in the literature (variously 17, 18.5 or 20). For patients who are unable to stand for measures of height and weight, anthropometric assessments of upper arm (mid-upper arm circumference) or lower leg (calf circumference) may be compared with normative data.

Percentage weight loss is calculated, either relative to premorbid body weight, or over a defined period of time such as 1, 3 or 6 months. This criterion is treated heterogeneously in screening tools, in the literature and in publications by various health authorities and expert groups: variously 5, 10 or 20% weight loss either in total or during a specified time frame is attributed a level of nutritional risk. Oedema, ascites, increased organ volume (i.e. hepatomegaly), and tumour burden including metastasis contribute to shifts in body weight in advanced cancer patients[2–4] and should be taken into account in the assessment of weight and weight change over time.

Rarely do any of the screening tools consider aspects of body composition; however, at least one nutrition screening tool designed for oncology, the Patient-Generated Subjective Global Assessment, includes a physical examination to detect muscle and adipose tissue wasting.

Biological criteria used in nutritional screening assessments are derived from routine laboratory data which may be collected in different care settings. The biological criteria used in nutritional assessment at the screening level largely relate to the acute-phase response, a complex series of reactions initiated in response to infection, physical trauma, or malignancy. The acute-phase response is characterized by leukocytosis, fever, alterations in the metabolism of many organs as well as changes in the plasma concentrations of various acute-phase proteins.[5] Acute phase proteins have been defined as any protein whose plasma concentrations increase [positive acute-phase proteins: fibrinogen, α_1-acid glycoprotein serum amyloid A, C-reactive protein (CRP)] or decrease (negative acute-phase proteins: albumin, transferrin) by at least 25% during an inflammatory disorder. CRP distinguishes groups with weight loss versus weight stable patients, and this is confirmed by correlational studies.[6–9] Many studies (five group comparisons, three correlational studies) have shown an association between low serum albumin[7–11] and weight loss. Other surrogate inflammatory markers, lymphocyte CD4/CD8 and HLA-DR expression on $CD14^+$ cells also discriminate between groups with or without weight loss.

The laboratory values associated with nutritional risk vary according to different authors: albumin (cut-off points variously <30, <32 or <35 g/l), transthyretin (prealbumin) (variously <110 or <180 mg/l) and C-reactive protein (variously >5 or >10 mg/l). Sometimes these variables have been used to calculate a score, such as the Nutritional Risk Index (NRI) attributed to Buzby,[12] or the Prognostic Inflammation Nutrition Index (PINI) a clinical assessment tool which aggregates serum CRP, α_1-acid glycoprotein, prealbumin, and albumin concentrations into a single score.[13–15]

$$\text{NRI} = 1.519 \times \text{albumin g/l} + 0.417\ (\text{current weight/usual weight} \times 100)$$

$$\text{PINI} = (\text{CRP mg/l} * \alpha_1\text{-acid glycoprotein})/(\text{albumin g/l} * \text{transthyretin g/l})$$

Nutritional risk factors associated with the underlying pathology and treatments

This broadly stated category may include a variety of parameters that are quite heterogeneously represented in the various screening tools. Although this list is not exhaustive, the presence of any of the following factors should be taken into account; old age, poor cognition, limited mobility, advanced disease stage, extensive tumour burden and metastases, the presence of fever, comorbid conditions associated with additional nutritional risk (i.e. compromised organ function, major stress, infection). A variety of medications may also contribute to poor food intake or altered metabolism (i.e. high dose corticosteroids).

Nutrition screening tools and algorithms

The elements described above are assembled to form nutrition screening tools but may not have been designed and validated specifically for oncology patients. There is no universal and agreed upon screening tool in nutritional oncology. Having standardized procedures in place for nutrition screening, triage and referral, within a given cancer care setting is perhaps more important than the specific identity of the screening tool employed. Most of the available tools are likely to be adequate, insofar as they all consider the same major categories of information. In some studies up to four nutritional screening tools have been applied to the same population of patients (i.e. Kyle *et al.*[16]) with the results showing relatively minor variation between the tools in the identification of patients at nutritional risk and in the prediction of clinical parameters such as length of stay in hospital, infectious and non-infectious complications in hospital and mortality. Many of the nutritional screening assessments have been translated into multiple languages.

The Oncology Nursing Society and the Oncology Nutrition Dietetics Practice Group of the American Dietetics Association suggest the use of the Patient-Generated Subjective Global Assessment (PG-SGA) or Mini Nutritional Assessment (MNA) for cancer patients. Another authority, the French Ministry of Health, recommends a screening algorithm (Figure 3.1) for the identification of malnutrition in hospitalized patients and the British Association for Parenteral and Enteral Nutrition favours the Malnutrition Universal Screening Tool (MUST). These instruments, which are described briefly below, appear to be diverse, but they are generally based on the same fundamental concepts and any would be useful in an oncology setting.

Patient-Generated Subjective Global Assessment (PG-SGA)[17]

This is an adaptation for oncology patients of the earlier SGA[18] which was originally validated as a screening tool for malnutrition in hospitalized patients. The PG-SGA is scored and incorporates questions relating intake, weight and nutritional risk factors, and is a mixture of patient report (weight history, food intake, functional status, symptoms affecting food intake) and assessments made by health care professionals (comorbid conditions, corticosteroid use, fever). The inclusion of a detailed scored physical examination including seven muscle groups, three adipose depots and oedema at three sites acknowledges the importance of body composition but limits the practical utility of this evaluation which is difficult to standardize across a wide variety of caregivers.

Mini Nutritional Assessment (MNA)

The MNA was designed and validated to provide a single, rapid assessment of nutritional status in elderly patients in outpatient clinics, hospitals, and nursing homes.[19] It is composed of simple measurements and brief questions to be completed in about 10 min by a health care professional. The MNA incorporates information relating to intake, weight and nutritional risk factors. BMI (or calf circumference), mid-arm circumference, and weight loss are considered. Questions concerning intake probe recent alterations in food intake, number of meals/day and quantity of fluids, high protein foods, and ability to eat independently. Nutritional risk factors include acute illness or psychological distress, reduced cognition, medications, pressure sores and ulcers. The sum of the MNA score distinguishes between elderly patients with adequate nutritional status, protein-calorie malnutrition and at risk of malnutrition.

Malnutrition Universal Screening Tool (MUST)

This is intended to be used by any category of health care worker. MUST contains three very simple elements, a score for BMI, a score for weight loss and a score for underlying disease condition combined with no oral intake for >5 days.[20] This instrument proposes useful alternatives for height (ulnar length, demispan, knee height) and BMI (mid-upper arm circumference) in patients for whom these measurements are impossible because they are unable to stand.

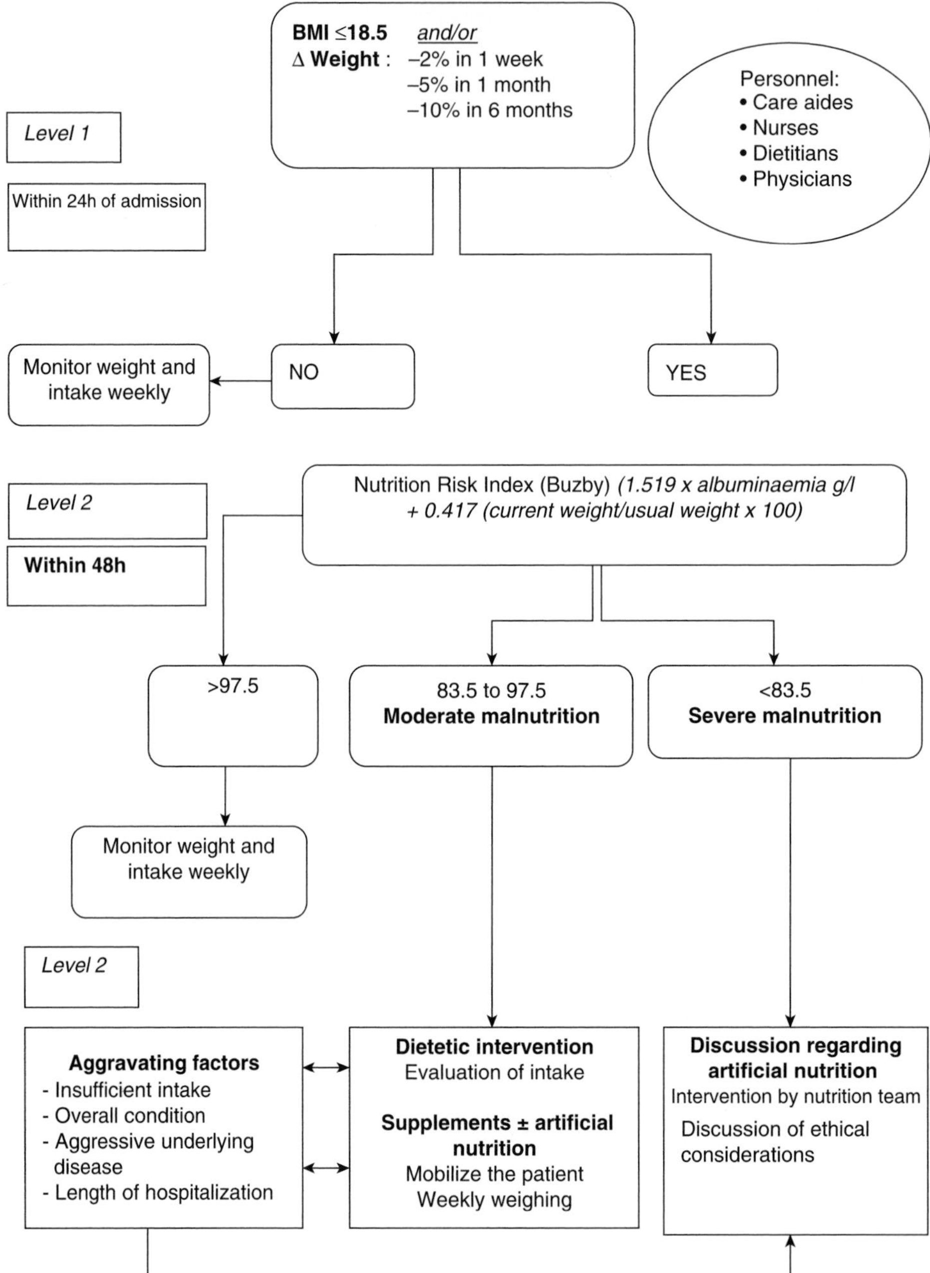

Fig. 3.1 Screening strategy for malnutrition in hospitalized patients. French Ministry of Health: National Nutrition Health Plan.

Nutrition screening algorithm, French Ministry of Health

The screening and assessment plan illustrated in Figure 3.1 is yet another example of a standardized instrument used to detect malnutrition and is intended for hospitalized patients.[21] The point of departure is identification of patients with severe weight loss or who are already underweight, and these patients are further stratified using the Nutrition Risk Index (see above) into groups requiring intervention or monitoring.

In-depth nutritional assessments

Further evaluation of nutritional status includes the same basic elements as at the screening level, but in greater depth. There are both real and perceived barriers to more detailed investigations of nutritional status, particularly in patients with more advanced disease. Patients may be elderly, frail, cognitively impaired, and may decline rapidly, so that much of their available energy may be devoted to immediate needs. These factors may explain why detailed nutritional assessments are less commonly used in clinical practice and reported in the literature than screening level evaluations. Fearon *et al.* have studied large groups of patients with pancreatic and oesophageal cancer, who are at risk for malnutrition.[22,23] Multiple regression analyses identified dietary intake <1500 kcal/day (estimate of effect, 38%), serum CRP concentrations (estimate of effect, 34%) and stage of disease (estimate of effect, 28%) as independent variables in determining degree of weight loss in oesophageal cancer patients. Importantly, these results suggest that all three of these elements make important contributions to weight loss, and underscore the value of conducting assessments of dietary intake and of biological factors.

Assessment of energy balance should include estimates of intake and expenditure

Assessment of energy expenditure: indirect calorimetry vs equations

Measurement of resting energy expenditure by indirect calorimetry is possible in multiple clinical settings, whereas measures of total energy expenditure (TEE) require specialized expertise and have rarely been reported for cancer populations.[24–26] Instead of indirect calorimetry, daily energy needs can be more conveniently estimated by a variety of equations for resting energy expenditure (REE; e.g. Harris–Benedict equation), but their accuracy is questionable.

Measuring total energy expenditure would have to include the energy consumed by physical activity plus the REE (the two major components of TEE). Patients with cancer might be expected to have a decline in their TEE because of decreased physical activity, yet simultaneously exhibit increased REE because of an acute-phase response. If there were an increased energy cost of cancer it would in theory be based on the difference between measured REE (by indirect calorimetry) and predicted REE (usually measured by using standard equations such as Harris–Benedict). Although handheld calorimetry is convenient and less burdensome than traditional systems such as metabolic carts and respiration chambers in patients with advanced cancer, the handheld devices may not be as accurate.[27,28] Nevertheless, they provide some advantage over equations that estimate basal energy needs,[29] and are less expensive, do not require trained personnel and are not as time-consuming as traditional indirect calorimetry systems. Their measures appear to be lower than traditional devices used in the research setting, but may provide an acceptable[30] alternative for patients.[31]

There is a variety of equations for predicting REE; the most commonly used is the Harris–Benedict equation (HBE), as follows for male and females:[32]

$$\text{Male: BMR (kcal/d)} = 66.4730 + 13.7516\ W + 5.0033\ H - 6.7550\ A$$

$$\text{Female: BMR (kcal/d)} = 655.955 + 9.5634\ W + 1.8496\ H - 4.6756\ A$$

where: BMR = basal metabolic rate; W = weight (kg); H = height (cm); A = age (years).

A large study of 714 newly detected cancer patients and 642 control subjects with non-malignant diseases underwent open-circuit indirect calorimetry using a ventilated hood system. Patients with oesophageal cancer, gastric cancer, pancreatic cancer and non-small cell lung cancer (NSCLC) had higher energy consumption than those with colon cancer. Although 47% of all cancer patients were hypermetabolic, 43% normometabolic and 10% hypometabolic, 25% of control subjects were also hypermetabolic. Overall, no significant difference was found in measured REE (mREE) between cancer patients and controls. However, in order to account for existing weight and muscle loss, as well as variations in height, REE was adjusted for fat-free mass (FFM) or for the predicted REE (pREE) by the Harris–Benedict equation. Calculated mREE/FFM and mREE/pREE were shown to be higher in cancer patients, revealing that REE was in fact elevated, especially those with stage IV disease. When REE data were further evaluated, patients were classified as hypometabolic (REE <90% of predicted), normometabolic (90–110% of predicted) or hypermetabolic (>110% of predicted). Three-quarters of gastric, pancreatic and oesophageal cancer patients, almost two-thirds of NSCLC and half of colon cancer patients were hypermetabolic.[33] An earlier study in NSCLC patients showed hypermetabolism correlated with a systemic inflammatory response (e.g. IL-6) and acute phase proteins (e.g CRP).[34] The fact that a considerable proportion of cancer patients are documented to be hypermetabolic raises a concern that standardized equations for estimating energy requirements may underestimate total energy needs. Even in patients with non-metastatic lung cancer, REE (adjusted for lean body mass) is significantly elevated compared with matched healthy controls.[35] This suggests that an evaluation of energy requirements is important early in the disease trajectory as well as in patients with advanced disease. A study comparing weight-stable (weight loss <2%) and weight-losing (>5%) cancer patients found that HBEs tended to underestimate REE in both groups.[36] Other studies have suggested that modified equations might also be innaccurate and could in fact overestimate energy needs. One such equation to estimate total daily energy expenditure[37] uses the HBE together with an 'injury' factor of 1.3. A small study of patients receiving anticancer therapy showed a modest overall 10% increase in REE compared with healthy control subjects. The authors suggested that an automatic 'injury factor' applied to the HBE may not be appropriate for cancer patients.[38]

A study in obese hospitalized cancer patients (BMI ≥30) used various equations for estimating REE such as the HBE, Mifflin–St Jeor, Ireton–Jones, 21 kcal/kg body weight, and 25 kcal/kg body weight. These were compared with measured energy expenditures by metabolic cart for ventilated patients and a handheld indirect calorimeter in non-ventilated patients. Compared with indirect calorimetry, the estimation strategies were inconsistent and inaccurate predictors of energy expenditure.[39]

Estimation of intake

Prospectively collected dietary records are the standard for evaluation of total energy and macronutrient intake,and for these three-day[40] collection periods seem to be the compromise generally taken between the length of the assessment and the frailty or vulnerability of the studied patients. Twenty-four-hour dietary recall and food frequency questionnaires are sometimes used as alternatives.[41–43] There are relatively few studies in which cancer patients completed a dietary record for the purposes of computing total caloric intake[44–45] and this seems generally very rare in clinical practice.

Extent of physiological reserves of energy and protein

Physiological reserves of energy and protein in human body can be estimated by assessing body composition. Several methods of body composition analysis are currently available and summarized in Table 3.1. Most commonly used methods to measure body composition in patients with

Table 3.1 Summary of body composition measurement methods

Modality	Premise	Advantages	Disadvantages
Hydrodensitometry (underwater weighing)	◆ Body volume is measured by underwater weighing and body density is calculated ◆ Estimates body fat and fat-free mass	◆ Reliable and valid for measuring body density and percentage body fat	◆ Does not differentiate fat-free mass components ◆ Relies on assumed densities of fat-free mass and fat mass compartments to determine percent body fat ◆ High subject burden
Air displacement plethysmography (Bod Pod)	◆ Body volume is determined by air displacement and body density is calculated ◆ Estimates body fat and fat-free mass	◆ Well suited for a broad segment of the population ◆ Good-to-excellent reliability and acceptable validity ◆ Fast, non-invasive	◆ Does not differentiate fat-free mass components ◆ Relies on assumed densities of fat-free mass and fat mass compartments to determine percentage body fat
In vivo neutron activation analysis	◆ Fast neutron source from a low radioactive field produces isotopic atoms that can be measured	◆ High precision and accuracy ◆ Capable of quantifying all the main atomic elements found *in vivo*	◆ High cost and limited availability ◆ Involves neutron adiation exposure potential danger during childhood and pregnancy
Dual-energy X-ray absorptiometry (DXA)	◆ Uses very low radiation X-rays of two different levels and the amount of energy absorbed is used to differentiate between soft tissue and bone. Fat tissue is then estimated from specific attenuation characteristics of soft tissues	◆ Differentiates fat, lean and bone tissue ◆ Safe for repeated measures ◆ High precision and accuracy ◆ Fast ◆ Regional measures of body composition can be obtained	◆ Differences within and between manufacturers ◆ Inability to differentiate compartments within fat and lean tissues
Biolectrical impedance analysis (BIA)	◆ Determines resistance and reactance from an electrical signal ◆ Fat-free mass has a higher water and electrolyte content, making it a good conductor ◆ Measures total body water which is then used to estimate fat-free mass and fat mass	◆ Portable ◆ Safe ◆ Low cost	◆ Small changes in hydration status can affect results ◆ Regression equations can be variable

(Continued)

Table 3.1 (Continued) Summary of body composition measurement methods

Modality	Premise	Advantages	Disadvantages
Computed tomography (CT)	◆ The X-ray attenuation through tissues is detected and an image is reconstructed. Adipose tissue, skeletal muscle, bone, visceral organs and brain can be identified by the different X-ray attenuation.	◆ Most accurate method to determine body composition at the tissue-organ level, specifically total and regional adipose tissue and skeletal muscle tissue ◆ Able to determine the muscle quality ◆ High image resolution ◆ Consistent image attenuation value within and between scans	◆ Large radiation dose ◆ High cost ◆ High technical skill ◆ Size of the patient (usually patients with a BMI >35 kg/m^2 cannot fit in the scanner)
Magnetic resonance imaging (MRI)	◆ When a magnetic field is generated, atomic protons behave like magnets and become aligned in the magnetic field. These protons are then activated by a radio-frequency wave, absorbing energy. The signal generated is used to develop regional and whole-body cross-sectional images ◆ Quantifies adipose tissue, skeletal muscle, and visceral organs	◆ Most accurate method to determine body composition at the tissue-organ level, specifically total and regional adipose tissue and skeletal muscle tissue ◆ No exposure to ionizing radiation ◆ Often used in children and adolescents ◆ Best method for multiple-image protocols for whole body and serial measurements	◆ High cost ◆ High technical skill ◆ Image quality affected by respiratory motion ◆ Size of the patient (usually patients with a BMI >35 kg/m^2 cannot fit in the scanner)
Anthropometry: skinfold thickness and circumferences	◆ Estimates tissue quantity using calipers ◆ Skinfold thickness can be used to calculate fat, fat-mass and muscle size	◆ Portable ◆ Low cost	◆ Need trained individuals ◆ Need proper instrument for a good accuracy and reliability ◆ Uses assumptions that the thickness of subcutaneous adipose tissue reflects a constant proportion of the total body fat and that subcutaneous adipose tissue has a constant compressibility ◆ Relatively insensitive measure ◆ Differences cannot be detected over the short term

cancer include skinfold thickness measurements,[46] bioelectrical impedance analysis (BIA),[47] dual-energy X-ray absorptiometry (DXA)[10] and computed tomography (CT) imaging analysis.[48] Skinfold thickness measurements together with body weight, BMI, and body surface area represent anthropometric methods and are both clinically practical and useful in research studies in large populations where cost/efficiency are an issue. In general, anthropometric methods are less accurate due to the underlying assumptions and indirect approach. A general problem with several of these techniques is that they may be unable to differentiate a unit of body weight into specific amounts of lean and fat tissues, a problem that imposes important limitations on detecting key components of wasting.[48] Muscle wasting can coexist with depletion of adipose tissue but may also coexist with obesity, and this independent behaviour of lean and adipose tissues makes body composition analyses essential to understanding the status of protein and energy reserves.

Image-based analysis such as DXA, CT and magnetic resonance imaging represent the gold standard for evaluating body composition and they share high precision and specificity. DXA is an appealing approach due to the relatively low radiation exposure and cost. Unfortunately, DXA cannot differentiate between the different subsets of fat and non-fat tissues, such as the separation of lean tissue into muscle, organs and tumours; and the separation of adipose tissue into intramuscular, visceral and subcutaneous compartments. Moreover, DXA may overestimate lean tissue in patients with large changes in hydration (>5%), which is often reported in patients with cancer.[48]

Computed tomography may be a method of choice for studying body composition in patients with malignant disease because CT imaging is often required for clinical assessment of the cancer. CT has excellent ability to discriminate individual tissues.[49] Muscle, adipose tissues, bone and organs can be quantified,[8,9] and the amount of fatty infiltration in muscle and organs can also be estimated with this technique. The major limitation of using CT analysis to assess body composition (radiation exposure) is not applicable in patients with cancer since CT images are routinely required for medical information to follow tumour growth and response to therapy. CT images can be used opportunistically to investigate body composition including changes over time for longitudinal studies.[4,50] Figure 3.2 provides a brief illustration of this approach. CT images are evaluated at a standard skeletal landmark, the third lumbar vertebra. The two illustrated patients have nearly identical BMI, but the cross-sectional area of the skeletal muscles highlighted (paraspinal muscles and muscles of the abdominal wall) are considerably different in these two individuals.

Wasting of lean tissues and especially skeletal muscle is an important component of cancer-associated weight loss. The assessment of these quantities requires the use of the image-based techniques listed above. Some reference values are available from large population-based studies of healthy individuals using DXA, for example for n = 2984 healthy 65-year-old Caucasian men and women. Newman *et al.*[51] reported mean (SD):

- whole-body lean (FFM) without bone (kg): men 54.8 (6.7); women 38.1 (5.1);
- lean (FFM) index without bone (kg/m^2): men 18.2 (1.8): women 15 (1.8);
- total appendicular skeletal muscle (kg): men 23.6 (3.2); women 15.5 (2.4);
- total appendicular skeletal muscle index (kg/m^2): men 7.8 (0.9); women 6.1 (0.8).

These values for otherwise healthy persons serve as a useful point of comparison for populations affected by cancer. Researchers studying the muscularity of human populations have coined a term, sarcopenia, to denote a reduced quantity of skeletal muscle which is significantly associated with elevated risks of physical disability and mortality. Expressed in units of total appendicular skeletal muscle, generally accepted cut-off points for sarcopenia are for men <7.26 kg/m^2 and for women <5.45 kg/m^2. These values are >2 SD below that typical of healthy adults.[52]

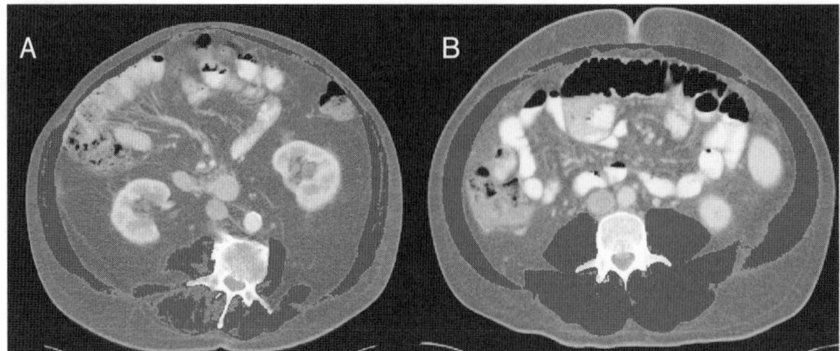

Fig. 3.2. Lumbar cross-sectional images of two male cancer patients with identical body mass index of 30.3 kg/m^2. Segmented tissue (dark grey ■) of interest is total lumbar skeletal muscle. Relative to patient B (skeletal muscle area of 211cm^2); patient A has a much smaller amount of lumbar skeletal muscle (159cm^2) and is classified as sarcopenic.

Sarcopenia was first characterized in the elderly, and is called the 'silent crippler' because of its association with risks of physical disability, falls, fractures and frailty. Sarcopenia is known to associate with extended hospital stays, infectious and non-infectious complications in hospitalized patients, and overall mortality. Sarcopenia is not restricted to people who are thin or wasted. The ageing process is often paralleled by decreases in muscle and increases in fat mass, which may culminate in sarcopenic obesity, a worst-case condition with the combined health risks of both obesity and muscle wasting. Recent studies[53] indicate increasing prevalence of sarcopenic obesity in elderly people in westernized countries.

Image-based body composition analysis is an important asset to the identification of cancer patients with significant erosion of the lean body mass and skeletal muscle. Prado *et al.* produced evidence that sarcopenia is common in obese patients with solid tumours,[54] and is associated with elevated risk of being partially or entirely bedridden. Sarcopenia was found to be an independent prognostic factor for increased mortality (i.e. a median survival of 10 months versus 21 months for non-sarcopenic patients.[55] Sarcopenic patients are also prone to severe toxicity during chemotherapy[56] necessitating reductions in the dose of drugs or treatment delays that ultimately may reduce treatment efficacy.

Biological criteria related to potential mechanisms of altered metabolism

The main stimulators of acute-phase protein production are the inflammation-associated cytokines, which are produced during inflammatory processes: interleukin (IL)-6, IL-1β, tumour necrosis factor-α (TNFα), interferon-γ, transforming growth factor-β (TGFβ) and possibly IL-8.[5] Many of these are known to have specific catabolic effects on skeletal muscle and adipose tissue.[57] To date, these cytokines have proved to be rather poor biomarkers in nutritional evaluation of cancer patients compared with C-reactive protein. IL-6 levels were lower in weight-stable versus weight-losing patients[58–61] whereas correlations of IL-6 with weight loss lacked significance in other studies.[11] Associations of several cytokines with weight loss were negative: for IL-8 in pancreatic, for IL-10, IL-12 in gastrointestinal cancer patients, and for TNF and other cytokines in other several tumours.[62–64]

There are other biomarkers potentially relevant to nutritional assessment of cancer patients, but this awaits more systematic evidence. A putative proteolysis-inducing factor appeared to distinguish pancreatic cancer patients with different degrees of weight loss; however, current evidence suggests no association of this factor with weight loss in advanced cancer patients.[65] Some studies showed that weight-losing patients had increased fasting insulin levels.[66] Data for leptin and ghrelin are equivocal, with both negative and positive results in studies where these were analysed in relation to weight loss.[67–71]

Risk factors associated with the underlying pathology and treatments

More detailed attention may be paid to risk factors for malnutrition in specific individuals. Stage and burden of disease are primary risks. In advanced disease stage, overall tumour burden, including metastases, may contribute in a quantitatively important fashion to overall energy expenditure. Lieffers *et al.*[4] recently quantified the extent of liver metastases in colorectal cancer patients and found an average accumulation of 0.7 kg disease burden during the last year of life. The estimated percentage of FFM occupied by the liver inclusive of metastases increased from 4.5% to 7.0% over this time. A positive linear relationship was demonstrated between the mass of the liver inclusive of metastases and whole-body resting energy expenditure ($r^2 = 0.35$, $P = 0.010$). Based on reports of specific metabolic rate of tumour tissue *in situ*, these authors estimate that increases in mass and proportion of liver and tumour (which have a high metabolic rate) may explain an increased energy expenditure of ~17 700 kcal over 3 months which contributes substantially to weight loss.

Risks of malnutrition in elderly and frail elderly have been considered, and these are generally applicable to cancer patients, for whom the median age at diagnosis is about 65 years. In the elderly, specific attention to protein intake is required to maximize protein synthesis and retention.[72] Depression is a significant independent factor explaining nutritional risk in the elderly, as is cognitive impairment,[73] and there are various issues associated with mobility, family and institutional contexts and food security that predispose many elderly to additional nutritional risks.

Nutrition assessment team

A wide range of professionals playing roles in cancer care will be involved at some level with nutritional assessment. These roles differ in the degree of contact with the patient and in the level of responsibility involved for nutritional assessment and care. In an interdisciplinary collaborative health care team, the levels and areas of responsibility must be clearly established. It is critical for all members of the team to understand the education, core competencies and scope of practice of different members.

Unless there is a clearly defined policy and delegation of authority for conducting screening and taking appropriate action, it is possible for individual patients to become extremely malnourished before interventions can be initiated.[74] (Please see Chapter 19 for more details.)

Role of the registered dietitian (RD)

The nutrition care process is facilitated if the multidisciplinary oncology team includes the dietitian as an integral team member.[75] The role of the RD is more specifically treated in Chapter 18. RDs with specific training in oncology dietetics are key members of the nutrition care continuum. A certification in Oncology Nutrition is available from the Commission on Dietetics Registration of the American Dietetic Association. The Oncology Nutrition Dietetics Practice Group (ON DPG) is an important resource and has developed standards of best practice outlined in books, videos, toolkits, a website, and list-serve using evidence-based resources.[76,77]

Role of the medical nutrition specialist (MNS)

Not all cases require MNS input, and the role of this specialized expertise is normally oriented towards a subset of specific cases. The MNS will have a role in the establishment of algorithms for screening and referral and in establishing practice guidelines in collaboration with RD and medical staff. Some of the issues and limitations of the implementation of clinical practice guidelines in nutrition have been discussed.[78,79]

The oncologist may encounter a malnourished patient for whom there is a clear course of action based on published recommendations. In situations where there is a base of scientific evidence for nutritional support (see below), available recommendations and clinical practice guidelines should be applied by the RD, oncologist or primary care physician.[80–82] MNS intervention is also unnecessary when there is evidence that the potential benefit from nutritional support is negligible or benefit is outweighed by the risk of complications. In these instances good palliative clinical practices should be defined, promoted and applied.[80–82]

Outside of these clearly defined areas, there are situations where the available scientific evidence has not clearly established the role of nutritional support and where treatment decisions are taken on a case-by-case basis. In these instances the experience and knowledge of the MNS are necessary. Patients with solid tumours undergoing radiation or chemotherapy, and those with cancers of the head and neck in particular, may benefit from MNS assessment.

Please refer to Parts 6 and 9 which address the clinical assessment and management of these patients in detail.

Conclusions

A hierarchy of screening level and more in-depth evaluations of nutritional status and nutritional risk provides the basis for timely nutritional intervention. The nutritional risk for cancer patients of different types and on different treatment regimens may pre-date the cancer diagnosis, and may evolve slowly or acutely throughout the disease progression. Standardized procedures for nutrition screening, triage and referral are required within cancer care settings, and the identity of members of the health care team responsible for nutritional assessment and intervention must be clearly established.

References

1. Perry GS, Byers TE, Mokdad AH, Serdula MK, Williamson DF (1995) The validity of self-reports of past body weights by U.S. adults. *Epidemiology*, **6**, 61–6.
2. Doyle D, Hanks G, Cherny NI, Calman K (eds) (2005) *Oxford Textbook of Palliative Medicine.* Oxford: Oxford University Press.
3. Honnor A (2008) Classification, aetiology and nursing management of lymphoedema. *Br J Nurs*, **17**(9), 576–86.
4. Lieffers JR, Mourtzakis M, Hall KD, McCargar LJ, Prado CM, Baracos VE (2009) A viscerally driven cachexia syndrome in patients with advanced colorectal cancer: contributions of organ and tumor mass to whole-body energy demands. *Am J Clin Nutr*, **89**(4), 1173–9.
5. Gabay C, Kushner I (1999) Acute-phase proteins and other systemic responses to inflammation. *N Engl J Med*, **340**(6), 448–54.
6. Scott HR, McMillan DC, Crilly A, McArdle CS, Milroy R (1996) The relationship between weight loss and interleukin 6 in non-small-cell lung cancer. *Br J Cancer*, **73**, 1560–2.
7. Martín F, Santolaria F, Batista N, *et al.* (1999) Cytokine levels (IL-6 and IFN-gamma), acute phase response and nutritional status as prognostic factors in lung cancer. *Cytokine*, **11**, 80–6.
8. Scott HR, McMillan DC, Forrest LM, Brown DJ, McArdle CS, Milroy R (2002) The systemic inflammatory response, WL, performance status and survival in patients with inoperable non-small cell lung cancer. *Br J Cancer*, **87**, 264–7.

9. Slaviero KA, Read JA, Clarke SJ, Rivory LP (2003) Baseline nutritional assessment in advanced cancer patients receiving palliative chemotherapy. *Nutr Cancer*, **46**, 148–57.
10. Fouladiun M, Korner U, Bosaeus I, Daneryd P, Hyltander A, Lundholm KG (2005) Body composition and time course changes in regional distribution of fat and lean tissue in unselected cancer patients on palliative care – correlations with food intake, metabolism, exercise capacity, and hormones. *Cancer*, **103**, 2189–98.
11. Kayacan O, Karnak D, Beder S, *et al.* (2006) Impact of TNF-alpha and IL-6 levels on development of cachexia in newly diagnosed NSCLC patients. *Am J Clin Oncol*, **29**, 328–35.
12. Buzby GP, Mullen JL, Matthews DC, Hobbs CL, Rosato EF (1980) Prognostic nutritional index in gastrointestinal surgery. *Am J Surg*, **139**(1), 160–7.
13. Ingenbleek Y, Carpentier YA (1985) A prognostic inflammatory and nutritional index scoring critically ill patients. *Int J Vitam Nutr Res*, **55**(1), 91–101.
14. Vehe KL, Brown RO, Kuhl DA, Boucher BA, Luther RW, Kudsk KA (1991) The prognostic inflammatory and nutritional index in traumatized patients receiving enteral nutrition support. *J Am Coll Nutr*, **10**(4), 355–63.
15. Walsh D, Mahmoud F, Barna B (2003) Assessment of nutritional status and prognosis in advanced cancer: interleukin-6, C-reactive protein, and the prognostic and inflammatory nutritional index. *Support Care Cancer*, **11**(1), 60–2.
16. Kyle UG, Kossovsky MP, Karsegard VL, Pichard C (2006) Comparison of tools for nutritional assessment and screening at hospital admission: a population study. *Clin Nutr*, **25**(3), 409–17.
17. Ottery FD (1996) Definition of standardized nutritional assessment and interventional pathways in oncology. Review. *Nutrition*, **12**(1 Suppl), S15–9.
18. Detsky AS, Baker JP, O'Rourke K, *et al.* (1987) Predicting nutrition-associated complications for patients undergoing gastrointestinal surgery. *J Parenter Enteral Nutr*, **11**(5), 440–6.
19. Vellas B, Guigoz Y, Garry PJ, *et al.* (1999) The Mini Nutritional Assessment (MNA) and its use in grading the nutritional state of elderly patients. *Nutrition*, **15**(2), 116–22.
20. Stratton RJ, Hackston A, Longmore D, *et al.* (2004) Malnutrition in hospital outpatients and inpatients: prevalence, concurrent validity and ease of use of the 'malnutrition universal screening tool' ('MUST') for adults. *Br J Nutr*, **92**(5), 799–808.
21. Antoun S, Baracos V (2009) [Malnutrition in cancer patient: when to have a specialized consultation?] *Bull Cancer*, **96**(5), 615–23.
22. Deans DA, Tan BH, Wigmore SJ, *et al.* (2009) The influence of systemic inflammation, dietary intake and stage of disease on rate of weight loss in patients with gastro-oesophageal cancer. *Br J Cancer*, **100**(1), 63–9.
23. Fearon KC, Voss AC, Hustead DS; Cancer Cachexia Study Group (2006) Definition of cancer cachexia: effect of weight loss, reduced food intake, and systemic inflammation on functional status and prognosis. *Am J Clin Nutr*, **83**(6), 1345–50.
24. Gibney E, Elia M, Jebb SA, Murgatroyd P, Jennings G (1997) Total energy expenditure in patients with small-cell lung cancer: results of a validated study using the bicarbonate–urea method. *Metabolism*, **46**(12), 1412–7.
25. Reilly JJ, Blacklock CJ, Dale E, Donaldson M, Gibson BE (1996) Resting metabolic rate and obesity in childhood acute lymphoblastic leukaemia. *Int J Obes Relat Metab Disord*, **20**(12), 1130–2.
26. Demark-Wahnefried W, Peterson BL, *et al.* (2001) Changes in weight, body composition, and factors influencing energy balance among premenopausal breast cancer patients receiving adjuvant chemotherapy. *J Clin Oncol*, **19**(9), 2381–9.
27. Fares S, Miller MD, Masters S, Crotty M (2005) Measuring energy expenditure in community-dwelling older adults: are portable methods valid and acceptable? *J Am Diet Assoc*, **108**(3), 544–8.
28. Reeves MM, Capra S, Bauer J, Davies PS, Battistutta D (2005) Clinical accuracy of the MedGem indirect calorimeter for measuring resting energy expenditure in cancer patients. *Eur J Clin Nutr*, **59**(4), 603–10.

29. Spears KE, Kim H, Behall KM, Conway JM (2009) Hand-held indirect calorimeter offers advantages compared with prediction equations, in a group of overweight women, to determine resting energy expenditures and estimated total energy expenditures during research screening. *J Am Diet Assoc*, **109**(5), 836–45.
30. Compher C, Hise M, Sternberg A, Kinosian BP (2005) Comparison between Medgem and Deltatrac resting metabolic rate measurements. *Eur J Clin Nutr*, **59**(10), 1136–41.
31. McDoniel SO (2007) Systematic review on use of a handheld indirect calorimeter to assess energy needs in adults and children. *Int J Sport Nutr Exerc Metab*, **17**(5), 491–500.
32. Harris JA, Benedict FG. (1918) A biometric study of human basal metabolism. *Proc Natl Acad Sci USA*, **4**(12), 370–373.
33. Cao DX, Wu GH, Zhang B, *et al.* (2010) Resting energy expenditure and body composition in patients with newly detected cancer. *Clin Nutr*. **29**(1), 72–7.
34. Staal-van den Brekel AJ, Dentener MA, Schols AM, Buurman WA, Wouters EF (1995) Increased resting energy expenditure and weight loss are related to a systemic inflammatory response in lung cancer patients. *J Clin Oncol*, **13**(10), 2600–5.
35. Jatoi A, Daly BD, Hughes VA, Dallal GE, Kehayias J, Roubenoff R (2001) Do patients with nonmetastatic non-small cell lung cancer demonstrate altered resting energy expenditure? *Ann Thorac Surg*, **72**(2), 348–51.
36. Johnson G, Sallé A, Lorimier G, *et al.* (2008) Cancer cachexia: measured and predicted resting energy expenditures for nutritional needs evaluation. *Nutrition*, **24**(5), 443–50.
37. Alpers D, Stenson W, Bier D (2002) *Manual of nutritional therapeutics*, 4th edn. Philadelphia: Lippincott Williams & Wilkins.
38. Reeves M, Battistuta D, Capra S, Bauer J, Davies P (2006) Resting energy expenditure and body composition in patients with newly detected cancer. *Nutrition*, **22**(6), 609–615.
39. Anderegg BA, Worrall C, Barbour E, Simpson KN, Delegge M (2009) Comparison of resting energy expenditure prediction methods with measured resting energy expenditure in obese, hospitalized adults. *J Parenter Enteral Nutr*, **2**, 168–75.
40. von Gruenigen V,Courneya K, Gibbons H, *et al.* (2008) Feasibility and effectiveness of a lifestyle intervention program in obese endometrial cancer patients. *Gynecol Oncol*, **109**(1), 19–26.
41. Cross AJ, Leitzmann MF, Subar AF, Thompson FE, Hollenbeck AR, Schatzkin A (2008) A prospective study of meat and fat intake in relation to small intestinal cancer. *Cancer Res*, **68**(22), 9274–9.
42. Wirfält E, Midthune D, Reedy J, *et al.* (2009) Associations between food patterns defined by cluster analysis and colorectal cancer incidence in the NIH-AARP diet and health study. *Eur J Clin Nutr*, **63**(6), 707–17.
43. Horn-Ross PL, Lee VS, Collins CN, *et al.* (2008) Dietary assessment in the California Teachers Study: reproducibility and validity. *Cancer Causes Control*, **19**(6), 595–603.
44. Isenring EA, Bauer JD, Capra S (2007) Nutrition support using the American Dietetic Association medical nutrition therapy protocol for radiation oncology patients improves dietary intake compared with standard practice. *J Am Diet Assoc*, **107**(3), 404–12.
45. Hutton JL, Martin L, Field CJ, *et al.* (2006) Dietary patterns in patients with advanced cancer: implications for anorexia-cachexia therapy. *Am J Clin Nutr*, **84**(5), 1163–70.
46. Harvie MN, Campbell IT, Thatcher N, Baildam A (2003) Changes in body composition in men and women with advanced nonsmall cell lung cancer (NSCLC) undergoing chemotherapy. *J Hum Nutr Diet*, **16**(5), 323–6.
47. Fearon KC, Von Meyenfeldt MF, Moses AG, Van Geenen R, Roy A, Gouma DJ (2003) Effect of a protein and energy dense N-3 fatty acid enriched oral supplement on loss of weight and lean tissue in cancer cachexia: a randomised double blind trial. *Gut*, **52**(10), 1479–86.
48. Prado CM, Birdsell L, Baracos V (2010) The emerging role of computerized tomography in assessing cancer cachexia. *Curr Opin Support Palliat Care*. **3**(4), 269–75.

49. Heymsfield SB, Wang Z, Baumgartner RN, Ross R (1997) Human body composition: advances in models and methods. *Annu Rev Nutr*, **17**, 527–58.
50. Cohn SH, Gartenhaus W, Sawitsky A, Rai K, Zanzi I, Vaswani A (1981) Compartmental body composition of cancer patients by measurement of total body nitrogen, potassium, and water. *Metabolism*, **30**(3), 222–9.
51. Newman AB, Kuoelian V, Visser M, *et al.* (2005) Sarcopenia: alternative definitions and associations with lower extremity function. *J Am Geriatric Sc*, **51**(11), 1602–9.
52. Rolland Y, Czerwinski S, Abellan Van Kan G, *et al.* (2008) Sarcopenia: its assessment, etiology, pathogenesis, consequences and future perspectives. *J Nutr Health Aging*, **12**(7), 433–50.
53. Prado CM, Lieffers JR, McCargar LJ, *et al.* (2008) Prevalence and clinical implications of sarcopenic obesity in patients with solid tumours of the respiratory and gastrointestinal tracts: a population-based study. *Lancet Oncology*, **9**(7), 629–35.
54. Bouchard DR, Dionne IJ, Brochu M (2009) Sarcopenic/obesity and physical capacity in older men and women: data from the Nutrition as a Determinant of Successful Aging (NuAge)—the Quebec Longitudinal Study. *Obesity*, **17**(11), 2082–8.
55. Prado CM, Baracos VE, McCargar LJ, *et al.* (2007) Body composition as an independent determinant of 5-fluorouracil-based chemotherapy toxicity. *Clin Cancer Res*, **13**(11), 3264–8.
56. Prado CMM, Baracos VE, McCargar LJ, *et al.* (2009) Sarcopenia as a determinant of chemotherapy toxicity and time to tumor progression in metastatic breast cancer patients receiving capecitabine treatment. *Clin Cancer Res*, **15**(8), 2920–6.
57. Baracos VE (2006) Cytokines and the pathophysiology of skeletal muscle atrophy. In: Anker SD, Hofbauer K (eds), *The Pharmacotherapy of Cachexia*. CRC Press. pp. 101–114.
58. van Bokhorst-De van der Schuer MA, von Blomberg-van der Flier BM, *et al.* (1998) Differences in immune status between well-nourished and malnourished head and neck cancer patients. *Clin Nutr*, **17**, 107–11.
59. Tas F, Oguz H, Argon A, *et al.* (2005) The value of serum levels of IL-6, TNF-alpha, and erythropoietin in metastatic malignant melanoma: serum IL-6 level is a valuable prognostic factor at least as serum LDH in advanced melanoma. *Med Oncol*, **22**, 241–6.
60. Shibata M, Nezu T, Kanou H, Abe H, Takekawa M, Fukuzawa M (2002) Decreased production of interleukin-12 and type 2 immune responses are marked in cachectic patients with colorectal and gastric cancer. *J Clin Gastroenterol*, **34**, 416–20.
61. Okada S, Okusaka T, Ishii H, *et al.* (1998) Elevated serum interleukin-6 levels in patients with pancreatic cancer. *Jpn J Clin Oncol*, **28**, 12–5.
62. Oka M, Yamamoto K, Takahashi M, *et al.* (1996) Relationship between serum levels of interleukin 6, various disease parameters and malnutrition in patients with esophageal squamous cell carcinoma. *Cancer Res*, **56**, 2776–80.
63. Jatoi A, Egner J, Loprinzi CL, *et al.* (2004) Investigating the utility of serum cytokine measurements in a multi-institutional cancer anorexia/WL trial. *Support Care Cancer*, **12**, 640–4.
64. Maltoni M, Fabbri L, Nanni O, *et al.* (1997) Serum levels of tumour necrosis factor alpha and other cytokines do not correlate with WL and anorexia in cancer patients. *Support Care Cancer*, **5**, 130–5.
65. Wieland BM, Stewart GD, Skipworth RJ, *et al.* (2007) Is there a human homologue to the murine proteolysis-inducing factor? *Clin Cancer Res*, **13**, 4984–92.
66. Gambardella A, Paolisso G, D'Amore A, Granato M, Verza M, Varricchio M (1993) Different contribution of substrates oxidation to insulin resistance in malnourished elderly patients with cancer. *Cancer*, **72**, 3106–13.
67. Wolf I, Sadetzki S, Kanety H, *et al.* (2006) Adiponectin, ghrelin, and leptin in cancer cachexia in breast and colon cancer patients. *Cancer*, **106**, 966–73.
68. Bolukbas FF, Kilic H, Bolukbas C, *et al.* (2004) Cancer serum leptin concentration and advanced gastrointestinal cancers: a case-controlled study. *BMC Cancer*, **4**, 29.

69. Moses AG, Dowidar N, Holloway B, Waddell I, Fearon KC, Ross JA (2001) Leptin and its relation to weight loss, ob gene expression and the acute-phase response in surgical patients. *Br J Surg*, **88**, 588–93.
70. Shimizu Y, Nagaya N, Isobe T, *et al.* (2003) Increased plasma ghrelin level in lung cancer cachexia. *Clin Cancer Res*, **9**, 774–8.
71. Huang Q, Fan YZ, Ge BJ, Zhu Q, Tu ZY (2007) Circulating ghrelin in patients with gastric or colorectal cancer. *Dig Dis Sci*, **52**, 803–9.
72. Symons TB, Sheffield-Moore M, Wolfe RR, Paddon-Jones D (2009) A moderate serving of high-quality protein maximally stimulates skeletal muscle protein synthesis in young and elderly subjects. *J Am Diet Assoc*, **109**(9), 1582–6.
73. Orsitto G, Fulvio F, Tria D, Turi V, Venezia A, Manca C (2009) Nutritional status in hospitalized elderly patients with mild cognitive impairment. *Clin Nutr*, **28**(1), 100–2.
74. Mirhosseini N, Fainsinger RL, Baracos V (2005) Parenteral nutrition in advanced cancer: indications and clinical practice guidelines. *J Palliat Med*, **8**(5), 914–8.
75. Anonymous (2008) Nutrition Care Process and Model Part 1: The 2008 Update. *J Am Diet Assoc*, **108**(7), 1116.
76. Robien K, Levin R, Pritchett E, Otto M; American Dietetic Association (2006) Standards of practice and standards of professional performance for registered dietitians (generalist, specialty, and advanced) in oncology nutrition care. *J Am Diet Assoc*, **106**(6), 946–951.
77. Oncology Nutrition Dietetic Practice Group website. Available at: http://www.oncologynutrition.org (accessed 23 October 2008).
78. Grimshaw JM, Russel IT (1993) Effect of clinical guidelines on medical practice: a systematic review of rigorous evaluation. *Lancet*, **342**, 1317–22.
79. Robinson MK, Trujillo EB, Mogensen KM, Rounds J, McManus K, Jacobs DO (2003) Improving nutritional screening of hospitalized patients: the role of prealbumin. *J Parenter Enteral Nutr*, **27**, 389–95.
80. Klein S, Kinney J, Jeejeebhoy K, *et al.* (1997) Nutrition support in clinical practice: review of published data and recommendations for future research directions. Summary of a conference sponsored by the National Institute of Health, American Society for Parenteral and Enteral nutrition, and American Society for Clinical Nutrition. *J Parenter Enteral Nutr*, **21**, 133–56.
81. Anonymous (1995) Conférence de consensus. Nutrition artificielle périopératoire en chirurgie programmée de l'adulte. *Nutr Clin Métabol*, **9**, 1–148.
82. Weimann A, Braga M, Harsanyi L, *et al.* (2006) ESPEN guidelines on enteral nutrition: surgery including organ transplantation. *Clin Nutr*, **25**, 224–44.

Part 2

Anorexia–cachexia syndrome

Chapter 4

Epidemiology of body weight and body weight loss and its relation to cancer

Egidio Del Fabbro and Vickie E. Baracos

Introduction

We use weight adjusted for stature (body mass index) and weight loss as primary criteria in nutritional evaluation. Assessment of cancer patients based on these criteria must take into account the demographics of body weight. In contemporary times the predominant theme is obesity. Although obesity and cachexia seem to be at opposite ends of the nutrition spectrum, they share some pathological mechanisms (e.g. increased inflammation[1]) and generally have a deleterious impact on survival. The epidemiology of obesity is, however, better characterized than cachexia, since 'overnutrition' has become a global health issue. Unhealthy diets and the related factors of obesity and physical inactivity have resulted in a rapid increase of obesity even in low-income countries.[2] There is also a newly found awareness that in some patients muscle wasting (in the form of sarcopenia) coexists with obesity.

Cachexia due to a variety of chronic illnessses may affect more than 5 million people in the USA alone,[3] but there are very few studies in the scientific literature investigating large population samples. More than 400 000 patients with cancer in the USA may suffer unintentional weight loss which requires management by health care providers. Obesity appears to affect about a third of adults in the USA, and one in five children/adolescents are overweight.[4] Since 1980, obesity prevalence has doubled in adults, and overweight prevalence has tripled in children.

This chapter will not address the epidemiology of other nutritional factors in the aetiology of cancer. The evidence for protective nutritional factors is discussed in other chapters (please see Chapters 25 and 27).

Definition challenges

Cachexia

Research is particularly challenging when there is no universally accepted definition of cachexia and a number of seemingly disparate diseases/comorbidities [including congestive heart failure (CHF), chronic obstructive pulmonary disease (COPD), chronic kidney disease (CKD), acquired immune deficiency syndrome, rheumatoid arthritis] are also associated with the condition. Standard criteria for defining cachexia are needed for measuring prevalence, determining quality of life outcomes and even resource allocation.[5,6] A retrospective US study of more than 8500 cancer patients estimated the proportion of cachexia patients using four different definitions[7] based on two sets of International Statistical Classification of Diseases codes (ICD-9), prescriptions for appetite stimulants or documented weight loss ≥5%. The two sets of ICD-9 codes were (i) ICD-9 code for cachexia (ICD-9-CM 799.4), (ii) ICD-9 code for cachexia, ICD-9-CM 783.0 for anorexia, ICD-9-CM 783.2x for abnormal weight loss, or ICD-9-CM 783.3 for feeding difficulties. The appetite stimulants included at least one prescription for megestrol acetate, oxandrolone, somatropin or dronabinol. The proportion assigned a diagnosis of cachexia varying from 2% (ICD-9 code 799.4) to 15% (weight loss ≥5%), with 23% meeting at least one of the definitions. These findings emphasize the need for a universal definition of cachexia and suggest that the ICD-9 codes appear to be particularly ineffective at identifying the condition.

Body mass index

Elderly patients are especially at risk for multiple comorbidities and are more vulnerable to muscle wasting caused by cachexia because of pre-existing age-related sarcopenia. The nutritional assessment of older people is difficult even when a simple measure such as body mass index (BMI; kg/m^2) is used, since body length is not a constant factor.[8] This leads to an error in calculation and overestimation of the BMI. Also, body weight and length are often estimated, rather than measured in older disabled people.[9] Similarly, in paediatric oncology patients, using BMI percentile alone to identify those at risk for malnutrition would categorize too many patients as being at risk.[10] Although there are many population studies using well-defined criteria for obesity, there are very few that evaluate body composition in patients with increased BMI. Using BMI alone as a measure of obesity or muscle wasting is flawed since body composition, particularly lean body mass, is not assessed. Because of the obesity epidemic in the developed world, more recent studies using BMI alone may be under-reporting patients with cachexia/sarcopenia. Currently, the diagnosis of obesity in adults is based on criteria from the World Health Organization (WHO) where normal range is BMI between 18.5 and 24.9, grade 1 overweight (between 25.0 and 29.9), grade 2 overweight (between 30.0 and 39.9), and grade 3 overweight ≥40.0.[11] Waist circumference of >35 inches for women and >40 inches for men has been added as a risk factor for diabetes, hypertension and cardiovascular disease to the USA National Institutes of Health guidelines on management of obesity.[12]

Cachexia in cancer patients

Early landmark studies

A study conducted from 1968 to 1970 at M. D. Anderson Hospital of 816 patients with solid tumours showed that the commonest cause of death was infection followed by organ failure. All patients underwent a complete postmortem examination and in 10% of cases no cause other than severe emaciation and/or electrolyte imbalance could be attributed.[13] A landmark study by DeWys *et al.*[14] in 1980 identified the high prevalence of weight loss in cancer patients and its association with decreased survival. More than 3000 patients enrolled in various Eastern Cooperative Oncology Group (ECOG) chemotherapy trials were included in the analysis. Median survival was significantly shorter in patients with weight loss, compared to patients without weight loss. Except for patients with pancreatic or gastric cancer, decreased weight correlated with poor performance status and, within each performance status category or tumour stage, weight loss was associated with decreased survival. Up to 70% of patients with breast cancer or acute lymphoblastic leukaemia had no evidence of weight loss, but about half of prostate cancer, colon cancer and lung cancer patients experienced weight loss, and 85% of gastric and pancreatic patients lost weight (one-third >10%). The study also suggested that any weight loss (0–5%) was associated with a poorer prognosis compared to no weight loss, especially in colorectal and prostate cancers. Furthermore the prognostic effect of weight loss was greater in patients with a more favourable prognosis (good performance status or early tumour stage). A smaller Italian study in 1982 of 280 patients with a variety of tumours and stages showed that weight loss was present in

25% of all patients with unresectable cancer.[15] Similarly to the study by DeWys *et al.*, specific cancers and advanced stage were more likely to be associated with weight loss. Patients with upper gastrointestinal tumours in particular had significantly decreased weight, serum albumin and triceps skinfold thickness. Any chemo- or radiotherapy was associated with an additional decrease in arm muscle circumference. Breast and cervix cancers were not associated with weight loss or other abnormal nutritional parameters. A subsequent study from the USA showed that two-thirds of 254 consecutive patients with a favourable performance status (ECOG 0–2) had lost ≥5% of their weight. Symptoms of abdominal fullness, altered taste, nausea/vomiting and dry mouth occurred more frequently in those with weight loss.[16]

Recent studies

Although cachexia is now recognized as a poor prognostic factor in patients with cancer, there have been few large studies since that by DeWys *et al.*

Outpatient

Preliminary findings of a recent, multicentre outpatient study[17] suggest that cachexia continues to be a major problem in patients with cancer. Italian investigators screened 1000 patients with solid tumours and found that almost 40% of patients had weight loss of ≥10% and more than one-third of patients had high risk scores on Nutritional Risk Screening.[18] The majority of patients with poor performance status and also those with pancreatic, stomach or oesophageal cancers had high risk scores. The median BMI was within normal range (23.3), but 90% of all patients reported some weight loss in the preceding 3 months. The majority also had symptoms of fatigue, anorexia or bowel disturbance (constipation or diarrhoea), and early satiety was a problem in more than one-third of patients.

Hospital patients

Studies investigating the prevalence of malnutrition in hospital populations often note that cancer is associated with weight loss and associated symptoms. In 502 consecutive hospitalized German patients the prevalence of malnutrition (based on clinical scores, anthropometry and bioimpedance analysis) was significantly higher in malignant than in non-malignant diseases (50.9 vs 21.0%).[19] The same group of investigators assessed nutrition in 1886 consecutive patients from multiple hospital sites by subjective global assessment (SGA) and anthropometric measurements including measured arm muscle area and fat. The highest prevalence of malnutrition was found in geriatric departments, followed by oncology, and was associated with a significantly longer hospital stay compared with well-nourished patients.[20] A large screening study of almost 7000 hospitalized or nursing home patients in The Netherlands by 91 teams of dietitians revealed that malnutrition was commoner in cancer than in non-cancer conditions. Malnutrition was defined as >10% unintentional weight loss during the past 6 months and baseline weight was based on patient 'recall'.[21] A multicentre prospective cohort study randomly selected 5051 adult patients admitted to hospital from the Middle East and Europe and screened them for nutritional risk using the Nutritional Risk Screening tool (NRS-2002). Thirty per cent of 492 cancer patients with solid tumours were at a nutritional risk, which was associated with higher complication rates, mortality and length of stay.[22]

Patients in developing countries may be at greater risk of weight loss.A multi-hospital Cuban study found that almost two-thirds of cancer patients were undernourished as measured by the SGA.[23]

Other smaller studies have evaluated the nutritional status of people with cancer, using screening tools such as the Scored Patient-Generated Subjective Global Assessment (PG-SGA) and also anthropometric measurements. A French observational cross-sectional survey on 477 patients with cancer at different stages showed that 30% had weight loss >10%.[24] Only 10% of the patients had a BMI less than normal, suggesting BMI alone is not a sufficiently sensitive indicator. Weight loss of ≥10% was associated with depression, digestive and head and neck tumours, chemotherapy, and male gender. A Spanish study using the PG-SGA in 781 patients with locally advanced or metastatic cancer found that 52% were moderately or severely malnourished and 97% required some form of nutritional intervention or recommendation[25] Again, the greatest weight loss was in cancers of the oesophagus (57%), stomach (50%) and larynx (47%). The median number of symptoms impeding food intake was 2, with anorexia affecting 42% of patients.

Cachexia and prognosis

Although the criteria used to define cachexia are variable in different studies, validation of the criteria usually encompasses the notion that they are predictive of cancer—specific outcomes, such as treatment toxicity, time to tumour progression and mortality.

A systematic review of prognostic factors in patients with recently diagnosed incurable cancer identified 53 studies testing associations between clinical or laboratory variables and survival time in adults with advanced solid tumours.[26] Weight loss, fatigue, anorexia, nausea, dyspnoea, pain, multiple comorbidities, poor performance status and impaired physical well-being were all associated with decreased survival. In 1555 consecutive patients with locally advanced or metastatic gastrointestinal carcinomas (oesophagus, stomach, pancreas, colorectal), weight loss at presentation was more common in men than women (51% versus 44%) and correlated with decreased tumour response, quality of life (QOL) and performance status.[27] Patients with weight loss received lower chemotherapy doses but developed more frequent and more severe dose-limiting toxicity (plantar–palmar syndrome and stomatitis) and on average received one month less treatment. Weight loss correlated with overall survival only in patients with colorectal and gastric cancer. Another UK study of 780 lung cancer patients enrolled for chemotherapy found that weight loss was reported by 59%, 58% and 76% of patients with small cell lung cancer (SCLC), non-small cell lung cancer (NSCLC) and mesothelioma, respectively.[28] Again, patients with weight loss had increased treatment toxicity and decreased survival. Those with weight loss and NSCLC or mesothelioma more frequently failed to complete at least three cycles of chemotherapy, and anaemia as a toxicity occurred more frequently in cachectic NSCLC patients. NSCLC and mesothelioma patients with weight loss had fewer symptomatic responses, and weight loss was an independent predictor of shorter overall survival for all types of lung cancer.

Some large population data sets are available for patients evaluated with standardized QOL assessments, and while they are not formally considered to be nutritional assessment tools, they do contain certain fields (i.e. appetite) related to nutrition. This information can be used to derive an estimate of prevalence of the included features and their prognostic value. A meta-analysis of 30 randomized controlled trials with Quality Of Life data for over 7400 patients found health-related QOL parameters such as appetite loss, physical functioning and pain provide significant prognostic value in addition to the sociodemographic variables (age and sex), and clinical variables (WHO performance status and distant metastases).[29] The data were derived from a single instrument, the QLQ-C30 (European Organization for Research and Training in Cancer Core Quality of Life Questionnaire). In another study of advanced lung cancer,[30] self-reported health-related quality of life questionnaires revealed dysphagia to be an independent prognostic factor for survival.

A systematic review[31] of 24 studies in terminally ill cancer patients found weight loss, dysphagia, anorexia and dyspnoea to be independent survival predictors for patients with a median survival of ≤3 months. A multicentre study prospectively evaluated variables for survival and QOL in patients who were no longer eligible for disease-specific therapy.[32] At the onset of this terminal phase of the disease trajectory, severity of nausea/emesis was associated independently with the length of survival. At later stages of their terminal disease, the presence of dyspnoea and weakness in patients who had digestive, breast, and genitourinary tumours was more predictive of shortened survival than the type of primary tumour. Since the anorexia–cachexia syndrome is associated with symptoms of nausea, early satiety, fatigue and dyspnoea (secondary to muscle wasting), these findings suggest that cachexia severity may be an important prognostic factor in patients with terminal cancer.

Obesity

Obesity is associated with changes in the physiology of adipose tissue, leading to insulin resistance, chronic inflammation and altered adipokine secretion. Several of these factors are involved in carcinogenesis and cancer progression including insulin resistance, decreased adiponectin levels and increased levels of leptin, plasminogen activator inhibitor-1, endogenous sex steroids, and chronic inflammation.[33] A prospective 16-year study of more than 900 000 US adults who were free of cancer at enrolment[34] found that people with BMI ≥40 had higher death rates from all cancers combined (52% higher for men and 62% higher for women) than people of normal weight. Increased BMI was associated with increased mortality in cancers of the oesophagus, colon and rectum, liver, gallbladder, pancreas, and kidney as well as non-Hodgkin lymphoma and multiple myeloma. Significant trends of increasing mortality with higher BMI were observed in men with gastric and prostate cancers and in women with cancers of the breast, uterus, cervix, or ovary. A population-based prospective study in Japan examining the relationship between BMI and the risk of incident cancer found that a higher BMI was associated with a higher risk of cancers of the colon, breast (postmenopausal), endometrium and gallbladder in women.[35] Unusually, there was no increased risk in Japanese men.

A large European cohort study[36] found that general and abdominal adiposity were independently related to the risk of death. The association of BMI with the risk of death was J-shaped, with higher risks of death observed in the lower and upper BMI categories than in the middle categories. Although a large prospective European study[37] of >368 000 people found that waist circumference and waist:hip ratio (indicators of abdominal obesity) were strongly associated with colon cancer risk in men and women, other studies from Sweden and Canada suggest there may be a gender difference with regard to the risk imparted by obesity. These cancers may also be quite specific for site and age, e.g. a large prospective study of more than 61 000 women demonstrated a positive association with obesity only for distal cancers among younger, premenopausal women in Sweden.[38] A Canadian prospective study of almost 90 000 women found that obesity (BMI ≥30) was associated with a twofold increased risk of colorectal cancer among premenopausal women. Data from the Framingham study in the USA indicate that the effect of BMI is stronger for men than for women and for cancers of the proximal colon. Waist circumference is a stronger predictor of colon cancer risk than is BMI, and central obesity is responsible for an increased risk of cancer of both the proximal and distal colon.[39]

Obesity not only increases the risk for incident breast cancer, it also adversely affects patients undergoing definitive treatment. A comprehensive literature review of 344 studies related to breast cancer and obesity concluded that women with breast cancer who are overweight or gain weight after diagnosis are at greater risk for recurrence and death.[40] A large retrospective study at a single institution compared overweight and obese groups with those of normal weight, and found a significant decrease in the achievement of a pathological complete response to neoadjuvant chemotherapy.

Obese patients appeared to have a significantly shorter survival time than did normal or underweight patients.[41]

Both ends of the nutrition spectrum appeared to have a significant effect on 4200 patients with Dukes' B and C colon cancer who underwent a median follow-up of 11 years after initial diagnosis and treatment.[42] Very obese patients (BMI ≥35) had greater risk of recurrence or secondary primary tumour, and both obese and underweight patients (BMI <18.5) had increased all-cause mortality when compared to normal weight (BMI = 18.5–24.9). Mortality in underweight patients was more often due to non-colon cancer-related causes than mortality in normal weight patients. The very obese had a greater risk of colon cancer recurrence and colon cancer deaths. A case–control study of 841 pancreatic cancer patients confirmed previous reports of an association between pancreatic cancer risk and obesity. Overweight patients were diagnosed with pancreatic cancer at a younger age than those with normal weight, and had poorer survival after their diagnosis.[43]

Despite the strong associations between obesity and cancer there are some inconsistent findings in specific cancers, e.g. although increased BMI seems to increase the risk for renal cell cancer, a large single-institution study showed that overweight patients had a significantly better 5-year survival after partial nephrectomy compared to those with BMI <25.[44]

There are other examples of risk factor paradox[45] in patients with very advanced illness that may also apply to advanced cancer patients. In non-cancer conditions such as CHF, COPD, CKD, and rheumatoid arthritis, traditional risk factors associated with 'overnutrition' such as cholesterol[46] and blood pressure[47] do not apply once patients have developed 'wasting'. This counter-intuitive concept is supported by epidemiological studies. For example, higher BMI, higher serum cholesterol concentration, and higher systolic blood pressure values are associated with better survival in patients on dialysis or with CHF.

Obesity and sarcopenia

Sarcopenia (depletion of skeletal muscle) can be defined as a muscle mass of >2 SD below that of healthy adults[48] and is associated with physical decline and mortality in non-cancer patients.[49] A large Canadian study of more than 2100 patients with either lung or gastrointestinal cancer showed that 15% were obese (BMI ≥30), and 15% of obese patients were also identified on computed tomography as being sarcopenic. Sarcopenic obesity was more likely in men, those aged ≥65 years, in patients with colon cancer, and it was associated with poorer performance status and decreased survival. The lean body mass of these obese patients was comparable to very underweight or emaciated patients.[50] Although there are few nutritional epidemiological studies conducted in patients referred for palliative care, a study from the Cleveland Clinic also suggested that pre-existing obesity could play an important role in concealing muscle wasting. Their palliative programme assessed the nutritional status of 352 consecutive cancer referrals. Whereas 71% had lost weight and 30% had significant muscle mass reduction (as measured by mid-arm muscle area) the BMI was normal or increased in most patients (suggesting that pre-cancer obesity was masking the loss of lean body mass).[51]

Biomarkers of survival in cachexia and obesity

A review[26] of patients recently diagnosed with incurable cancer found that anaemia, thrombocytopenia, hypoalbuminaemia and elevated serum levels of alkaline phosphatase and lactate dehydrogenases were associated with shorter survival. C-Reactive protein (CRP) was also associated with decreased survival although the studies were noted to be small. CRP has been included in recent definitions of cachexia based on tools such as the Glasgow Prognostic Score which identifies patients who are likely to develop cachexia, respond poorly to treatment, and have decreased survival.[52] As expected, the review also noted measures of tumour bulk such as number of metastases, number of metastatic sites, or tumour volume were associated with survival.

Genetic factors could influence the increased risk for incident cancer, poor response to therapy or increased mortality in patients with either obesity or cachexia.

Particular single nucleotide polymorphisms (SNPs) that code for proteins involved in biological processes related to inflammation show promise in identifying patients who are at risk.

Patients with pancreatic cancer homozygous for allele 2 of the interleukin (IL)-1β gene had significantly shorter survival,[53] higher IL-1β production, and significantly higher CRP levels than other groups. The authors speculated that this may reflect the role of IL-1β in inducing an acute-phase protein response and cachexia in cancer. A subsequent study[54] evaluated the roles of host cytokines in systemic inflammation and prognosis of 203 patients with oesophagogastric cancer. IL-6 and the IL-10 gene polymorphisms were associated with elevated CRP levels and decreased survival. Tumour necrosis factor (TNF)-α AA genotype was also associated with reduced survival, but not with inflammation. An earlier study in patients with advanced pancreatic cancer did not find an association between TNF polymorphisms, inflammation and cachexia.[55] A more recent study of Chinese patients with pancreatic cancer[56] indicated that an IL-6 allele is associated with increased susceptibility to cachexia and decreased survival.

Data analysed from 9919 individuals who participated in two large community-based cohort studies[57] in the USA showed statistically significant associations between cancer-related mortality and two SNPs (a peroxisome proliferator-activated receptor-γ, and TNFα). A prospective study of incident colorectal cases and matched controls suggested that polymorphisms in IL-10, CRP and other genes related to immune response or obesity and its metabolic sequelae may be associated with risk of colorectal cancer.[58] Recently, a case–control study of obese individuals with a polymorphic variant of the insulin-like growth factor type I receptor gene were found to have significantly increased risk for oesophageal adenocarcinoma.[59]

Conclusion

With the changing patterns in global obesity, more current research is required into the epidemiology of cachexia, and more sophisticated evaluations of body composition will be necessary to unmask underlying muscle loss in overweight patients. The impact of these individual factors and their combination on incident cancer, response to therapy and prognosis[60] needs to be clarified.

References

1. Nguyen XM, Lane J, Smith BR, Nguyen NT (2009) Changes in inflammatory biomarkers across weight classes in a representative US population: a link between obesity and inflammation. *J Gastrointest Surg*, **13**(7), 1205–12.
2. Popkin BM (2007) Understanding global nutrition dynamics as a step towards controlling cancer incidence. *Nature Reviews Cancer*, **7**, 61–7.
3. Morley JE, Thomas DR, Wilson MM (2006) Cachexia: pathophysiology and clinical relevance. *Am J Clin Nutr*, **83**(4), 735–43.
4. Ogden CL, Carroll MD, Curtin LR, McDowell MA, Tabak CJ, Flegal KM (2006) Prevalence of overweight and obesity in the United States, 1999–2004. *J Am Med Assoc*, **295**(13), 1549–55.
5. Evans WJ, Morley JE, Argilés J, *et al.* (2008) Cachexia: a new definition. *Clin Nutr*, **27**(6), 793–9.
6. Bozzetti F, Mariani L (2009) Defining and classifying cancer cachexia: a proposal by the SCRINIO Working Group. *J Parenter Enteral Nutr*, **33**(4), 361–7.

7. Fox KM, Brooks JM, Gandra SR, Markus R, Chiou CF (2009) Estimation of cachexia among cancer patients based on four definitions. *J Oncol*, 693458 [Epub ahead of print].
8. Van Hoeyweghen RJ, De Leeuw IH, Vandewoude MF (1992) Creatinine arm index as alternative for creatinine height index. *Am J Clin Nutr*, **56**, 611–5.
9. Vandewoude M (2009) Nutritional assessment in geriatric cancer patients. *Support Care Cancer* [Epub ahead of print].
10. Nething J, Ringwald-Smith K, Williams R, Hancock ML, Hale GA (2007) Establishing the use of body mass index as an indicator of nutrition risk in children with cancer. *J Parenter Enteral Nutr*, **31**(1), 53–7.
11. Anonymous (1995) Physical status: the use and interpretation of anthropometry: report of a WHO expert committee. *WHO Tech Rep Ser*, **854**, 1–452.
12. Anonymous (1998) *Clinical guidelines on the identification, evaluation, and treatment of overweight and obesity in adults.* Bethesda, MD: US Department of Health and Human Services, Public Health Service.
13. Inagaki J, Rodriguez V, Bodey GP (1974) Proceedings: causes of death in cancer patients. *Cancer*, **33**(2), 568–73.
14. DeWys WD, Begg C, Lavin PT, *et al.* (1980) Prognostic effect of weight loss prior to chemotherapy in cancer patients. *Am J Med*, **69**(4), 491–7.
15. Bozzetti F, Migliavacca S, Scotti A *et al.* (1982) Impact of cancer, type, site, stage and treatment on the nutritional status of patients. *Ann Surg*, **196**, 170–9.
16. Grosvenor M, Bulcavage L, Chlebowski RT (1989) Symptoms potentially influencing weight loss in a cancer population. Correlations with primary site, nutritional status, and chemotherapy administration. *Cancer*, **63**(2), 330–4.
17. Bozzetti F, SCRINIO Working Group (2009) Screening the nutritional status in oncology: a preliminary report on 1,000 outpatients. *Support Care Cancer*, **17**(3), 279–84.
18. Kondrup J, Rasmussen HH, Hamberg O, Stanga Z, ad hoc ESPEN Working Group (2003) Nutrition risk screening (NRS 2002): a new method based on an analysis of controlled clinical trials. *Clin Nutr*, **22**, 321–6.
19. Pirlich M, Schütz T, Kemps M, *et al.* (2003) Prevalence of malnutrition in hospitalized medical patients: impact of underlying disease. *Dig Dis*, **21**(3), 245–51.
20. Pirlich M, Schütz T, Norman K, *et al.* (2006) The German hospital malnutrition study. *Clin Nutr*, **25**(4), 563–72.
21. Kruizenga HM, Wierdsma NJ, van Bokhorst MA, *et al.* Screening of nutritional status in The Netherlands. *Clin Nutr* **22**(2), 147–52.
22. Sorensen J, Kondrup J, Prokopowicz J, *et al.* EuroOOPS: an international, multicentre study to implement nutritional risk screening and evaluate clinical outcome. *Clin Nutr*, **27**(3), 340–9.
23. Barreto Penié J, Cuban Group for the Study of Hospital Malnutrition (2005) State of malnutrition in Cuban hospitals. *Nutrition*, **21**(4), 487–97.
24. Nourissat A, Mille D, Delaroche G, *et al.* Estimation of the risk for nutritional state degradation in patients with cancer: development of a screening tool based on results from a cross-sectional survey. *Ann Oncol*, **18**(11), 1882–6.
25. Segura A, Pardo J, Jara C, *et al.* An epidemiological evaluation of the prevalence of malnutrition in Spanish patients with locally advanced or metastatic cancer. *Clin Nutr*, **24**(5), 801–14.
26. Hauser CA, Stockler MR, Tattersall MH (2006) Prognostic factors in patients with recently diagnosed incurable cancer: a systematic review. *Support Care Cancer*, **10**, 999–1011.
27. Andreyev HJ, Norman AR, Oates J, Cunningham D (1998) Why do patients with weight loss have a worse outcome when undergoing chemotherapy for gastrointestinal malignancies? *Eur J Cancer*, **34**(4), 503–9.
28. Ross PJ, Ashley S, Norton A, *et al.* (2004) Do patients with weight loss have a worse outcome when undergoing chemotherapy for lung cancers? *Br J Cancer*, **90**(10), 1905–11.

29. Quinten C, Coens C, Mauer M, *et al.* (2009) Baseline quality of life as a prognostic indicator of survival: a meta-analysis of individual patient data from EORTC clinical trials. *Lancet Oncol*, **10**(9), 865–71.
30. Efficace F, Bottomley A, Smit EF, *et al.* (2006) Is a patient's self-reported health-related quality of life a prognostic factor for survival in non-small-cell lung cancer patients? A multivariate analysis of prognostic factors of EORTC study 08975. *Ann Oncol*, **17**(11), 1698–704.
31. Viganò A, Dorgan M, Buckingham J, Bruera E, Suarez-Almazor ME (2000) Survival prediction in terminal cancer patients: a systematic review of the medical literature. *Palliat Med*, **14**(5), 363–74.
32. Vigano A, Donaldson N, Higginson IJ, Bruera E, Mahmud S, Suarez-Almazor M (2004) Quality of life and survival prediction in terminal cancer patients: a multicenter study. *Cancer*, **101**(5), 1090–8.
33. van Kruijsdijk RC, van der Wall E, Visseren FL (2009) Obesity and cancer: the role of dysfunctional adipose tissue. *Cancer Epidemiol Biomarkers*, Prev **18**(10), 2569–78.
34. Calle EE, Rodriguez C, Walker-Thurmond K, Thun MJ (2003) Overweight, obesity, and mortality from cancer in a prospectively studied cohort of U.S. adults. *N Engl J Med*, **348**(17), 1625–38.
35. Kuriyama S, Tsubono Y, Hozawa A (2005) Obesity and risk of cancer in Japan. *Int J Cancer*, **113**(1), 148–57.
36. Pischon T, Boeing H, Hoffmann K, *et al.* (2008) General and abdominal adiposity and risk of death in Europe. *N Engl J Med*, **359**(20), 2105–20.
37. Pischon T, Lahmann PH, Boeing H, *et al.* (2006) Body size and risk of colon and rectal cancer in the European Prospective Investigation into Cancer and Nutrition (EPIC). *J Natl Cancer Inst*, **98**(13), 920–31.
38. Terry P, Giovannucci E, Bergkvist L, Holmberg L, Wolk A (2001) Body weight and colorectal cancer risk in a cohort of Swedish women: relation varies by age and cancer site. *Br J Cancer*, **85**, 346–9.
39. Moore LL, Bradlee ML, Singer MR, *et al.* (2004) BMI and waist circumference as predictors of lifetime colon cancer risk in Framingham Study adults. *Int J Obes Relat Metab Disord*, **28**(4), 559–67.
40. Chlebowski RT, Aiello E, McTiernan A (2002) Weight loss in breast cancer patient management. *J Clin Oncol*, **20**,1128–43.
41. Litton JK, Gonzalez-Angulo AM, Warneke CL, *et al.* (2008) Relationship between obesity and pathologic response to neoadjuvant chemotherapy among women with operable breast cancer. *J Clin Oncol*, **26**, 4072–7.
42. Dignam JJ, Polite BN, Yothers G, *et al.* (2006) Body mass index and outcomes in patients who receive adjuvant chemotherapy for colon cancer. *J Natl Cancer Inst*, **98**(22), 1647–54.
43. Li D, Morris JS, Liu J, *et al.* (2009) Body mass index and risk, age of onset, and survival in patients with pancreatic cancer. *J Am Med Assoc*, **301**(24), 2553–62.
44. Schrader AJ, Rustemeier J, Rustemeier JC, *et al.* (2009) Overweight is associated with improved cancer-specific survival in patients with organ-confined renal cell carcinoma. *J Cancer Res Clin Oncol*, **135**(12), 1693–9.
45. Kalantar-Zadeh K, Horwich TB, Oreopoulos A, *et al.* (2007) Risk factor paradox in wasting diseases. *Curr Opin Clin Nutr Metab Care*, **10**(4), 433–42.
46. Kilpatrick RD, McAllister CJ, Kovesdy CP, *et al.* (2007) Association between serum lipids and survival in hemodialysis patients and impact of race. *J Am Soc Nephrol*, **18**, 293–303.
47. Kalantar-Zadeh K, Abbott KC, Kronenberg F, *et al.* (2006) Epidemiology of dialysis patients and heart failure patients. *Semin Nephrol*, **26**, 118–33.
48. Baumgartner RN, Koehler KM, Gallagher D, *et al.* (1998) Epidemiology of sarcopenia among the elderly in New Mexico. *Am J Epidemiol*, **147**(8), 755–63.
49. Roubenoff R (2003) Sarcopenia: effects on body composition and function. *J Gerontol A Biol Sci Med Sci*, **58**(11), 1012–7.
50. Prado CM, Lieffers JR, McCargar LJ, *et al.* (2008) Prevalence and clinical implications of sarcopenic obesity in patients with solid tumours of the respiratory and gastrointestinal tracts: a population-based study. *Lancet Oncol*, **9**(7), 629–35.

51. Sarhill N, Mahmoud F, Walsh D, *et al.* (2003) Evaluation of nutritional status in advanced metastatic cancer. *Support Care Cancer*, **11**(10), 652–9.
52. McMillan, DC (2009) Systemic inflammation, nutritional status and survival in patients with cancer. *Curr Opin Clin Nutr Metab Care*, **12**(3), 223–6.
53. Barber MD, Powell JJ, Lynch SF, Fearon KC, Ross JA (2004) A polymorphism of the interleukin-1 beta gene influences survival in pancreatic cancer. *Br J Cancer*, **90**(10), 1905–11.
54. Deans C, Rose-Zerilli M, Wigmore S, *et al.* (2007) Host cytokine genotype is related to adverse prognosis and systemic inflammation in gastro-oesophageal cancer. *Ann Surg Oncol*, **14**(2), 329–39.
55. Barber MD, Powell JJ, Lynch SF, Gough NJ, Fearon KC, Ross JA (1999) Two polymorphisms of the tumour necrosis factor gene do not influence survival in pancreatic cancer. *Clin Exp Immunol*, **117**(3), 425–9.
56. Zhang D, Zhou Y, Wu L, *et al.* (2008) Association of IL-6 gene polymorphisms with cachexia susceptibility and survival time of patients with pancreatic cancer. *Ann Clin Lab Sci*, **38**(2), 113–9.
57. Gallicchio L, Chang HH, Christo DK (2009) Single nucleotide polymorphisms in obesity-related genes and all-cause and cause-specific mortality: a prospective cohort study. *BMC Med Genet*, **10**, 103.
58. Tsilidis KK, Helzlsouer KJ, Smith MW, *et al.* (2009) Association of common polymorphisms in IL10, and in other genes related to inflammatory response and obesity with colorectal cancer. *Cancer Causes Control*, **20**(9), 1739–51.
59. MacDonald K, Porter GA, Guernsey DL, Zhao R, Casson AG (2009) A polymorphic variant of the insulin-like growth factor type I receptor gene modifies risk of obesity for esophageal adenocarcinoma. *Cancer Epidemiol*, **33**(1), 37–40.
60. Maltoni M, Caraceni A, Brunelli C, *et al.* (2005) Prognostic factors in advanced cancer patients: evidence-based clinical recommendations—a study by the Steering Committee of the European Association for Palliative Care. *J Clin Oncol*, **23**(25), 6240–8.

Chapter 5

Mechanisms of primary cachexia

Vickie E. Baracos and Henrique A. Parsons

The aetiology of cancer cachexia and other wasting syndromes is not clearly understood; however, most experts point to a variety of contributing factors.[1–4] These are categorized as either primary or secondary. The primary component refers to the direct effects of the tumour and the host response to the presence of the tumour. The secondary component is conceived by most authors as a group of symptoms that pose barriers to food intake, above and beyond the presence of anorexia. This component is often termed secondary cachexia and more specifically secondary nutrition impact symptoms: nausea, vomiting, constipation, diarrhoea, defecation after meal (also called dumping syndrome), pain including epigastric and abdominal pain as well as at other sites, dyspnoea, fatigue, anxiety/depression, sense of hopelessness, stomatitis, dysgeusia, dental problems, difficulty chewing, dysosmia, xerostomia, thick saliva, and dysphagia. MacDonald *et al.*[5] emphasize that many of these are potentially treatable causes of poor food intake, and that close attention should be paid to their management. The causes and management of several of these symptoms are treated in detail in Chapters 13–16.

Here, we will discuss the mechanisms of primary cachexia.

Direct role of the tumour mass

Cancer, weight loss and malnutrition are regarded as evolving together. This general notion is encompassed in nutritional assessment by evaluation of disease stage and determination of whether the disease is stable or progressive. Advanced disease stage, multiple sites of metastasis and progressive disease are regarded as risk factors for weight loss and malnutrition.

The exact contribution of tumour to negative energy balance has rarely been assessed, although it is known that tumour tissue is energetically demanding. Lieffers *et al.*[6] hypothesized that unresectable hepatic metastases may represent an important burden of high metabolic rate tissue; importantly, ~50% of all colorectal cancer patients develop this complication[7] which has been associated with weight loss.[8,9] Lieffers *et al.*[6] used several approaches to investigate this question. A serial computed tomography (CT) image analysis in subjects who died of colorectal cancer was used to demonstrate that liver metastases increased exponentially during progressive disease. Eleven months from death, liver weight inclusive of metastases was 2.3 ± 0.7 kg, and by 1 month from death, liver plus metastases weight increased by 0.7 to 3.0 ± 1.5 kg. Concurrent to this progressive disease, loss of muscle (4.2 kg) and fat (3.5 kg) occurred. The estimated percentage of fat-free mass occupied by the liver increased from 4.5% to 7.0% ($P < 0.001$) with this expansion of metastatic disease burden. The most rapid loss of peripheral tissue and gain of liver and metastases occurred within 3 months of death. A positive linear relationship was demonstrated between the estimated mass of liver plus metastases and measured whole-body resting energy expenditure ($r^2 = 0.35$, $P = 0.010$) and they further estimated that tumour may explain an incremental total energy expenditure of ~17 700 kcal during the last 3 months of life. During this same time period 3.5 kg of fat mass was lost, equivalent to approximately 30 000 kcal total energy content.

The importance of these results is that they allow for some quantitative understanding of how much the tumour might contribute to cachexia-associated weight loss. Central to this issue is the magnitude of tumour burden, and the specific metabolic rate of the tumour. There are few available data in the literature derived from direct measurements; however, a value of 200–300 kcal/day per kg of tumour tissue seems a likely range of specific metabolic rate based on available information.[6] The role of tumour burden is often not exactly quantifiable in early disease, and especially after tumour resection or in tumours responding to radiation or systemic therapy, the contributions of the tumour to energy balance overall may well be trivial. By contrast, in metastatic disease and in progressive disease unresponsive to therapy, the tumour could become a dominant player in negative energy balance.

Tumour-derived catabolic mediators for proteolysis and lipolysis

The idea that tumours may produce specific and unusual catabolic factors has been championed by M. Tisdale, who produced reports in the early 1990s of novel proteolysis-inducing and lipid-mobilizing factors produced by mouse tumours which induced cachexia in their hosts. The lipid-mobilizing factor was subsequently shown to be identical to zinc-α_2-glycoprotein, and our understanding of its role in adipose tissue biology continues to evolve.[10] The proteolysis-inducing factor role in human cancer cachexia is still controversial and will be further discussed in the following sections.[11,12]

Lipid-mobilizing factor: zinc-α_2-glycoprotein

Lipid-mobilizing factors (LMFs) have been related to weight loss and fat mobilization for many years in animal and cell line studies.[13–17] Todorov *et al.* purified an LMF with characteristics of an already known protein, zinc-α_2-glycoprotein (ZAG), from a cachexia-inducing murine tumour cell line (MAC16) and from the urine of cachectic patients.[18] Bing and Trayhurn have provided a succinct review of the role of ZAG in cancer cachexia.[10] Structurally, ZAG belongs to the class I MHC family. It is overexpressed by several types of malignant tumour, such as breast, prostate and bladder cancers, and ZAG levels are elevated in physiological fluids of some cancer patients.[10] ZAG has the characteristics of an LMF: it induces lipolysis in adipocytes *in vitro* and ZAG-induced weight loss after systemic treatment in animals is exclusively due to loss of fat mass.[19]

Currently ZAG is considered to be an adipokine produced by adipose tissue and is involved locally in the regulation of fat mass, based on work in experimental studies. There are preliminary reports that ZAG mRNA and protein expression are upregulated in adipose tissue of patients with cancer cachexia,[10] but a great deal more work is required to establish its overall role in humans exhibiting cancer-associated lipolysis.[20]

Proteolysis-inducing factor

Proteolysis-inducing factor (PIF) is a glycoprotein first isolated from the already cited MAC16 cachexia-inducing tumour in mice.[21] A similar molecule was found in the urine of cancer patients with cachexia, and was absent in patients with similar cancers and no cachexia. The human molecule, when administered into mice, was able to cause significant weight loss without decrease in food or water intake.[22] The excretion of PIF in the urine of cachectic cancer patients was shown by other groups. Wang *et al.* showed that PIF was present in the majority of 19 samples from advanced pancreatic cancer patients but absent in all 19 samples from healthy controls.[23] Williams *et al.* showed in a prospective study with 36 advanced gastrointestinal cancers that patients who excreted PIF in the urine evolved with weight loss, as opposed to patients with undetectable urinary PIF.[24] More recent studies have cast some doubt on the role of PIF in cancer cachexia.[11,12]

Jatoi's group was not able to replicate the findings from Williams *et al.* in a sample of 41 advanced oesophageal/gastric cancers[25] and Monitto[26] found that tumour xenografts overexpressing human PIF protein did not induce cachexia *in vivo*. Recently, the murine monoclonal antibody against PIF was found to be an ineffective tool for the study of PIF in humans, because of poor specificity and, in particular, strong reactivity toward human albumin and immunoglobulins.

Central nervous system involvement

The central nervous system (CNS) is a key site for physiological control of appetite, however because of the overall lack of even basic knowledge of which specific controls are altered in cancer anorexia, there is for the moment no clear basis for the development of a new therapeutic strategy directed at appetite control in the brain.

The hypothalamus functions as the interface between peripheral adiposity and energy signals and the control of food intake and body weight. The peripheral adiposity signs integrated by the hypothalamus include the levels of leptin (mostly produced by adipocytes), insulin (produced by the exocrine pancreas), and ghrelin.[27] Insulin will decrease appetite centrally, but has an anabolic effect on peripheral muscle. Leptin levels have a more intense effect on energy intake than insulin. Increasing leptin levels drive a reduction of energy intake.[28,29] While it might be hypothesized that leptin has a role in the genesis of cachexia, this remains to be adequately tested in animal models or humans. Leptin receptor abundance was characterized by immunohistochemistry in experimental animals [30] and a few data for leptin levels in peripheral blood of cancer patients[31,32] exist. Importantly none of these investigations have tested the sensitivity of leptin responses in relevent populations of neurons involved in appetite and metabolic control, the leptin responsiveness of appetite in the whole body or used specific interventions such as over-expression or genetic ablation of leptin receptors in tumor models to characterize the role of leptin in cancer anorexia.

The energy information received by the hypothalamus includes lipid-derived fuels, which serve to signal a catabolic (i.e. non-esterified fatty acids) or anabolic energy status.[33] The driving force for energy intake is therefore the accumulation (signal to reduce energy intake) or reduction (signal to increase energy intake) of intracellular malonyl-coenzyme-A.[34] In animal models, it has been recently shown by Celik *et al.* that decreased levels of malonyl-coenzyme-A might contribute to the acceleration of lipolysis in cancer cachexia. Further studies are needed to demonstrate this effect in humans.[35]

Several factors form the entero-endocrine component of the regulation of food intake, including ghrelin, peptide YY, cholecystokinin and GLP-1. As for leptin, these remain uncharacterized or poorly characterized in cancer cachexia,with an important lack of assesment of the sensitivity of appetite controls to these factors. Ghrelin is secreted primarily by the stomach, and is the only known circulating orexigenic hormone in humans. Elevated serum levels are found in patients with cancer cachexia, suggesting 'ghrelin resistance'. Ghrelin has a number of other effects that might influence the development of cachexia, including the modulation of sympathetic activation, decreasing proinflammatory cytokine release, improving GI motility, and stimulating growth hormone release via vagal afferents. Ghrelin is a vasodilator, improves cardiac function and appears to exert an anabolic action on skeletal muscle. The therapeutic potential of ghrelin and ghrelin mimetics is discussed in Chapter 8 (anabolic hormones). Gastric ghrelin crossing the blood–brain barrier (or locally produced hypothalamic ghrelin) is likely to increase appetite by stimulating orexigenic neuropeptides. Resistance to these actions may be mediated by proinflammatory cytokines and could be a key limitation to the therapeutic application of ghrelin in cancer anorexia. Cholecystokinin, a key signal for satiety, merits investigation in cancer cachexia, in light of its potential contribution to inappropriately high or early satiety.

Two transductional pathways exist in the hypothalamus as different neuron populations and respond to the peripheral signals, expressing neuropeptides as described in Chapter 2. The orexigenic pathway has neurons expressing the neuropeptite Y (NPY) and agouti-related protein (AgRP). The anorexigenic pathway's neurons express pro-opiomelanocortin (POMC).[27] Neuropeptide Y has been studied in animal models for cancer cachexia, but conclusive evidence of its role is still lacking. Chance and Balasubramaniam, for example, showed that rats with cancer anorexia had alterations in NPY receptor mechanisms.[36] Another group showed that rats with cancer cachexia have defective NPY innervation in the hypothalamus.[37] Furthermore, NPY pathways recover after tumor ablation.[38,39]

The transductional neurons cited interact with other second-order neuronal pathways, and even though several studies already showed the relationship between increased serotoninergic neurotransmission and cancer anorexia/cachexia, further research is still needed.

Cancer inflammation–hypercatabolism syndrome

Inflammation is the single most important theme consistently emerging from both animal and human studies in cancer cachexia.[40,41] More broadly, cachexia is associated with a number of disease states, including acute inflammatory processes associated with critical illness and chronic inflammatory diseases, such as cancer, congestive heart failure, chronic obstructive pulmonary disease, and human immunodeficiency virus infection. In the view of many researchers and clinical experts, a primary requirement for the development of cachexia is the presence of an inflammatory process.[42,43] The presence of a chronic inflammatory state seems to account for seemingly disparate aberrations, including changes in the hypothalamic–pituitary axis, dysautonomia, hypermetabolism, oxidative stress, decreased muscle protein synthesis, and increased ubiquitin-proteosome-mediated muscle proteolysis together with other metabolic changes such as insulin resistance.[1,3,5,44–52] Through its effect on multiple organs and tissues, chronic inflammation leads to the pathophysiologicL profile accounting for anorexia–cachexia.

Catabolic–proinflammatory cytokines promote skeletal muscle wasting and loss of adipose tissue

Of the proinflammatory cytokines, tumour necrosis factor (TNF)-α interleukin (IL)-1β and IL-6, and interferon (IFN)-γ are currently thought to be the principal catabolic actors in skeletal muscle (Figure 5.1). In 1983 IL-1 was the first cytokine reported to act on skeletal muscle, inducing catabolism,[53] and in 1986 TNFα action as a 'cachectin' was described.[54] Both of these cytokines and Il-6[44,55–58] have been extensively studied in skeletal muscle and adipose tissue. The actions of cytokines such as TNFα are catabolic (i.e. cause induction of proteolysis) and concurrently inhibit anabolism (i.e. TNFα + IFNγ strongly reduces myosin expression).[59] The proinflammatory cytokines potentiate each others' actions and a variety of potent synergies on muscle have been demonstrated. These include TNFα + IFNγ for protein catabolism,[59] TNFα + IFNγ + endotoxin (LPS) for cytokine receptor induction, and TNFα + IFNγ + LPS for nitric oxide synthesis and insulin resistance.[60,61]

With regards to skeletal muscle wasting, TNFα is extensively studied in animals. Hamster ovarian cells transfected with a human TNFα gene and transplanted into normal animals can trigger a cachexia-like syndrome.[62] TNFα increases muscle breakdown,[63] interferes with cell cycle exit and represses the accumulation of transcripts encoding muscle-specific genes in differentiating myoblasts.[64–66] TNFα also activates nuclear factor kappa B (NFκB), inducing the ubiquitin–proteassome pathway, the most important pathway leading to protein degradation.[67] However,

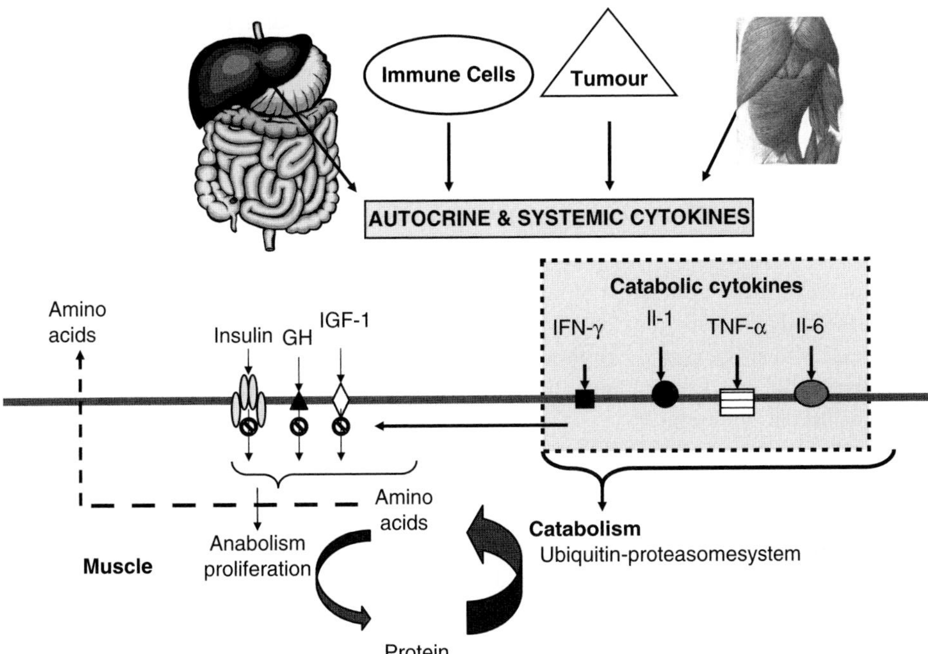

Fig. 5.1 Cytokine action on skeletal muscle. Cytokines acting on muscle originate in various tissues. Cytokines promote protein degradation as well as resistance to the anabolic actions of growth hormone (GH), insulin and insulin-like growth factor (IGF)-1. IFN, interferon; IL-1, interleukin-1; TNF, tumour necrosis factor.

NFκB-driven skeletal muscle degradation via the generation of reactive oxygen species (ROS) is dependent on several intermediaries[68] and oxidative stress caused by other reasons may drive proteolysis by itself in the absence of TNFα.[69] Also, the muscle regulatory factor MyoD, which induces muscle-specific transcription, is degraded in response to NFκB induced by TNFα. TNFα also induces the reduction of lipids in adipose tissue by two mechanisms: inhibition of the transcription of lipoprotein lipase,[70,71] or by direct stimulation of lipolysis.[72] As regards human clinical studies, a role for TNFα in cancer cachexia has been hypothesized because of significant serum levels of TNFα in advanced pancreatic cancer patients, and the inverse correlation between these levels and body weight.[73] However, other groups are not able to reproduce these findings, showing no correlation between TNFα levels and appetite or weight loss.[74,75]

In muscle, Il-6 is hypothesized to be related to protein degradation via hyperexpression of cathepsins and ubiquitins.[76] Experimentally, IL-6 appears to have a major role in muscle wasting[59] and cachexia, even though some studies have not been able demonstrate IL-6-induced wasting in mice.[77] Several groups are dedicating efforts to understand the effects of IL-6 in muscle wasting. In the adipose arena, it is speculated that IL-6 might play a role in the aetiology of fat loss via its proinflammatory effects, leading to catabolism. TNFα induces IL-6 secretion, and both play important roles in the acute-phase response. However, IL-6 alone exerts no effect on appetite or energy intake, as reported by Espat *et al.*[77] The combination of proinflammatory cytokines seems to be more important in the pathogenesis of cachexia than any single cytokine.

IL-1has a very similar effect on mice's adipose tissue as TNFα, helping drive body weight loss and anorexia.[78] However, a clinical study of 61 advanced cancer patients showed that levels of IL-1 did not correlate with weight loss.[74] Once again, it suggests cachexia in humans may depend on the actions of cytokine combinations or local cytokine production (which is not accurately reflected by serum levels).

INF-γ levels also did not correlate with weight loss[74] and low levels of this cytokine were associated with shorter survival in advanced lung cancer patients.[79] Further research is also needed to understand the role of INF-γ in cancer cachexia.

Loci of inflammation and cytokine production in the tumour-bearing host

Inflammation and the production of inflammatory mediators can originate in a wide variety of sites in the body of a cancer patient, including the tumour, immune cells of the host such as mononuclear phagocytes and lymphocytes, gastrointestinal tract and liver, peripheral tissues including skeletal muscle and adipose tissue, as well as from secondary conditions such as infection or comorbid conditions.[80]

In addition to the production of proinflammatory cytokines by tumour cells *per se*, the recruitment and infiltration of macrophages in the tumour environment (tumour-associated macrophages) are a significant source inflammatory cytokines, chemokines and angiogenesis-promoting factors, matrix metalloproteinases, prostanoids and ROS. The production of these mediators is associated with enhanced tumour growth and angiogenesis.[81,82] The tumour and its environment are only one of many sources of inflammation in the tumour-bearing host.

One interesting hypothesis concerning the aetiology of cachexia is the central role of the gut.[83] In this view, altered passage of bacterial endotoxins into the blood may occur as a consequence of a loss of gut integrity and barrier function. Loss of gut integrity has been described after a variety of chemotherapy treatments[84,85] and this may be a relatively common occurrence as the majority of systemic drug treatments have some degree of intestinal toxicity. Translocated endotoxins present a potent stimulus for cytokine production by mononuclear cells. Increased endotoxaemia might be a potent trigger of the systemic inflammatory response which is involved in the pathogenesis of the cachexia syndrome.

The production of cytokines in muscle cells has been clearly demonstrated and this is a likely source of cytokines in the tumour-bearing state. Isolated myocytes and myotubes in the absence of any other cell type produce proinflammatory cytokines and respond to them through locally expressed receptor proteins.[44,60] Frost and Lang[86] suggest that this muscle cytokine axis qualifies its inclusion as a component of the innate immune system, along with phagocytes, such as neutrophils and macrophages, its classically identified cellular components. The presence of toll-like receptor (TLR)-2 and -4 in skeletal muscle permits muscle response to lipopolysaccharide (LPS) from Gram-negative bacteria and LPS stimulates muscle to produce numerous effectors including early and late-phase cytokines as well as nitric oxide. These findings, coupled with the earlier demonstration of TNFα, IL-6, IL-1 and IFNγ receptors in muscle,[61] provide convincing evidence for the afferent limb of the innate immune system in muscle. In addition, the efferent limb of the system is also present in myocytes as evidenced by the dose- and time-dependent increase in the expression of cytokines, such as TNFα, IL-1 and IL-6, in response to endotoxin.

Owing to their age, cancer patients typically have a number of comorbid conditions that may be associated with inflammation.[87] Many of these are also associated with involuntary weight loss and muscle wasting, such as chronic heart failure, pulmonary diseases, ulcers, arthritis and renal disease. In addition to these chronic inflammatory conditions, cancer patients are susceptible to infections. Pereira *et al.*[88] in a survey of advanced cancer patients in a palliative care unit, showed that 55 of 100 patients were diagnosed with a total of 74 separate infections of which 54 were culture positive. These infections involved the urinary tract (39.2%), the respiratory tract (36.5%), skin and subcutaneous tissues (12.2%), and blood (5.4%). Together, these chronic and acute conditions add to the overall burden of inflammation in cancer patients.

Anti-inflammatory therapy for cancer cachexia

The causal role of inflammation in cancer cachexia has been clearly established in many animal models. The participation of proinflammatory cytokines including IL-1β, IL-6, TNFα, and IFNγ are proven by changing cytokine production or activity using experimental approaches such as passive immunization with antibodies to cytokines, cytokine receptor antagonists, receptor knockout mice or animals overexpressing soluble receptor isoforms.[89–92] Drugs such as pentoxyfylline and cyclo-oxygenase inhibitors[93–96] affecting cytokine production have been used in clinical trials with varying levels of success.

Loss of trophic influence on skeletal muscle

Insulin resistance, lack of physical activity, and low levels of testosterone in males is a trio of culprits suggested to be important in the failure of muscle protein anabolism in cancer patients.

Experimental studies demonstrate the resistance of skeletal muscle anabolism to insulin in tumour-bearing rats.[97,98] Studies of metabolic responses to insulin in humans require complex infusions under basal and insulin-stimulated conditions and are done less frequently in humans and rarely in cancer patients.[99] However, the insulin resistance of protein synthesis has been clearly demonstrated in elderly, obese and type II diabetic humans[100–102] and, given the prevalence of these comorbidities in cancer patients and the ability of inflammation to render muscle insulin-resistant,[58] it seems a reasonable conjecture that insulin resistance contributes to cancer-associated muscle wasting.

It has been known for a very long time that physical activity is a potent trophic factor for skeletal muscle and that lack of activity induces loss of muscle and of functional capacity. The results of Kortebein *et al.*[103,104] demonstrate a striking propensity for muscle loss and depression of protein synthesis during 10 days of bed rest in healthy elderly subjects, compared with younger individuals. Together with loss of muscle, all measures of lower extremity strength were significantly lower after bed rest including isotonic knee extensor strength (–13.2%), stair-climbing power (–14%), and maximal aerobic capacity (–12%). Interestingly, after bed rest, the amount of daily time that the subjects spent being inactive increased significantly by 7%, which suggests the potential for further losses. These types of effects may be exacerbated in advanced cancer patients, who on average spend 35 days in hospital during the year preceding their death.[105]

Hypogonadism appears to be a widespread problem in elderly men, obesity, the metabolic syndrome, and cancer. Hypogonadism may be mediated at the hypothalamic level by cytokines and drugs leading to decreased gonadotrophin-releasing hormone production. Testicular production of testosterone may also be diminished by the direct effect of certain chemotherapeutic agents and cytokines such as IL-6. Drugs commonly used in cancer patients such as opioid analgesics, megestrol acetate, and corticosteroids are associated with hypogonadal testosterone levels. A study examining the prevalence of hypogonadism in the primary care setting found that higher age, liver disease, and cancer were associated with especially low testosterone levels (<1.0 ng/mL).[106] Hypogonadism results in a loss of primary anabolic influence on skeletal muscle and is one of the reasons for androgen replacement therapy, a therapy which has been considered extensively in the elderly.[107] Risk factors for developing hypogonadism in cancer patients include old age, alkylating agents and high-dose chemotherapy with autologous stem cell support, radiation, and comorbidities (chronic kidney or obstructive pulmonary disease, human immunodeficiency virus, type II diabetes mellitus).[108–110]

Multifactorial nature of cancer cachexia

Most experts describe cancer cachexia as being multifactorial, meaning that in any given individual, any (or all) of the mechanisms of primary and/or secondary cachexia can be involved. This poses a significant problem for the treatment of cachexia, since all of these numerous possible causes must be evaluated in order to be included or excluded in the treatment plan. The difficult task from a therapeutic perspective is to correctly apportion the blame to the most significant factors in each individual. These can be tremendously varied since intense weight loss could be due to extensive tumour burden or severe inflammation or to a secondary condition such as renal failure or severe dysgeusia, or any combination of these types of factors. Treatment for cancer cachexia has not yet achieved this level of specificity, and up to now the vast majority of randomized clinical trials of cachexia therapy have investigated the use of a single agent (and sometimes one with a highly specific action such as a monoclonal antibody to a cytokine), in unselected cancer patients presenting with involuntary weight loss of unknown aetiology.[111] More extensive characterization of the underlying aetiology would benefit individual patients requiring intervention, and would improve the clarity of conclusions that could be drawn from clinical trials.

References

1. Delano MJ, Moldawer LL (2006) The origins of cachexia in acute and chronic inflammatory diseases. *Nutr Clin Pract*, **21**(1), 68–81.
2. Laviano A, Meguid MM, Inui A, Muscaritoli M, Rossi-Fanelli F (2005) Therapy insight: cancer anorexia–cachexia syndrome—when all you can eat is yourself. *Natl Clin Pract Oncol*, **2**(3), 158–65.
3. Baracos VE (2006) Cancer-associated cachexia and underlying biological mechanisms. *Annu Rev Nutr*, **26**, 435–61.
4. Elia M (1997) Tissue distribution and energetics in weight loss and undernutrition. In: Kinney J, Tucker H (eds), *Physiology, Stress, and Malnutrition: Functional Correlates, Nutritional Interventions*, pp. 383–411. Philadelphia: Lippincott–Raven.
5. MacDonald N, Easson AM, Mazurak VC, Dunn GP, Baracos VE (2003) Understanding and managing cancer cachexia. *J Am Coll Surg*, **197**(1), 143–61.
6. Lieffers JR, Mourtzakis M, Hall KD, McCargar LJ, Prado CM, Baracos VE (2009) A viscerally driven cachexia syndrome in patients with advanced colorectal cancer: contributions of organ and tumor mass to whole-body energy demands. *Am J Clin Nutr*, **89**(4), 1173–9.
7. Taylor I (2008) Adjuvant chemotherapy after resection of liver metastases from colorectal cancer. *Eur J Cancer*, **44**(9), 1198–201.
8. Fordy C, Glover C, Henderson DC, Summerbell C, Wharton R, Allen-Mersh TG (1999) Contribution of diet, tumour volume and patient-related factors to weight loss in patients with colorectal liver metastases. *Br J Surg*, **86**(5), 639–44.
9. Zibari GB, Riche A, Zizzi HC, *et al.* (1998) Surgical and nonsurgical management of primary and metastatic liver tumors. *Am Surg*, **64**(3), 211–20; discussion 20–1.
10. Bing C, Trayhurn P (2009) New insights into adipose tissue atrophy in cancer cachexia. *Proc Nutr Soc*, **68**(4), 385–92.
11. Stewart GD, Skipworth RJ, Ross JA, Fearon K, Baracos VE (2008) The dermcidin gene in cancer: role in cachexia, carcinogenesis and tumour cell survival. *Curr Opin Clin Nutr Metab Care*, **11**(3), 208–13.
12. Wieland BM, Stewart GD, Skipworth RJ, *et al.* (2007) Is there a human homologue to the murine proteolysis-inducing factor? *Clin Cancer Res*, **13**(17), 4984–92.
13. Kitada S, Hays EF, Mead JF (1981) Characterization of a lipid mobilizing factor from tumors. *Prog Lipid Res* **20**, 823–6.

14. Kitada S, Hays EF, Mead JF (1980) A lipid mobilizing factor in serum of tumor-bearing mice. *Lipids*, **15**(3), 168–74.
15. Kitada S, Hays EF, Mead JF, Zabin I (1982) Lipolysis induction in adipocytes by a protein from tumor cells. *J Cell Biochem*, **20**(4), 409–16.
16. Costa G, Holland JF (1962) Effects of Krebs-2 carcinoma on the lipide metabolism of male Swiss mice. *Cancer Res*, **22**, 1081–3.
17. Taylor DD, Gercel-Taylor C, Jenis LG, Devereux DF (1992) Identification of a human tumor-derived lipolysis-promoting factor. *Cancer Res*, **52**(4), 829–34.
18. Todorov PT, McDevitt TM, Meyer DJ, Ueyama H, Ohkubo I, Tisdale MJ (1998) Purification and characterization of a tumor lipid-mobilizing factor. *Cancer Res*, **58**(11), 2353–8.
19. Russell ST, Zimmerman TP, Domin BA, Tisdale MJ (2004) Induction of lipolysis in vitro and loss of body fat in vivo by zinc-alpha2-glycoprotein. *Biochim Biophys Acta*, **1636**(1), 59–68.
20. Tisdale MJ (2009) Zinc-alpha2-glycoprotein in cachexia and obesity. *Curr Opin Support Palliat Care*, **3**(4), 288–93.
21. Todorov P, Cariuk P, McDevitt T, Coles B, Fearon K, Tisdale M (1996) Characterization of a cancer cachectic factor. *Nature*, **379**(6567), 739–42.
22. Cariuk P, Lorite MJ, Todorov PT, Field WN, Wigmore SJ, Tisdale MJ (1997) Induction of cachexia in mice by a product isolated from the urine of cachectic cancer patients. *Br J Cancer*, **76**(5), 606–13.
23. Wang Z, Corey E, Hass GM, *et al.* (2003) Expression of the human cachexia-associated protein (HCAP) in prostate cancer and in a prostate cancer animal model of cachexia. *Int J Cancer*, **105**(1), 123–9.
24. Williams ML, Torres-Duarte A, Brant LJ, Bhargava P, Marshall J, Wainer IW (2004) The relationship between a urinary cachectic factor and weight loss in advanced cancer patients. *Cancer Invest*, **22**(6), 866–70.
25. Jatoi A, Foster N, Wieland B, *et al.* (2006) The proteolysis-inducing factor: in search of its clinical relevance in patients with metastatic gastric/esophageal cancer. *Dis Esophagus*, **19**(4), 241–7.
26. Monitto CL, Dong SM, Jen J, Sidransky D (2004*) Characterization of a human homologue of proteolysis-inducing factor and its role in cancer cachexia. Clin Cancer Res,* **10**, 5862–9.
27. Schwartz MW, Woods SC, Porte D, Jr, Seeley RJ, Baskin DG (2000) Central nervous system control of food intake. *Nature*, **404**(6778), 661–71.
28. Havel PJ (2001) Peripheral signals conveying metabolic information to the brain: short-term and long-term regulation of food intake and energy homeostasis. *Exp Biol Med (Maywood)*, **226**(11), 963–77.
29. Meier U, Gressner AM (2004) Endocrine regulation of energy metabolism: review of pathobiochemical and clinical chemical aspects of leptin, ghrelin, adiponectin, and resistin. *Clin Chem*, **50**(9), 1511–25.
30. Chance WT, Sheriff S, Moore J, Peng F, Balasubramaniam A (1998) Reciprocal changes in hypothalamic receptor binding and circulating leptin in anorectic tumor-bearing rats. *Brain Res*, **803**(1–2), 27–33.
31. Wolf I, Sadetzki S, Kanety H, *et al.* (2006) Adiponectin, ghrelin, and leptin in cancer cachexia in breast and colon cancer patients. *Cancer*, **106**(4), 966–73.
32. Mantovani G, Maccio A, Mura L, *et al.* (2000) Serum levels of leptin and proinflammatory cytokines in patients with advanced-stage cancer at different sites. *J Mol Med*, **78**(10), 554–61.
33. Kahler A, Zimmermann M, Langhans W (1999) Suppression of hepatic fatty acid oxidation and food intake in men. *Nutrition*, **15**(11–12), 819–28.
34. Loftus TM, Jaworsky DE, Frehywot GL, *et al.* (2000) Reduced food intake and body weight in mice treated with fatty acid synthase inhibitors. *Science*, **288**(5475), 2379–81.
35. Celik A, Kano Y, Tsujinaka S, *et al.* (2009) Decrease in malonyl-CoA and its background metabolic alterations in murine model of cancer cachexia. *Oncol Rep*, **21**(4), 1105–11.
36. Chance WT, Balasubramaniam A, Fischer JE (1995) Neuropeptide Y and the development of cancer anorexia. *Ann Surg*, **221**(5), 579–87; discussion 87–9.

37. Makarenko IG, Meguid MM, Gatto L, Chen C, Ugrumov MV (2003) Decreased NPY innervation of the hypothalamic nuclei in rats with cancer anorexia. *Brain Res*, **961**(1), 100–8.
38. Makarenko IG, Meguid MM, Gatto L, *et al.* (2005) Normalization of hypothalamic serotonin (5-HT 1B) receptor and NPY in cancer anorexia after tumor resection: an immunocytochemical study. *Neurosci Lett*, **383**(3), 322–7.
39. Ramos EJ, Suzuki S, Meguid MM, *et al.* (2004) Changes in hypothalamic neuropeptide Y and monoaminergic system in tumor-bearing rats: pre- and post-tumor resection and at death. *Surgery*, **136**(2), 270–6.
40. MacDonald N (2007) Cancer cachexia and targeting chronic inflammation: a unified approach to cancer treatment and palliative/supportive care. *J Support Oncol*, **5**(4), 157–62; discussion 64–6, 83.
41. Stephens NA, Skipworth RJ, Fearon KC (2008) Cachexia, survival and the acute phase response. *Curr Opin Support Palliat Care*, **2**(4), 267–74.
42. Evans WJ, Morley JE, Argiles J, *et al.* (2008) Cachexia: a new definition. *Clin Nutr*, **27**(6), 793–9.
43. Fearon KC, Voss AC, Hustead DS (2006) Definition of cancer cachexia: effect of weight loss, reduced food intake, and systemic inflammation on functional status and prognosis. *Am J Clin Nutr*, **83**(6), 1345–50.
44. Baracos VE (2005) Cytokines and the pathophysiology of skeletal muscle atrophy. In: Anker SD, Hofbauer K (eds), *The Pharmacotherapy of Cachexia*, pp. 101–14. Boca Raton, FL: CRC Press.
45. Bedard S, Marcotte B, Marette A (1997) Cytokines modulate glucose transport in skeletal muscle by inducing the expression of inducible nitric oxide synthase. *Biochem J*, **325**(Pt 2), 487–93.
46. de Alvaro C, Teruel T, Hernandez R, Lorenzo M (2004) Tumor necrosis factor alpha produces insulin resistance in skeletal muscle by activation of inhibitor kappaB kinase in a p38 MAPK-dependent manner. *J Biol Chem*, **279**(17), 17070–8.
47. Filippatos GS, Anker SD, Kremastinos DT (2005) Pathophysiology of peripheral muscle wasting in cardiac cachexia. *Curr Opin Clin Nutr Metab Care*, **8**(3), 249–54.
48. Frost RA, Lang CH (2004) Alteration of somatotropic function by proinflammatory cytokines. *J Anim Sci*, **82**(E-Suppl), E100–09.
49. Lang CH, Hong-Brown L, Frost RA (2005) Cytokine inhibition of JAK-STAT signaling: a new mechanism of growth hormone resistance. *Pediatr Nephrol*, **20**(3), 306–12.
50. Lundholm K, Daneryd P, Korner U, Hyltander A, Bosaeus I (2004) Evidence that long-term COX-treatment improves energy homeostasis and body composition in cancer patients with progressive cachexia. *Int J Oncol*, **24**(3), 505–12.
51. Lundholm K, Gelin J, Hyltander A, *et al.* (1994) Anti-inflammatory treatment may prolong survival in undernourished patients with metastatic solid tumors. *Cancer Res*, **54**(21), 5602–6.
52. Ramos EJ, Suzuki S, Marks D, Inui A, Asakawa A, Meguid MM (2004) Cancer anorexia-cachexia syndrome: cytokines and neuropeptides. *Curr Opin Clin Nutr Metab Care*, **7**(4), 427–34.
53. Baracos V, Rodemann HP, Dinarello CA, Goldberg AL (1983) Stimulation of muscle protein degradation and prostaglandin E2 release by leukocytic pyrogen (interleukin-1). A mechanism for the increased degradation of muscle proteins during fever. *N Engl J Med*, **308**(10), 553–8.
54. Beutler B, Cerami A (1986) Cachectin and tumour necrosis factor as two sides of the same biological coin. *Nature*, **320**(6063), 584–8.
55. Bruce CR, Dyck DJ (2004) Cytokine regulation of skeletal muscle fatty acid metabolism: effect of interleukin-6 and tumor necrosis factor-alpha. *Am J Physiol Endocrinol Metab*, **287**(4), E616–21.
56. Haddad F, Zaldivar F, Cooper DM, Adams GR (2005) IL-6-induced skeletal muscle atrophy. *J Appl Physiol*, **98**(3), 911–7.
57. Dennis RA, Trappe TA, Simpson P, *et al.* (2004) Interleukin-1 polymorphisms are associated with the inflammatory response in human muscle to acute resistance exercise. *J Physiol*, **560**(Pt 3), 617–26.
58. Rieusset J, Bouzakri K, Chevillotte E, *et al.* (2004) Suppressor of cytokine signaling 3 expression and insulin resistance in skeletal muscle of obese and type 2 diabetic patients. *Diabetes*, **53**(9), 2232–41.

59. Acharyya S, Ladner KJ, Nelsen LL, *et al.* (2004) Cancer cachexia is regulated by selective targeting of skeletal muscle gene products. *J Clin Invest*, **114**(3), 370–8.

60. Zhang Y, Pilon G, Marette A, Baracos VE (2000) Cytokines and endotoxin induce cytokine receptors in skeletal muscle. *Am J Physiol Endocrinol Metab*, **279**(1), E196–205.

61. Fernandez-Celemin L, Pasko N, Blomart V, Thissen JP (2002) Inhibition of muscle insulin-like growth factor I expression by tumor necrosis factor-alpha. *Am J Physiol Endocrinol Metab*, **283**(6), E1279–90.

62. Oliff A, Defeo-Jones D, Boyer M, *et al.* (1987) Tumors secreting human TNF/cachectin induce cachexia in mice. *Cell*, **50**(4), 555–63.

63. Llovera M, Garcia-Martinez C, Lopez-Soriano J, *et al.* (1998) Protein turnover in skeletal muscle of tumour-bearing transgenic mice overexpressing the soluble TNF receptor-1. *Cancer Lett*, **130**(1–2), 19–27.

64. Pajak B, Orzechowska S, Pijet B, *et al.* (2008) Crossroads of cytokine signaling—the chase to stop muscle cachexia. *J Physiol Pharmacol*, **59**(Suppl 9), 251–64.

65. Guttridge DC, Mayo MW, Madrid LV, Wang CY, Baldwin AS Jr (2000) NF-kappaB-induced loss of MyoD messenger RNA: possible role in muscle decay and cachexia. *Science*, **289**(5488), 2363–6.

66. Szalay K, Razga Z, Duda E (1997) TNF inhibits myogenesis and downregulates the expression of myogenic regulatory factors myoD and myogenin. *Eur J Cell Biol*, **74**(4), 391–8.

67. Lecker SH, Solomon V, Mitch WE, Goldberg AL (1999) Muscle protein breakdown and the critical role of the ubiquitin–proteasome pathway in normal and disease states. *J Nutr*, **129**(1S Suppl), 227S–37S.

68. Woo CH, Eom YW, Yoo MH, *et al.* (2000) Tumor necrosis factor-alpha generates reactive oxygen species via a cytosolic phospholipase A2-linked cascade. *J Biol Chem*, **275**(41), 32357–62.

69. Mastrocola R, Reffo P, Penna F, *et al.* (2008) Muscle wasting in diabetic and in tumor-bearing rats: role of oxidative stress. *Free Radic Biol Med*, **44**(4), 584–93.

70. Price SR, Olivecrona T, Pekala PH (1986) Regulation of lipoprotein lipase synthesis in 3T3-L1 adipocytes by cachectin. Further proof for identity with tumour necrosis factor. *Biochem J*, **240**(2), 601–4.

71. Price SR, Olivecrona T, Pekala PH (1986) Regulation of lipoprotein lipase synthesis by recombinant tumor necrosis factor—the primary regulatory role of the hormone in 3T3-L1 adipocytes. *Arch Biochem Biophys*, **251**(2), 738–46.

72. Ryden M, Arvidsson E, Blomqvist L, Perbeck L, Dicker A, Arner P (2004) Targets for TNF-alpha-induced lipolysis in human adipocytes. *Biochem Biophys Res Commun*, **318**(1), 168–75.

73. Karayiannakis AJ, Syrigos KN, Polychronidis A, Pitiakoudis M, Bounovas A, Simopoulos K (2001) Serum levels of tumor necrosis factor-alpha and nutritional status in pancreatic cancer patients. *Anticancer Res*, **21**(2B), 1355–8.

74. Maltoni M, Fabbri L, Nanni O, *et al.* (1997) Serum levels of tumour necrosis factor alpha and other cytokines do not correlate with weight loss and anorexia in cancer patients. *Support Care Cancer*, **5**(2), 130–5.

75. Socher SH, Martinez D, Craig JB, Kuhn JG, Oliff A (1988) Tumor necrosis factor not detectable in patients with clinical cancer cachexia. *J Natl Cancer Inst*, **80**(8), 595–8.

76. Tsujinaka T, Fujita J, Ebisui C, *et al.* (1996) Interleukin 6 receptor antibody inhibits muscle atrophy and modulates proteolytic systems in interleukin 6 transgenic mice. *J Clin Invest*, **97**(1), 244–9.

77. Espat NJ, Auffenberg T, Rosenberg JJ, *et al.* (1996) Ciliary neurotrophic factor is catabolic and shares with IL-6 the capacity to induce an acute phase response. *Am J Physiol*, **271**(1 Pt 2), R185–90.

78. Moldawer LL, Andersson C, Gelin J, Lundholm KG (1988) Regulation of food intake and hepatic protein synthesis by recombinant-derived cytokines. *Am J Physiol*, **254**(3 Pt 1), G450–6.

79. Martin F, Santolaria F, Batista N, *et al.* (1999) Cytokine levels (IL-6 and IFN-gamma), acute phase response and nutritional status as prognostic factors in lung cancer. *Cytokine*, **11**(1), 80–6.

80. Medzhitov R (2008) Origin and physiological roles of inflammation. *Nature*, **454**(7203), 428–35.

81. Ono M (2008) Molecular links between tumor angiogenesis and inflammation: inflammatory stimuli of macrophages and cancer cells as targets for therapeutic strategy. *Cancer Sci*, **99**(8), 1501–6.
82. Dinarello CA (2006) The paradox of pro-inflammatory cytokines in cancer. *Cancer Metastasis Rev*, **25**(3), 307–13.
83. Pirlich M, Norman K, Lochs H, Bauditz J (2006) Role of intestinal function in cachexia. *Curr Opin Clin Nutr Metab Care*, **9**(5), 603–6.
84. Bow EJ, Meddings JB (2006) Intestinal mucosal dysfunction and infection during remission-induction therapy for acute myeloid leukaemia. *Leukemia*, **20**(12), 2087–92.
85. Blijlevens NM, Donnelly JP, de Pauw BE (2005) Prospective evaluation of gut mucosal barrier injury following various myeloablative regimens for haematopoietic stem cell transplant. *Bone Marrow Transplant*, **35**(7), 707–11.
86. Frost RA, Lang CH (2005) Skeletal muscle cytokines: regulation by pathogen-associated molecules and catabolic hormones. *Curr Opin Clin Nutr Metab Care*, **8**(3), 255–63.
87. Lund L, Jacobsen J, Norgaard M, *et al.* (2009) The prognostic impact of comorbidities on renal cancer, 1995 to 2006: a Danish population based study. *J Urol*, **182**(1), 35–40; discussion 40.
88. Pereira J, Watanabe S, Wolch G (1998) A retrospective review of the frequency of infections and patterns of antibiotic utilization on a palliative care unit. *J Pain Sympt Manag*, **16**(6), 374–81.
89. Combaret L, Ralliere C, Taillandier D, Tanaka K, Attaix D (1999) Manipulation of the ubiquitin–proteasome pathway in cachexia: pentoxifylline suppresses the activation of 20S and 26S proteasomes in muscles from tumor-bearing rats. *Mol Biol Rep*, **26**(1–2), 95–101.
90. Enomoto A, Rho MC, Fukami A, Hiraku O, Komiyama K, Hayashi M (2004) Suppression of cancer cachexia by 20S,21-epoxy-resibufogenin-3-acetate—a novel nonpeptide IL-6 receptor antagonist. *Biochem Biophys Res Commun*, **323**(3), 1096–102.
91. Fujita J, Tsujinaka T, Yano M, *et al.* (1996) Anti-interleukin-6 receptor antibody prevents muscle atrophy in colon-26 adenocarcinoma-bearing mice with modulation of lysosomal and ATP-ubiquitin-dependent proteolytic pathways. *Int J Cancer*, **68**(5), 637–43.
92. Llovera M, Garcia-Martinez C, Lopez-Soriano J, *et al.* (1998) Role of TNF receptor 1 in protein turnover during cancer cachexia using gene knockout mice. *Mol Cell Endocrinol*, **142**(1–2), 183–9.
93. Hitt A, Graves E, McCarthy DO (2005) Indomethacin preserves muscle mass and reduces levels of E3 ligases and TNF receptor type 1 in the gastrocnemius muscle of tumor-bearing mice. *Res Nurs Health*, **28**(1), 56–66.
94. McCarthy DO, Whitney P, Hitt A, Al-Majid S (2004) Indomethacin and ibuprofen preserve gastrocnemius muscle mass in mice bearing the colon-26 adenocarcinoma. *Res Nurs Health*, **27**(3), 174–84.
95. Ross JA, Fearon KC (2002) Eicosanoid-dependent cancer cachexia and wasting. *Curr Opin Clin Nutr Metab Care*, **5**(3), 241–8.
96. Strelkov AB, Fields AL, Baracos VE (1989) Effects of systemic inhibition of prostaglandin production on protein metabolism in tumor-bearing rats. *Am J Physiol*, **257**(2 Pt 1), C261–9.
97. Asp ML, Tian M, Wendel AA, Belury MA (2010) Evidence for the contribution of insulin resistance to the development of cachexia in tumor-bearing mice. *Int J Cancer* **126**(3), 756–63.
98. Daneryd P, Hafstrom L, Svanberg E, Karlberg I (1995) Insulin sensitivity, hormonal levels and skeletal muscle protein metabolism in tumour-bearing exercising rats. *Eur J Cancer*, **31A**(1), 97–103.
99. Pisters PW, Cersosimo E, Rogatko A, Brennan MF (1992) Insulin action on glucose and branched-chain amino acid metabolism in cancer cachexia: differential effects of insulin. *Surgery*, **111**(3), 301–10.
100. Pereira S, Marliss EB, Morais JA, Chevalier S, Gougeon R (2008) Insulin resistance of protein metabolism in type 2 diabetes. *Diabetes*, **57**(1), 56–63.
101. Chevalier S, Marliss EB, Morais JA, Lamarche M, Gougeon R (2005) Whole-body protein anabolic response is resistant to the action of insulin in obese women. *Am J Clin Nutr*, **82**(2), 355–65.

102. Morais JA, Gougeon R, Pencharz PB, Jones PJ, Ross R, Marliss EB (1997) Whole-body protein turnover in the healthy elderly. *Am J Clin Nutr*, **66**(4), 880–9.

103. Kortebein P, Ferrando A, Lombeida J, Wolfe R, Evans WJ (2007) Effect of 10 days of bed rest on skeletal muscle in healthy older adults. *J Am Med Assoc*, **297**(16), 1772–4.

104. Kortebein P, Symons TB, Ferrando A, *et al.* (2008) Functional impact of 10 days of bed rest in healthy older adults. *J Gerontol A Biol Sci Med Sci*, **63**(10), 1076–81.

105. Fassbender K, Fainsinger R, Brenneis C, Brown P, Braun T, Jacobs P (2005) Utilization and costs of the introduction of system-wide palliative care in Alberta, 1993–2000. *Palliat Med*, **19**(7), 513–20.

106. Schneider HJ, Sievers C, Klotsche J, *et al.* (2009) Prevalence of low male testosterone levels in primary care in Germany: cross-sectional results from the DETECT study. *Clin Endocrinol (Oxf)*, **70**(3), 446–54.

107. Bassil N, Alkaade S, Morley JE (2009) The benefits and risks of testosterone replacement therapy: a review. *Ther Clin Risk Manag*, **5**(3), 427–48.

108. Kiserud CE, Fossa A, Bjoro T, Holte H, Cvancarova M, Fossa SD (2009) Gonadal function in male patients after treatment for malignant lymphomas, with emphasis on chemotherapy. *Br J Cancer*, **100**(3), 455–63.

109. Yau I, Vuong T, Garant A, *et al.* (2009) Risk of hypogonadism from scatter radiation during pelvic radiation in male patients with rectal cancer. *Int J Radiat Oncol Biol Phys*, **74**(5), 1481–6.

110. Fraser LA, Morrison D, Morley-Forster P, *et al.* (2009) Oral opioids for chronic non-cancer pain: higher prevalence of hypogonadism in men than in women. *Exp Clin Endocrinol Diabetes*, **117**(1), 38–43.

111. Yavuzsen T, Davis MP, Walsh D, LeGrand S, Lagman R (2005) Systematic review of the treatment of cancer-associated anorexia and weight loss. *J Clin Oncol*, **23**(33), 8500–11.

Part 3

Treatment of primary cachexia

Chapter 6

Conducting clinical research in cancer cachexia

Henrique A. Parsons and Eduardo Bruera

Introduction

As a research topic, cancer-related cachexia has not attracted the attention of a large number of investigators for several reasons. First, because it was historically misinterpreted as a normal and inexorable part of late stages of chronic diseases. Second, the limited success of clinical research on aggressive nutritional interventions during the 1980s[1] contributed to a decrease in interest in cachexia research over time. Third, practical issues such as the lack of a clear-cut definition, variable inception points for clinical trials, and the complex methodology involved in assessing appetite, body composition, and nutritional status in a population of frail and highly symptomatic patients also have traditionally driven researchers away from this topic.

There has been limited amount of research on the epidemiology, pathophysiology, and treatment of cancer-related cachexia. Therefore, the evidence base for the management of the syndrome is weak,[2] which is deleterious for the quality of life of these very ill patients. In this chapter we discuss some of the challenges and opportunities in conducting cachexia research.

Participants

Patients with cancer-related cachexia have multiple sources of physical and psychosocial distress. They frequently have multiple symptoms related not only to the cachexia syndrome, but to the underlying cancer itself. These include pain, nausea, fatigue, lack of appetite, depression, anxiety, insomnia, and others.[3,4] Even though a significant proportion of cancer patients might have some degree of cachexia at the time of cancer diagnosis,[5] overt cachexia is generally noted towards more advanced phases of the disease, where symptoms are usually more severe.[6–8]

In addition, the patient population to be studied will usually be under cancer treatment with chemotherapy, radiotherapy, and surgery—treatment modalities known to cause significant distress. Several symptoms might be caused by or worsen by chemotherapy, including nausea and vomiting (with a direct effect on appetite), fatigue, and neuropathic pain, among others.[9] Radiotherapy might also be cause of side-effects which might impair these patients' quality of life, ranging from topical side-effects that might cause pain or, in the case of head and neck cancers for example, inability to eat, to systemic side-effects such as fatigue.[10] Patients with cancer undergoing surgery are prone to have symptoms because of the procedure itself, and in the cases of gastrointestinal cancers, for example, feeding tubes or draining/decompression tubes might be needed, impairing their ability to eat for a considerable period of time.[11] All these, while concurrent causes to secondary cachexia, are also factors impairing these patients' ability to take part in cachexia research studies.

Cachexia is frequently detected towards the late stages of the underlying disease. Therefore, it is logical to expect a very short average lifespan for these patients, making it difficult for them to participate in extended longitudinal interventional trials. These facts make it challenging to accrue patients in studies about cachexia, since they might be too ill to participate, or their lifespan might not allow for standard outcome observations. In addition to the severe physical suffering, patients with cachexia also experience significant psychological distress related to eating issues, body image concepts, and other factors,[12,13] which also impair their willingness to participate in protocol research.

Mostly due to its complex multifactorial aetiology, there is no consensual and widely accepted definition of cachexia.[14] This also reduces the ability of researchers to identify appropriate participants for studies in such a syndrome.[15] The section on 'Outcomes' below will discuss this issue in more detail.

Clinical investigators have dealt with the challenges of the patient population by adapting their experimental designs to best fit the aforementioned issues. Clinical trials should be as short as possible as a way of minimizing patient drop-outs due to clinical worsening. Early access to patients potentially eligible for clinical trials can be secured by approaching these patients when they arrive for early treatment with the medical oncology, surgical oncology, or radiation oncology teams rather than when they develop signs and symptoms of cachexia. Assessments should be simplified as much as possible to minimize the burden on these already symptomatic patients. Finally, sample size calculations should take into consideration a significant number of drop-outs due to clinical deterioration.

The homogeneity of the underlying cancer diagnosis of participants in cachexia clinical trials is important. In those cases in which the primary outcome might be differentially influenced by the underlying cancer (for example, studies on the impact of cachexia on overall survival, side-effects, or response to treatment), the patient sample has to be as homogeneous as possible, with patients with similar diagnosis, at similar stages of the disease at the time of study entry, and with similar past and current antineoplastic treatments, in order to avoid confounding. Study populations with heterogeneous underlying cancer diagnoses, stages of disease, or with multiple different treatments with the common denominator of cachexia are still suitable for symptomatic or body composition-related studies.

Outcomes

The main variable used to decide the result of a study is called the primary outcome.[16] The clear and precise anticipated determination of one single primary outcome is always advisable,[17] as studies with multiple primary outcomes are likely to fail.[16] It is clear from the previous section that the primary outcome is the most important force driving not only patient sample characteristics but also the study methodology.

With regards to methodology determination, studies aiming to observe symptoms might have very short duration (days to weeks), while studies aiming at survival duration or response to cancer treatment will need significantly longer duration (months or even years). For example, in a clinical trial on the effects of fish oil on appetite, the symptomatic primary outcome chosen allowed the shorter duration of the trial.[18] However, another study aiming to explore changes in body composition among cancer patients had a very long follow-up time (up to 62 months).[19]

The determination of the primary outcome is also very important because it determines the sample size needed for an adequately powered study. The power of a study might be understood as the ability of detecting a difference between two groups in the study sample when such a difference exists in the underlying population from which given study sample was drawn.[20] Usually sample size calculations are undertaken considering acceptable an 80% power level. In the determination of the primary outcome, it is fundamental to clearly define what an effect size of clinical significance is, since it will also be considered in the sample size calculation.[16] For example, if the primary outcome is weight gain, one has to determine what is a clinically significant weight gain for the purpose of the study (a specific percentage of the baseline weight or an amount in kilograms, for instance). In a randomized controlled trial with appetite as primary outcome, a difference of at least 15 mm in an appetite visual analogic scale was considered clinically significant based on the experience obtained from another study.[18,21] In another study, the primary outcome was weight gain, and it was considered as clinically significant when ≥2 kg, also based on data previously obtained.[22,23]

Several outcomes might be studied in cachexia research. The following paragraphs will highlight some of the most common assessments applied in the field. Notice that details on the specific measurements are not provided here since they would fall out of the scope of this chapter. All methods are described in detail elsewhere in this book.

Body composition measurements

Body composition measurements are widely used and may provide very useful information about muscularity and fat deposits. Simple anthropometric measurements such as the determination of body weight or the body mass index (BMI; kg/m^2; which is considered a surrogate for the amount of body fat)[24] are widely used. BMI is generally accepted, is considered a good surrogate for malnutrition (when <20 kg/m^2),[25] is part of the most recent cancer cachexia definition,[26] but is not free of criticisms, for example, for not taking into consideration changes in fat:muscle ratio that happen as a result of ageing, racial specificities, and intense physical training.[27] Better estimations of body fat and muscularity can be obtained by the measurement of skinfold thicknesses (such as the widely used triceptal skinfold) and body circumferences (such as the mid-upper arm circumference), but are very dependent on the operator and the equipment (well-calibrated calipers and standardized tape measures).[28–31] Near-infrared interactance also provides a good estimation of the body composition, being a fast and reliable method that uses portable equipment, but this is not yet widely available and has conversion equations validated only for healthy subjects.[32] Bioelectric impedance is one of the most widely used and available methods to estimate body composition, even though suffers from the lack of portability of the most adequate equipment.[33,34] Dual-energy X-ray absorptiometry (DXA) is probably the most widely accepted method for the determination of body composition. However, it is expensive, not widely available, and provides accurate measurements only in well-hydrated patients (which might pose a problem for advanced cancer patients who frequently are dehydrated).[35–37] The gold standard for body composition determination is the impractical and expensive underwater weighting method, which has to be conducted in special facilities under controlled conditions, and might not be a feasible option for very sick advanced cancer patients.[38,39] The estimation of total body potassium, which is characteristic of the muscular compartment, also provides a good estimate of muscularity and might be used as an outcome in cachexia research.[40] More recently, imaging methods have been arising as alternatives to more expensive and complex assessments of body composition. Computed tomography and magnetic resonance images, frequently obtained in the course of cancer treatment, might be used to determine the fat/muscle contents by relatively simple imaging analysis procedures.[41,42]

Other clinical assessments

Several clinical features might be of interest in cachexia research. The assessment of **symptoms** such as anorexia, nausea, vomiting, and fatigue, for example, might be undertaken by the use of validated scales such as the Edmonton Symptom Assessment System, which comprises

10 common symptoms in patients with advanced cancer which are rated in individual 0–10 scales anchored from 'no symptom at all' to 'worst imaginable symptom' and is widely used and validated in the advanced cancer setting.[43,44] The use of visual analogue scales for specific symptoms is also usually accepted and has been used in a variety of cachexia studies.[45,46] Specific tools for assessment of fatigue are available and might be used when appropriate; some examples are the Functional Assessment of Chronic Illness Therapy—Fatigue (FACIT-F)[47,48] and the Revised Piper Fatigue Scale.[49] Assessment of **muscular strength** might be needed depending on the focus of the study, and this can be done by the use of dynamometers.[50] **Physical function** might be assessed by the use of several widely accepted scales such as the Eastern European Collaborative Oncology Group (ECOG),[51] and the Karnofsky Performance Status Scales.[52] Since cachexia might significantly impair patients' **quality of life** (QoL), validated assessments for QoL assessment might be used, such as the European Organization for Research and Treatment of Cancer—Quality of Life Questionnaire (EORTC-QLQ30)[53] or the Functional Assessment of Cancer Therapy—General (FACT-G) scale.[47] **Response to antineoplastic therapies** has to be assessed in a standardized, validated system such as the Response Evaluation Criteria in Solid Tumors (RECIST),[54] or others for specific types of cancers.

The assessment of **food intake** might also be applied in cachexia research. The use of food diaries (usually ranging from 3 to 7 days) is extremely helpful in determining eating patterns, preferences, and diet deficiencies.[55,56] In addition, the subjective assessment of the nutritional status is possible using validated questionnaires such as the Subjective Global Assessment (SGA) and the Patient-Generated Subjective Global Assessment (PG-SGA), which are specific for cancer patients.[57–60]

Study design

Several study designs may be applied to obtain answers to research questions. Figure 6.1 summarizes the type of study designs.[61,62] The choice of the most adequate study design is complicated in the setting of cachexia research. Even though longitudinal interventional studies (such as prospective randomized placebo-controlled studies) generally draw attention in most fields of medical research, it is difficult to conduct such studies in this particular setting, due to the very special characteristics of the patient population.

Shorter, straightforward cross-sectional observational studies such as surveys on attitudes and beliefs or observation of patient characteristics such as symptoms and/or body composition, for example, are easier and less prone to suffer from participant drop-out than longitudinal studies

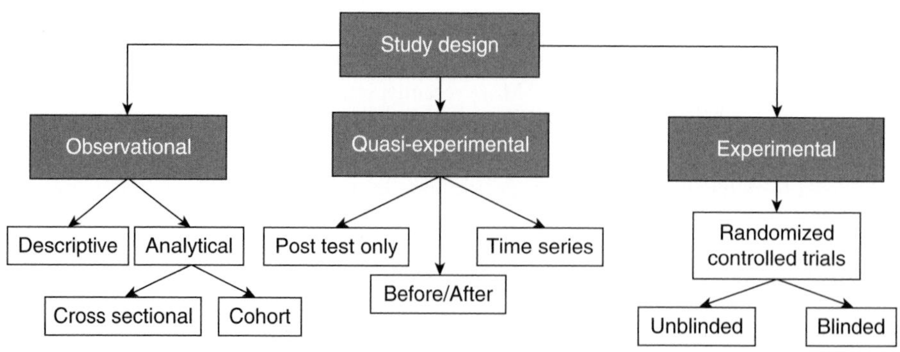

Fig. 6.1 Types of clinical research study.

with multiple assessments over time. It is important to notice that due to the very poor health of the study populations, studies longer than two weeks are prone to have very high drop-out rates (>30%), especially when conducted with patients with overt cachexia and in very advanced stages of their cancers.

On the other hand, the characterization of the natural history of cachexia would require longer, multi-assessment studies. Due to the multifactorial nature of cancer cachexia and to the evolving role of different factors over time, it is important that longer studies be conducted with appropriate inception points so that early cancer patients are not combined with patients with advanced malignancies due to the different roles played by different factors such as inflammatory cytokines and other tumour by-products, side-effects of therapies, and the overall symptom burden on cancer cachexia. In the following paragraphs, we provide examples of the very different studies already conducted in the field of cancer cachexia.

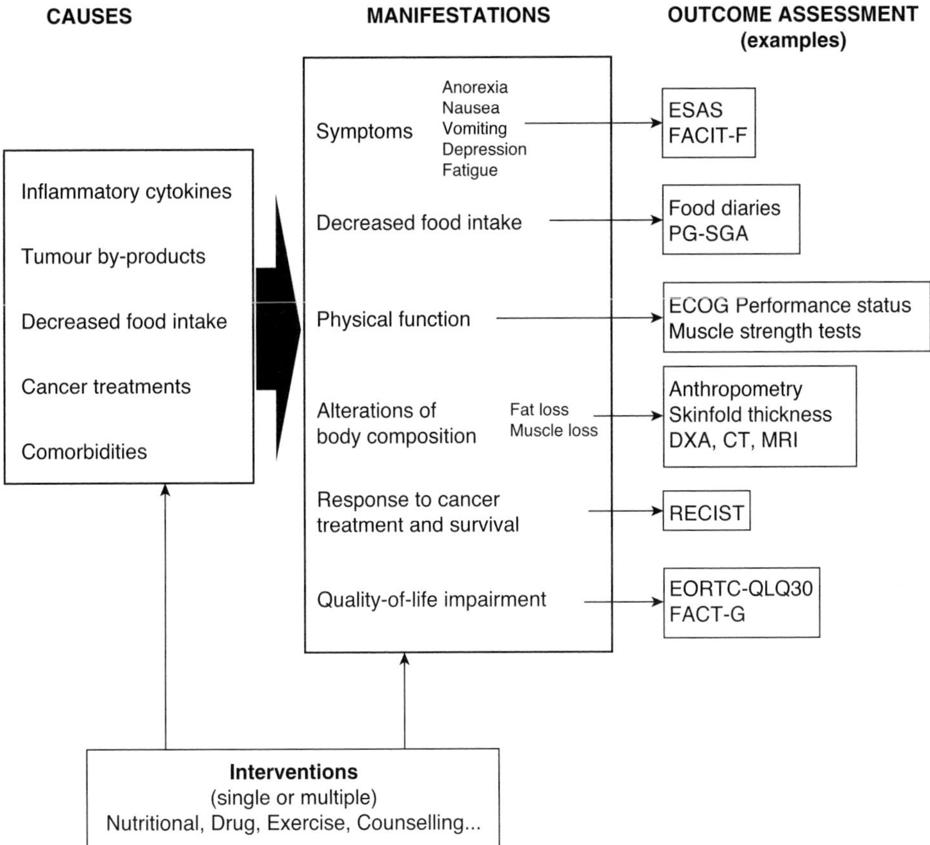

Fig. 6.2 A conceptual model for research interventions in cancer cachexia. ESAS, Edmonton Symptom Assessment System; FACIT-F, Functional Assessment of Chronic Illness Therapy—Fatigue; PG-SGA, Patient-Generated Subjective Global Assessment; ECOG, Eastern European Collaborative Oncology Group; DXA, dual-energy X-ray absorptiometry; CT, computed tomography; MRI, magnetic resonance imaging; RECIST, Response Evaluation Criteria In Solid Tumours; EORTC-QLQ30, European Organization for Research and Treatment of Cancer—Quality of Life Questionnaire; FACT-G, Functional Assessment of Cancer Therapy—Global.

Clinical trials: randomized controlled trials

Clinical trials are experiments with humans as subjects.[63] Randomized controlled trials (RCTs) are studies in which patients are assigned (based solely on chance) to two or more groups to receive different interventions and are observed over time for the occurrence of a predetermined outcome.[64] RCTs are considered the gold standard for the decision for or against utilizing a therapy in clinical practice.[65] Despite the inherent methodological difficulties, clinical trials have been and are necessary to establish the effectiveness of pharmacological and non-pharmacological interventions in the cachexia setting.

One of the first drugs studied in depth for the treatment of cancer cachexia-related symptoms was the megestrol acetate. In a randomized, double-blind, placebo-controlled trial with 133 participants, Loprinzi *et al.* were able to show significant improvement in appetite, food intake, and also weight gain among patients who took 800 mg of megestrol acetate daily compared with those who took placebo, with no clinically significant toxicities.[66] The same group has conducted a randomized trial comparing four doses of megestrol acetate in 342 patients and showed that there is a positive dose–response relationship for the drug, but suggested starting the use with the lower doses due to the inconvenience and cost of the higher-dose regimens.[67] Our group has conducted another randomized, double-blind, placebo-controlled cross-over trial with 53 patients to test the efficacy of megestrol acetate in a lower dose (160 mg/day) on symptoms of cancer cachexia. This study also showed significant improvement in appetite among patients who took the drug compared with those who took placebo, although no nutritional parameters were altered.[21] A prospective randomized open-label trial tested the efficacy of two different doses (160 mg/day and 320 mg/day) of megestrol acetate in 122 cancer anorexia–cachexia syndrome patients and found that the lower dose is as effective as the higher, confirming previous findings.[68]

Corticosteroids were also studied by several groups in the cancer cachexia setting as appetite stimulants. Willox *et al.* conducted a randomized, double-blind, placebo-controlled cross-over trial in 61 unselected cancer patients to investigate the efficacy of 15 mg daily of prednisolone on weight, appetite, and other symptoms and were able to show significant improvements in appetite and well-being.[69] Our group conducted a randomized, double-blind, placebo-controlled cross-over trial testing whether methylprednisolone 32 mg/day was able to improve several symptoms in a sample of 40 terminally ill cancer patients. This study also showed an improvement in several symptoms, including appetite, in the group which received methylprednisolone.[70]

Nutritional interventions are of interest in the cancer cachexia setting and several such studies have been conducted, with results pointing towards the limited effect of aggressive nutrition strategies in cancer cachexia.[71,72] Intensive oral nutrition was studied in a randomized controlled trial in which 180 advanced cancer patients were randomly assigned to one of three groups: no nutritional intervention, standard nutritional counselling, and 'augmented' nutritional counselling. Participants were followed for around 12 weeks and evaluated for several treatment-related factors. No difference was found between groups with regards to survival, toxicities, and response to oncological therapy.[73] Randomized controlled trials on parenteral nutrition focused on survival, toxicities, and response to oncological therapies, and the majority did not show clinically significant improvements in the advanced cancer setting.[1]

Among nutritional interventions, the use of eicosapentaenoic acid has been studied by several groups. Our group has conducted a randomized, double blind, placebo controlled trial to understand whether 2 weeks of oral administration of fish oil was able to increase appetite in advanced cancer patients with anorexia and weight loss. The predicted sample size was of 91 participants, but a drop-out rate of 31% was responsible for reducing the final evaluable sample size to 30 patients per group accrued in a 17-month period. Patients on the fish oil group did not show difference in the appetite changes compared with the placebo group.[18] Another study had shown similar results in another randomized, double-blind, placebo-controlled protocol to assess whether an eicosapentaenoic acid formulation used orally for 8 weeks was able to increase weight and lean body mass in 81 cancer patients with cachexia. The drop-out rate was also very high (around 50%), and the study was unable to detect significant improvement in body weight or lean body mass after 8 weeks of treatment.[22]

A very recent randomized, double-blind, placebo-controlled study by Jatoi *et al.* to study whether infliximab improved or stabilized weight loss in elderly or poor performance status lung cancer patients was closed earlier than predicted because of lack of effectiveness and unacceptable side effect profile (patients receiving infliximab showed significantly reduced QoL and increased fatigue).[74] The same group had similar results in another randomized, double-blind, placebo-controlled trial testing etanarecept versus placebo in 63 advanced cancer patients, and no benefit was perceived.[75] These are important examples of the importance of randomized controlled trials in the understanding of the disease, since both drugs are ultimately tumour necrosis factor blockers.

Quasi-experimental studies

Quasi-experimental studies are those in which an intervention is tested, but no randomization of the patient sample is used.[61,76] Such studies might have only one group of patients, and each participant serves as its own control (internal comparison) by observing the outcome before and after the implementation of the study intervention. They also might draw conclusions from the comparison of outcomes between multiple groups in which each one receives different interventions (given that no randomization exists, for example, if a researcher wants to determine the difference in survival of cachetic patients seen at hospitals with and without dedicated cachexia clinics). Mixed designs including internal and external controlling are also valuable.[61,62]

One study which exemplifies a quasi-experimental study with both internal and external controls in cachexia research is a prospective study on the effects of thalidomide on cancer cachexia conducted by our group.[77] Thirty-seven patients were treated with thalidomide 100 mg daily at bedtime and symptoms were assessed at baseline and after 10 days. The study showed statistically significant improvement in several symptoms when comparing patients at the two timepoints (internal controls). External controlling was performed by comparing the sample of patients who took thalidomide with a sample of 28 patients who took megestrol acetate as part of a previously conducted study.[21] The external comparison showed that patients who used thalidomide had significantly greater improvement in nausea, appetite, and sensation of well-being.[21]

Observational studies

Very frequently due to ethical issues and resource limitations, experimental and quasi-experimental studies are not feasible.[63] In observational studies, no intervention is put in place by the investigator.[61] Rather, features already present in patients at the time of study entry (specific demographic characteristics, previous recent or distant exposure to specific factors or presence of a given disease, for example) are considered reasons to enter patients in a study sample and/or to determine allocation to one or another study group.[63] The observation of the outcome might happen at the time of study entry only with the objective of describing the sample at that point, and studies designed that way are called cross-sectional.

One example of a cross-sectional study in cachexia is the one undertaken by Hartmuller *et al.* on the views of cancer patients and their health care providers about nutrition. In all, 873 health care professionals and 653 patients were surveyed with the objective of determining concerns related to nutrition in cancer patients and to study the content of printed materials related to the matter. The researchers were able to better understand patients' concerns and also to show that current practices were not focused on patients' concerns.[78]

Case–control studies are observational studies in which patients are allocated to different groups according to the presence or absence of a specific characteristic (for example, cachexia) for the purpose of comparing study groups with regards to a predetermined outcome or outcomes, with cases being the participants with the characteristic and controls the ones without it.[63]

A group in Sweden has conducted secondary analysis of a previously generated database on nutritional state and energy metabolism of 1332 patients in order to determine if long term use of the cyclo-oxygenase (COX) blocker indomethacin was associated with beneficial effects in energy homeostasis, cardiovascular activity, and body composition in a group of weight-losing cancer patients. A total of 299 weight-losing cancer patients were found in the database. Among those, 151 patients had been treated with indomethacin. These were matched to 145 cancer patients who did not have indomethacin or any other non-steroidal anti-inflammatory drug. By comparing the two groups, the researchers were able to show that resting energy expenditure was significantly lower and that caloric intake, body fat, and body weight were significantly higher among weight-losing cancer patients treated with indomethacin as compared to those not using it. The study provided preliminary data on the potential usefulness of COX blockers in the treatment of cancer cachexia.[79]

Another case–control study focused on details of the loss of muscularity among 19 patients with cancer cachexia compared with matched healthy volunteers. The study included muscle biopsies, muscle imaging and spectroscopy, all of which could be done in a single encounter with the research team, and are likely to provide important insights on the management of cancer cachexia.[80] Another group in Sweden was recently able to tackle the issue of fat mass loss in cachexia with a simple cross-sectional study with a sample of 23 cancer patients and 5 subjects without cancer in which subcutaneous fat and blood samples were obtained and analysed for specific markers. They found that it is likely that the fat loss in cachexia is due to lipolysis more than to other mechanisms (such as reduced lipogenesis), which might prove to be useful in the development of further treatments for the syndrome.[81]

Sometimes the observation of the outcome might also be done prospectively. This can be achieved in cohort studies. In this case, patients are entered in the study based on specific characteristics and they are followed up over time and frequently assessed for the development of the outcome in question.[63] A group from Germany selected 227 patients with confirmed ductal adenocarcinoma of the pancreas who underwent surgery and performed assessments of body composition, function, comorbidities, and surgery complications before and after surgery and then every 6 months until death. Patients were grouped according to the presence or absence of cachexia (defined as unintended weight loss >10% of the pre-illness stable weight). The study was able to show that cachexia impacts survival and performance status.[82]

Other methods

Basic science/laboratory studies

Through the 1990s and the beginning of the twenty-first century, cancer cachexia has experienced enormous progress with regards to the understanding of the mechanisms of the syndrome. This was possible due to the expansion of the basic research focusing on several aspects of the syndrome such as muscle and fat metabolism, inflammatory pathways, appetite, and food intake regulation, for example.[83] Exploring the details about basic science methodologies lies beyond the scope of this chapter. However, the combination of classical study designs with basic science is able to generate very useful evidence. For example, Eley *et al.* have recently shown, using a case–control design with a sample of 15 gastric adenocarcinoma patients and nine healthy controls, that phosphorylation of dsRNA-dependent protein kinase might be an important initiator of muscle loss in patients with cancer.[84]

Qualitative studies

Qualitative methodology employs descriptive and inductive methodologies with the intent of profoundly understanding specific problems happening with patients. Qualitative studies are time-consuming and labour intensive, so are restricted to small samples. Therefore, they suffer from a lack of generalizability, but are especially useful to generate preliminary data and to help in the development of outcome assessment techniques.[85]

One recent study from Ireland was able to gather a great amount of data on various aspects of suffering caused by cancer cachexia among 15 patients and 12 family members by using a qualitative interview approach with very limited subject contact (only one or two encounters, with no follow-up required).[12] Impact on body image and other aspects of cancer cachexia were also studied using a qualitative approach with only one subject–interviewer encounter in a sample of 12 patients in England, and provided important and useful information on the care of such patients.[86]

Interventions

Several interventions have been hypothesized as potentially effective in improving cachexia, but very few monotherapy modalities have been successful. In reality, only corticosteroids and progestational agents have consistent evidence supporting their role in the cachexia syndrome, and even in these cases, specifically acting on the anorexia component for a short period of time.[87,88]

Given the complexity of the manifestations of the syndrome, it is easy to note that the successful treatment of the cachexia syndrome will necessarily include the management of several distinct physical and psychological components. The very few successes of monotherapy and the vertiginous progress of the basic research on the pathophysiology of cachexia shifted the research focus to combined modalities including several agents targeting different aspects of the syndrome.[89] However, even though combinations of drugs might be the way to achieve success in the treatment of cachexia, the development of studies with drug combinations is significantly more challenging, because of the potential drug interactions and combination of side-effects.

Careful study design is mandatory in order to allow for the maximum benefit of each component being tested with the least frequency of side-effects. Factorial designs including one new agent at a time might be one way to tackle the issue, but in the cachexia patient population this might not be practical due to the long predicted follow up time.[90] Innovative data analysis techniques such as Bayesian inference also might be considered, in order to be able to detect specific contributions of multiple interventions.[91]

It is advisable also to consider psychosocial interventions for cachexia including patients and family members, due to the reported impact of the syndrome in both populations.[12,86] The selection of adequate controls and placebos is even more complex in this field, and attention must be paid to the use of validated techniques and for the determination of adequate outcome assessments and clinically significant effect sizes, to avoid the conduction of underpowered studies. As with pharmacological interventions, and perhaps even more so, the formation of a multidisciplinary team is mandatory for the successful conduction of psychosocial research in cachexia.

Administrative/practical issues

The conduction of biomedical research is not feasible without the implementation of effective multidisciplinary teamwork since the conception of the study. Individuals with experience in clinical trial design (or in the specific design intended for the study) and content specialists with background on the specifics of the study (i.e. body composition, symptoms, QoL) will allow for a sound study design. The biostatistician also has to be involved from the conception of the study, which will allow not only his/her complete understanding of the study dynamics but also the incorporation of his/her comments and ideas and, more importantly, the determination of adequate sample sizes and randomization mechanisms, if appropriate. Ideally, even the data analysis should be at least drafted during the study design. This allows for the detection of fatal flaws in design such as missing variables or errors in measurement procedures. The presence of an oncologist with experience in the cancer which is going to be studied in cases of single-type studies or at least with experience in advanced cancer management is also very important. The research nurse or research coordinator presence is also required from the beginning of the study design. These are the persons who will be 'in the field' with the participants, and their insights on practical matters are extremely valuable in helping to avoiding problems that would otherwise only surface when the study is actually activated and accruing participants (such as the need for excessive frequent clinic visits, or the disproportionate length of some of the assessments). Data entry/data analysis personnel should also be represented in the team, and also very useful is the inclusion in the team of a research regulations expert person, who is able to identify regulatory issues even before they appear and to provide feedback on the correct regulatory procedures needed to be performed according to the study specifics.

Meetings involving the research team should be conducted at regular intervals during the performance of the study in order to identify possible problematic issues or concerns. Small problems detected promptly will trigger early corrective actions without causing too much trouble for the whole study. Issues with inclusion/exclusion criteria, timeframes for assessments, and minor recurrent deviations from the protocol are frequent, especially just after activation, and might turn into larger problems if not corrected as soon as possible. Alterations in the study protocol might be implemented based on these team meetings in order to improve the study and ultimately allow fast accrual and timely study completion. During the regular meetings, data entry should be checked with the responsible party and, if needed, audits should be arranged in order to keep data entry as current and accurate as possible in comparison with the data gathered in the field. Ideally, there should be no or negligible (not more than a few days) delay between data acquisition and data entry. Another very important point to be checked during the regular meetings is the actual versus projected accrual and retention of participants. Drop-out rates of around 30% are very worrisome and might invalidate a study if not promptly corrected by whatever necessary means, including protocol changes and inclusion of collaborator sites when possible. The participation of the principal investigator or his/her representative in these meetings is also extremely advisable, since he/she functions as the leader of the team and is ultimately the responsible for the study.

References

1. Koretz RL (1984) Parental nutrition: is it oncologically logical? *J Clin Oncol*, **2**(5), 534–8.
2. Baracos VE (2006) More research needed on the treatment of the cancer anorexia/cachexia syndrome. *J Support Oncol*, **4**(10), 508–9.
3. Andrew I, Kirkpatrick G, Holden K, Hawkins C (2008) Audit of symptoms and prescribing in patients with the anorexia–cachexia syndrome. *Pharm World Sci*, **30**(5), 489–96.

4. Dalal S, Bruera E, del Fabbro E (2008) Association between CRP and symptoms in patients assessed at a cachexia clinic (CC) with involuntary weight loss (IWL). *Res Forum Eur Assoc Palliative Care*, 523.
5. Bruera E (1997) ABC of palliative care. Anorexia, cachexia, and nutrition. *Br Med J*, **315**(7117), 1219–22.
6. Walsh D, Donnelly S, Rybicki L (2000) The symptoms of advanced cancer: relationship to age, gender, and performance status in 1,000 patients. *Support Care Cancer*, **8**(3), 175–9.
7. Tan BH, Fearon KC (2008) Cachexia: prevalence and impact in medicine. *Curr Opin Clin Nutr Metab Care*, **11**(4), 400–7.
8. Anker SD, Ponikowski P, Varney S, *et al.* (1997) Wasting as independent risk factor for mortality in chronic heart failure. *Lancet*, **349**(9058), 1050–3.
9. Peters BG (1994) An overview of chemotherapy toxicities. *Top Hosp Pharm Manag*, **14**(2), 59–88.
10. Lawrence TS, Haken RKT, Giaccia A (2008) Principles of radiation oncology. In: DeVita Jr VT, Lawrence TS, Rosenberg SA (eds), *Cancer: Principles and Practice of Oncology*, vol. 1, pp. 331–32. Philadelphia, PA: Lippincott, Williams & Wilkins.
11. Strasser F (2004) Pathophysiology of the anorexia/cachexia syndrome. In: Doyle D, Hanks G, Cherny N, Calman K (eds), *Oxford Textbook of Palliative Medicine*, pp. 520–33. New York: Oxford University Press.
12. Reid J, McKenna H, Fitzsimons D, McCance T (2009) The experience of cancer cachexia: a qualitative study of advanced cancer patients and their family members. *Int J Nurs Stud*, **46**(5), 606–16.
13. Lesko LM (1989) Psychosocial issues in the diagnosis and management of cancer cachexia and anorexia. *Nutrition*, **5**(2), 114–6.
14. Fearon KC, Voss AC, Hustead DS (2006) Definition of cancer cachexia: effect of weight loss, reduced food intake, and systemic inflammation on functional status and prognosis. *Am J Clin Nutr*, **83**(6), 1345–50.
15. Dahele M, Fearon KC (2004) Research methodology: cancer cachexia syndrome. *Palliat Med*, **18**(5), 409–17.
16. Bennett MI (2007) Principles of designing clinical trials in palliative care. In: Addington-Hall JM, Bruera E, Higginson IJ, Payne S (eds), *Research Methods in Palliative Care*, pp. 13–26. New York: Oxford University Press.
17. Gebski V, Marschner I, Keech AC (2002) Specifying objectives and outcomes for clinical trials. *Med J Aust*, **176**(10), 491–2.
18. Bruera E, Strasser F, Palmer JL, *et al.* (2003) Effect of fish oil on appetite and other symptoms in patients with advanced cancer and anorexia/cachexia: a double-blind, placebo-controlled study. *J Clin Oncol*, **21**(1), 129–34.
19. Fouladiun M, Korner U, Bosaeus I, Daneryd P, Hyltander A, Lundholm KG (2005) Body composition and time course changes in regional distribution of fat and lean tissue in unselected cancer patients on palliative care—correlations with food intake, metabolism, exercise capacity, and hormones. *Cancer*, **103**(10), 2189–98.
20. Whitley E, Ball J (2002) Statistics review 4: sample size calculations. *Crit Care*, **6**(4), 335–41.
21. Bruera E, Ernst S, Hagen N, *et al.* (1998) Effectiveness of megestrol acetate in patients with advanced cancer: a randomized, double-blind, crossover study. *Cancer Prev Control*, **2**(2), 74–8.
22. Fearon KC, Barber MD, Moses AG, *et al.* (2006) Double-blind, placebo-controlled, randomized study of eicosapentaenoic acid diester in patients with cancer cachexia. *J Clin Oncol*, **24**(21), 3401–7.
23. Simons JP, Aaronson NK, Vansteenkiste JF, *et al.* (1996) Effects of medroxyprogesterone acetate on appetite, weight, and quality of life in advanced-stage non-hormone-sensitive cancer: a placebo-controlled multicenter study. *J Clin Oncol*, **14**(4), 1077–84.
24. World Health Organization (2000) *Obesity: Preventing and Managing the Global Epidemic*. Geneva: WHO.

25. Thoresen L, Fjeldstad I, Krogstad K, Kaasa S, Falkmer UG (2002) Nutritional status of patients with advanced cancer: the value of using the subjective global assessment of nutritional status as a screening tool. *Palliat Med*, **16**(1), 33–42.
26. Evans WJ, Morley JE, Argiles J, *et al.* (2008) Cachexia: a new definition. *Clin Nutr*, **27**(6), 793–9.
27. Prentice AM, Jebb SA (2001) Beyond body mass index. *Obes Rev*, **2**(3), 141–7.
28. Lohman TG (1981) Skinfolds and body density and their relation to body fatness: a review. *Hum Biol*, **53**(2), 181–225.
29. Wang J, Thornton JC, Kolesnik S, Pierson RN Jr (2000) Anthropometry in body composition. An overview. *Ann NY Acad Sci*, **904**, 317–26.
30. Lohman TG, Roche AF, Martorell R (1991) *Anthropometric Standardization Reference Manual.* Champaign, IL: Human Kinetics Books.
31. Heymsfield SB, McManus C, Smith J, Stevens V, Nixon DW (1982) Anthropometric measurement of muscle mass: revised equations for calculating bone-free arm muscle area. *Am J Clin Nutr*, **36**(4), 680–90.
32. Franssila-Kallunki A (1992) Comparison of near-infrared light spectroscopy, bioelectrical impedance and tritiated water techniques for the measurement of fat-free mass in humans. *Scand J Clin Lab Invest*, **52**(8), 879–85.
33. Chumlea WC, Baumgartner RN (1990) Bioelectric impedance methods for the estimation of body composition. *Can J Sport Sci*, **15**(3), 172–9.
34. Matthie JR (2008) Bioimpedance measurements of human body composition: critical analysis and outlook. *Expert Rev Med Devices*, **5**(2), 239–61.
35. Plank LD (2005) Dual-energy X-ray absorptiometry and body composition. *Curr Opin Clin Nutr Metab Care*, **8**(3), 305–9.
36. Andreoli A, Scalzo G, Masala S, Tarantino U, Guglielmi G (2009) Body composition assessment by dual-energy X-ray absorptiometry (DXA). *Radiol Med*, **114**(2), 286–300.
37. Pietrobelli A, Wang Z, Formica C, Heymsfield SB (1998) Dual-energy X-ray absorptiometry: fat estimation errors due to variation in soft tissue hydration. *Am J Physiol*, **274**(5 Pt 1), E808–16.
38. Heymsfield SB, Wang ZM (1993) Measurement of total-body fat by underwater weighing: new insights and uses for old method. *Nutrition*, **9**(5), 472–3.
39. Jones PR, Norgan NG (1974) Proceedings: A simple system for the determination of human body density by underwater weighing. *J Physiol* **239**(2), 71P–73P.
40. Wang Z, Zhu S, Wang J, Pierson RN, Jr, Heymsfield SB (2003) Whole-body skeletal muscle mass: development and validation of total-body potassium prediction models. *Am J Clin Nutr*, **77**(1), 76–82.
41. Mourtzakis M, Prado CM, Lieffers JR, Reiman T, McCargar LJ, Baracos VE (2008) A practical and precise approach to quantification of body composition in cancer patients using computed tomography images acquired during routine care. *Appl Physiol Nutr Metab*, **33**(5), 997–1006.
42. Prado CM, Birdsell LA, Baracos VE (2010) The emerging role of computerized tomography in assessing cancer cachexia. *Curr Opin Support Palliat Care*, **3**(4), 269–75.
43. Bruera E, Kuehn N, Miller MJ, Selmser P, Macmillan K (1991) The Edmonton Symptom Assessment System (ESAS): a simple method for the assessment of palliative care patients. *J Palliat Care*, **7**(2), 6–9.
44. Chang VT, Hwang SS, Feuerman M (2000) Validation of the Edmonton Symptom Assessment Scale. *Cancer*, **88**(9), 2164–71.
45. Wewers ME, Lowe NK (1990) A critical review of visual analogue scales in the measurement of clinical phenomena. *Res Nurs Health*, **13**(4), 227–36.
46. Stubbs RJ, Hughes DA, Johnstone AM, *et al.* (2000) The use of visual analogue scales to assess motivation to eat in human subjects: a review of their reliability and validity with an evaluation of new hand-held computerized systems for temporal tracking of appetite ratings. *Br J Nutr*, **84**(4), 405–15.
47. Cella DF, Tulsky DS, Gray G, *et al.* (1993) The Functional Assessment of Cancer Therapy scale: development and validation of the general measure. *J Clin Oncol*, **11**(3), 570–9.

48. Cella DF (1997) *Manual of the Functional Assessment of Chronic Illness Therapy (FACIT) Measurement System*, Version 4. Evanston, IL: Evanston Northwestern Healthcare and Northwestern University.
49. Piper BF, Dibble SL, Dodd MJ, Weiss MC, Slaughter RE, Paul SM (1998) The revised Piper Fatigue Scale: psychometric evaluation in women with breast cancer. *Oncol Nurs Forum*, **25**(4), 677–84.
50. Smidt GL, Rogers MW (1982) Factors contributing to the regulation and clinical assessment of muscular strength. *Phys Ther*, **62**(9), 1283–90.
51. Oken MM, Creech RH, Tormey DC, *et al.* (1982) Toxicity and response criteria of the Eastern Cooperative Oncology Group. *Am J Clin Oncol*, **5**(6), 649–55.
52. Schag CC, Heinrich RL, Ganz PA (1984) Karnofsky performance status revisited: reliability, validity, and guidelines. *J Clin Oncol*, **2**(3), 187–93.
53. Sprangers MA, Cull A, Bjordal K, Groenvold M, Aaronson NK (1993) The European Organization for Research and Treatment of Cancer. Approach to quality of life assessment: guidelines for developing questionnaire modules. EORTC Study Group on Quality of Life. *Qual Life Res*, **2**(4), 287–95.
54. Eisenhauer EA, Therasse P, Bogaerts J, *et al.* (2009) New response evaluation criteria in solid tumours: revised RECIST guideline (version 1.1). *Eur J Cancer*, **45**(2), 228–47.
55. Bruera E, Chadwick S, Cowan L, *et al.* (1986) Caloric intake assessment in advanced cancer patients: comparison of three methods. *Cancer Treat Rep*, **70**(8), 981–3.
56. Posner BM, Martin-Munley SS, Smigelski C, *et al.* (1992) Comparison of techniques for estimating nutrient intake: the Framingham Study. *Epidemiology*, **3**(2), 171–7.
57. Makhija S, Baker J (2008) The Subjective Global Assessment: a review of its use in clinical practice. *Nutr Clin Pract*, **23**(4), 405–9.
58. Baker JP, Detsky AS, Wesson DE, *et al.* (1982) Nutritional assessment: a comparison of clinical judgement and objective measurements. *N Engl J Med*, **306**(16), 969–72.
59. Bauer J, Capra S, Ferguson M (2002) Use of the scored Patient-Generated Subjective Global Assessment (PG-SGA) as a nutrition assessment tool in patients with cancer. *Eur J Clin Nutr*, **56**(8), 779–85.
60. Ottery FD (1994) Rethinking nutritional support of the cancer patient: the new field of nutritional oncology. *Semin Oncol*, **21**(6), 770–8.
61. Kleinbaum DG, Kupper LL, Morgenstern H (1982) Types of epidemiologic research. In: Kleinbaum DG, Kupper LL, Morgenstern H (eds), *Epidemiologic Research: Principles and Quantitative Methods*, pp. 40–50. New York: Van Nostrand Reinhold.
62. Constantini M, Higginson IJ (2007) Experimental and quasi experimental designs. In: Addington-Hall JM, Bruera E, Higginson IJ, Payne S (eds), *Research Methods in Palliative Care*, pp. 84–97. New York: Oxford University Press.
63. Rothmann KJ, Greenland S (1998) Types of epidemiologic studies. In: Rothmann KJ, Greenland S (eds), *Modern Epidemiology*, 2nd edn, pp. 67–78. Philadelphia, PA: Lippincott, Williams & Wilkins.
64. Weiss NS (1998) Clinical epidemiology. In: Rothmann KJ, Greenland S (eds), *Modern Epidemiology*, 2nd edn, pp. 519–28. Philadelphia, PA: Lippincott, Williams & Wilkins.
65. Phillips B, Ball C, Sackett D, *et al.* (2009) *Levels of Evidence*. Oxford: Oxford Centre for Evidence Based Medicine. www.cebm.net/levels_of_evidence.asp.
66. Loprinzi CL, Ellison NM, Schaid DJ, *et al.* (1990) Controlled trial of megestrol acetate for the treatment of cancer anorexia and cachexia. *J Natl Cancer Inst*, **82**(13), 1127–32.
67. Loprinzi CL, Michalak JC, Schaid DJ, *et al.* 1993) Phase III evaluation of four doses of megestrol acetate as therapy for patients with cancer anorexia and/or cachexia. *J Clin Oncol*, **11**(4), 762–7.
68. Gebbia V, Testa A, Gebbia N (1996) Prospective randomised trial of two dose levels of megestrol acetate in the management of anorexia–cachexia syndrome in patients with metastatic cancer. *Br J Cancer*, **73**(12), 1576–80.
69. Willox JC, Corr J, Shaw J, Richardson M, Calman KC, Drennan M (1984) Prednisolone as an appetite stimulant in patients with cancer. *Br Med J (Clin Res Ed)*, **288**(6410), 27.

70. Bruera E, Roca E, Cedaro L, Carraro S, Chacon R (1985) Action of oral methylprednisolone in terminal cancer patients: a prospective randomized double-blind study. *Cancer Treat Rep*, **69**(7–8), 751–4.
71. Bozzetti F (2003) Home total parenteral nutrition in incurable cancer patients: a therapy, a basic humane care or something in between? *Clin Nutr*, **22**(2), 109–11.
72. Koretz RL (2007) Should patients with cancer be offered nutritional support: does the benefit outweigh the burden? *Eur J Gastroenterol Hepatol*, **19**(5), 379–82.
73. Evans WK, Nixon DW, Daly JM, *et al.* (1987) A randomized study of oral nutritional support versus ad lib nutritional intake during chemotherapy for advanced colorectal and non-small-cell lung cancer. *J Clin Oncol* **5**(1), 113–24.
74. Jatoi A, Ritter HL, Dueck A, *et al.* (2009)A placebo-controlled, double-blind trial of infliximab for cancer-associated weight loss in elderly and/or poor performance non-small cell lung cancer patients (N01C9). *Lung Cancer*, 2009 Aug 7 [Epub ahead of print].
75. Jatoi A, Dakhil SR, Nguyen PL, *et al.* (2007) A placebo-controlled double blind trial of etanercept for the cancer anorexia/weight loss syndrome: results from N00C1 from the North Central Cancer Treatment Group. *Cancer*, **110**(6), 1396–403.
76. Campbell DT, Stanley JC (1963) *Experimental and Quasi-experimental Designs for Research*, 1st edn. Chicago, IL: Rand McNally.
77. Bruera E, Neumann CM, Pituskin E, Calder K, Ball G, Hanson J (1999) Thalidomide in patients with cachexia due to terminal cancer: preliminary report. *Ann Oncol* **10**(7), 857–9.
78. Hartmuller VW, Desmond SM (2004) Professional and patient perspectives on nutritional needs of patients with cancer. *Oncol Nurs Forum*, **31**(5), 989–96.
79. Lundholm K, Daneryd P, Korner U, Hyltander A, Bosaeus I (2004) Evidence that long-term COX-treatment improves energy homeostasis and body composition in cancer patients with progressive cachexia. *Int J Oncol*, **24**(3), 505–12.
80. Weber MA, Krakowski-Roosen H, Schroder L, *et al.* (2009) Morphology, metabolism, microcirculation, and strength of skeletal muscles in cancer-related cachexia. *Acta Oncol*, **48**(1), 116–24.
81. Ryden M, Agustsson T, Laurencikiene J, *et al.* (2008) Lipolysis—not inflammation, cell death, or lipogenesis—is involved in adipose tissue loss in cancer cachexia. *Cancer*, **113**(7), 1695–704.
82. Bachmann J, Heiligensetzer M, Krakowski-Roosen H, Buchler MW, Friess H, Martignoni ME (2008) Cachexia worsens prognosis in patients with resectable pancreatic cancer. *J Gastrointest Surg*, **12**(7), 1193–201.
83. Gordon JN, Green SR, Goggin PM (2005) Cancer cachexia. *Q J Med*, **98**(11), 779–88.
84. Eley HL, Skipworth RJ, Deans DA, Fearon KC, Tisdale MJ (2008) Increased expression of phosphorylated forms of RNA-dependent protein kinase and eukaryotic initiation factor 2alpha may signal skeletal muscle atrophy in weight-losing cancer patients. *Br J Cancer*, **98**(2):443–9.
85. Maly RC (2000) Qualitative research for the study of cancer and age. *Hematol Oncol Clin North Am*, **14**(1), 79–88, ix.
86. Hinsley R, Hughes R (2007) 'The reflections you get': an exploration of body image and cachexia. *Int J Palliat Nurs*, **13**(2), 84–9.
87. Berenstein EG, Ortiz Z (2005) Megestrol acetate for the treatment of anorexia–cachexia syndrome. *Cochrane Database Syst Rev* (2), CD004310.
88. Gagnon B, Bruera E (1998) A review of the drug treatment of cachexia associated with cancer. *Drugs* **55**(5), 675–88.
89. Fearon KC (2008) Cancer cachexia: developing multimodal therapy for a multidimensional problem. *Eur J Cancer*, **44**(8), 1124–32.
90. Montgomery AA, Peters TJ, Little P (2003) Design, analysis and presentation of factorial randomised controlled trials. *BMC Med Res Methodol*, **3**, 26.
91. Ashby D (2006) Bayesian statistics in medicine: a 25 year review. *Stat Med*, **25**(21), 3589–631.

Chapter 7

Appetite stimulants

Florian Strasser and David Blum

Introduction

The regulation of appetite is highly complex and influenced by peripheral neurohormonal signals, central neurotransmitters and other factors. Appetite is controlled centrally in the nucleus arcuatus of the hypothalamus and the nucleus tractus solitarius of the brainstem.[1] Appetite regulation has mainly been studied in animals and information in advanced cancer patients is scarce. Although the use of appetite stimulants in clinical practice is mostly empirical, an increase in appetite can be achieved by pharmacological and non-pharmacological interventions.

Nutritional counselling increases energy and protein intake[2] during radiotherapy, and even 3 months after completion, individualized nutritional counselling is capable of sustaining a significant impact on quality of life (QoL). Just as adjustment in dietary patterns can be an effective behavioural intervention, the control of symptoms, such as pain, anxiety or constipation, can also improve appetite stimulation.[3] Interestingly, despite a poor appetite, patients with advanced cancer may retain the motivation and ability to eat, as long as the intake of food does not provoke nausea.[4] For these patients, nutritional counselling could be helpful in assisting family members to understand that a shift to conscious control (i.e. overeating) is necessary.

Corticosteroids and progestins are the most commonly used appetite stimulants in clinical practice, even though their mechanism of action is unclear. The following discussion will focus primarily on the effect of these medications and newer agents on appetite.

Corticosteroids

In addition to other indications, corticosteroids are widely used as an appetite stimulant in advanced cancer care. Their exact mechanism of action remains unclear but may include effects on mood (euphoria), an anti-inflammatory action, or modulation of orexigenic hormones in the hypothalamus. Many studies show an improvement in appetite, food intake and QoL in advanced cancer patients.

A meta-analysis listed six double-blind randomized controlled trials with a total of 647 patients using various corticosteroids, including methylprednisolone, prednisolone and dexamethasone.[5] Doses ranged from 300 mg to 1200 mg for methylprednsiolone and study duration from 6 to 12 weeks. Although appetite and QoL improved in two studies, a significant increase in body weight was not shown compared with placebo, and the benefits diminished over time.[6]

Moertel *et al.* showed a significant increase in appetite in patients with advanced gastrointestinal cancer after 4 weeks.[7] There was no difference between 3 mg vs 6 mg of dexamethasone and no weight gain. In another trial Willox *et al.* showed an increase in appetite with 5 mg prednisolone after 2 weeks.[8] Prospective randomized trials of oral methylprednisolone (16 mg daily) and intravenous methylprednisolone[9] (125 mg) in advanced cancer patients also had positive effects on appetite and food intake.[10]

Unfortunately, corticosteroids have a wide range of adverse effects. Apart from improving the symptoms of anorexia they can worsen cachexia due to muscle myopathy, insulin resistance and immune suppression. The risk of adrenal insufficiency due to withdrawal must also be taken into consideration.

In general corticosteroids are only recommended to alleviate symptoms and appetite at the end of life, but not to treat cachexia *per se*.

Progestins

Side-effects of weight gain and increased appetite are observed when synthetic progestins are used to treat hormone-sensitive tumours. Several prospective controlled randomized trials have investigated the role of progestins in cancer cachexia. Two systematic reviews[11,12] and a Cochrane meta-analysis suggested[13] a beneficial effect of progestins [megestrol acetate (MA) and medroxy-progesterone] on body weight and appetite. Unfortunately no effect on lean body mass (LBM) and no clear benefit on QoL was demonstrated. One study comparing MA with corticosteroids showed better appetite than fluoxymesterone and less toxicity than dexamethasone.[14] There appears to be a dose-dependent effect on appetite ranging from 160 mg up to 1600 mg. It is recommended to start with the lowest doses and titrate up to 800 mg[15] since some of the adverse effects such as thromboembolism may increase with higher doses, especially in combination with chemotherapy. There is also the potential for other side-effects including oedema, adrenal insufficiency, and profound gonadal suppression in males.[16]

An MA nanocrystal oral suspension designed to optimize drug delivery is approved for acquired immune deficiency syndrome (AIDS) patients but its role in patients with cancer is yet to be determined.

Several pilot studies combining MA with celecoxib or nutritional supplements[17] have yielded promising preliminary results. This approach, using a combination of agents, is discussed in Chapter 11.

Most studies of MA for appetite stimulation were undertaken in patients with advanced incurable cancer, including some with untreated cancer.[18] No subgroup analyses were performed for cancer type, either in the systematic reviews or trials. There are studies evaluating the use of progestins in specific tumour types including patients with gastrointestinal malignancies,[19,20] small cell lung cancer,[21] head and neck cancer[22] or patients receiving pelvic irradiation.[23]

If the cachexia syndrome is subdivided into three stages, namely early, manifest or late cachexia, there are limited data for the use of progestins in any of the three different stages. In the late irreversible stage, there may be limited benefit from MA, because of the impact of other symptoms. On the other hand, Rowland *et al.* found no benefit of progestins in pre-cachetic patients receiving chemotherapy. Therefore MA can only be recommended in manifest cachexia when anorexia is the predominant symptom. The costs and possible adverse effects of therapy with progestins also have to be taken into account.

Cannabinoids

Extracts from the plant *Cannabis sativa* have been used for recreational and therapeutic purposes throughout history. Cannabinoids are the active compounds that act on the CB1 and CB2 cell surface receptors which are expressed in the brain, and on various other tissues. Their endogenous ligands the endocannabinoids may be important in the natural regulation of appetite.

Dronabinol (δ-9THC) is a synthetic cannabinoid approved as an anti-emetic drug and as an appetite stimulant in AIDS wasting. Although cannabinoids improved appetite in advanced AIDS[24,25] and showed promising phase II results[26] in cancer cachexia, a recent large clinical trial in advanced cancer patients was disappointing.[27] The multicentre randomized trial compared the effects of cannabis extract (CE), δ-9-tetrahydrocannabinol (THC), and placebo on appetite and QoL. There were no differences between the three groups.

An earlier trial compared MA and dronabinol, or both agents, for appetite stimulation. There was an improvement with MA and no further benefit with the combination of agents.[28] Besides a significant increase in reports of male impotence with MA, adverse effects including neurocortical dysfunction and thromboembolism were similar in both groups

Although the endocannabinoid system may be important in appetite regulation, the large trials so far have been negative, perhaps because of a negative influence on gastrointestinal motility which neutralizes the positive effect on appetite. The use of cannabinoids may be an option in selected cachectic patients experiencing chronic nausea, but having no cognitive decline and no evidence of delirium.

Antidepressants and antihistamines

Weight gain is a common side-effect of antidepressants. A study with mirtazapine in 45 patients with advanced cancer showed only appetite stimulation in week 1 but not in week 2.[29]

Other trials are ongoing (Table 7.2)[30] although it may be difficult to determine the mechanism of appetite stimulation in view of its therapeutic effect on mood, anxiety and nausea. The atypical neuroleptic drug olanzapine has been used successfully in anorexia nervosa and preliminary results from a phase I study for cancer cachexia are promising.[31] Olanzapine may stimulate appetite by several mechanisms including raising ghrelin levels.

Cyproheptadine, a serotonin and histamine antagonist, was associated with weight gain in open-label trials of patients with advanced cancer. In a placebo-controlled phase III trial, cyproheptadine showed mild effect on appetite, but no effect on body weight.[32] Due to its sedating side-effects, clinical use is limited.

Prokinetics

Prokinetics are widely used anti-emetic drugs in cancer care. They are useful in patients with impaired upper gastrointestinal motility and early satiety, a common symptom of cancer cachexia. Even though metoclopramide showed positive effects on early satiety and chronic nausea,[33] an improvement in appetite and weight gain has not been demonstrated.

Melanocortin receptor antagonists

In animal trials, blockade of the melanocortin system resulted in improvement in appetite and body mass.[34] Various antagonists are under development but large clinical trials are still lacking.

Table 7.1 Dosage of commonly used appetite stimulants

Corticosteroids	
Dexamethasone	4 mg
Prednisolone	10 mg
Methylprednisolone	125 mg
Progestins	
Megestrol acetate and medroxyprogesterone acetate	160–800 mg
Cannabinoids	
Dronabinol	5 mg

Ghrelin and ghrelin mimetics

Ghrelin is a natural hormone produced by gastric endocrine cells which increases appetite, gastrointestinal motility and reduces inflammation. Ghrelin and several ghrelin mimetics have been evaluated in preliminary trials. A multicentre, double-blind, placebo-controlled phase II trial of a ghrelin mimetic (RC-1291) showed positive results in terms of lean body mass, handgrip strength and QoL. Chapter 8 discusses the potential benefits and mechanisms of ghrelin and ghrelin mimetics.

Anti-inflammatory approaches

There is growing evidence for an effect on appetite by using an anti-inflammatory approach.[35]

The effect of immune modulation on the anorexia–cachexia syndrome is discussed further in Chapter 9.

n-3 Fatty acids (eicosapentaenoic acid)

Eicosapentaenoic acid (EPA) is a polyunsaturated acid found in fish oil. It suppresses proinflammatory cytokines and in three phase II trials EPA produced weight stabilization in weight-losing pancreatic cancer patients.[36,37,38]

A 2-week trial of 60 patients receiving fish-oil capsules or placebo (olive oil) did not show a difference in terms of appetite or QoL and many patients were unable to swallow more than 10 fish oil capsules per day.[39]

The first multicentre placebo-controlled trial with an EPA-containing oral supplement was negative for the primary endpoint LBM.[40] However, in a subgroup analysis a significant correlation was noticed between weight gain and supplement intake, as well as blood levels of EPA and the EPA intake. Patients who were able to drink one or two cans of EPA supplements profited in terms of weight gain.

A large trial including 421 patients with cancer cachexia compared the effect of an EPA nutritional supplement plus placebo versus MA plus placebo versus a combination of both. The addition of EPA supplements showed no benefits in terms of non-fluid weight gain, appetite, survival or QoL.

A Cochrane review including five trials involving 587 patients concluded that there is insufficient evidence for an advantage of EPA or EPA-containing protein-enriched oral supplements for improvement of weight, QoL, or associated symptoms of cachexia.[41] Conversely, a systematic review of 17 studies judged by an expert panel concluded that administration of EPA improved (evidence grade B) weight, appetite, and QoL in patients with advanced cancer and cachexia.[42]

Due to conflicting and inconsistent results the general use of EPA cannot be recommended. An interim report of a trial comparing pharmacological nutritional support containing EPA to various other regimens has not been encouraging. In spite of these results, selected patients receiving comprehensive multidisciplinary cachexia treatment may still derive benefit if they are able to ingest enough EPA to reach adequate blood levels.

Non-steroidal anti-rheumatic agents

Although there is some evidence that non-steroidal anti-rheumatic agents improve cachexia due to their effects on systemic inflammatory response in patients with advanced cancer, their effect on appetite stimulation appears to be variable.

In 72 gastrointestinal cancer patients, ibuprofen plus MA was superior to MA plus placebo at maintaining weight and QoL despite no significant change in appetite between the two groups.[43]

Thalidomide

Thalidomide is an immunomodulatory and anti-inflammatory agent, which improved weight, arm muscle mass, and patient-perceived physical functioning in 50 pancreatic cancer patients with cachexia.[44] There was no specific assessment of appetite in this trial or another open-label trial of patients with oesophageal cancer. Despite improvements in lean body mass, caloric intake was unchanged suggesting that thalidomide produced a peripheral anticatabolic effect. An earlier open-label 10-day trial of 100 mg thalidomide significantly increased appetite scores and other symptoms including insomnia and nausea. Thalidomide is discussed further in Chapter 9.

Conclusions

Pharmacological treatment is only effective when used as part of a comprehensive treatment plan. Many orexigenic agents have been studied in recent years, with limited success. New agents (Table 7.2) such as ghrelin and ghrelin mimetics exhibit early promise, but further studies are needed to demonstrate improved clinical outcomes and establish safety.

Table 7.2 Experimental therapeutics/ongoing trials

Intervention target	Investigator	Trial design and status	Source information	Patient population
Infliximab ± placebo	Jatoi A	Phase III RCT, infliximab treatment discontinued effective after 3 years, May 2005	NCT00040885	Unresectable NSCLC, docetaxel chemotherapy; planned $n = 220$
Etanercept vs placebo	Jatoi A	RCT, 2 arms	Cancer 2007	Incurable malignancy; $n = 63$
Etanercept vs placebo	Thomas CR	RCT phase II–III, start May 2001	NCT00127387	Advanced lung, prostate, or bone metastasis radiation therapy of at least 4000 Gy over 4 weeks; planned $n = 54$
Celecoxib vs placebo	Lai V	Phase II pilot study	Head Neck 2008	Head and neck or gastroin-testinal cancer; $n = 11$
Celecoxib vs placebo	Lawrence D	RCT, phase III, study withdrawn before recruitment	NCT00093678	Metastatic or local unre-sectable tumour, support-ive care only rather than active cancer treatment; planned $n = 296$
VT-122 (propranolol and etodolac), two doses	Guarino RA	Pilot, open label, start Jan 2007	NCT00527319	NSCLC IV not on chemotherapy; planned $n = 60$
Thalidomide vs placebo	Gordon JN	Phase II RCT	Gut 2005	Advanced pancreatic cancer; $n = 50$
Thalidomide vs placebo	Bruera E	Phase II RCT, start Sep 2006	NCT00379353	Cancer, chemotherapy allowed; planned $n = 62$
Thalidomide	Wilkes EA	RCT, completed	ISRCTN45162540	Inoperable oesophageal cancer; planned $n = 12$

(Continued)

Table 7.2 (Continued) Experimental therapeutics/ongoing trials

Intervention target	Investigator	Trial design and status	Source information	Patient population
Thalidomide vs placebo	Green S	RCT, completed	ISRCTN51456701	Advanced upper gastrointestinal adenocarcinoma, no chemotherapy or radiation therapy; planned *n* = 180
Mirtazapine vs placebo	Dalal S	RCT, start Jan 2007	NCT00488072	Advanced cancer; planned *n* = 98
Mirtazapine	Kirkova J	Open label, no placebo, dose escalating	Cachexia Conf. 2007	Advanced cancer; *n* = 45
Mirtazapine	Riechelmann R	Phase II, open-label, no placebo	MASCC 2007	Gastrointestinal cancer; *n* = 15
Haelan (fermented soy product)	Guo Y	Phase II, start Oct 2007	NCT00558558	Advanced solid tumour; planned *n* = 32
N-Acetylcysteine vs placebo	Hildebrandt W	Phase II, start Dec 2003	NCT00196885	Gastrointestinal or bronchial cancer, patients undergoing resistance training; planned *n* = 60
Antioxidant-deficient diet vs normal diet	Couch M	RCT, phase I, start May 2007	NCT00486304	Oropharyngeal cancer, patients receiving chemoradiation therapy (CRT); planned *n* = 15
Atorvastatin	Castro M	Pilot-dose-escalating study	MASCC 2006	Solid tumours, CRP >10 μg/ml; *n* = 25
Melatonin vs placebo	Del Fabbro E	RCT, placebo, start Jun 2006	NCT00513357	Solid gastrointestinal tumours or lung cancer; planned *n* = 126
Ghrelin natural intravenous	Strasser F	Phase I/II RCT, placebo-controlled	Br J Cancer 2008	Mixed solid tumour; *n* = 21
RC-1291 (anamorelin) vs placebo	Kumor K	Phase II RCT, start Sep 2006	NCT00378131	Incurable advanced cancer; planned *n* = 36
Anamorelin (RC-1291) (2 doses) vs placebo	Garcia JM	Phase II, 3-arm RCT, start Feb 2008	NCT00622193	NSCLC, stage IIIB or IV; planned *n* = 228
Anamorelin vs placebo	Polvino WJ	Phase II RCT	MASCC 2007	Advanced cancer, mostly lung and colorectal; *n* = 82
Olanzapine	Kurzrock R	Phase I dose-finding pilot study, start Oct 2006	NCT00489593	Advanced cancer; planned *n* = 57
Nicotine inhaler vs placebo	Jatoi A	Pilot study, RCT, start Dec 2003	NCT00425906	Incurable malignancy, malignant bowel obstruction, on strict 'nothing per os' status over the next 48 h; planned *n* = 20

RCT, randomized controlled trial; NSCLC, non-small cell lung cancer.

References

1. Davis MP, Dreicer R, Walsh D, Lagman R, LeGrand SB (2004) Appetite and cancer-associated anorexia: a review. *J Clin Oncol*, **22**(8), 1510–7.
2. Ravasco P, Monteiro Grillo I, Camilo M (2007) Cancer wasting and quality of life react to early individualized nutritional counselling! *Clin Nutr*, **26**(1), 7–15.
3. Strasser F, Bruera ED (2002) Update on anorexia and cachexia. *Hematol Oncol Clin North Amer*, **16**, 589–617.
4. Shragge JE, Wismer WV, Olson KL, Baracos VE (2007) Shifting to conscious control: psychosocial and dietary management of anorexia by patients with advanced cancer. *Palliat Med*, **21**(3), 227–33.
5. Yavuzsen T, Davis MP, Walsh D, LeGrand S, Lagman R (2005) Systematic review of the treatment of cancer-associated anorexia and weight loss. *J Clin Oncol*, **23**, 8500–11.
6. Popiela T, Lucchi R, Giongo F (1989) Methylprednisolone as an appetite stimulant in patients with cancer. *Eur J Cancer Clin Oncol*, **25**, 1823.
7. Moertel CG, Schutt AJ, Reitemeier RJ, Hahn RG (1974) Corticosteroid therapy of preterminal gastrointestinal cancer. *Cancer*, **33**, 1607.
8. Willox JC, Corr J, Shaw J, *et al.* (1984) Prednisolone as an appetite stimulant in patients with cancer. *Br Med J (Clin Res Ed)*, **288**, 27.
9. Della Cuna GR, Pellegrini A, Piazzi M (1989) Effect of methylprednisolone sodium succinate on quality of life in preterminal cancer patients: a placebo-controlled, multicenter study. *Eur J Cancer Clin Oncol*, **25**, 1817–21.
10. Bruera E, Roca E, Cedaro L, *et al.* Action of oral methylprednisolone in terminal cancer patients: a prospective randomized double-blind study. *Cancer Treat Rep*, **69**, 751.
11. Maltoni M, Nanni O, Scarpi E, *et al.* High-dose progestins for the treatment of cancer anorexia–cachexia syndrome: a systematic review of randomised clinical trials. *Ann Oncol*, **12**(3), 289–300.
12. Ruiz-Garcia V, Juan O, Perez Hoyos S, *et al.* (2002) Megestrol acetate: a systematic review usefulness about the weight gain in neoplastic patients with cancer. *Med Clinica*, **119**(5), 166-70.
13. Berenstein EG, Ortiz Z (2005) Megestrol acetate for the treatment ofanorexia–cachexia syndrome. *Cochrane Database Syst Rev*, **18**(2).
14. Loprinzi CL, Kugler JW, Sloan JA (1999) Randomized comparison of megestrol acetate versus dexamethasone versus fluoxymesterone for the treatment of cancer anorexia/cachexia. *J Clin Oncol*, **17**, 3299–306.
15. Loprinzi, CL, Michalak, JC, Schaid, DJ, *et al.* (1993) Phase III evaluation of four doses of megestrol acetate as therapy for patients with cancer anorexia and/or cachexia. *J Clin Oncol*, **11**, 762.
16. Dev R, Del Fabbro E, Bruera E (2007) Association between megestrol acetate treatment and symptomatic adrenal insufficiency and hypogonadism in male patients with cancer. *Cancer*, **110**, 1173.
17. Cerchietti LC, Navigante AH, Peluffo GD, *et al.* (2007) Effects of celecoxib, medroxyprogesterone, and dietary intervention on systemic syndromes in patients with advanced lung adenocarcinoma: a pilot study. *J Pain Sympt Manag*, **27**, 85–95.
18. Vadell C, Seguí MA, Giménez-Arnau JM, *et al.* (1998) Anticachectic efficacy of megestrol acetate at different doses and versus placebo in patients with neoplastic cachexia. *Am J Clin Oncol*, **21**(4), 347–51.
19. Kornek GV, Schenk T, Ludwig H, *et al.* (1996) Placebo-controlled trial of medroxyprogesterone acetate in gastrointestinal malignancies and cachexia. *Onkologie*, **19**, 164–8.
20. McMillan DC, Wigmore SJ, Fearon KC, *et al.* (1999) A prospective study of megestrol acetate and ibuprofen in gastrointestinal cancer patients with weight loss. *Br J Cancer*, **79**, 495–500.
21. Rowland KM, Loprinzi CL, Shaw EG, *et al.* (1996) Randomized double blind placebo controlled trial of cisplatin and etoposide plus megestrol acetate/placebo in extensive stage small cell lung cancer: A North Central Cancer Treatment Group study. *J Clin Oncol*, **14**, 135–41.

22. Chen HC, Leung SW, Wang CJ, Sun LM, Fang FM, Hsu JH (1999) Effect of megestrol acetate and propulsid on nutritional improvement in patients with head and neck cancers undergoing radiotherapy. *Radiother Oncol*, **3**(1), 75–9.
23. Lai YL, Fang FM, Yeh CY (1994) Management of anorexic patients in radiotherapy: aprospective andomized comparison of megestrol and prednisolone. *J Pain Sympt Manag*, **9**(4), 265–8.
24. Beal JE, Olson R, Laubenstein L, *et al.* (1995) Dronabinol as a treatment for anorexia associated with weight loss in patients with AIDS. *J Pain Symptom Manage*, **10**, 89.
25. Beal JE, Olson R, Lefkowitz L, *et al.* (1997) Long-term efficacy and safety of dronabinol for acquired immunodeficiency syndrome-associated anorexia. *J Pain Sympt Manag*, **14**, 7.
26. Nelson K, Walsh D, Deeter P, Sheehan F (1994) A phase II study of delta-9-tetrahydrocannabinol for appetite stimulation in cancer-associated anorexia. *J Palliat Care*, **10**, 14–18.
27. Strasser F, Luftner D, Possinger K, *et al.* (2008) Comparison of orally administered cannabis extract and delta-9-tetrahydrocannabinol in treating patients with cancer-related anorexia-cachexia syndrome: a multicenter, phase III, randomized, double-blind, placebo-controlled. *J Clin Oncol*, **24**, 3394.
28. Jatoi A, Windschitl HE, Loprinzi CL, *et al.* (2002) Dronabinol versus megestrol acetate versus combination therapy for cancer-associated anorexia: a North Central Cancer Treatment Group study. *J Clin Oncol*, **20**, 567.
29. Kirkova J, Davis MP, Walsh D, Lagman R, Bennani-Baitit N, Seyidova-Khoshknabi D (2007) Mirtazapine and appetite in advanced cancer. 4th Cachexia Conference, Tampa. Abstract 470.
30. Riechelmann R, Tannock I, Rodin G, Zimmermann C (2007) Phase II trial of mirtazapine for cancer-related cachexia/anorexia. *Support Care Cancer*, **15**, 775, 197.
31. Braiteh F, Dalal S, Khuwaja A, David H, Bruera E, Kurzrock R (2008) Phase I pilot study of the safety and tolerability of olanzapine (OZA) for the treatment of cachexia in patients with advanced cancer *J Clin Oncol*, **26** (15S), 20529.
32. Kardinal CG, Loprinzi CL, Schaid DJ, *et al.* (1990) A controlled trial of cyproheptadine in cancer patients with anorexia and/or cachexia. *Cancer*, **65**, 2657.
33. Bruera E, Belzile M, Neumann C, *et al.* (2000) A double-blind, crossover study of controlled-release metoclopramide and placebo for the chronic nausea and dyspepsia of advanced cancer. *J Pain Sympt Manag*, **19**, 427.
34. Joppa MA, Gogas KR, Foster AC, Markison S (2007) Central infusion of the melanocortin receptor antagonist agouti-related peptide (AgRP(83-132)) prevents cachexia-related symptoms induced by radiation and colon-26 tumors in mice. *Peptides*, **28**, 636–42.
35. Laviano A, Meguid MM, Yang ZJ, Gleason JR, Cangiano C, Rossi Fanelli F (1996) Cracking the riddle of cancer anorexia. *Nutrition*, **12**(10), 706–10.
36. Jadad AR, Moore CA, Carroll D, *et al.* (1996) Assessing the quality of reports on randomized clinical trials: Is blinding necessary? *Control Clin Trials*, **17**, 1–12.
37. Mantovani G, Macciò A, Madeddu C, *et al.* (2008) Randomized phase III clinical trial of five different arms of treatment for patients with cancer cachexia: interim results. *Nutrition*, **24**(4), 305–13.
38. Read JA, Beale PJ, Volker DH, Smith N, Childs A, Clarke SJ (2007) Nutrition intervention using an eicosapentaenoic acid - containing supplement in patients with advanced colorectal cancer. Effects on nutritional and inflammatory status: a phase II trial. *Support Care Cancer*, **15**, 301–7.
39. Bruera E, Strasser F, Palmer JL, *et al.* (2003) Effect of fish oil on appetite and other symptoms in patients with advanced cancer and anorexia/cachexia: a double-blind, placebo-controlled study. *J Clin Oncol*, **21**(1), 129–34.
40. Fearon KC, Barber MD, Moses AG, *et al.* (2006) Double-blind, placebo-controlled, randomized study of eicosapentaenoic acid diester in patients with cancer cachexia. *J Clin Oncol*, **24**, 3401–7.
41. Dewey A, Baughan C, Dean T, Higgins B, Johnson I (2007) Eicosapentaenoic acid (EPA, an omega-3 fatty acid from fish oils) for the treatment of cancer cachexia. *Cochrane Database Syst Rev* (1).

42. Colomer R, Moreno-Nogueira JM, Garcia-Luna PP, *et al.* (2007) N-3 fatty acids, cancer and cachexia: a systematic review of the literature. *Br J Nutr*, **97**, 823–31.
43. McMillan DC, Wigmore SJ, Fearon KC, *et al.* (1999) A prospective randomized study of megestrol acetate and ibuprofen in gastrointestinal cancer patients with weight loss. *Br J Cancer*, **79**, 495–500.
44. Gordon JN, Trebble TM, Ellis RD, *et al.* (2005) Thalidomide in the treatment of cancer cachexia: a randomised placebo controlled trial. *Gut*, **54**, 540–5.

Chapter 8

Anabolic hormones

Jose Garcia

Introduction

Nutritional status of individuals with cancer is determined by the balance between two opposing processes: anabolism, defined as the constructive phase of metabolism, and catabolism that involves breaking down large molecules with the objective of releasing energy. These two processes are regulated by several hormones that work synergistically to adjust body weight to different scenarios by changing appetite, energy expenditure and utilization.

Androgens

Testosterone is a hormone necessary for normal growth, development, and the maintenance of secondary sexual characteristics in men. Approximately 95% of testosterone is produced in the testes and adrenal glands in men; whereas in women testosterone is synthesized in the ovaries and adrenal glands. The production and maintenance of normal testosterone levels is regulated by gonadotrophin-releasing hormone (GnRH) that is synthesized in the hypothalamus and regulates the release of luteinizing hormone (LH) and follicle-stimulating hormone (FSH) by the pituitary, which in turn regulate testosterone production in the gonads. Testosterone circulates in the blood either freely (unbound, 2%), loosely bound to albumin (38%), or tightly bound to sex-hormone-binding globulin (SHBG, 60%). The portion of testosterone that is bound to albumin can bind the androgen receptor in target tissues. The albumin-bound testosterone together with the free fraction of testosterone is known as bioavailable testosterone or 'free and weakly bound testosterone'.

Testosterone production is characterized by a prominent diurnal rhythm with highest levels in the morning and a nadir in the late afternoon.[1] Hence, up to 15% of healthy young individuals have testosterone levels below the normal range in a 24 h period.[2] Also, 30% of patients with a low testosterone level have a normal level upon retesting[3] and therefore current guidelines recommend checking early morning testosterone levels and to do so on two separate occasions.[4]

Several chronic conditions including cancer have been associated with an increase in SHBG levels,[5] that leads to falsely elevated total testosterone levels. In these settings, a bioavailable testosterone level should be measured by a reliable method, such as liquid chromatography and tandem mass spectrometry, or calculated based on total testosterone and SHBG concentrations. Free testosterone measurements by analogue plate methods are affected by alterations in SHBG and are inaccurate; therefore they should be avoided.[6]

Androgens exert both direct and indirect anabolic effects on muscle. Testosterone and other androgens directly increase muscle mass and strength by augmenting the synthesis of myosin, the main contractile protein in muscle,[7] and perhaps by also upregulating the expression of the androgen receptor.[8] Other indirect mechanisms include antiglucocorticoid effects, and interactions with the growth hormone (GH)/insulin like growth factor-1 (IGF-1) axis since testosterone treatment increases muscle IGF-1 levels.[9]

In men, the failure of the testis to produce physiological levels of testosterone is known as hypogonadism. Primary hypogonadism results from testicular failure; secondary hypogonadism results from hypothalamic or pituitary dysfunction. Non-cancer patients with hypogonadism present with low libido, sexual dysfunction, depressed mood, fatigue, osteoporosis, sarcopenia and weakness.[10,11] These symptoms are also commonly seen in patients with cancer.[12–16] Many types of cancer and cancer therapies are frequently associated with sexual dysfunction and estimates of sexual dysfunction after cancer treatments have ranged from 40% to 100%.[17] Unfortunately, even in the presence of these symptoms testosterone levels are rarely checked in male cancer patients and this diagnosis is often missed.

The prevalence of hypogonadism in male cancer patients may be as high as 90%[5] and it is probably a multifactorial process. Moreover, we have reported an association between hypogonadism and poor appetite on numerical rating scale[5] and Strasser *et al.* found testosterone levels to be associated with mood, fatigue and other symptoms related to anorexia and cachexia.[18]

Several other chronic diseases including human immunodeficiency virus (HIV) infection, chronic obstructive lung disease, congestive heart failure and liver disease also are associated with hypogonadism. This has led to the hypothesis that downregulation of the gonadal axis in these settings may be part of a normal adaptive response to illness (eugonadal sick syndrome). Medications including opioids, megestrol and chemotherapeutic agents are known to cause hypogonadism. Platinum-based drugs induce primary hypogonadism due to a direct toxic effect in the gonads that is dose dependent.[19] The prevalence of hypogonadism has been reported to be as high as 29% in patients receiving these agents. However, in most of these studies hypogonadism was defined as an LH level above the upper limit of normal and most patients had normal total testosterone (TT) and SHBG levels.[20,21] Opioids are almost universally used in the cancer population and they also can cause secondary hypogonadism.[22,23] Rajagopal *et al.*[24] reported low TT levels in 18 out of 20 cancer survivors who were receiving high dose opioids orally (≥200 mg of morphine equivalent daily dose for ≥1 year) compared with 8 of 20 matched cancer survivors who had not received opioids, suggesting that hypogonadism is common in cancer survivors, and even more so in those requiring high doses of opioids. Megestrol acetate, a drug commonly prescribed off-label for the treatment of cancer-cachexia, is known to centrally suppress testosterone production.[25] Glucocorticoids also can induce hypogonadism by inhibiting gonadotrophin secretion[26] and by directly interfering with androgen production at the testicular or adrenal level.[27]

Current evidence suggests that a proinflammatory state may be responsible for many of the symptoms associated with cancer and hypogonadism.[28–31] Several cytokines are increased in cancer patients and these cytokines also may regulate the hypothalamic–pituitary–gonadal axis. Interleukin (IL)-6 administration induced prolonged suppression of testosterone levels in healthy men.[32] Testosterone replacement therapy (TRT) has been shown to reduce cytokine levels in hypogonadal men[33] and to reduce inflammatory markers in subjects with rheumatoid arthritis.[34]

Testosterone

The prevalence of hypogonadism in men increases with age, and treatment with exogenous testosterone is indicated in those subjects that are symptomatic and have no contraindication to TRT.[35] There are no clear guidelines for the diagnosis of low testosterone levels in women in the general population and most experts advise against its use because of the lack of a well-established clinical syndrome and lack of efficacy and safety data.[36] In men, TRT is likely to improve libido, mood, muscle mass and strength, and prevent osteoporosis.[37] Although testosterone replacement in the cancer patient has not been systematically evaluated and there are no specific guidelines in this setting, it seems reasonable to treat symptomatic subjects with confirmed hypogonadism regardless of whether they have cancer or not.

Contraindications to TRT include subjects with breast, prostate or other hormone-responsive cancer,[38] subjects with a palpable prostate nodule or a prostatic-specific antigen (PSA) >3 ng/mL, polycythaemia, severe heart failure, untreated sleep apnoea or symptomatic benign prostatic hyperplasia. Multiple formulations exist and the decision on which one to use should be made on a case-by-case basis according to the side-effect profile, patient's preference and availability. The goal of treatment should be to restore testosterone levels to mid-normal levels. Proper monitoring during therapy includes a thorough physical examination, a rectal examination, and questioning the patients for side-effects of prostatism such as urgency, weak stream and incomplete emptying of the bladder. Laboratory monitoring should include measurements of haemoglobin levels, and prostatic-specific antigen (PSA) after 3 months and yearly thereafter. If the PSA increases above the upper limit of normal or if it rises by >1.4 ng/mL during the first year or >0.8 ng/mL in 2 years or if a prostate nodule is palpated at any time, the patient should be referred for prostate biopsy and testosterone discontinued.[4] It is also important to remind patients that the suppression in gonadotrophins often caused by androgen therapy will probably suppress spermatogenesis and may lead to infertility.

Selective androgen receptor modulators (SARMs)

Testosterone exerts its action by activating the androgen receptor (AR). Depending on the target tissue, activation of this receptor will induce androgenic effects (prostate growth, acne, deepening of the voice, terminal hair growth, and clitoromegaly in women) or anabolic effects (increased muscle and bone mass and strength). In theory, a purely anabolic SARM with no androgenic action will be beneficial in the setting of cancer because it would allow us to maximize the effect on bone and muscle without the side-effects on prostate, skin and hair follicle. Most importantly, women could be treated without the virilizing effects that preclude the use of testosterone. Several synthetic steroidal compounds have been developed to separate these effects (i.e. oxandrolone, nandrolone); however, its clinical use has been limited by poor tissue selectivity and liver toxicity. Non-steroidal compounds with better oral bioavailability, higher specificity for the AR and more tissue-specific activity are being developed and some of them have already entered clinical studies.

In the setting of cancer cachexia, several preliminary reports[39] have shown an improvement in lean body mass, muscle strength and performance scores with good tolerability using the SARMs oxandrolone and more recently ostarine. However, further studies are needed to confirm these reports.

Growth hormone, ghrelin and ghrelin mimetics or growth hormone secretagogue receptor

Growth hormone

Growth hormone (GH) exerts its anabolic actions mainly by increasing IGF-1 levels. IGF-1 is synthesized primarily in the liver and circulates bound to several proteins known as insulin-like growth factor binding proteins or IGFBPs. The most common IGFBP in humans is IGFBP-3. GH also stimulates the production of IGF-1 in other tissues including muscle and it is said that GH also has some effects that are not mediated through IGF-1. Individuals with GH deficiency typically have increased fat mass, and decreased muscle mass and strength, energy levels and quality of life. Furthermore, these parameters improve with GH administration[40] confirming the anabolic nature of this hormone. GH is released from the pituitary gland in a pulsatile fashion, so evaluation of GH axis often involves provocative tests [i.e. arginine + growth hormone-releasing hormone (GHRH) stimulation test] and measurements of the more stable marker IGF-1.

Cancer subjects have reduced circulating IGF-1 levels in the presence of increased GH secretion suggesting a state of 'GH resistance'. This is expected in cachectic subjects since malnutrition and weight loss from other causes are also associated with GH resistance and low IGF-1 levels. However, these changes also have been reported in cancer subjects before the development of malnutrition suggesting that other mechanisms, perhaps an increase in proinflammatory cytokines, may play a role in this setting.[41]

Activation of the GH–IGF-1 axis has been used therapeutically in other wasting conditions such as HIV-induced wasting with some success. In this setting, GH treatment has been shown to increase body weight, nitrogen balance and lean body mass (LBM), also improving function as measured by treadmill work output.[42] Treatment with IGF-1 was not as effective as GH therapy and it was limited by hypoglycaemia.[43]

GH therapy is associated with several side-effects that tend to be dose-related. Most common side-effects include fluid retention (5–18%) and carpal tunnel syndrome (2%). Other side-effects are less common and can be transient such as hypertension and hyperglycaemia. Rare side-effects include retinopathy and gynaecomastia. In non-cancer individuals, there is the concern that increasing GH and IGF-1 levels can lead to the development of cancer. This has not been confirmed in clinical studies.[44] Nevertheless, GH or IGF-1 therapies are currently contraindicated in patients with an active cancer.[45]

In a small trial where 10 patients receive three daily injections of GH, a significant increase in GH and IGF-1 levels was detected along with a decrease in protein breakdown as evidenced by 24 h urea nitrogen measurements. Nitrogen balance was significantly improved in those subjects with a body weight ≥90% of their ideal body weight.[46] Although these results were promising, the lack of further evidence for GH use precludes its use outside controlled clinical trials at this time.

Ghrelin and growth hormone secretagogue receptor agonists (ghrelin mimetics)

In 1981, a new series of compounds that stimulated GH secretion through a non-classical pathway were identified.[47] Using a reverse pharmacology approach, the receptor responsible for these compounds' activity was identified in 1996 and named growth hormone secretagogue receptor (GHS-R).[48] Ghrelin, a 28-amino-acid peptide secreted mainly from the stomach, was subsequently isolated in 1999 as the endogenous ligand for the GHS-R.[49,50] In addition to its GH-secretagogue activity,[51] ghrelin was found to be an important orexigenic hormone.[52] It reduces fat oxidation and increases adiposity.[53] Recently, it was unambiguously demonstrated through experiments on GHS-R-knockout mice that the GHS-R mediates ghrelin's GH-releasing and orexigenic properties.[54]

Fasting plasma ghrelin levels are inversely related to body mass index (BMI), and they increase with weight loss induced by caloric restriction.[55,56] Subjects with anorexia nervosa also have substantially elevated fasting levels of ghrelin that return to normal when body weight is normalized.[57] Individuals with congestive heart failure-induced cachexia[58] and cancer-induced cachexia[28] have been reported to have increased levels of ghrelin. The increase in active ghrelin levels is likely to be a compensatory response to weight loss. However, it does not seem sufficient to restore appetite and body weight in this setting.

Several groups are currently working on the hypothesis that this 'resistance' to the orexigenic effects of ghrelin in this setting can be overcome by exogenous administration of this hormone. Because ghrelin is a peptide with a half-life of 30 min, its efficacy in humans is limited unless administered parenterally as a continuous infusion. Ghrelin mimetics (also known as growth hormone secretagogues) are non-peptidic, orally available, small molecules that have a long half-life allowing for once-a-day administration. These compounds have been in clinical trials for more than a decade. Our group and others have demonstrated their safety and efficacy in non-cancer patients.[59,60]

Activation of GHS-R by these ghrelin mimetics induces GH secretion,[61,62] increases food intake and body weight.[60,63] In non-cancer patients, GHS increase body weight and reverse the negative nitrogen balance induced by starvation independently of their orexigenic effects. These findings suggest that ghrelin's effects are not entirely mediated through an increase in appetite and that other mechanisms, such as a decrease in energy expenditure, are involved.[64] Ghrelin administration decreases energy expenditure in non-cancer human and animal models.[65,66] In two small groups of cancer patients, a single infusion of ghrelin was well tolerated, increasing appetite and food intake in one of the studies[67] but not in the other.[68]

Another useful feature of ghrelin is its potential anti-inflammatory action. Ghrelin administration can antagonize the effects of cytokines on appetite and body weight. Ghrelin administration blunts the anorectic effect of IL-1 and increases food intake and body weight in animals with cancer cachexia.[69,70] *In vitro* and *in vivo* studies also show that ghrelin decreases IL-6 and TNF-α production.[71]

More recently, an oral ghrelin mimetic, anamorelin, administered over a 12-week period in a randomized, placebo-controlled trial to subjects with various cancer types, increased total body mass and exhibited a trend toward increased lean mass.[72] In this study, IGF-1 and IGFBP-3 levels were increased suggesting that the 'GH resistance' reported in this setting can be overcome by administration of this compound.

As with GH therapy, a central question is the safety of these compounds, given the potential for increasing IGF-1 levels and causing tumour progression. When whole-animal tumour growth studies have been conducted to evaluate the effect of increasing GH tone, the results have generally indicated a beneficial effect.[73–75] Although *in vitro* studies suggest that IGF-1 may have oncogenic potential, there have been reports indicating the therapeutic potential of the major binding protein, IGFBP-3, in attenuating oncogenic behaviour by binding IGF-1 or through direct, IGF-independent actions. Consequently, it may be that the balanced effect of a GH-based intervention to increase both IGF-1 and IGFBP-3 may be responsible, in part, for some of the apparent discrepancies. Hanada *et al.*[70] tested the effects of ghrelin in a different model of tumour-induced cachexia. In this experiment, cachexia was reversed by the administration of ghrelin and tumour size remained unchanged, decreasing the tumour:carcass ratio.

More importantly, anamorelin administration to humans was well tolerated in our preliminary studies where approximately 40 subjects were exposed to the drug for 3 months. Tumour progression rates as reported by the providers were not different from those in placebo and survival was not affected. Further studies on the safety and efficacy of this compound, including its effect on the rate of tumour progression, are needed.

References

1. Diver MJ, Imtiaz KE, Ahmad AM, Vora JP, Fraser WD (2003) Diurnal rhythms of serum total, free and bioavailable testosterone and of SHBG in middle-aged men compared with those in young men. *Clin Endocrinol (Oxf)*, **58**, 710–17.
2. Spratt DI, O'Dea LS, Schoenfeld D, Butler J, Rao PN, Crowley WF Jr (1988) Neuroendocrine–gonadal axis in men: frequent sampling of LH, FSH, and testosterone. *Am J Physiol*, **254**, E658–66.
3. Swerdloff RS, Wang C, Cunningham G, *et al.* (2000) Long-term pharmacokinetics of transdermal testosterone gel in hypogonadal men. *J Clin Endocrinol Metab*, **85**, 4500–10.

4. Bhasin S, Cunningham GR, Hayes FJ, *et al.* (2006) Testosterone therapy in adult men with androgen deficiency syndromes: an endocrine society clinical practice guideline. *J Clin Endocrinol Metab*, **91**, 1995–2010.
5. Garcia JM, Li H, Mann D, *et al.* (2006) Hypogonadism in male patients with cancer. *Cancer*, **106**, 2583–91.
6. Wang C, Catlin DH, Demers LM, Starcevic B, Swerdloff RS (2004) Measurement of total serum testosterone in adult men: comparison of current laboratory methods versus liquid chromatography–tandem mass spectrometry. *J Clin Endocrinol Metab*, **89**, 534–43.
7. Brodsky IG, Balagopal P, Nair KS (1996) Effects of testosterone replacement on muscle mass and muscle protein synthesis in hypogonadal men—a clinical research center study. *J Clin Endocrinol Metab*, **81**, 3469–75.
8. Sheffield-Moore M, Urban RJ, Wolf SE, *et al.* (1999) Short-term oxandrolone administration stimulates net muscle protein synthesis in young men. *J Clin Endocrinol Metab*, **84**, 2705–11.
9. Urban RJ, Bodenburg YH, Gilkison C, *et al.* (1995) Testosterone administration to elderly men increases skeletal muscle strength and protein synthesis. *Am J Physiol*, **269**, E820–6.
10. Hijazi RA, Cunningham GR (2005) Andropause: is androgen replacement therapy indicated for the aging male? *Annu Rev Med*, **56**, 117–37.
11. Shores MM, Sloan KL, Matsumoto AM, Moceri VM, Felker B, Kivlahan DR (2004) Increased incidence of diagnosed depressive illness in hypogonadal older men. *Arch Gen Psychiatry*, **61**, 162–7.
12. Bruera E, Carraro S, Roca E, Cedaro L, Chacon R (1984) Association between malnutrition and caloric intake, emesis, psychological depression, glucose taste, and tumor mass. *Cancer Treat Rep*, **68**, 873–6.
13. MacDonald N, Alexander HR, Bruera E (1995) Cachexia–anorexia–asthenia. *J Pain Sympt Manag*, **10**, 151–5.
14. Argiles JM, Busquets S, Felipe A, Lopez-Soriano FJ (2005) Molecular mechanisms involved in muscle wasting in cancer and ageing: cachexia versus sarcopenia. *Int J Biochem Cell Biol*, **37**, 1084-1104.
15. Chatterjee R, Kottaridis PD, McGarrigle HH, Linch DC (2002) Management of erectile dysfunction by combination therapy with testosterone and sildenafil in recipients of high-dose therapy for haematological malignancies. *Bone Marrow Transpl*, **29**, 607–10.
16. Llobera J, Esteva M, Rifa J, *et al.* (2000) Terminal cancer. duration and prediction of survival time. *Eur J Cancer*, **36**, 2036–43.
17. Derogatis LR, Kourlesis SM (1981) An approach to evaluation of sexual problems in the cancer patient. *CA Cancer J Clin*, **31**, 46–50.
18. Strasser F, Palmer JL, Schover LR, *et al.* (2006) The impact of hypogonadism and autonomic dysfunction on fatigue, emotional function, and sexual desire in male patients with advanced cancer: a pilot study. *Cancer*, **107**, 2949–57.
19. Gerl A, Muhlbayer D, Hansmann G, Mraz W, Hiddemann W (2001) The impact of chemotherapy on Leydig cell function in long term survivors of germ cell tumors. *Cancer*, **91**, 1297–1303.
20. Howell SJ, Shalet SM (2001) Testicular function following chemotherapy. *Hum Reprod Update*, **7**, 363–9.
21. Kenney LB, Laufer MR, Grant FD, Grier H, Diller L (2001) High risk of infertility and long term gonadal damage in males treated with high dose cyclophosphamide for sarcoma during childhood. *Cancer*, **91**, 613–21.
22. Paice JA, Penn RD, Ryan WG (1994) Altered sexual function and decreased testosterone in patients receiving intraspinal opioids. *J Pain Sympt Manag*, **9**, 126–31.
23. Abs R, Verhelst J, Maeyaert J, *et al.* (2000) Endocrine consequences of long-term intrathecal administration of opioids. *J Clin Endocrinol Metab*, **85**, 2215–22.
24. Rajagopal A, Vassilopoulou-Sellin R, Palmer JL, Kaur G, Bruera E (2004) Symptomatic hypogonadism in male survivors of cancer with chronic exposure to opioids. *Cancer*, **100**, 851–8.

25. Dev R, Del Fabbro E, Bruera E (2007) Association between megestrol acetate treatment and symptomatic adrenal insufficiency with hypogonadism in male patients with cancer. *Cancer*, **110**, 1173–7.
26. Sakakura M, Takebe K, Nakagawa S (1975) Inhibition of luteinizing hormone secretion induced by synthetic LRH by long-term treatment with glucocorticoids in human subjects. *J Clin Endocrinol Metab*, **40**, 774–9.
27. MacAdams MR, White RH, Chipps BE (1986) Reduction of serum testosterone levels during chronic glucocorticoid therapy. *Ann Intern Med*, **104**, 648–51.
28. Garcia JM, Garcia-Touza M, Hijazi RA, *et al.* (2005) Active ghrelin levels and active to total ghrelin ratio in cancer-induced cachexia. *J Clin Endocrinol Metab*, **90**, 2920–926.
29. Tisdale MJ (2002) Cachexia in cancer patients. *Nat Rev Cancer*, **2**, 862–71.
30. Pfitzenmaier J, Vessella R, Higano CS, Noteboom JL, Wallace D Jr, Corey E (2003) Elevation of cytokine levels in cachectic patients with prostate carcinoma. *Cancer*, **97**, 1211–16.
31. Lee BN, Dantzer R, Langley KE, *et al.* (2004) A cytokine-based neuroimmunologic mechanism of cancer-related symptoms. *Neuroimmunomodulation*, **11**, 279–92.
32. Tsigos C, Papanicolaou DA, Kyrou I, Raptis SA, Chrousos GP (1999) Dose-dependent effects of recombinant human interleukin-6 on the pituitary–testicular axis. *J Interferon Cytokine Res*, **19**, 1271–6.
33. Malkin CJ, Pugh PJ, Jones RD, Kapoor D, Channer KS, Jones TH (2004) The effect of testosterone replacement on endogenous inflammatory cytokines and lipid profiles in hypogonadal men. *J Clin Endocrinol Metab*, **89**, 3313–8.
34. Cutolo M, Balleari E, Giusti M, Intra E, Accardo S (1991) Androgen replacement therapy in male patients with rheumatoid arthritis. *Arthritis Rheum*, **34**, 1–5.
35. Morley JE, Charlton E, Patrick P, *et al.* (2000) Validation of a screening questionnaire for androgen deficiency in aging males. *Metabolism*, **49**, 1239–42.
36. Wierman ME, Basson R, Davis SR, *et al.* (2006) Androgen therapy in women: an Endocrine Society Clinical Practice guideline. *J Clin Endocrinol Metab*, **91**, 3697–710.
37. Wang C, Swedloff RS, Iranmanesh A, *et al.* (2000) Transdermal testosterone gel improves sexual function, mood, muscle strength, and body composition parameters in hypogonadal men. Testosterone Gel Study Group. *J Clin Endocrinol Metab*, **85**, 2839–53.
38. Fowler JE Jr, Whitmore WF Jr (1981) The response of metastatic adenocarcinoma of the prostate to exogenous testosterone. *J Urol*, **126**, 372–5.
39. Boughton B (2003 Drug increases lean tissue mass in patients with cancer. *Lancet Oncol*, **4**, 135.
40. Hoffman AR, Kuntze JE, Baptista J, *et al.* (2004) Growth hormone (GH) replacement therapy in adult-onset GH deficiency: effects on body composition in men and women in a double-blind, randomized, placebo-controlled trial. *J Clin Endocrinol Metab*, **89**, 2048–56.
41. Crown AL, Cottle K, Lightman SL, *et al.* (2002) What is the role of the insulin-like growth factor system in the pathophysiology of cancer cachexia, and how is it regulated? *Clin Endocrinol (Oxf)*, **56**, 723–33.
42. Schambelan M, Mulligan K, Grunfeld C, *et al.* (1996) Recombinant human growth hormone in patients with HIV-associated wasting. A randomized, placebo-controlled trial. Serostim Study Group. *Ann Intern Med*, **125**, 873–82.
43. Mulligan K, Schambelan M (2002) Anabolic treatment with GH, IGF-I, or anabolic steroids in patients with HIV-associated wasting. *Int J Cardiol*, **85**, 151–9.
44. Tuffli GA, Johanson A, Rundle AC, Allen DB (1995) Lack of increased risk for extracranial, nonleukemic neoplasms in recipients of recombinant deoxyribonucleic acid growth hormone. *J Clin Endocrinol Metab*, **80**, 1416–22.
45. Molitch ME, Clemmons DR, Malozowski S, *et al.* (2006) Evaluation and treatment of adult growth hormone deficiency: an Endocrine Society Clinical Practice Guideline. *J Clin Endocrinol Metab*, **91**, 1621–34.

46. Tayek JA, Brasel JA (1995) Failure of anabolism in malnourished cancer patients receiving growth hormone: a clinical research center study. *J Clin Endocrinol Metab*, **80**, 2082–7.
47. Momany FA, Bowers CY, Reynolds GA, Chang D, Hong A, Newlander K (1981) Design, synthesis, and biological activity of peptides which release growth hormone, *in vitro*. *Endocrinology*, **108**, 31–9.
48. Howard AD, Feighner SD, Cully DF, *et al.* (1996) A receptor in pituitary and hypothalamus that functions in growth hormone release. *Science*, **273**, 974–7.
49. Kojima M, Hosoda H, Date Y, Nakazato M, Matsuo H, Kangawa K (1999) Ghrelin is a growth-hormone-releasing acylated peptide from stomach. *Nature*, **402**, 656–60.
50. Smith RG, Van der Ploeg LH, Howard AD, *et al.* (1997) Peptidomimetic regulation of growth hormone secretion. *Endocr Rev*, **18**, 621–45.
51. Takaya K, Ariyasu H, Kanamoto N, *et al.* (2000) Ghrelin strongly stimulates growth hormone release in humans. *J Clin Endocrinol Metab*, **85**, 4908–11.
52. Wren AM, Seal LJ, Cohen MA, *et al.* (2001) Ghrelin enhances appetite and increases food intake in humans. *J Clin Endocrinol Metab*, **86**, 5992.
53. Tschop M, Smiley DL, Heiman ML (2000) Ghrelin induces adiposity in rodents. *Nature*, **407**, 908–13.
54. Sun Y, Wang P, Zheng H, Smith RG (2004) Ghrelin stimulation of growth hormone release and appetite is mediated through the growth hormone secretagogue receptor. *Proc Natl Acad Sci USA*, **101**, 4679–84.
55. Shiiya T, Nakazato M, Mizuta M, *et al.* (2002) Plasma ghrelin levels in lean and obese humans and the effect of glucose on ghrelin secretion. *J Clin Endocrinol Metab*, **87**, 240–4.
56. Cummings DE, Weigle DS, Frayo RS, *et al.* (2002) Plasma ghrelin levels after diet-induced weight loss or gastric bypass surgery. *N Engl J Med*, **346**, 1623–30.
57. Soriano-Guillen L, Barrios V, Campos-Barros A, Argente J (2004) Ghrelin levels in obesity and anorexia nervosa: effect of weight reduction or recuperation. *J Pediatr*, **144**, 36–42.
58. Nagaya N, Uematsu M, Kojima M, *et al.* (2001) Elevated circulating level of ghrelin in cachexia associated with chronic heart failure: relationships between ghrelin and anabolic/catabolic factors. *Circulation*, **104**, 2034–8.
59. Svensson J, Lonn L, Jansson J-O, *et al.* (1998) Two-month treatment of obese subjects with the oral growth hormone (GH) secretagogue MK-677 increases GH secretion, fat-free mass, and energy expenditure. *J Clin Endocrinol Metab*, **83**, 362–9.
60. Garcia JM, Polvino WJ (2007) Effect on body weight and safety of RC-1291, a novel, orally available ghrelin mimetic and growth hormone secretagogue: results of a phase I, randomized, placebo-controlled, multiple-dose study in healthy volunteers. *Oncologist*, **12**, 594–600.
61. Takaya K, Ariyasu H, Kanamoto N, *et al.* (2000) Ghrelin strongly stimulates growth hormone release in humans. *J Clin Endocrinol Metab*, **85**, 4908–11.
62. Garcia JM, Polvino WJ (2009) Pharmacodynamic hormonal effects of anamorelin, a novel oral ghrelin mimetic and growth-hormone secretagogue in healthy volunteers. *Growth Horm IGF-1 Res*, **19**(3), 267–73.
63. Wren AM, Small CJ, Abbott CR, *et al.* (2001) Ghrelin causes hyperphagia and obesity in rats. *Diabetes*, **50**, 2540–7.
64. Murphy MG, Plunkett LM, Gertz BJ, *et al.* (1998) MK-0677, an orally active growth hormone secretagogue reverses diet-induced catabolism. *J Clin Endocrinol Metab*, **83**, 320–5.
65. Vestergaard ET, Djurhuus CB, Gjedsted J, *et al.* (2008) Acute effects of ghrelin administration on glucose and lipid metabolism. *J Clin Endocrinol Metab*, **93**, 438–44.
66. Jatoi A, Daly BD, Hughes VA, Dallal GE, Kehayias J, Roubenoff R (2001) Do patients with nonmetastatic non-small cell lung cancer demonstrate altered resting energy expenditure? *Ann Thorac Surg*, **72**, 348–51.
67. Neary NM, Small CJ, Wren AM, *et al.* (2004) Ghrelin increases energy intake in cancer patients with impaired appetite: acute, randomized, placebo-controlled trial. *J Clin Endocrinol Metab*, **89**, 2832–6.

68. Strasser F, Lutz TA, Maeder MT, *et al.* (2008) Safety, tolerability and pharmacokinetics of intravenous ghrelin for cancer-related anorexia/cachexia: a randomised, placebo-controlled, double-blind, double-crossover study. *Br J Cancer*, **98**, 300–8.
69. Asakawa A, Inui A, Kaga T, *et al.* (2001) Ghrelin is an appetite-stimulatory signal from stomach with structural resemblance to motilin. *Gastroenterology*, **120**, 337–45.
70. Hanada T, Toshinai K, Kajimura N, *et al.* (2003) Anti-cachectic effect of ghrelin in nude mice bearing human melanoma cells. *Biochem Biophys Res Commun*, **301**, 275–9.
71. Dixit VD, Schaffer EM, Pyle RS, *et al.* (2004) Ghrelin inhibits leptin- and activation-induced proinflammatory cytokine expression by human monocytes and T cells. *J Clin Invest*, **114**, 57–66.
72. Garcia JM, Graham, C, Kumor K, Polvino W (2007) A Phase II, randomized, placebo-controlled, double blind study of the efficacy and safety of RC-1291 for the treatment of cancer-cachexia. *J Clin Oncol*, **25**, S25.
73. Wolf RF, Ng B, Weksler B, Burt M, Brennan MF (1994) Effect of growth hormone on tumor and host in an animal model. *Ann Surg Oncol*, **1**, 314–20.
74. Bartlett DL, Charland S, Torosian MH (1994) Growth hormone, insulin, and somatostatin therapy of cancer cachexia. *Cancer*, **73**, 1499–1504.
75. Bartlett DL, Stein TP, Torosian MH (1995) Effect of growth hormone and protein intake on tumor growth and host cachexia. *Surgery*, **117**, 260–7.

Chapter 9

Immune modulators

Egidio Del Fabbro

Introduction

Because basic research suggests that cytokines play an important role in the pathogenesis of cachexia, several clinical studies have used immune modulators either as single agents or in combination therapy. Some of the most promising treatments are discussed in this chapter, while combination therapy for cachexia is discussed in Chapter 11. The role of immune modulators earlier in the disease trajectory is less well defined. Attenuating the side-effects of chemo- and radiation therapy [by melatonin or tumour necrosis factor (TNF)-α inhibitors] and improving surgical outcomes (with immunonutrition) are potential uses of immune modulators in concert with disease-specific therapy. Immune modulators also exhibit an anti-tumour effect experimentally, suggesting that their clinical benefit (e.g. improved appetite and lean body mass) may be partially derived from activity against the disease itself. Certain haematological malignancies respond to interleukin (IL)-6 inhibitors, and systematic reviews indicate that non-steroidal anti-inflammatory drugs (NSAIDs) may be effective for secondary or even primary colorectal prevention.[1]

This chapter divides therapies into two broad categories, namely, non-specific and specific immune modulators. As single agents, melatonin, NSAIDs, fish oil, and thalidomide all have immune-modulating effects and improve selected clinical outcomes in cachexia trials. Specific nutritional supplements and proinflammatory cytokine inhibitors have also shown promise in preliminary studies.

Other therapies not discussed in this chapter could modulate the inflammatory response, but do not specifically target cytokines or the immune system. These include ghrelin, testosterone, megestrol acetate and even non-pharmacological therapies such as exercise. Their effects on inflammation and clinical outcomes are discussed within their relevant chapters.

Cinical relevance of cytokines in cancer cachexia

Although cytokines are important in the pathogenesis of cancer cachexia and could prove to be useful therapeutic targets, the relationship between serum cytokines and clinical outcomes is inconsistent. Compared to non-cachectic cancer patients, those with early cachexia display elevated TNFα serum levels and reactive oxygen species.[2] A study of pancreatic cancer patients at M. D. Anderson Cancer Center examined the association between serum levels of cytokines and clinical outcomes.[3] Higher IL-6, IL-10, and IL-8 levels were associated with poor performance status and/or weight loss, compared to healthy volunteers. A more recent study in patients with advanced prostate cancer examined the serum levels of TNFα, IL-1β, IL-6, IL-8, and prostate-specific antigen (PSA) in normal donors, patients with organ-confined cancer, patients with advanced cancer without cachexia, and patients with advanced cancer and cachexia.[4] Levels of TNFα, IL-6, and IL-8 were elevated in patients with advanced prostate cancer and cachexia, compared to those without cachexia. In the cachectic patients, there was no correlation between PSA levels and any of the cytokine levels. Another prospective study in newly diagnosed non-small cell lung cancer (NSCLC) patients[5] assessed the impact of TNFα and IL-6 levels on developing cachexia. IL-6 was increased, and correlated with poor nutritional status, impaired performance status and shorter survival.

Other investigators have not found significant correlations between proinflammatory serum cytokines and weight loss.[6] A recent study of NSCLC[7] patients with weight loss ≥10% compared to those with <10% showed that TNFα and IL-6 levels did not differ between groups. A Japanese study in cachectic gastric and colorectal patients found that production of IL-12 was lowest in the patients with distant metastasis and cachexia but levels of IL4, IL-6, and IL-10 did not differ significantly.[8] Lastly, a multi-institutional cachexia trial found little clinical utility in measuring serum cytokines.[9] Baseline serum IL-6 predicted a diminished survival only after adjustment for age and cancer site, whereas no correlations were observed between serum cytokine concentrations (IL-6, TNFα, IL-1) and changes in weight or appetite.

In pancreatic cancer, the presence of an acute-phase response identifies a group of patients who are often markedly hypermetabolic. Falconer *et al.* showed that the serum concentration of TNF and IL-6 does not correlate with the presence of an acute-phase response in cachectic patients, whereas rates of cytokine production by peripheral blood mononuclear cells were significantly greater in patients with such a response.[10] Local rather than systemic cytokine production may therefore be important in regulating the acute-phase response. A recent study comparing cancer patients with and without cachexia to non-cancer patients found that plasma levels of TNFα were not significantly elevated in cachectic patients, and no correlation was found between TNFα and weight loss or appetite scores. The authors suggested that TNF may act in a paracrine rather than an endocrine fashion, and that serum levels may not accurately reflect tissue concentrations.[11]

Other reasons for the inconsistent relationship between cachexia and serum cytokine levels include differences in tumour phenotype, tumour stage, type of cytokine assays, or a genetic variation in the immune response.[12] In future, a genetic predisposition to systemic inflammation and cachexia could be identified through gene polymorphisms, allowing treatment to be initiated earlier, thereby improving the chances of a therapeutic response. Possible candidates under investigation include single nucleotide polymorphisms of IL-6, TNF and IL-1.

Non-specific immune modulators

Melatonin

Melatonin is a lipophilic, pleiotropic hormone which modulates multiple mechanisms promoting cachexia, including inflammation, autonomic failure and malabsorption. Melatonin also has antimitotic, antioxidant and antiangiogenic activity, and may prevent chemotherapy and radiation side-effects. Initially believed to be synthesized exclusively in the pineal gland and primarily involved as a circadian messenger of light and dark, melatonin is now recognized to have multiple actions[13] and is synthesized in widely diverse tissues. The retina, thymus, airway epithelium, bone marrow, gut, ovary, testicles, lymphocytes and skin all have the capacity to synthesize melatonin.[14] Melatonin has no physiological barriers, has a wide distribution, and in the peripheral circulation is primarily derived from nocturnal secretion by the pineal gland. Melatonin is synthesized in even greater quantities by the gastrointestinal system[15] (up to 400-fold), possibly in response to feeding. This locally produced melatonin (from the gut or other organs) is likely to be consumed by tissues in the near environs as a protective mechanism for oxidative stress caused by toxins, infection and radiation.

Animal models have provided some insight into melatonin's potential for attenuating the decline in appetite and muscle wasting. In cachectic animals the pineal gland is less responsive to stimulation by noradrenaline.[16] Melatonin supplementation stimulates appetite in animals,[17] and its presence in the digestive tract is associated with intestinal transit and nutrient absorption.[18] In addition, melatonin may prevent muscle dysfunction caused by inflammatory conditions and attenuate the myopathy produced by catabolic conditions such as hyperthyroidism.[19]

In humans, changes in melatonin secretion are associated with increased cancer risk, cancer progression, and also with symptom burden. Altered levels of melatonin are found in patients with a variety of solid tumours, including breast, prostate, endometrial, lung, gastric and colorectal cancers. Based on this research, melatonin supplementation could modulate several mechanisms associated with cachexia, including the pro inflammatory response, gastrointestinal dysfunction and symptom distress.

One of the first clinical studies of melatonin[20] evaluated its effect as a preventive therapy for cachexia. Patients with a variety of metastatic solid tumours were randomized to either supportive care alone or supportive care plus melatonin for a period of 3 months. Weight loss >10% occurred less often in the melatonin group, and symptoms of depression and performance status tended to improve from baseline. These clinical benefits were accompanied by a significant decrease in serum levels of TNFα.

In a subsequent trial, 1400 patients with untreatable solid tumours who had received at least one cycle of chemotherapy and no prior biological therapy were randomized to supportive care alone or supportive care plus 20 mg of melatonin at night.[21] Although no inflammatory markers were reported, cachexia, weakness, anorexia and depression occurred more frequently in the group receiving supportive care alone.

In several more recent trials, the same group of investigators demonstrated decreased symptoms, improved survival, and fewer adverse effects for melatonin combined with chemotherapy compared to chemotherapy alone. The encouraging results from these studies are limited by methodological issues such as the lack of blinding and absence of placebo controls. In an attempt to corroborate some of these findings, a North American multicentre trial of radiation therapy for brain metastases, added 20 mg of melatonin to conventional therapy. Although melatonin was again well tolerated, no survival benefit[22] was demonstrated and unfortunately changes in symptom severity, appetite, or weight were not reported.

Despite the ongoing debate about the merits of melatonin supplementation, a systematic review[23] of 10 randomized controlled trials and a meta-analysis concluded that exogenous melatonin consistently reduced the risk of death at 1 year across all doses and all types of solid tumours. The numbers needed to treat were small, ranging between one and five, but the lack of any double-blind placebo-controlled trials was noted to be a limitation.

Side-effects

The risk of side-effects is an important consideration in patients who may be debilitated by their disease. Fortunately, melatonin appears to have few adverse effects, even at doses of 20 mg daily. Although doses higher than 50 mg may cause side-effects that include fatigue and drowsiness, up to 300 mg daily in non-cancer conditions does not appear to increase daytime sleepiness.[24] No severe adverse effects were reported in a systematic review, nor in a randomized, double-blind placebo-controlled trial of 28 days' duration in normal volunteers receiving a dose of 10 mg at night. Polysomnography and frequent hepatic, renal, and endocrine laboratory monitoring revealed no abnormalities.[25] Another systematic review of melatonin for the treatment of jet-lag concluded that the risk of side-effects was low.[26]

Finally, melatonin may be particularly effective in reducing the side-effects of some cancer therapies. Animal models indicate that combining melatonin with chemotherapy will diminish side-effects such as cardiac and neurotoxicity, and that the prophylactic use of melatonin may be radioprotective.[27]

Although melatonin shows great potential in animal models and preliminary clinical trials for attenuating cachexia and symptom distress, further research may be hindered by regulatory issues,[28] lack of funding and meagre industry interest. Although at least one double-blind trial of melatonin for appetite in advanced cancer patients is underway in the USA, many more placebo-controlled trials are needed to confirm the numerous clinical benefits ascribed to melatonin.

Non-steroidal anti-inflammatory medications

These appear to modulate the aberrant inflammatory response considered the dominant mechanism causing cachexia. The tumour–host interaction produces elevated levels of proinflammatory cytokines, including TNF, interferon (IFN)-γ and IL-6, which specifically target the thick filaments[11] of myofibrils, leading to muscle wasting. NSAIDs decrease the production of proinflammatory cytokines such as IL-6 in animal models of cachexia[29] and experiments on tumour-bearing rats suggest that indomethacin[30] may inhibit TNF and ubiquitin-mediated pathways of protein degradation. Meloxicam, a relatively selective COX-2 inhibitor, attenuates the protein degradation caused by proteolysis-inducing factor (PIF) in mouse myoblasts.[31] Although NSAIDs reverse muscle loss in both animal models and preliminary studies in humans, it must be acknowledged that at least some of their impact on cachexia may be a result of their antitumour effect. In this respect, NSAIDs are similar to thalidomide and melatonin.

A retrospective case–control study of cachectic cancer patients revealed that long term indomethacin[32] use preserved body fat and decreased the acute-phase-reactant C-reactive protein (a useful surrogate marker of IL-6). Significant weight gain, but no decline in serum cytokine levels, occurred in patients with head and neck or gastrointestinal cancer[33] treated with celecoxib (200 mg twice daily). Although there were no significant improvements in lean body mass compared to placebo in this small prospective study, two other open-label trials showed that celecoxib in combination with a progestin and calorie-dense supplements increased weight and lean body mass. These multimodality trials are discussed in greater detail in Chapter 11. In the only large randomized double-blind trial of an NSAID for cachexia, ibuprofen (400 mg three times a day) plus megestrol acetate (MA) or MA alone was administered for 12 weeks to patients with gastrointestinal cancer. Patients receiving MA alone experienced a median 2.8 kg weight loss, whereas those receiving MA/ibuprofen experienced a median 2.3 kg weight increase.[34] Quality of life was improved and the acute-phase response was diminished (demonstrated by a decrease in CRP level) in the group receiving ibuprofen.

Side-effects

The most common adverse reactions associated with NSAIDs are gastrointestinal (GI) complaints which occur in up to 16% of patients in controlled clinical trials. Although minor GI symptoms such as dyspepsia are common, symptomatic upper GI ulcers, perforation or bleeding occur in approximately 1% of patients treated with ibuprofen for 3–6 months. Risk factors[35] for peptic ulcers include advanced age, concomitant use of corticosteroids and high doses of NSAIDs. GI side-effects are not as common in patients receiving <2400 mg of ibuprofen daily. Rarely, acute renal failure and hepatic dysfunction are reported, and NSAIDs can decrease the tubular excretion of methotrexate resulting in increased toxicity.

NSAIDs affect prothrombin times when co-administered with warfarin. More selective COX-2 inhibitors (e.g. celecoxib, meloxicam) should be used[36] if anticoagulants are unavoidable.

Non-selective NSAIDs inhibit platelet aggregation and are to be avoided in those with counts <20. There are ongoing trials to determine the relative risks of COX-2 selective inhibitors versus older NSAIDs as regards gastrointestinal and cardiovascular events. Although the selective COX-2 inhibitors reduce gastrointestinal ulcer complications[37] (bleeding, perforation, or obstruction) compared with traditional NSAIDs, their cardiovascular safety has been questioned.[38] Rofecoxib, diclofenac and indomethacin were problematic in a meta-analysis[39] of observational studies, although it seems that all NSAIDs (except naproxen) may increase cardiovascular risk (especially at higher doses). As regards cancer survivors in particular, a placebo-controlled trial to reduce recurrence of colorectal cancer showed that rofecoxib was associated with an increased frequency of adverse cardiovascular events.[40]

Thalidomide

Thalidomide, a derivative of glutamic acid, has a complex mechanism of action that is not yet completely understood. Thalidomide[41] is lipid-soluble, crosses the blood–brain barrier, and is absorbed from the gastrointestinal tract slowly. It is not metabolized appreciably by the liver and does not influence the cytochrome P450 enzyme system. There is evidence that thalidomide inhibits angiogenesis and modulates the inflammatory response by downregulating production of TNFα, IL-6, COX-2 and transcription of nuclear factor kappa B (NFκB).[42] In an animal model of cancer cachexia, thalidomide attenuated the loss of skeletal muscle.[43]

Thalidomide has activity against a number of solid and haematological malignancies (especially in combination therapy), and is effective for a wide range of inflammatory diseases such as rheumatoid arthrits, Crohn's, leprosy and cutaneous lupus. Thalidomide reverses cachexia in non-cancer patients at doses between 100 and 200 mg daily. Human immunodeficiency virus (HIV) patients with aphthous ulcers gain weight[44] and those with acquired immune deficiency syndrome (AIDS)-related cachexia regain fat-free mass.[45] A randomized placebo-controlled trial of patients with active pulmonary tuberculosis[46] found that those on thalidomide gained weight and that their serum levels of TNFα declined. Patients with metastatic cancer, poor appetite and weight loss of >5% who were given low dose thalidomide[47] (100 mg/day) experienced improved appetite, caloric intake and sense of well-being. Although no assessment of appetite scores or lean body mass was performed, 2 weeks of thalidomide (300 mg/day) treatment significantly reduced serum levels of C-reactive protein and IL-6 in patients with renal cancer and cachexia.[48] Two weeks of thalidomide (200 mg/day) in patients with oesophageal cancer[49] reversed lean body mass loss, and although sedation was experienced by all, daytime somnolence was transitory and disappeared after 2 or 3 days.

A randomized placebo-controlled trial[50] of 50 patients with pancreatic cancer showed that thalidomide (200 mg/day) was well tolerated and effective at attenuating loss of weight and lean body mass after 4 weeks of therapy. There were no significant differences in quality of life, survival, strength or physical function between thalidomide and placebo. The relatively high dose of thalidomide used in this study may explain the lack of significant improvement in subjective outcomes, or perhaps maximum benefit occurred prior to the assessment at 4 weeks.

Other researchers are investigating the effect of thalidomide in combination[51] with multimodal therapy and also as a single agent for symptom clusters. Symptoms within a cluster are usually related to one another, their intensity scores often correlate and they may share a common biological mechanism (e.g. inflammation). Thalidomide may be an effective therapy for the cachexia symptom cluster (anorexia, nausea, fatigue and weight loss) and for other symptoms such as pain and insomnia.

Side-effects

Thalidomide administration in pregnant women is absolutely contraindicated and access to thalidomide in the USA requires participation in the System for Thalidomide Education and Prescription Safety (STEPS) Program. Teratogenesis can be seen even with a single dose of 100 mg, and its use in the 1950s as a sedative and as an anti-emetic for morning sickness resulted in thousands of birth defects, including absent or hypoplastic limbs, dysplasia and absent internal organs. Thalidomide for the treatment of multiple myeloma and other malignancies usually requires doses ≥300 mg daily and for a longer duration than used in cachexia studies. In patients with metastatic renal cancer, fewer than one-third of patients were able to tolerate the maximum dose of 400 mg/day because of side-effects of somnolence, constipation, fatigue and paraesthesia. The risk of developing peripheral neuropathy increases in combination with neurotoxic chemotherapy and with high cumulative doses of thalidomide. Although high dose thalidomide can cause severe side-effects, doses of 50–100 mg are well tolerated in patients with advanced cancer. Patients develop no signs of neurotoxicity, daytime somnolence is transitory (for 2 or 3 days), and constipation responds to osmotic laxatives.

Immunonutrition in cancer patients

Specific nutritional supplements such as arginine, glutamine, nucleic acids, antioxidants and ω-3 oils (as single agents and in combination) have the potential to modulate the immune system. In acutely ill patients, meta-analyses find that immunonutrition results in fewer infectious complications and reduced length of hospital stay. Although many of these studies are noted to be of poor methodological quality and fail to show a clear clinical benefit, in some patients (such as those with acute respiratory distress syndrome) enteral formulas with fish oils, borage oils and antioxidants are recommended.[52]

Interventions incorporating these agents have been applied to cancer patients in diverse clinical settings, ranging from patients with minimal malnutrition receiving preoperative therapy to those with advanced disease and cachexia. Most of the trials in surgical patients have used a specific combination of enteral supplements perioperatively. A recent randomized trial of patients with oral and laryngeal cancer showed that an enteral formula enhanced with arginine, ribonucleic acid and ω-3 fatty acid (given within 12 h of surgery and continued for at least 7 days) resulted in fewer wound infections than a control group.[53] No significant differences in IL-6, C-reactive protein (CRP) and TNFα were detected between the groups. The timing, duration and composition of the enteral immunonutrition mixture may all play a role in influencing outcomes. Surgical wound infection and the postoperative inflammatory response decreased in oesophagectomy patients receiving perioperative immunonutrition compared to those on postoperative enteral formulas.[54] A randomized trial of patients with gastrointestinal cancer and weight loss <10% revealed that oral supplementation for 5 days before surgery was as effective as preoperative treatment plus postoperative jejunal infusion with the same enriched formula.[55] Although both strategies of immunonutrition appeared to be superior to conventional enteral feeding, the same group of investigators reported that malnourished patients (≥10% weight loss) experienced fewer complications with perioperative immunonutrition.[56] A recent prospective randomized study of well-nourished patients undergoing resection for gastrointestinal cancer failed to demonstrate any advantage of routine postoperative enteral or parenteral immunonutrition.[57] Differences in the nutritional status of the patient population and the composition of the enteral mixtures might account for the lack of benefit compared to earlier trials.

Systematic reviews have tried to define the role of immunonutrition in cancer patients undergoing surgery. A systematic review of immunonutrition for patients undergoing surgery for head and neck cancer showed a reduction in length of hospital stay but no change in clinical complications.[58] Another review of surgery for gastrointestinal cancer suggested that preoperative oral immunonutrition is associated with a 50% decrease in postoperative complications in non-severely malnourished patients.[59] Of all the individual components in immunonutrition formulas, fish oil has been tested most frequently in cachexia studies.

Fish oil

The benefits of n-3 fatty acids in fish oil may be linked to their substitution of n-6 arachidonic acid within inflammatory cell membrane phospholipids. Proinflammatory eicosanoids from n-6 arachidonic acid (e.g. leukotriene B_4, thromboxane A_2, prostaglandin E_2) are decreased, and the production of other eicosanoids (e.g. thromboxane A_3, prostaglandin E_3, leukotriene B_5) from n-3 fatty acids is facilitated.[48] Overall, the administration of n-3 fatty acids to animals and humans produces variable effects on cytokines, with some studies reporting increased TNFα, IL-6 and IL-1 production and others reporting a decline. Clinical studies in humans have examined the role of n-3 fatty acids for primary cancer prevention, for enteral support perioperatively, and as therapy for cachexia. Results from a 22-year prospective study suggest that fish and long chain n-3 fatty acids from fish may decrease the risk for colorectal cancer.[60] ω-6 and ω-3 polyunsaturated fatty acids may play opposing roles in inflammation-driven colorectal carcinogenesis,[61] and in a large US prospective cohort the relationship of these polyunsaturated fatty acids with colorectal cancer risk was evaluated. Unexpectedly, the ratio of total ω-6 to total ω-3 intake was not associated with colorectal cancer risk in either sex, although in women, total ω-6 and marine ω-3 intake appeared to be associated with higher and lower risk.

Preliminary trials of oral nutritional supplements containing EPA in patients with advanced pancreatic cancer[62] improved lean body mass and increased physical activity. This initial success was tempered by the disappointing outcomes of more recent trials utilizing single agent ω-3 fish oil. Two weeks of 3 g eicosapentaenoic acid (EPA) plus docosahexaenoic acid (DHA) had no effect on weight, appetite, or fatigue compared to placebo in patients with advanced cancer. An attempt at improving outcomes by using very high doses (7.5 g EPA plus DHA) in a subsequent study, achieved weight stabilization or gain in a small but definite subset of patients, but many patients were affected by gastrointestinal side-effects such as nausea, and excessive belching.[63] A larger multicentre, placebo-controlled trial of >500 weight-losing patients with advanced gastrointestinal or lung cancer showed no statistically significant benefit from single agent EPA (2–4 g) in the treatment of cancer cachexia.[64] A Cochrane review also concluded that there is insufficient evidence to support the use of oral fish oil (on its own or in the presence of other treatments) for the management of the cachexia–anorexia syndrome in patients with advanced cancer.[65] A systematic review examined the efficacy and potential benefits of EPA supplementation in patients with cancer.[66] EPA supplementation appeared to improve survival, complications and inflammatory markers such as TNF and IFN (but not CRP) in patients undergoing bone marrow transplant (BMT). Outcomes in other groups (e.g. those undergoing surgery or receiving palliative care) either did not benefit from EPA supplementation or study results were inconsistent.

Despite these negative studies in patients with advanced cancer, fish oil may prove to be useful in subsets of patients depending on tumour type, stage or the duration of therapy. A second systematic review suggested that supplementation with 1.5 g daily of EPA and/or DHA for prolonged periods (8 weeks) in pancreatic and upper digestive tract cancers seemed to be associated with improvements in various clinical, biochemical and quality-of-life parameters.[67]

The immune-modulating effects of ω-3 oils are complex, influenced by other dietary factors, and may be more effective in combination therapy. The use of ω-3 oils as a component of enteral immunonutrition for cancer patients was discussed earlier in this chapter. Recently a murine model of cachexia exhibited decreased levels of proinflammatory cytokines after a combination of fish oil, specific oligosaccharides, and leucine were added to the diet. The authors concluded that a combination of these supplements was needed to produce synergism and improved immune competence.[68] At least two small trials in advanced cancer patients with cachexia suggest that some clinical benefit may be obtained when fish oil is combined with other immune modulators and nutritional supplementation.[14,68]

Other immune modulators

Arginine

Both arginine and its product nitric oxide influence T-cell-mediated immunity, cytokine induction and macrophage-mediated tumour toxicity. Plasma arginine concentrations are decreased in all tumour types, including breast and colonic cancer, even without weight loss.[69] A study investigating the effects of arginine on tumour cell behaviour showed that arginine decreased cell growth but had no significant effect on the invasive potential of malignant cells.[70] Dogs with lymphoma randomized to a diet of fish oil and arginine had a better disease-free interval and survival time than those fed an otherwise identical control diet.[71] In small clinical trials of patients with either cancer or HIV cachexia, arginine combined with glutamine and β-hydroxy β-methylbutyric acid increased lean body mass without significant side-effects. In a larger recent trial using the same combination, only 37% of patients completed the 8-week study and no significant difference in lean body mass was demonstrated compared with an isonitrogenous, isocaloric control mixture. The reasons for these inconsistent results and high patient drop-out rate are unclear.

Glutamine

Although glutamine is a non-essential amino acid, it is a preferred energy fuel for cells with rapid turnover, such as lymphocytes, enterocytes, and malignant cells. Consumption of glutamine is probably increased in catabolic states such as cachexia. Concerns about stimulating cancer growth are mitigated by studies demonstrating an antineoplastic effect,[72] and a review of catabolic patients suggests that glutamine may enhance antineoplastic therapies.[73] Glutamine supplementation enhances lymphocyte function and reduces gut permeability of patients during chemoradiation, and in animal models of cancer it attenuates protein loss.[74] The combination of glutamine with other amino acids such as arginine is addressed above and in Chapter 11.

Curcumin

Cumin, a plant-derived dietary ingredient with NFκB and tumour inhibitory properties in humans,[75] may benefit cachectic patients. Preliminary studies in animal models have not demonstrated any significant anticachectic effect.[76]

Specific immune modulators

Inhibitors of proinflammatory cytokines

IL-6

In animal studies,[77] a monoclonal antibody to IL-6 attenuated cachexia and decreased the tumour burden in melanoma. In prostate xenografts, cachexia improved independently of the tumour when IL-6 was inhibited. A review[78] of six clinical trials that used monoclonal antibodies (mAb) to IL-6 in patients with multiple myeloma, renal cell carcinoma, and B-lymphoproliferative disorders, suggested that anti-IL-6 mAb treatment was well tolerated with no serious adverse effects. CRP levels were decreased in all patients and the incidence of cachexia declined.

Activation of NFκB causes profound muscle wasting in mice, resembling clinical cachexia.[79] Compared with placebo, an NFκB inhibitor, dehydroxymethylepoxyquinomicin, ameliorated the loss of body weight,[80] serum albumin and gastrocnemius muscle weight when administered to tumour-bearing mice but has not been tested in humans.

TNFα

TNFα inhibition with monoclonal antibodies appears to be ineffective as a single therapy for the treatment of cachexia in humans. Both etanercept and infliximab have been evaluated in placebo-controlled trials. The addition of infliximab[81] to gemcitabine for the treatment of pancreatic cancer did not improve lean body mass or quality-of-life scores compared with gemcitabine alone. A higher dose of infliximab did improve fatigue scores compared with a lower dose or placebo. A multicentre trial compared etanercept (25 mg s.c. twice weekly) to placebo in patients with solid tumours who had lost more than 5% of their ideal body weight. Weight gain and appetite improvement was minimal in both treatment arms and no patient gained ≥10% of their baseline weight.[82] Although the median survival was comparable, TNF inhibition continues to be explored for its potential antitumour effect. An earlier study showed that the combination of docetaxel and etanercept allowed for the maintenance of chemotherapy dose-intensity while reducing the incidence of fatigue.[83] Unfortunately no assessment of appetite or lean body mass was performed in this trial.

Anti-inflammatory cytokines

Anti-inflammatory cytokines such as IL-4, IL-10 and IL-12 may prove useful for cachexia therapy but have yet to be evaluated for this purpose in humans. Administration of IL-15[84] or IL-12 to animal models with cancer cachexia reduces skeletal muscle wasting by downregulating the ubiquitin–proteasome pathway. In a tumour model, murine IL-12 suppresses the induction of cancer cachexia[85] and also inhibits tumour growth.

Conclusion

Non-specific immune modulators such as thalidomide generate increased muscle mass in preliminary studies of patients with cancer cachexia. Melatonin and NSAIDs also show promise but their benefits need to be confirmed in larger placebo-controlled trials. Although IL-6 and TNF are thought to be important in the pathogenesis of cachexia, their usefulness as therapeutic targets in humans is not yet established.

References

1. Dubé C, Rostom A, Lewin G, *et al.* (2007) U.S. Preventive Services Task Force. The use of aspirin for primary prevention of colorectal cancer: a systematic review prepared for the U.S. Preventive Services Task Force. *Ann Intern Med*, **146**(5), 365–75.
2. Fortunati N, Manti R, Birocco N, *et al.* (2007) Pro-inflammatory cytokines and oxidative stress/antioxidant parameters characterize the bio-humoral profile of early cachexia in lung cancer patients. *Oncol Rep*, **18**(6), 1521–7.
3. Ebrahimi B, Tucker SL, Li D, Abbruzzese JL, Kurzrock R (2004) Cytokines in pancreatic carcinoma: correlation with phenotypic characteristics and prognosis *Cancer*, **101**(12), 2727–36.
4. Pfitzenmaier J, Vessella R, Higano CS, Noteboom JL, Wallace D Jr, Corey E (2003) Elevation of cytokine levels in cachectic patients with prostate carcinoma. *Cancer*, **97**(5), 1211–6.

5. Martin F, Santolaria F, Batista N, *et al.* (1999) Cytokine levels (IL-6 and IFN-gamma), acute phase response and nutritional status as prognostic factors in lung cancer. *Cytokine*, **11**(1), 80–6.
6. Maltoni M, Fabbri L, Nanni O, *et al.* (1997) Serum levels of tumour necrosis factor alpha and other cytokines do not correlate with weight loss and anorexia in cancer patients. *Support Care Cancer*, **5**(2), 130–5.
7. Kayacan O, Karnak D, Beder S, *et al.* (2006) Impact of TNF-alpha and IL-6 levels on development of cachexia in newly diagnosed NSCLC patients. *Am J Clin Oncol*, **29**(4), 328–35.
8. Shibata M, Nezu T, Kanou H, Abe H, Takekawa M, Fukuzawa M (2002) Decreased production of interleukin-12 and type 2 immune responses are marked in cachectic patients with colorectal and gastric cancer. *J Clin Gastroenterol*, **34**(4), 416–20.
9. Jatoi A, Egner J, Loprinzi CL, *et al.* (2004) Investigating the utility of serum cytokine measurements in a multi-institutional cancer anorexia/weight loss trial. *Support Care Cancer*, **12**(9), 640–4.
10. Falconer JS, Fearon KC, Plester CE, Ross JA, Carter DC (1994) Cytokines, the acute-phase response, and resting energy expenditure in cachectic patients with pancreatic cancer. *Ann Surg*, **219**(4), 325–31.
11. Garcia JM, Garcia-Touza M, Hijazi RA, *et al.* (2005) Active ghrelin levels and active to total ghrelin ratio in cancer-induced cachexia. *J Clin Endocrinol Metab*, **90**(5), 2920–6.
12. Tan BH, Deans DA, Skipworth RJ, Ross JA, Fearon KC (2008) Biomarkers for cancer cachexia: is there also a genetic component to cachexia? *Support Care Cancer*, **16**(3), 229–34.
13. Reiter RJ, Tan DX, Manchester LC, Terron M, Flores LJ Koppisepi S (2007) Medical implications of melatonin: receptor-mediated and receptor-independent actions. *Adv Med Sci*, **52**, 11–28.
14. Tan DX, Manchester LC, Terron M, Flores LJ, Reiter RJ (2006) One molecule, many derivatives: a never-ending interaction of melatonin with reactive oxygen and nitrogen species? *J Pin Res*, **42**(1), 28–42.
15. Bubenik GA (2006) Gastrointestinal melatonin: localization, function, and clinical relevance. *Dig Dis Sci*, **47**(10), 2336–48.
16. Ferreira AC, Martins E Jr, Afeche SC, Cipolla-Neto J, Costa Rosa LF (2004) The profile of melatonin production in tumour-bearing rats. *Life Sci*, **75**(19), 2291–302.
17. Raghavendra V, Kulkarni SK (2000) Melatonin reversal of DOI-induced hypophagia in rats; possible mechanism by suppressing 5-HT(2A) receptor-mediated activation of HPA axis. *Brain Res*, **860**(1–2), 112–8.
18. Motilva V, Cabeza J, Alarcón de la Lastra C (2002) New issues about melatonin and its effects on the digestive system. *Curr Pharm Des*, **7**(10), 909–31.
19. Oner J, Ozan E (2003) Effects of melatonin on skeletal muscle of rats with experimental hyperthyroidism. *Endocr Res*, **29**(4), 445–55.
20. Lissoni P, Paolorossi F, Tancini G, *et al.* (1996) Is there a role for melatonin in the treatment of neoplastic cachexia? *Eur J Cancer*, **8**, 1340–3.
21. Lissoni P (2002) Is there a role for melatonin in supportive care? *Support Care Cancer*, **10**(2), 110–6.
22. Berk L, Berkey B, Rich T (2007) Randomized phase II trial of high-dose melatonin and radiation therapy for RPA class 2 patients with brain metastases (RTOG 0119). *Int J Radiat Oncol Biol Phys*, **68**(3), 852–7.
23. Mills EJ, Wu P, Seely D, Guyatt G (2005) Melatonin in the treatment of cancer: a systematic review of randomized controlled trials and meta-analysis. *J Pineal Res*, **39**(4), 360–6.
24. Weishaupt JH, Bartels C, Pölking E (2006) Reduced oxidative damage in ALS by high-dose enteral melatonin treatment. *J Pineal Res*, **41**(4), 313–23.
25. Seabra MLV, Bignotto M, Pinto LR, *et al.* (2000) Randomized, double-blind clinical trial, controlled with placebo, of the toxicology of chronic melatonin treatment. *J Pineal Res*, **29**, 193–200.
26. Herxheimer A, Petrie KJ (2002) Melatonin for the prevention of jet lag. *Cochrane Database Syst Rev* (2).

27. Vijayalaxmi, Reiter RJ, Tan DX, *et al.* (2004) Melatonin as a radioprotective agent: a review. *Int J Radiat Oncol Biol Phys*, **59**, 639–53.

28. Watson M (2006) Harmful impact of EU clinical trials directive ... and so has trial of melatonin in cancer related weight loss .... *Br Med J*, **332**(7542), 666.

29. Davis TW, Zweifel BS, O'Neal JM (2004) Inhibition of cyclooxygenase-2 by celecoxib reverses tumor-induced wasting. *J Pharmacol Exp Ther*, **308**(3), 929–34.

30. Hitt A, Graves E, McCarthy DO (2005) Indomethacin preserves muscle mass and reduces levels of E3 ligases and TNF receptor type 1 in the gastrocnemius muscle of tumor-bearing mice. *Res Nurs Health*, **28**(1), 56–66.

31. Hussey HJ, Tisdale MJ (2000) Effect of the specific cyclooxygenase-2 inhibitor meloxicam on tumour growth and cachexia in a murine model. *Int J Cancer*, **87**(1), 95–100.

32. Lundholm K, Daneryd P, Körner U, Hyltander A, Bosaeus I (2004) Evidence that long-term COX-treatment improves energy homeostasis and body composition in cancer patients with progressive cachexia. *Int J Oncol*, **24**(3), 505–12.

33. Lai V, George J, Richey L *et al.* (2008) Results of a pilot study of the effects of celecoxib on cancer cachexia in patients with cancer of the head, neck, and gastrointestinal tract. *Head Neck*, **30**(1), 67–74.

34. McMillan DC, Wigmore SJ, Fearon KC (1999) A prospective randomized study of megestrol acetate and ibuprofen in gastrointestinal individual with cancers with weight loss. *Br J Cancer*, **79**(3–4), 495–500.

35. Wolfe M, Lichtenstein D, Singh G (1999) Gastrointestinal toxicity of nonsteroidal antiinflammatory drugs. *N Engl J Med*, **340**(24), 1888–99.

36. Knijff-Dutmer EA, Postma MJ, van der Palen J, Brouwers JR, van de Laar MA (2004) Incremental cost-effectiveness of cyclooxygenase 2-selective versus nonselective nonsteroidal anti-inflammatory drugs in a cohort of coumarin users: a pharmacoeconomic analysis linked to a case–control study. *Clin Ther*, **26**(7), 1160–7.

37. Schnitzer TJ, Burmester GR, Mysler E, *et al.* (2004) TARGET Study Group. Comparison of lumiracoxib with naproxen and ibuprofen in the Therapeutic Arthritis Research and Gastrointestinal Event Trial (TARGET), reduction in ulcer complications: randomised controlled trial. *Lancet*, **364**(9435), 665–74.

38. Drazen JM (2005) COX-2 inhibitors—a lesson in unexpected problems. *N Engl J Med*, **352**(11), 1131–2.

39. McGettigan P, Henry D (2006) Cardiovascular risk and inhibition of cyclooxygenase: a systematic review of the observational studies of selective and nonselective inhibitors of cyclooxygenase 2. *J Am Med Assoc*, **296**(13), 1633–44.

40. Kerr DJ, Dunn JA, Langman MJ, *et al.* (2007) Rofecoxib and cardiovascular adverse events in adjuvant treatment of colorectal cancer. *N Engl J Med*, **357**(4), 360–9.

41. Davis MP, Dickerson ED (2001) Thalidomide: dual benefits in palliative medicine and oncology. *Am J Hosp Palliat Care*, **18**(5), 347-51.

42. Franks ME, Macpherson GR, Figg WD (2004) Thalidomide. *Lancet*, **363**(9423), 1802–11.

43. Liu KH, Liao LM, Ro LS, Wu YL, Yeh TS (2008) Thalidomide attenuates tumor growth and preserves fast-twitch skeletal muscle fibers in cholangiocarcinoma rats. *Surgery*, **143**(3), 375–83.

44. Jacobson JM, Greenspan JS, Spritzler J, *et al.* (1997) Thalidomide for the treatment of oral aphthous ulcers in patients with HIV infection. *N Engl J Med*, **22**(336), 1487–93.

45. Kaplan G, Thomas S, Fierer DS, *et al.* (2000) Thalidomide for the treatment of AIDS-associated wasting. *AIDS Res Hum Retroviruses*, **16**, 1345–55.

46. Tramontana JM, Utaipat U, Molloy A, *et al.* (1995) Thalidomide treatment reduces tumor necrosis factor alpha production and enhances weight gain in patients with pulmonary tuberculosis. *Mol Med*, **1**, 384–97.

47. Bruera E, Neumann CM, Pituskin E, *et al.* (1999) Thalidomide in patients with cachexia due to terminal cancer: preliminary report. *Ann Oncol*, **10**, 857–9.
48. Kedar I, Mermershtain W, Ivgi H (2004) Thalidomide reduces serum C-reactive protein and interleukin-6 and induces response to IL-2 in a fraction of metastatic renal cell cancer patients who failed IL-2-based therapy. *Int J Cancer*, **110**(2), 260–5.
49. Khan ZH, Simpson EJ, Cole AT (2003) Oesophageal cancer and cachexia:the effect of short-term treatment with thalidomide on weight loss and lean body mass. *Aliment Pharmacol Ther*, **17**, 677–82.
50. Gordon JN, Trebble TM, Ellis RD, *et al.* (2005) Thalidomide in the treatment of cancer cachexia: a randomized placebo controlled trial. *Gut*, **54**, 540–5.
51. Mantovani G, Macciò A, Madeddu C, *et al.* (2008) Randomized phase III clinical trial of five different arms of treatment for patients with cancer cachexia: interim results. *Nutrition*, **24**(4), 305–13.
52. Jones NE, Heyland DK (2008) Pharmaconutrition: a new emerging paradigm. *Curr Opin Gastroenterol*, **24**(2), 215–22.
53. Casas-Rodera P, Gómez-Candela C, Benítez S, *et al.* (2008) Immunoenhanced enteral nutrition formulas in head and neck cancer surgery: a prospective, randomized clinical trial. *Nutr Hosp*, **23**(2), 105–10.
54. Takeuchi H, Ikeuchi S, Kawaguchi Y, *et al.* (2007) Clinical significance of perioperative immunonutrition for patients with esophageal cancer. *World J Surg*, **31**(11), 2160–7.
55. Gianotti L, Braga M, Nespoli L, Radaelli G, Beneduce A, Di Carlo V (2002) A randomized controlled trial of preoperative oral supplementation with a specialized diet in patients with gastrointestinal cancer. *Gastroenterology*, **122**(7), 1763–70.
56. Braga M, Gianotti L, Nespoli L, Radaelli G, Di Carlo V (2002) Nutritional approach in malnourished surgical patients: a prospective randomized study. *Arch Surg*, **137**(2), 174–80.
57. Klek S, Kulig J, Sierzega M, *et al.* (2008) The impact of immunostimulating nutrition on infectious complications after upper gastrointestinal surgery: a prospective, randomized, clinical trial. *Ann Surg*, **248**(2), 212–20.
58. Stableforth WD, Thomas S, Lewis SJ (2009) A systematic review of the role of immunonutrition in patients undergoing surgery for head and neck cancer. *Int J Oral Maxillofac Surg*, **38**(2), 103–10.
59. Senesse P, Assenat E, Schneider S, *et al.* (2008) Nutritional support during oncologic treatment of patients with gastrointestinal cancer: who could benefit? *Cancer Treat Rev*, **34**(6), 568–75.
60. Hall MN, Chavarro JE, Lee IM, Willett WC, Ma J (2008) A 22-year prospective study of fish, n-3 fatty acid intake, and colorectal cancer risk in men. *Cancer Epidemiol Biomarkers Prev*, **17**(5), 1136–43.
61. Daniel CR, McCullough ML, Patel RC, *et al.* (2008) Dietary intake of ω-6 and ω-3 fatty acids and risk of colorectal cancer in a prospective cohort of U.S. men and women. *Cancer Epidemiol Biomarkers Prev*, **18**(2),516–25.
62. Wigmore SJ, Barber MD, Ross JA, Tisdale MJ, Fearon KC (2000) Effect of oral eicosapentaenoic acid on weight loss in patients with pancreatic cancer. *Nutr Cancer*, **36**,177–184.
63. Burns CP, Halabi S, Clamon G, *et al.* (2004) Phase II study of high-dose fish oil capsules for patients with cancer-related cachexia. *Cancer*, **101**(2), 370–8.
64. Fearon KC, Barber MD, Moses AG, *et al.* (2006) Double-blind, placebo-controlled, randomized study of eicosapentaenoic acid diester in patients with cancer cachexia. *J Clin Oncol*, **24**(21), 3401–7.
65. Dewey A, Baughan C, Dean T, Higgins B, Johnson E (2007) Eicosapentaenoic acid (EPA, an omega-3 fatty acid from fish oils) for the treatment of cancer cachexia. *Cochrane Database Syst Rev*, **24**(1)
66. Elia M, Van Bokhorst-de van der Schueren MA, Garvey J, *et al.* (2006) Enteral (oral or tube administration) nutritional support and eicosapentaenoic acid in patients with cancer: a systematic review. *Int J Oncol*, **28**(1), 5–23.
67. Colomer R, Moreno-Nogueira J, García-Luna P, *et al.* (2007) n-3 Fatty acids, cancer and cachexia: a systematic review of the literature. *Br J Nutr*, **97**, 823–31.

68. Faber J, Vos P, Kegler D, *et al.* (2008) Beneficial immune modulatory effects of a specific nutritional combination in a murine model for cancer cachexia. *Br J Cancer*, **99**(12), 2029–36.
69. Cerchietti LC, Navigante AH, Castro MA (2006) Effects of eicosapentaenoic and docosahexaenoic n-3 fatty acids from fish oil and preferential Cox-2 inhibition on systemic syndromes in patients with advanced lung cancer. *Nutr Cancer*, **59**(1), 14–20.
70. Vissers YL, Dejong CH, Luiking YC, Fearon KC, von Meyenfeldt MF, Deutz NE (2006) Plasma arginine concentrations are reduced in cancer patients: evidence for arginine deficiency? *Am J Clin Nutr*, **81**(5), 1142–6.
71. Nanthakumaran S, Brown I, Heys SD, Schofield AC (2009) Inhibition of gastric cancer cell growth by arginine: molecular mechanisms of action. *Clin Nutr*, **28**(1), 65–70.
72. Ogilvie GK, Fettman MJ, Mallinckrodt CH, *et al.* (2000) Effect of fish oil, arginine, and doxorubicin chemotherapy on remission and survival time for dogs with lymphoma: a double-blind, randomized placebo-controlled study. *Cancer*, **88**(8), 1916–28.
73. Kaufmann Y, Spring P, Klimberg VS (2008) Oral glutamine prevents DMBA-induced mammary carcinogenesis via upregulation of glutathione production. *Nutrition*, **24**(5), 462-9.
74. Sacks GS (1999) Glutamine supplementation in catabolic patients. *Ann Pharmacother*, **33** (1999), 348–354.
75. Yoshida S, Kaibara A, Ishibashi N, Shirouzu K (2001) Glutamine supplementation in cancer patients. *Nutrition*, **17**(9), 766–8.
76. Dhillon N, Aggarwal BB, Newman RA, *et al.* (2008) Phase II trial of curcumin in patients with advanced pancreatic cancer. *Clin Cancer Res*, **14**(14), 4491–9.
77. Busquets S, Carbó N, Almendro V, Quiles MT, López-Soriano FJ, Argilés JM (2001) Curcumin, a natural product present in turmeric, decreases tumor growth but does not behave as an anticachectic compound in a rat model. *Cancer Lett*, **167**(1), 33–8.
78. Zaki MH, Nemeth JA, Trikha M (2004) CNTO 328, a monoclonal antibody to IL-6, inhibits human tumor-induced cachexia in nude mice. *Int J Cancer*, **111**(4), 592–5.
79. Trikha M, Corringham R, Klein B, Rossi JF (2003) Targeted anti-interleukin-6 monoclonal antibody therapy for cancer: a review of the rationale and clinical evidence. *Clin Cancer Res*, **9**(13), 4653–65.
80. Cai D, Frantz JD, Tawa NE, *et al.* (2004) IKKbeta/NF-kappaB activation causes severe muscle wasting in mice. *Cell*, **119**(2), 285–98.
81. Kuroda K, Horiguchi Y, Nakashima J, *et al.* (2004) Prevention of cancer cachexia by a novel nuclear factor κB inhibitor in prostate cancer. *Clin Cancer Res*, **11**(15), 5590–4.
82. Wiedenmann B, Malfertheiner P, Friess H, *et al.* (2008) A multicenter, phase II study of infliximab plus gemcitabine in pancreatic cancer cachexia. *J Support Oncol*, **6**(1), 18–25.
83. Jatoi A, Dakhil SR, Nguyen PL, *et al.* (2007) A placebo-controlled double blind trial of etanercept for the cancer anorexia/weight loss syndrome: results from N00C1 from the North Central Cancer Treatment Group. *Cancer*, **110**(6), 1396–403.
84. Monk JP, Phillips G, Waite R, *et al.* (2006) Assessment of tumor necrosis factor alpha blockade as an intervention to improve tolerability of dose-intensive chemotherapy in cancer patients. *J Clin Oncol*, **24**(12), 1852–9.
85. Argilés JM, Busquets S, López-Soriano FJ (2005) The pivotal role of cytokines in muscle wasting during cancer. *Int J Biochem Cell Biol*, **37**(10), 2036–46.
86. Mori K, Fujimoto-Ouchi K, Ishikawa T, Sekiguchi F, Ishitsuka H, Tanaka Y (1996) Murine interleukin-12 prevents the development of cancer cachexia in a murine model. *Int J Cancer*, **67**(6), 849–55.

Chapter 10

Autonomic system modulators

Nada Fadul

Introduction

The autonomic nervous system (ANS) innervates all major internal organs. Autonomic nervous dysfunction is common in patients with advanced cancer. There is ample evidence to support the role of the ANS in symptom production, and even survival in non-cancer populations such as diabetes mellitus and heart failure. The impact of the ANS on disorders such as fatigue and cachexia is less certain. This chapter discusses the role of the ANS and its modulation of cancer cachexia as well as evidence generated from other patient populations.

The ANS regulates involuntary internal organ functions and maintains homeostasis via the sympathetic and parasympathetic nervous systems.[1] The sympathetic system is responsible for energy consumption during stress,[2] originates from the thoracolumbar ganglia and its effects are mediated by the neurotransmitter norepinephrine. The parasympathetic system on the other hand originates from the craniosacral ganglia and is responsible for energy production, e.g. from digestion.[3] Acetylcholine is the preganglionic neurotransmitter for both divisions of the ANS, the postganglionic neurotransmitter of the parasympathetic neurons and the neurotransmitter for the sudomotor functions of the sympathetic nervous system.[4]

Autonomic failure in patients with advanced cancer

Autonomic dysfunction (AD) is a common problem affecting the majority of patients with advanced cancer.[5,6] Despite its high incidence, AD is among the least recognized and understood complications of cancer. There is evidence AD has a negative impact on survival and quality of life in diabetes[7] and may be associated with poor quality of life and increased inflammation in cancer patients. AD is characterized by unbalanced cholinergic and/or noradrenergic output to the periphery, and can involve the entire ANS with dysfunction of one or more organ systems (e.g. cardiovascular, gastrointestinal, genitourinary, sudomotor, or ocular). ANS vasomotor, visceromotor, and sensory fibres innervate every organ in the body including many organs that are dually innervated, receiving fibres from the parasympathetic and sympathetic divisions of the ANS.

The reported incidence of AD in patients with advanced cancer exceeds 80%.[5] A study of 50 patients with advanced cancer evaluated autonomic function using five bedside cardiovascular tests, and found evidence of AD in all participants. Only 35% of the cardiovascular reflex tests performed were normal or borderline normal. AD was first described in patients with bronchogenic carcinoma but can occur in other primary malignancies including lymphoma, leukaemia, and pancreatic, prostatic, breast, ovarian, and testicular carcinomas.

The aetiology of AD in cancer patients can be multifactorial[8] including local invasion of the vagus nerve by tumour,[9] proinflammatory cytokines (e.g. interleukin-1 and tumor necrosis factor-α),[10] chemotherapies (especially platinum, paclitaxel and vinca alkaloids),[11,12] radiation therapy,[13] and cachexia.

Paraneoplastic autonomic dysfunction is a distinct syndrome described in cancer. This autoimmune-mediated disorder is associated with paraneoplastic onconeural autoantibodies such as anti-Hu antibodies. The syndrome typically presents as chronic gastrointestinal pseudo-obstruction or orthostatic hypotension and usually occurs in association with other paraneoplastic syndromes. The most commonly associated tumours are small cell lung cancer, ovarian, and thymomas. At the onset of the neurological syndrome, the primary tumour is often undetectable or at early stages of development.

Role of autonomic dysfunction in cachexia in cancer patients

Autonomic dysfunction has been implicated in the pathogenesis of cachexia in cancer patients and other populations. The exact mechanism by which autonomic dysfunction might lead to cachexia is not yet fully understood but several hypotheses are proposed. Disturbances in the parasympathetic division of the ANS are associated with gastrointestinal dysmotility, gastroparesis and chronic constipation. They are all known to be factors contributing to the anorexia–cachexia syndrome. In addition, recent evidence has linked the vagus nerve to the regulation of inflammatory cytokines. Vagal dysfunction may therefore contribute to a proinflammatory state, thought to be a major mechanism producing cachexia. There is also increased adrenergic transmission and activation of the sympathetic nervous system in advanced cancer which encourages an elevated basal metabolic rate and weight loss. Other mechanisms include the mediation of leptin effects.[14] In the next section we will describe the different mechanisms though which ANS dysfunction can contribute to cachexia, and the evidence for using ANS modulators.

Disorders of cholinergic transmission

Gastrointestinal dysmotility

Gastroparesis is a common syndrome in cancer patients and characterized by delayed gastric emptying in the absence of mechanical obstruction.[15] Symptoms of gastroparesis include chronic nausea, anorexia, early satiety and abdominal bloating. Although many patients present with this symptom cluster, the symptoms can also occur individually. Gastroparesis can contribute to cachexia in cancer patients through decreased food intake, nausea, and food aversion.

There is good evidence to suggest a role for autonomic dysfunction and gastroparesis in the gastrointestinal symptoms of advanced cancer. A study comparing healthy volunteers to patients with advanced cancer experiencing unexplained chronic nausea found clinical and electrographic evidence of autonomic dysfunction in 16 out of 23 cancer patients and none in the healthy subjects.[1] Patients with unexplained nausea and anorexia had significantly delayed gastric emptying compared to healthy subjects.[9] Radiographic evidence of reduced upper gastrointestinal motility is present in patients with advanced cancer and can be improved by a metoclopramide infusion.[16] Delayed gastric emptying is also detected in up to 80% of patients with pancreatic cancer and associated with a high prevalence of symptoms.[17] These findings suggest that visceral autonomic disturbances lead to gastric dysmotility and symptoms associated with the anorexia–cachexia syndrome. The management of gastroparesis in patients with cancer cachexia is beyond the scope of this chapter and is discussed in chapter 15.

Cholinergic anti-inflammatory pathway

In addition to controlling internal visceral organ function, recent evidence suggests an important role for the vagus nerve in regulating systemic inflammation. A 'cholinergic anti-inflammatory pathway' exists involving higher brain structures, including the hypothalamus, brain nuclei and neural networks, which are associated with the generation of brain-derived anti-inflammatory output through the nucleus tractus solitarius, and efferent vagus nerve.[18] Stimulation of the efferent vagus nerve activates the release of acetylcholine (ACh), which binds nicotinic cholinergic receptors (α7nAChR) on resident macrophages, and inhibits the synthesis of tumour necrosis factor (TNF)-α at a post-transcriptional level.[19] Vagus nerve stimulation also inhibits production of interleukin (IL)-1, IL-8 and high mobility group box (HMGB)-1.[20] Pharmacological and electrical stimulation of the vagus nerve releases ACh which enables binding to α7nAChR. This receptor–ligand interaction then inhibits nuclear factor kappa B (NFκB) translocation to the nucleus, thereby decreasing proinflammatory cytokine production. NFκB is a key transcription factor for the synthesis of TNF and other cytokines. Vagus nerve signalling modulates cytokine production, and improves disease endpoints in experimental models of sepsis, ischaemia, haemorrhagic shock, myocardial ischaemia, ileus, experimental arthritis, and pancreatitis.[21–23]

The data support the role of the ANS in regulation of systemic inflammation both in the acute and chronic states. Modalities that augment cholinergic transmission and α7nAChR agonists might have a therapeutic application in patients with cancer-related cachexia. Anti-inflammatory agents that specifically target the cholinergic anti-inflammatory system, for example semapimod,[24] have shown promise in conditions such as Crohn's disease and collagen-induced arthritis. A phase I study demonstrating the safety of the compound is completed in patients with melanoma and renal cell cancer and phase II trials for psoriasis and Crohn's disease are ongoing. Currently, preclinical and early clinical studies are underway for a variety of indications, including congestive heart failure and pancreatitis.[25]

Disorders of adrenergic transmission

The sympathetic nervous system regulates lipid metabolism and energy consumption. High muscle sympathetic nerve activity contributes to lipid peroxidation and a reduced tendency to gain weight.[26] In addition, precedents from congestive heart failure and other diseases characterized by sympathetic activation show a close relationship between sympathetic activation and systemic inflammation.[27]

Sympathetic overactivity and lipid oxidation

Several studies suggest that sympathetic nervous system activity has an effect on the lipid oxidation rate. Administration of the β_2-adrenergic agonist terbutaline for 2 weeks in non-cancer patients causes an increase in lipid oxidation, whereas administration of the β-antagonist propranolol caused a decrease in lipid oxidation.[28] Norepinephrine infusion increases whole-body oxygen consumption by almost 10%, the rate of muscle uptake of non-esterified fatty acids and β-hydroxybutyrate several-fold, and the activity of the triglyceride–fatty acid cycle increases 4-fold after norepinephrine administration.[29] The evidence for a stimulatory effect of the sympathetic nervous system on lipid oxidation[30] and the relationship between lipid oxidation and weight loss suggest that lipid oxidation may contribute to the higher rates of weight loss in individuals with high sympathetic nervous system activity.

Adrenoreceptors modulate fat and skeletal muscle

β-Adrenoreceptor agonists

β-Adrenoceptors play an important regulatory role in cardiovascular, respiratory, metabolic, and reproductive function. Three subtypes of β-adrenoceptors have been identified and cloned: β_1-, β_2-, and β_3-adrenoceptors. Although the role of β-adrenoceptor signalling in cardiovascular function is well documented, their anabolic effect on skeletal muscle has been identified more recently. Skeletal muscle contains a significant proportion of β-adrenoceptors, which are mostly of the β_2-subtype, but 7–10% are β_1-adrenoceptors.

The effects of β-adrenoceptors on skeletal muscles are mediated through the phosphoinositide-3 kinase (PI3K)–AKT pathway. The PI3K–AKT signalling pathway is implicated in protein synthesis, gene transcription, cell proliferation, and cell survival.[31] Stimulation of the β-adrenoceptor signalling pathway results in AKT phosphorylation and subsequent activation of the mammalian target of rapamycin (mTOR).[32] Although there are three distinct isoforms of AKT, the predominant skeletal muscle isoform is AKT1.[33] Multiple skeletal muscle AKT1 pathways are activated following β-adrenoceptor stimulation, and these lead predominantly to skeletal muscle hypertrophy.

β-Adrenoceptor agonists (β-agonists) are traditionally used for the treatment of bronchial asthma. In the past two decades research has revealed β-agonists also have the ability to increase skeletal muscle mass and decrease body fat, the so-called 'repartitioning effect'.[34] This combination of muscle hypertrophy and decreased body fat is desirable in the livestock industry for improving feed efficiency and meat quality.[35] Because of their potent muscle anabolic actions, the effects of β-agonist administration have been examined in animal models and humans in the hope of discovering a new therapeutic strategy for cachexia.[36,37] β-Agonists also are able to enhance muscle repair and restore muscle function after injury or following reconstructive surgery. Moreover, β-agonists have been used by athletes to increase muscle strength.[38]

Clenbuterol and fenoterol are powerful muscle anabolic agents when used in animal studies at relatively high doses. They are not as potent when used at therapeutic doses for treating bronchial asthma.[39] In addition to their anabolic effect, these agents exert a powerful lipolytic effect secondary to their thermogenic properties.[40]

Although studies show beneficial effects of β-agonists, they are inconsistent. Clenbuterol administered to tumour-bearing adult mice did not improve body composition, whereas growing animals had increased quadriceps muscle mass and increased food intake.[41] A newer generation β-agonist, formoterol, reversed muscle wasting in tumour-bearing rats through increased protein synthesis and inhibition of muscle proteolysis.[42] Although chronic heart failure patients treated with salbutamol for 3 weeks demonstrated no improvement in quadriceps muscle mass, or strength, their respiratory muscle strength increased and side-effects were similar to placebo.[43] The potency of salbutamol (less than clenbuterol) or the fairly low dose used in the study may explain the relative lack of anabolic effect. At higher doses β-agonists could produce undesirable side-effects, including increased heart rate (tachycardia) and muscle tremor, thereby limiting their therapeutic potential.

β-Blockers

β-Blockers may be effective treatment for cardiovascular autonomic dysfunction in non-cancer patients, and improve gastrointestinal[44] tract dysfunction in animal models. TNF injected into rats increases sympathetic outflow to brown adipose tissue, resulting in elevated temperatures and oxygen consumption. These effects are inhibited by administration of propranolol.[45]

A few clinical studies in cancer patients and in non-cancer conditions such as congestive heart failure (CHF) and burns suggest a potential role for β-blockers

A pilot study indicated that β-blockers increase total body-fat content in patients with CHF and weight loss,[46] possibly by modulating sympathetic activity. Severe burns produce a hypermetabolic response with increased energy expenditure, release of substrate from protein and fat stores and persistent muscle proteolysis for many months. Propranolol given to children with severe burns[47] reverses muscle catabolism, attenuates the hypermetabolic state and decreases proinflammatory cytokines.[48] Both atenolol and propranolol decrease resting energy expenditure (REE) in patients with solid tumours[49] who experience cachexia. A 6-day administration of propranolol to elderly cancer patients with an elevated REE rectified the AD and promoted a decline in REE.[50]

β-Blockers exhibit the potential for modulating several important aspects of neurohormonal dysfunction in advanced cancer, including sympathetic activation, elevated REE, and proinflammatory cytokine production. Paradoxically, β-agonists may also prove to be useful for increasing lean body mass in certain cachectic patients. Some patients may derive greater benefit from the antihypermetabolic effects of β-blockers whereas others may respond more readily to the β-agonist-induced anabolic effects on skeletal muscle. More clinical trials are needed to identify the patient characteristics that would predict a response to either of these interventions.

References

1. Bruera E, Chadwick S, Fox R, Hanson J, MacDonald N (1986) Study of cardiovascular autonomic insufficiency in advanced cancer patients. *Cancer Treat Rep*, **70**(12), 1383–7.
2. Kamath MV, Halton J, Harvey A, Turner-Gomes S, McArthur A, Barr RD (1998) Cardiac autonomic dysfunction in survivors of acute lymphoblastic leukemia in childhood. *Int J Oncol*, **12**(3),635–40.
3. Morrow GR, Angel C, Dubeshter B (1992) Autonomic changes during cancer chemotherapy induced nausea and emesis. *Br J Cancer Suppl*, **19**, S42–5.
4. Mousa AR, Al-Din AN (1985) Neurological and cardiac complications of carcinoma of the breast. Case report. *Acta Neurol Scand*, **72**(5), 518–21.
5. Strasser F, Palmer JL, Schover LR, *et al.* (2006) The impact of hypogonadism and autonomic dysfunction on fatigue, emotional function, and sexual desire in male patients with advanced cancer: a pilot study. *Cancer*, **107**(12), 2949–57.
6. Walsh D, Nelson KA (2002) Autonomic nervous system dysfunction in advanced cancer. *Support Care Cancer*, **10**(7), 523–8.
7. Low PA, Benrud-Larson LM, Sletten DM, *et al.* (2004) Autonomic symptoms and diabetic neuropathy: a population-based study. *Diabetes Care*, **27**(12), 2942–7.
8. Nelson K, Walsh D, Sheehan F (2002) Cancer and chemotherapy-related upper gastrointestinal symptoms: the role of abnormal gastric motor function and its evaluation in cancer patients. *Support Care Cancer*, **10**(6), 455–61.
9. Thomas WE, Fletcher MS. Neoplastic autovagotomy causing gastric stasis (1979). *Postgrad Med J*, **55**(644), 411–6.
10. Emch GS, Hermann GE, Rogers RC (2002) Tumor necrosis factor-alpha inhibits physiologically identified dorsal motor nucleus neurons in vivo. *Brain Res*, **951**(2), 311–5.
11. Quasthoff S, Hartung HP (2002) Chemotherapy-induced peripheral neuropathy. *J Neurol*, **249**(1), 9–17.
12. Roca E, Bruera E, Politi PM, *et al.* (1985) Vinca alkaloid-induced cardiovascular autonomic neuropathy. *Cancer Treat Rep*, **69**(2), 149–51.
13. Adams MJ, Lipsitz SR, Colan SD, *et al.* (2004) Cardiovascular status in long-term survivors of Hodgkin's disease treated with chest radiotherapy. *J Clin Oncol*, **22**(15), 3139–48.
14. Takabatake N, Nakamura H, Minamihaba O, *et al.* (2001) A novel pathophysiologic phenomenon in cachexic patients with chronic obstructive pulmonary disease: the relationship between the circadian rhythm of circulating leptin and the very low-frequency component of heart rate variability. *Am J Resp Crit Care Med*, **163**(6), 1314–9.
15. Kassander P (1958) Asymptomatic gastric retention in diabetics (gastroparesis diabeticorum). *Ann Intern Med*, **48**(4), 797–812.
16. Nelson KA, Walsh TD, Sheehan FG, O'Donovan PB, Falk GW (1993) Assessment of upper gastrointestinal motility in the cancer-associated dyspepsia syndrome. *J Palliat Care*, **9**(1), 27–31.

17. Shivshanker K, Bennett RW Jr, Haynie TP (1983) Tumor-associated gastroparesis: correction with metoclopramide. *Am J Surg*, **145**(2), 221–5.
18. Tracey KJ (2004) Physiology and immunology of the cholinergic antiinflammatory pathway. *J Clin Invest*, **117**(2), 289–96.
19. Borovikova LV, Ivanova S, Zhang M, *et al.* (2000) Vagus nerve stimulation attenuates the systemic inflammatory response to endotoxin. *Nature*, **405** (6785), 458–62.
20. Wang H, Liao H, Ochani M, *et al.* (2004) Cholinergic agonists inhibit HMGB1 release and improve survival in experimental sepsis. *Nat Med*, **10**(11), 1216–21.
21. Altavilla D, Guarini S, Bitto A, *et al.* (2006) Activation of the cholinergic anti-inflammatory pathway reduces NF-kappab activation, blunts TNF-alpha production, and protects againts splanchic artery occlusion shock. *Shock*, **25**(5), 500–6.
22. Mioni C, Bazzani C, Giuliani D, *et al.* (2005) Activation of an efferent cholinergic pathway produces strong protection against myocardial ischemia/reperfusion injury in rats. *Crit Care Med*, **33**(11), 2621–8.
23. van Westerloo DJ, Giebelen IA, Florquin S, *et al.* (2006) The vagus nerve and nicotinic receptors modulate experimental pancreatitis severity in mice. *Gastroenterology*, **130**(6),1822–30.
24. Bernik TR, Friedman SG, Ochani M, *et al.* (2002) Pharmacological stimulation of the cholinergic anti-inflammatory pathway. *J Exp Med*, **195**(6), 781–8.
25. Sitaraman SV, Hoteit M, Gewirtz AT (2003) Semapimod. Cytokine. *Curr Opin Invest Drugs*, **4**(11), 1363–8.
26. Snitker S, Tataranni PA, Ravussin E (1998) Respiratory quotient is inversely associated with muscle sympathetic nerve activity. *J Clin Endocrinol Metab*, **83**(11), 3977–9.
27. Anker SD, Coats AJ (1999) Cardiac cachexia: a syndrome with impaired survival and immune and neuroendocrine activation. *Chest*, **115**(3), 836–47.
28. Acheson KJ, Ravussin E, Schoeller DA, *et al.* (1988) Two-week stimulation or blockade of the sympathetic nervous system in man: influence on body weight, body composition, and twenty four-hour energy expenditure. *Metabolism*, **37**(1), 91–8.
29. Kurpad AV, Khan K, Calder AG, Elia M (1994) Muscle and whole body metabolism after norepinephrine. *Am J Physiol*, **266**(6 Pt 1), 877–84.
30. Tataranni PA, Young JB, Bogardus C, Ravussin E (1997) A low sympathoadrenal activity is associated with body weight gain and development of central adiposity in Pima Indian men. *Obes Res*, **5**(4), 341–7.
31. Bodine SC, Stitt TN, Gonzalez M, *et al.* (2001) Akt/mTOR pathway is a crucial regulator of skeletal muscle hypertrophy and can prevent muscle atrophy in vivo. *Nature Cell Biol*, **3**(11), 1014–9.
32. Kline WO, Panaro FJ, Yang H, Bodine SC (2007) Rapamycin inhibits the growth and muscle-sparing effects of clenbuterol. *J Appl Physiol*, **102**(2), 740–7.
33. Nader GA (2005) Molecular determinants of skeletal muscle mass: getting the “AKT” together. *Int J Biochem Cell Biol*, **37**(10), 1985–96.
34. Emery PW, Rothwell NJ, Stock MJ, Winter PD (1984) Chronic effects of beta 2-adrenergic agonists on body composition and protein synthesis in the rat. *Biosci Rep*, **4**(1), 83–91.
35. Sillence MN (2004) Technologies for the control of fat and lean deposition in livestock. *Vet J*, **167**(3), 242–57.
36. Carter WJ, Dang AQ, Faas FH, Lynch ME (1991) Effects of clenbuterol on skeletal muscle mass, body composition, and recovery from surgical stress in senescent rats. *Metabolism*, **40**(8), 855–60.
37. Maltin CA, Delday MI, Watson JS, *et al.* (1993) Clenbuterol, a beta-adrenoceptor agonist, increases relative muscle strength in orthopaedic patients. *Clin Sci (Lond)*, **84**(6), 651–4.
38. Prather ID, Brown DE, North P, Wilson JR (1998) Clenbuterol: a substitute for anabolic steroids? *Med Sci Sports Exerc*, **27**(8), 1118–21.

39. Malinowski K, Kearns CF, Guirnalda PD, Roegner V, McKeever KH (2004) Effect of chronic clenbuterol administration and exercise training on immune function in horses. *J Anim Sci*, **82**(12), 3500–7.

40. Arch JR, Kaumann AJ (1993) Beta 3 and atypical beta-adrenoceptors. *Med Res Rev*, **13**(6), 663–729.

41. Hyltander A, Svaninger G, Lundholm K (1993) The effect of clenbuterol on body composition in spontaneously eating tumour-bearing mice. *Biosci Rep*, **13**(6), 325–31.

42. Busquets S, Figueras MT, Fuster G, *et al.* (2004) Anticachectic effects of formoterol: a drug for potential treatment of muscle wasting. *Cancer Res*, **64**(18), 6725–31.

43. Harrington D, Chua TP, Coats AJ (2000) The effect of salbutamol on skeletal muscle in chronic heart failure. *Int J Cardiol*, **3**, 257–65.

44. Taha MO, Fraga MM, Guimaraes FA, Jurkiewicz A, Caricati-Neto A (2006) Atenolol attenuates autonomic dysfunction of rat jejunum. *Transplant Proc*, **38**(6), 1784–8.

45. Coombes RC, Rothwell NJ, Shah P, Stock MJ (1987) Changes in thermogenesis and brown fat activity in response to tumour necrosis factor in the rat. *Biosci Rep*, **7**(10), 791–9.

46. Lainscak M, Keber I, Anker SD (2006) Body composition changes in patients with systolic heart failure treated with beta-blockers: a pilot study. *Int J Cardiol*, **106**(3), 319–22.

47. Herndon DN, Hart DW, Wolf SE, Chinkes DL, Wolfe RR (2001) Reversal of catabolism by beta-blockade after severe burns. *N Engl J Med*, **345**(17), 1223–9.

48. Jeschke MG, Finnerty CC, Kulp GA, Przkora R, Mlcak RP, Herndon DN (2008) Combination of recombinant human growth hormone and propranolol decreases hypermetabolism and inflammation in severely burned children. *Pediatr Crit Care Med*, **9**(2), 209–16.

49. Hyltander A, Daneryd P, Sandstrom R, Korner U, Lundholm K (2002) Beta-adrenoceptor activity and resting energy metabolism in weight losing cancer patients. *Eur J Cancer*, **36**(3), 330–4.

50. Gambardella A, Tortoriello R, Pesce L, Tagliamonte MR, Paolisso G, Varricchio M (1999) Intralipid infusion combined with propranolol administration has favorable metabolic effects in elderly malnourished cancer patients. *Metabolism*, **48**(3), 291–7.

Chapter 11

Multimodality therapy

Egidio Del Fabbro

Introduction

Cachexia is characterized by involuntary weight loss, regardless of caloric intake. An aberrant inflammatory response due to a tumour–host interaction is probably the dominant mechanism impairing synthesis and increasing degradation of muscle and fat. In addition to the peripheral cytokine-mediated catabolic effects, neurohormonal dysfunction leads to ghrelin, testosterone and cortisol abnormalities, sympathetic activation, and altered hypothalamic sensitivity to orexigenic and anorexigenic peptides.

Moreover, the loss of appetite experienced by many patients can be exacerbated by symptoms such as severe pain, early satiety and depression.

A better understanding of these complex mechanisms has inspired several multimodality treatment strategies for the cancer anorexia–cachexia syndrome (CACS). Past efforts to treat cachexia with nutritional or medical interventions may have failed because they were directed at appetite stimulation alone (usually with a single therapeutic agent), and were not accompanied by therapy to reverse the underlying catabolic process. A more effective approach might be comprehensive multifaceted therapy targeting different pathophysiological mechanisms simultaneously. A theoretical model of multimodal therapy for cachexia is shown in Figure 11.1. Although there may be debate about the composition or relative importance of these interventions, the model illustrates the rationale for multimodality treatment.

Personalized multimodal model

The treatment goal for most patients is to maintain physical function and independence. For some individuals, the psychosocial aspects of the CACS such as altered body image and the inability to enjoy meals with family members may carry greater importance. Depending on these individual variations in patient goals, treatment plans should be tailored appropriately.

Ideally, the treatment should also be modified to target the pathophysiology affecting individual patients, since the contribution of the different mechanisms of cachexia may vary. For example, not all patients have an elevated resting energy expenditure (some may be hypo- or eumetabolic), and for many with cancer cachexia, poor appetite is a common, but not universal symptom. Currently, laboratory tests such as C-reactive protein (CRP) and testosterone identify those patients with a proinflammatory state or hypogonadism, respectively, while resting energy expenditure (REE) can be measured by bedside indirect calorimetry. Specific interventions that are used in response to these markers include non-steroidal anti-inflammatory drugs (NSAIDs) for an elevated CRP >10 mg/l, beta-blockers for elevated REE, and testosterone replacement for hypogonadic males. Note, however, that there is only preliminary evidence that these medications are effective for cancer cachexia. Additional clinical and biological markers are needed to better identify individuals who may respond to specific interventions. Biomarkers for cachexia

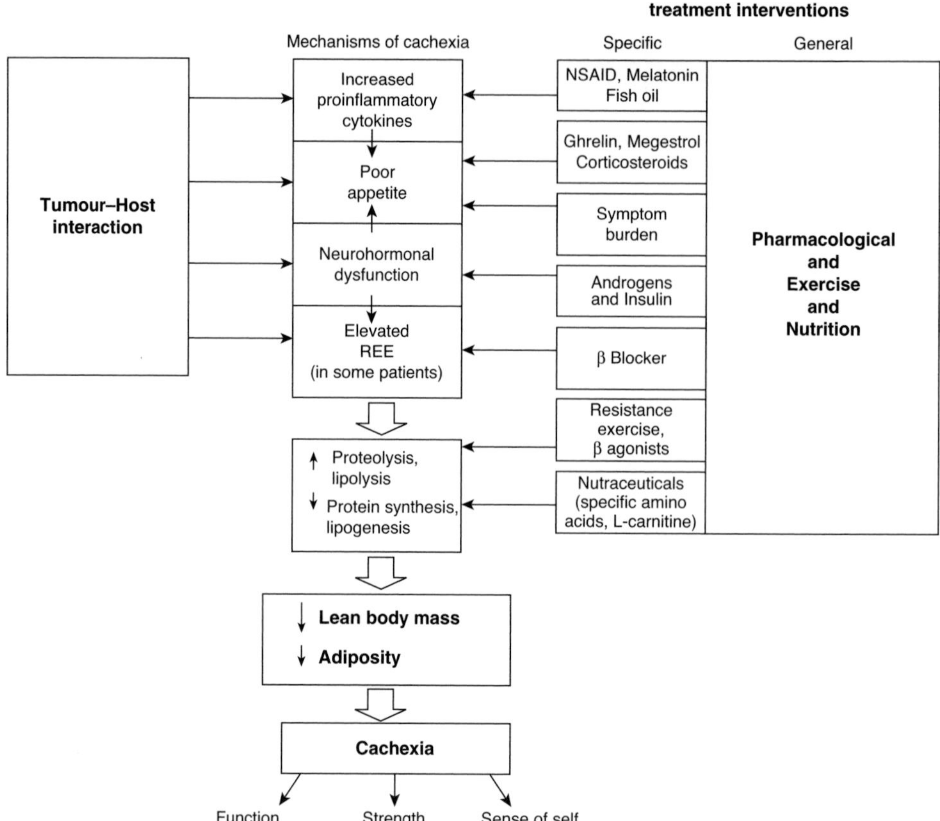

Fig. 11.1 Multimodality treatment model. NSAID, non-steroidal anti-inflammatory drug; REE, resting energy expenditure.

are in their infancy, but in future could facilitate earlier intervention, more effective individualized therapeutic regimens, and fewer unnecessary side-effects. Proinflammatory cytokines, reactive oxygen species,[1] and single-nucleotide polymorphisms[2] are examples of markers that might aid in creating the biological profiles of cachectic patients.

Of course, a single intervention 'targeting' multiple mechanisms of cachexia would be ideal and potentially effective for a broad range of patients. Unfortunately, some currently available medications such as progestins may modulate one pathway favourably while encouraging other potentially harmful mechanisms. For example, although progestins can decrease proinflammatory cytokines and improve appetite, they are associated with endocrine abnormalities such as hypogonadism and hypoadrenalism.[3] Other single interventions for cachexia under investigation such as ghrelin, melatonin and exercise, might affect more than one mechanism favourably (e.g. inflammatory as well as neurohormonal pathways).

A number of studies have used diverse combinations of pharmacological and non-pharmacological therapies with varying success. So far, psychosocial interventions have not been utilized in multimodal cachexia trials, but could play a crucial role in modifying eating habits and behavioural comorbidities. Ultimately, the combination therapy targeting the various mechanisms of cachexia should possess additive or synergistic properties and attenuate the side-effects of individual medications. The following discussion will focus on the evidence for individual interventions and their use in combination therapies.

Inflammation modulators

A pharmacological agent that modulates inflammation is included in virtually every treatment regimen using multiple interventions.

Non-steroidal anti-inflammatory drugs

Many NSAIDs, including celecoxib, ibuprofen and indomethacin, have been used in combination with other pharmacological agents to treat cachexia. NSAIDs may exert their influence via a number of mechanisms including inhibition of prostaglandins,[4] decreased production of interleukin (IL)-6 and other proinflammatory cytokines and the induction of peroxisome proliferator-activated receptor-γ.

Three preliminary trials combining NSAIDs with progestins (either medroxyprogesterone or megestrol acetate) showed an increase in weight[5] or lean body mass.[6,7] The two regimens using a selective cyclo-oxygenase-2 inhibitor also added a calorie-dense nutritional supplement or antioxidants/polyphenols to the intervention. The only prospective randomized study of an NSAID in combination with a progestin revealed that ibuprofen (1200 mg daily in divided doses) and megestrol increased lean body mass and improved quality of life compared to megestrol alone. Notably, individuals on combination therapy did not appear to be at greater risk of major haemorrhage than those on megestrol alone (800 mg daily).

A small 6-week prospective study compared celecoxib (200 mg twice daily) in combination with fish oil[8] to fish oil alone (6 g daily in divided doses). Those receiving combination therapy had significantly lower CRP levels and greater muscle strength than patients receiving fish oil. Both groups were provided with a food supplement equivalent to 20% of the basal metabolic rate. NSAIDs should always be used with caution because of the potential adverse effects (see Chapter 9).

Fish oil and melatonin

A small trial combining melatonin and fish oil in patients with gastrointestinal tumours produced stabilization of weight loss compared to either agent alone.[9] Although a synergistic effect was postulated, there was no change in the level of serum cytokines with the combination treatment.

Since many combination regimens include NSAIDs, adding medications with the potential for attenuating side-effects would be a significant advantage. Both fish oil and melatonin may enhance the anti-inflammatory action of NSAIDs, while melatonin also provides gastro-protection against NSAIDs in animal models. Unfortunately there are no other studies evaluating the effects of these two agents in combination.

Thalidomide

Thalidomide has immune modulatory and antiangiogenic properties. As a single agent, thalidomide has improved appetite and lean body mass in small studies of patients with cachexia. Preliminary results[10] suggest that lean body mass may respond to combination therapy with L-carnitine, a progestin and enriched high-protein nutritional supplementation [containing eicosapentanoic acid (EPA) and branched chain amino acids]. The use of fairly low dose megestrol acetate (320 mg daily) and thalidomide (200 mg daily) in this study may have avoided the increased risk of thromboembolism associated with higher doses. Combination therapy seems to be more effective than any single agent.

Hormonal therapy

Endocrine homeostasis is disrupted in cachexia and advanced cancer, resulting in various hormone deficiencies, hormone resistance and loss of circadian rhythm.

Progestational agents to stimulate appetite

The need for a pharmacological agent to increase appetite should be considered as an option in any multimodal therapy model (Figure 11.1). The satiety centre within the hypothalamus is under the influence of orexigenic and anorexigenic hormones, and individuals with cancer cachexia often experience altered sensitivity to these hormones, possibly induced by proinflammatory cytokines such as IL-1. Medroxyprogesterone and megestrol acetate seem to improve appetite by modulating IL-1, although the exact mechanism of action is not clear. Even so, caution needs to be exercised since there is a risk of thromboembolism at higher doses and evidence of clinically significant suppressive effects by progestins on the adrenal glands and testes.

Large randomized studies comparing megestrol to combination therapy with either fish oil or terahydrocannabinol have shown no benefit compared to megestrol alone. The trials were of short duration (4 weeks) and outcomes of lean body mass and physical function were not assessed. A few smaller non-randomized studies successfully combined progestins (megestrol acetate and medroxyprogesterone) with NSAIDs (celecoxib or ibuprofen) to increase appetite, weight and lean body mass.[5,6] These benefits need to be confirmed in larger randomized studies.

Hormone replacement therapies

Insulin

Cachexia is typically associated with insulin resistance, and so exogenous administration may benefit cachectic individuals. Although insulin decreases appetite centrally, it has peripheral anabolic effects particularly with regard to fat metabolism. A Swedish study[11] randomized patients with gastrointestinal malignancy to receive insulin plus best available palliative support (BAPS) or BAPS alone. Once daily, long-acting insulin was started at 4 units/day with a stepwise increase of 2 units/week to a total of 10–16 units/day. BAPS comprised a multimodal regimen of anti-inflammatories (indomethacin), recombinant erythropoietin for prevention of anaemia, and specialized nutritional care oral supplements plus home parenteral nutrition if intake declined to <80% of expected levels. The addition of insulin to the multimodal regimen did not produce weight gain or improve function but did show an unexplained survival benefit.

Testosterone

Low testosterone is associated with poor appetite[12] in individuals with cancer, yet no randomized testosterone replacement trials have been conducted in patients with CACS. Testosterone replacement is known to raise ghrelin levels and increase insulin sensitivity in non-cancer conditions. Replacement of testosterone could produce similar benefits in patients with cancer, particularly when combined with multimodal therapy.

Ghrelin

The potent, naturally occurring orexigenic hormone ghrelin (or ghrelin agonists) could be used in future multimodal trials to overcome ghrelin 'resistance' in cachectic cancer patients. Ghrelin and ghrelin agonists may also have other immune modulatory and metabolic benefits, but their safety and efficacy as single agents need to be confirmed (please refer to Chapter 8).

Modulating elevated metabolic rate

Beta-blockers improve survival and modulate body composition[13] in individuals with congestive heart failure, and they attenuate weight loss in catabolic conditions such as burns.[14] A small study of cachectic patients with solid tumours showed that beta-blockers decrease resting energy metabolism.[15] These medications could benefit specific cancer patients who are hypermetabolic or have increased sympathetic activity. Neuropsychychiatric side-effects of beta-blockers such as insomnia and depression might arise as a result of decreasing the endogenous production of melatonin. Adding exogenous melatonin to beta-blocker therapy may provide both therapeutic benefit and attenuate the side-effects of beta-blockers. Although there are no published studies using beta-blockers for cancer cachexia as part of multimodality therapy, there are ongoing trials of NSAIDs in combination with beta-blockers.

Symptoms contributing to poor oral intake

Uncontrolled symptoms such as pain, depression, nausea, early satiety and severe constipation may contribute to poor caloric intake. The majority of cachectic patients with weight loss have at least two of these symptoms.[16] Please refer to Chapter 12.

Non-pharmacological multimodality therapies

Exercise

Multiple studies show that exercise attenuates the fatigue experienced by individuals with cancer. Unfortunately there are few studies evaluating the effect of exercise on appetite, weight, and body mass. Animal models suggest that high intensity exercise training increases the lifespan of tumour-bearing rats, promotes a reduction in tumour mass, and prevents indicators of cachexia such as reduced food intake and weight loss.[17]

Resistance exercise in combination with testosterone has a greater anabolic[18] action than either intervention alone in age-related cachexia. In human immunodeficiency virus (HIV)-associated wasting, the combination of resistance training and testosterone in eugonadal men increases muscle mass.[19] Sadly, there are no single-intervention studies examining the effect of either testosterone replacement or exercise on cachexia symptoms, function or weight loss in patients with advanced cancer. Exercise has the potential to be an important component of multimodal therapy by modulating expression of cytokines and acting in concert with anabolic hormones to improve strength and function.[20]

Nutrition

Relying on caloric intake alone, at the expense of other mechanisms causing metabolic cachexia, will not improve lean body mass or function. Nonetheless, patients may overestimate their daily caloric intake. Sometimes they are unable to appreciate the magnitude of a 'starvation' component contributing to their cachexia. Nutritionists are able to identify and make recommendations to those patients who have insufficient caloric intake. Although individualized nutritional counselling has not been evaluated in the context of a multimodal strategy, this low risk intervention is able to improve quality-of-life[21] outcomes and should be used in the comprehensive management of cachectic cancer patients. An example of one approach is to provide calorie-dense enteral supplementation to patients as an initial strategy if <90% of their expected calories are consumed, and then parenteral nutrition once intake declines to <80%.[11] These nutritional interventions are also combined with multimodal pharmacological therapies. Other multimodality interventions have added a calorie-dense oral supplement empirically to their pharmacological therapy.[3,4]

Another strategy is to increase specific substrates within the daily diet. These include essential and non-essential amino acids, as well as branched chain amino acids and ω-3 fatty acids. In patients with advanced pancreatic cancer an energy- and protein-dense oral supplement enriched with n-3 fatty acid EPA was associated with a significant increase in physical activity, despite no gain in weight or lean body mass.[22] Specific amino acids, e.g. HMB, L-arginine and glutamine, promote protein synthesis and increased lean body mass in cachectic patients. Two small placebo-controlled trials in HIV patients and in patients with cancer cachexia revealed gains in muscle within 4 weeks. These two promising trials were followed by a more recent multi-institutional study showing no advantage of the amino acid combination compared to placebo.[23]

Antioxidants and polyphenols in multimodal trials are thought to decrease reactive oxygen species and modify the proinflammatory environment. When given in combination with progestins, celecoxib and n-3 fatty acids (EPA and docosahexaenoic acid) lean body mass and quality of life improved in patients with cachexia after 4 months.[6] In preliminary trials, patients given L-carnitine supplementation gained weight and experienced diminished fatigue and depression. L-Carnitine appears to have few side-effects, minimal drug interactions and is being evaluated in combination with thalidomide and a progestin.[10]

Despite some promising preliminary studies the evidence for supplementation of amino acids or other substrates is not clear, unless there is a documented specific deficiency.

Conclusion

The specific therapies used in combination for cachexia might vary greatly until larger trials are able to confirm the efficacy of a particular multimodality intervention. Despite the variations in composition, all multimodal regimens share a common purpose in simultaneously modulating the major mechanisms causing cachexia. Most of the regimens include individual agents that have improved clinical outcomes in single intervention trials. Implementing a multimodal strategy successfully (especially one that includes exercise) requires early identification of patients with CACS. Modulating the aberrant inflammatory response and restoring endocrine homeostasis early in the disease trajectory offers the best prospect for improving lean body mass and function. A greater awareness of the CACS by clinicians and the development of biomarkers will facilitate timely diagnosis and initiation of therapy. Finally, multimodality therapies for cachexia need to be without significant side-effects and must be introduced against a background of 'best supportive care' which includes optimal symptom management.

References

1. Fortunati N, Manti R, Birocco N, *et al.* (2007) Pro-inflammatory cytokines and oxidative stress/antioxidant parameters characterize the bio-humoral profile of early cachexia in lung cancer patients. *Oncol Rep*, **18**(6), 1521–7.
2. Tan BH, Deans DA, Skipworth RJ, Ross JA, Fearon KC (2008) Biomarkers for cancer cachexia: is there also a genetic component to cachexia? *Support Care Cancer*, **16**(3), 229–34.
3. Dev R, Del Fabbro E, Bruera E (2007) Association between megestrol acetate treatment and symptomatic adrenal insufficiency with hypogonadism in male patients with cancer. *Cancer*, **110**(6), 1173–7.
4. Peluffo GD, Stillitani I, Rodríguez VA, Diament MJ, Klein SM (2004) Reduction of tumor progression and paraneoplastic syndrome development in murine lung adenocarcinoma by nonsteroidal anti-inflammatory drugs. *Int J Cancer*, **110**(6), 825–30.

5. Cerchietti LC, Navigante AH, Peluffo GD, *et al.* (2004) Effects of celecoxib, medroxyprogesterone, and dietary intervention on systemic syndromes in patients with advanced lung adenocarcinoma: a pilot study. *J Pain Sympt Manag*, **27**(1), 85–95.
6. Mantovani G, Macciò A, Madeddu C, *et al.* (2006) A phase II study with antioxidants, both in the diet and supplemented, pharmaconutritional support, progestagen, and anti-cyclooxygenase-2 showing efficacy and safety in patients with cancer-related anorexia/cachexia and oxidative stress. *Cancer Epidemiol Biomarkers Prev*, **15**(5), 1030–4.
7. McMillan DC, Wigmore SJ, Fearon KC, O'Gorman P, Wright CE, McArdle CS (1999) A prospective randomized study of megestrol acetate and ibuprofen in gastrointestinal cancer patients with weight loss. *Br J Cancer*, **79**(3–4), 495–500.
8. Cerchietti LC, Navigante AH, Castro MA (2007) Effects of eicosapentaenoic and docosahexaenoic n-3 fatty acids from fish oil and preferential Cox-2 inhibition on systemic syndromes in patients with advanced lung cancer. *Nutr Cancer*, **59**(1), 14–20.
9. Persson C, Glimelius B, Rönnelid J, Nygren P (2005) Impact of fish oil and melatonin on cachexia in patients with advanced gastrointestinal cancer: a randomized pilot study. *Nutrition*, **21**(2), 170–8.
10. Mantovani G, Macciò A, Madeddu C, *et al.* (2008) Randomized phase III clinical trial of five different arms of treatment for patients with cancer cachexia: interim results. *Nutrition*, **24**(4), 305–13.
11. Lundholm K, Körner U, Gunnebo L, *et al.* (2007) Insulin treatment in cancer cachexia: effects on survival, metabolism, and physical functioning. *Clin Cancer Res*, **13**, 2699–2706.
12. Garcia JM, Li H, Mann D, *et al.* (2006) Hypogonadism in male patients with cancer. *Cancer*, **106**(12), 2583–91.
13. Lainscak M, Keber I, Anker SD (2006) Body composition changes in patients with systolic heart failure treated with beta blockers: a pilot study. *Int J Cardiol*, **106**(3), 319–22.
14. Herndon DN, Hart DW, Wolf SE, Chinkes DL, Wolfe RR (2001) Reversal of catabolism by beta-blockade after severe burns. *N Engl J Med*, **345**(17), 1223–9.
15. Hyltander A, Daneryd P, Sandström R, Körner U, Lundholm K (2000) Beta-adrenoceptor activity and resting energy metabolism in weight losing cancer patients. *Eur J Cancer*, **36**(3), 330–4.
16. Del Fabbro E, Dalal S, Delgado M, Freer G, Bruera E (2007) Secondary vs. primary cachexia in patients with advanced cancer. *J Clin Oncol, ASCO Ann Meeting Proc Part I*, **25**(18S), 9128.
17. Bacurau AV, Belmonte MA, Navarro F, *et al.* (2007) Effect of a high-intensity exercise training on the metabolism and function of macrophages and lymphocytes of walker 256 tumor bearing rats. *Exp Biol Med*, **232**(10), 1289–99.
18. Lambert CP, Sullivan DH, Freeling SA, Lindquist DM, Evans WJ (2002) Effects of testosterone replacement and/or resistance exercise on the composition of megestrol acetate stimulated weight gain in elderly men: a randomized controlled trial. *J Clin Endocrinol Metab*, **87**(5), 2100–6.
19. Grinspoon S, Corcoran C, Parlman K, *et al.* (2000) Effects of testosterone and progressive resistance training in eugonadal men with AIDS wasting. A randomized, controlled trial. *Ann Intern Med*, **133**(5), 348–55.
20. Lewis MI, Fournier M, Storer TW, *et al.* (2007) Skeletal muscle adaptations to testosterone and resistance training in men with COPD. *J Appl Physiol*, **103**(4), 1299–310.
21. Ravasco P, Monteiro Grillo I, Camilo M (2007) Cancer wasting and quality of life react to early individualized nutritional counseling. *Clin Nutr*, **26**(1), 7–15.
22. Moses AW, Slater C, Preston T, Barber MD, Fearon KC (2004) Reduced total energy expenditure and physical activity in cachectic patients with pancreatic cancer can be modulated by an energy and protein dense oral supplement enriched with n-3 fatty acids. *Br J Cancer*, **90**(5), 996–1002.
23. Berk L, James J, Schwartz A, *et al.* (2008) A randomized, double-blind, placebo-controlled trial of a beta-hydroxyl beta-methyl butyrate, glutamine, and arginine mixture for the treatment of cancer cachexia (RTOG 0122). *Support Care Cancer*, **16**(10), 1179–88.

Part 4

Treatment of nutrition impact symptoms

Chapter 12

Classification of cancer cachexia and secondary nutrition impact symptoms

Florian Strasser

Classification

Cachexia, defined as involuntary loss of weight of a certain degree affects most cancer patients with advanced incurable disease. It has a substantial negative impact on physical function, quality of life, anticancer treatment response and survival.[1]

The key cause is so called primary cachexia, which is a complex catabolic state, associated with anorectic mediators of the neurohormonal system, proinflammatory cytokines, and metabolic alterations including, but not limited, to insulin resistance and wasting of muscle issue.[2]

Additionally, in clinical practice advanced cancer patients may lose protein from body fluids because of paracentesis,[3] they may experience muscle wasting from prolonged bed rest or inactivity[4] and their muscles may atrophy after corticosteroid treatment,[5] or comorbid catabolic states such as hypothyroidism. This phenomenon can be conceptualized as secondary cachexia.

With regards to delivery of sufficient energy, protein, and other relevant nutrients, patients with advanced incurable cancer face many challenges that interfere with their appetite and ability to eat. Also, the patients' ability to cope with advanced progressive cancer, and understand the necessary changes to their eating habits,[6] may further impact the response to dietary needs. All these factors can be summarized as 'secondary nutrition impact symptoms' (S-NIS). While this concept is a clinical reality, systematic research is still quite limited and so far is restricted to nutritional screening instruments, and head and neck cancer patients.

Detection of S-NIS in clinical practice

It seems important to distinguish three types of symptoms (Box 12.1):

1) Symptoms directly associated with the mechanisms of primary cachexia are usually related to poor appetite. They include 'decreased central drive to eat', 'missing reward after eating', 'smell and taste abnormalities' (which are not associated with toxicity of anticancer treatment or specific nutrition deficits), and 'early satiety' (in absence of constipation). These symptoms are a reflection of the inflammatory downregulation of hypothalamic appetite stimulation and also of gastrointestinal motility.
2) Symptoms which reflect the impact of the cachexia syndrome on patients' functioning (e.g. physical fatigue) and the emotional distress related to loss of weight and function. Although fatigue is a hallmark of the consequence of cachexia, the cause of fatigue in patients with advanced cancer may be multifactorial.[7]
3) The so-called S-NIS are those symptoms resulting in a decreased ability to take food orally and/or affecting appetite. S-NIS can be reversible (for example, severe pain, dyspnoea or constipation) or irreversible (for example, malignant bowel obstruction). It is conceptually important to divide these three symptom domains from each other.

Box 12.1 Symptoms in cachexia assessment: 'a family of distinct characters'

1 Symptoms mirroring the pathogenesis of cachexia
 Early satiety, appetite loss, no desire to eat, weakness

2 Symptoms and syndromes impacting nutritional intake
 Nausea
 Vomiting
 Constipation
 Diarrhoea
 Defecation after meal
 Pain
 Dyspnoea
 Fatigue
 Anxiety/depression
 Sense of hopelessness
 Stomatitis
 Dysgeusia
 Dental problems
 Difficulty chewing
 Dysosmia
 Xerostomia
 Thick saliva
 Dysphagia
 Epigastric pain
 Abdominal pain

3 Symptoms reflecting the impact of cachexia
 Fatigue, eating-related distress

Data supporting the S-NIS concept

A recent systematic literature review on S-NIS (analysing 234 papers from >14 000 citations) identified seven papers clearly measuring energy and/or protein intake and defining S-NIS. Of head and neck cancer patients with radiation induced symptoms, such as swallowing discomfort or oral dryness, depression and taste disturbances, S-NIS correlated with impaired oral nutritional intake.[8] In 66 patients with various solid tumours the severity of chemosensory complaints was related to oral nutritional intake;[9] another study of 40 patients with colorectal cancer found no association of nausea with oral nutrition intake.[10] A more recent paper explored the use of a single dose of palonosetron with nutritional intake and found an improvement of oral intake after good nausea control.[11] With regards to the endpoint of weight loss, a study of 399 oesophageal and head and neck cancer patients found a clear correlation of mucositis and dysphagia with weight loss.[12]

Assessment of S-NIS

For the assessment of S-NIS, the Patient-Generated Subjective Global Assessment (PG-SGA) asks about the presence or absence of 'problems that have prevented me from eating enough during the past 2 weeks'. The list includes symptoms such as appetite, nausea, vomiting, constipation, diarrhoea, mouth sores, dry mouth, taste problems, smell, swallowing problems, early fullness, and pain.

The patients are asked about the presence or absence of symptoms, but do not rate the relative impact on nutritional intake. Patients may report the presence of such symptoms without necessarily stating that they impact nutritional intake.

Several groups are therefore developing semiquantitative checklists to measure S-NIS, and to explore the impact of the S-NIS assessment on the clinical management of cachexia. For example, a question regarding constipation might be framed as follows: 'Do you have decreased appetite or ability to eat because of constipation (i.e. better appetite after having a bowel movement?)'. In clinical care it is also important to estimate the reversibility of the S-NIS since there are readily available therapeutic options for the majority of these symptoms.

In addition to appropriate nutritional assessment and counselling,[13] good clinical practice seems to demand we ask our patients about their symptoms and determine whether they affect appetite and oral nutritional intake. Practice guidelines regarding the assessment of S-NIS should be developed and implemented as standard of care for advanced cancer patients.

Treatment of S-NIS

For the treatment of S-NIS the best palliative cancer care assessment and treatment of these symptoms is appropriate[14] and will be discussed in the ensuing chapters. The monitoring of nutritional intake and the symptoms related to eating should become an integral part of the multidisciplinary management[15] of cancer cachexia.

References

1. Tan BH, Fearon KC (2008) Cachexia: prevalence and impact in medicine. *Curr Opin Clin Nutr Metab* Care, **11**(4), 400–7.
2. Tisdale MJ (2009) Mechanisms of cancer cachexia. *Physiol Rev*, **89**(2), 381–410.
3. Mercadante S, Intravaia G, Ferrera P, Villari P, David F (2008) Peritoneal catheter for continuous drainage of ascites in advanced cancer patients. *Support Care Cancer*, **16**(8), 975–8.
4. Kortebein P, Symons TB, Ferrando A, *et al.* (2008) Functional impact of 10 days of bed rest in healthy older adults. *J Gerontol A Biol Sci Med Sci*, **63**(10), 1076–81.
5. Ma K, Mallidis C, Bhasin S, Mahabadi V, *et al.* (2003) Glucocorticoid-induced skeletal muscle atrophy is associated with upregulation of myostatin gene expression. *Am J Physiol Endocrinol Metab*, **285**(2), 363–71.
6. Hutton JL, Martin L, Field CJ, *et al.* (2006) Dietary patterns in patients with advanced cancer: implications for anorexia–cachexia therapy. *Am J Clin Nutr*, **84**(5), 1163–70.
7. Strasser F (2008) Diagnostic criteria of cachexia and their assessment: decreased muscle strength and fatigue. *Curr Opin Clin Nutr Metab Care*, **11**(4), 417–21.
8. Ravasco P, Monteiro-Grillo I, Marques Vidal P, Camilo ME (2005) Impact of nutrition on outcome: a prospective randomized controlled trial in patients with head and neck cancer undergoing radiotherapy. *Head Neck*, **27**(8), 659–68.
9. Hutton JL, Baracos VE, Wismer WV (2007) Chemosensory dysfunction is a primary factor in the evolution of declining nutritional status and quality of life in patients with advanced cancer. *J Pain Sympt Manag*, **33**(2), 156–65.

10. Fordy C, Glover C, Henderson DC, Summerbell C, Wharton R, Allen-Mersh TG (1999) Contribution of diet, tumour volume and patient-related factors to weight loss in patients with colorectal liver metastases. *Br J Surg*, **86**(5), 639–44.
11. Lorusso V, Spedicato A, Petrucelli L, Saracino V, Giampaglia M, Perrone T (2009) Single dose of palonosetron plus dexamethasone to control nausea, vomiting and to warrant an adequate food intake in patients treated with highly emetogenic chemotherapy (HEC). *Support Care Cancer.*
12. Bieri S, Bentzen SM, Huguenin P, *et al.* (2003) Early morbidity after radiotherapy with or without chemotherapy in advanced head and neck cancer. Experience from four nonrandomized studies. *Strahlenther Onkol*, **179**(6), 390–5.
13. Halfdanarson TR, Thordardottir E, West CP, Jatoi A (2008) Does dietary counseling improve quality of life in cancer patients? A systematic review and meta-analysis. *J Support Oncol* **6**(5), 234–7.
14. Ferris F, Bruera E, Cherny N, *et al.* (2009) Palliative cancer care a decade later: accomplishments, the need, next steps—from the American Society of Clinical Oncology. *J Clin Oncol*, **27**(18), 3052–8.
15. Fearon KC (2008) Cancer cachexia: developing multimodal therapy for a multidimensional problem. *Eur J Cancer*, **44**(8), 1124–32.

Chapter 13

Oral complications

Carla Ida Ripamonti, Nicla La Verde, Gabriella Farina, Marina Chiara Garassino

Introduction

Cancer can damage the oral cavity, either directly as in head–neck cancer, or indirectly, by reducing immunocompetence, and favouring the development of oral infections. Additionally, treatments such as chemotherapy, surgery and particularly radiotherapy can cause complications such as mucositis, infection, salivary gland dysfunction (i.e. xerostomia, sialadenitis), taste dysfunction (dysgeusia, ageusia), muscular fibrosis, cutaneous fibrosis, and trismus. Patients could also experience halitosis, abscess and fistulae formation, bleeding, osteoradionecrosis, soft tissue necrosis, or osteonecrosis of the jaw.

Oral complications impair nutrition and facilitate malnutrition, anorexia, and cachexia. In addition, the psychological impact may be enormous because the oral cavity plays such an important role in communication, social life, and the pleasures associated with eating. Oral health is important in all phases of the oncological illness because of its key role in nutrition, communication and, generally, in patient's quality of life.

The aim of the chapter is to provide the tools for maintaining good oral hygiene, preventing the onset of oral problems and managing them effectively when they arise.

Oral hygiene

Oral hygiene is a universal prevention strategy and should be considered part of 'good clinical practice' in patient care, at any phase of their disease.[1] Good oral hygiene is essential to reduce infection risk, to improve quality of life and maintain a good nutritional status. Since 3000 BC the Sumerians have left gold or silver toothpicks in their graves and Hippocrates emphasized the importance of removing food deposits from the teeth. Despite a lack of evidence, the value of basic oral care in maintaining mucosal health, function, and reducing the risk of complications, such as caries, periodontal disease or infections, is accepted by clinicians.[2] Dental plaque, as well as decayed and missing teeth, are more common among oncological patients than healthy patients,[3] and when systematically applied, oral care protocols have the potential to decrease the incidence, severity, and duration of oral disorders.[4] Oral care needs a multidisciplinary approach for patient education and the implementation of related clinical treatments. Before starting an oncological treatment, such as chemotherapy or radiotherapy, an evaluation of dental status is necessary, especially in head–neck cancer patients. Professional cleaning by a dental hygienist may help remove potential sources of oral problems, such as tooth decay, dental plaque, loose dentures, and sharp-edged or broken teeth, which increase the risk of mucosal ulceration.[3]

A Panel of experts has developed a set of guidelines for oral health care to prevent mucositis in cancer patients.[2] Patients should have baseline and ongoing oral assessments, that include patient self-reports and professional examinations. Patients must be evaluated both for preventive and therapeutic oral care regimens and should receive a standardized oral care protocol, that includes systematic oral hygiene through brushing, flossing, bland rinses, and moisturizers. The Panel recommended an interdisciplinary approach to oral care that includes all the professionals involved in cancer patient care, i.e. physicians, dentists, dental hygienists, nurses,[5] dietitians, and pharmacists. The correct oral hygiene procedures are summarized in Box 13.1.[6–8]

Mucositis

The treatment of solid malignancies with either cytotoxics or radiotherapy (or both) is becoming increasingly more effective, but it is associated with several side-effects. These include disruption in the function and integrity of the mouth which may result in severe ulceration (oral mucositis) and fungal infection (oral candidiasis). These complications can produce oral discomfort and pain, poor nutrition, delays in drug administration, increased hospital stay, and for some patients life-threatening infection (septicaemia). Dysphagia can decrease the intake of both liquids and solid food, so that enteral nutrition through a nasogastric tube or percutaneous gastrostomy may be required, in order to prevent or limit severe weight loss.

In some cancer patients inflammation of the oral mucosa (mucositis) occurs with a higher incidence. About 90% of head–neck cancer patients develop mucositis during concomitant radio-chemotherapy treatment.[9] Mucositis typically manifests initially as erythema with ulceration developing later.[10] Systemic infections may occur because the injured mucosa is susceptible to microbial colonization. Sonis *et al.*[11] proposed a four-phase model illustrating the physiopathology of mucositis:

1. Inflammatory/vascular phase (CT-RT-induced release of tumour necrosis factor (TNF)-α and interleukin-1).
2. Epithelial phase (epithelial thinning due to the suppression of the epithelial basal layer).
3. Ulcerative/bacteriological phase (bacterial colonization with release of cytokines and nitric oxide).
4. Healing phase (regeneration of epithelium).

Box 13.1 Oral hygiene procedures

- Personal dental health care should be performed after every meal, by brushing teeth for at least 2 min, with a soft-bristle toothbrush. The brush should be tilted at a 45° angle against the gumline and it should be swept or rolled away from the gumline, with an up-and-down motion to clean the inside surfaces of the front teeth, thus removing plaque and debris.
- Dental floss is useful to remove food and dental plaque from teeth. The floss must be inserted between the teeth and scraped along the teeth sides, especially close to the gums.
- The toothbrush should be regularly replaced, at least every 2 months.
- In spite of the lack of evidence, a bland rinse can be used as an anti-inflammatory and antiseptic device; some studies have assessed the efficacy of chlorhexidine or sodium bicarbonate moistures.[6,7] No rinse has been shown to be superior to the other; therefore, the choice is only based on clinical assessment and the patient's preference. Alcohol-containing mouth rinses are not recommended because they may cause oral burning or bad taste, and because they produce acetaldehyde, a toxic catabolic compound.[8]

Local pain is the most important symptom and pain severity generally correlates with the severity of mucositis. Pain is aggravated by drinking, eating and with poor oral hygiene. Topical anaesthetics and non-opioid systemic analgesic drugs may fail to relieve oral discomfort. Opioid analgesics are often required, but may cause adverse effects, including nausea, vomiting, constipation, confusion, and drowsiness.

A grading system for oral mucositis has been developed, although the most widely used is the common toxicity criteria scale of the National Cancer Institute (Table 13.1).[12]

Different pharmacological approaches have been employed to reduce the severity of mucositis. Sutherland *et al.*[13] carried out a meta-analysis, by dividing the different drugs into three classes: direct cytoprotectors, indirect cytoprotectors and antibacterials (either broad spectrum or small spectrum). More recently, Stokman *et al.*[14] performed a meta-analysis concerning the different therapeutic strategies in the prevention of radio-chemotherapy-induced oral cavity mucositis. Slow-release antibiotics, mucosal cooling procedures, granulocytic growth factors (granulocyte macrophage colony-stimulating factor: GM-CSF) and amifostine proved to be the most efficient strategies. Studies with the recombinant human keratinocyte growth factor, palifermin, showed efficacy in preventing mucositis after stem cell transplantation.[15] Its use during radiotherapy for head and neck cancer is under current investigation.

Regardless of the possible methodological limitations of each single study, no strategy was able to completely prevent all the mucositis-associated symptoms and no correlation was established between the reduction of the bacterial charge in the oral cavity and mucositis prevention.

Some phase II studies indicate a possible benefit from decontamination of the bacterial flora in the oral cavity[16] but no randomized phase III trial has shown it to be effective in radio-chemotherapy-induced mucositis.[17] A recent small randomized trial of intravenous L-alanyl-L-glutamine versus placebo showed a reduction in the incidence of oral mucositis due to radio-chemotherapy in head and neck cancer patients; but the efficacy of this protector agent needs further validation.[18]

Several guidelines and systematic reviews[19] concerning the treatment and prevention of oral mucositis have been published, including recommendations by the Multinational Association of Supportive Cancer Care (MASCC).

It is important to underline that correct management requires patient education and regular assessment of the condition's evolution by the entire multidisciplinary team. All patients must use a soft toothbrush on a regular basis; those with a higher risk of mucositis should also undergo a visit to a dentist before starting treatment.[20] The available trials only offer weak recommendations about the use of agents to prevent mucositis. Benzydamine, an anti-inflammatory drug, may be useful to prevent radiation-induced mucositis in those patients receiving moderate-dose radiation. Benzydamine reduces the concentration of TNF and is effective in reducing the intensity and duration of mucosal damage.[21]

Table 13.1 Toxicity criteria scale of the National Cancer Institute

Grade	Clinical features
0	None
1	Painless ulcers, erythema or mild soreness
2	Painful erythema, oedema, or ulcers, can eat orally
3	Painful erythema, oedema, or ulcers, cannot eat orally
4	Requires enteral or parenteral support

The efficacy of chlorhexidine, sucralfate[22] and antimicrobial lozenges[23] are not confirmed in trials. For patients who undergo 5-fluorouracil (5FU)-based chemotherapy, oral cryotherapy 20–30 min before treatment may prevent 5FU-associated mucositis.[24] In patients receiving high dose chemotherapy with or without total body irradiation a dose of 60 mg/kg/day keratinocyte growth factor-1 (palifermin) 3 days before conditioning treatment and for 3 days after transplantation may significantly reduce mucositis.[25] Acyclovir and its analogues may be used in selected patients although not routinely, whereas GM-CSFs are not recommended.[26]

Oral infections

Oral infections are common events in cancer patients because of many promoting factors that either directly or indirectly contribute to their development.

The malignancy (e.g. leukaemia), medications (chemotherapy, antibiotics, corticosteroids), lifestyle habits (smoking or alcohol consumption), or other systemic conditions (diabetes, dehydration) can induce immunodeficiency. Local factors can also favour oral infections including poor oral hygiene, modifications in oral microbiological environment, xerostomia, and head–neck radiotherapy.

The oral microbial population in cancer patients is different from that of healthy subjects. One study demonstrated that 83% of cancer patients are positive for yeasts, 49% are colonized by coliforms and 28% by coagulase-positive staphylococci.[27]

Fungi, bacteria and viruses are responsible for infected oral mucositis. Diagnosis is usually clinical and treatments are typically empirical, although cultural or cytological isolations are warranted.

Fungal infections

The most common oral infections have a fungal aetiology and *Candida albicans* is the principal pathogen; it is a commensal, but in about 30–83% of advanced cancer patients it becomes a pathogen.[28,29] Besides *C. albicans*, *Candida glabrata* and *Candida dubliniensis* have been isolated in the oral cavity of advanced cancer patients (46%, 18% and 5%, respectively).[30]

Clinical manifestations of *C. albicans* infections include acute pseudomembranous candidiasis (thrush) presenting as yellowish-white plaques; acute atrophic candidiasis, causing dysgeusia, pain and tongue atrophy; chronic atrophic candidiasis, with erythema and oedema, frequent in denture carriers; chronic hyperplasic candidiasis with plaque resembling leukoplakia; angular cheilitis, that presents with erythema and painful cracks at the corners of the mouth.

Limited candida infection can be successfully treated with nystatin oral suspension (100 000 U/ml, 4–6 ml every 6 h.[31] Since chlorhexidine may inactivate nystatin, the combination must be avoided.[32] Miconazole gel is used as topical treatment, especially for angular cheilitis and can be applied up to four times a day, mainly within the first 48 h. If the infection extends into the pharynx, systemic treatment is required, usually with the azole group which includes ketoconazole, fluconazole, and itraconazole. Use of ketoconazole (200 mg daily) is limited because of the risk of side-effects, such as liver toxicity, nausea and vomiting. Fluconazole, 100 mg once daily for at least 10 days, is usually selected for its good tolerability and broad spectrum of activity.[33,34] Itraconazole also has a broad spectrum of activity, is well tolerated, at 100–200 mg daily, and should be taken immediately after a meal because absorption is better at a low pH. Since the azole compounds inhibit cytochrome P450, the interaction with other drugs (including methadone and fentanyl) must be carefully monitored.[35]

As for the efficacy of systemic antifungal prophylaxis, a Cochrane review concluded that drugs absorbed by the gastrointestinal tract prevent oral candidiasis in patients receiving anticancer treatments, but the decision to use antifungal agents for prevention or treatment of superficial oral infections requires further consideration of the risks versus benefits (toxicity, costs, development of microbial drug resistance).[36]

Bacterial infections

Bacterial oral infections are very frequent in the general population and include tooth decay, abscesses or gingivitis. Cancer patients are at higher risk because their mechanical defences are reduced, favouring infection by commensal bacteria. Salivary composition alterations, xerostomia, hypercaloric carbohydrate-based diets and poor hygiene can produce a microenvironment which encourages bacterial growth. Typical clinical presentations include: gingivitis, periodontitis, and dental abscess. These infections are treated with antibiotics, such as amoxicillin/clavulanic acid, and may require dental procedures.

Bacterial mucositis is quite rare, with staphylococci generally the aetiological agents. Although dental infections may be the initial foci of bacteraemia in haematological patients undergoing myeloablative therapy,[37,38] the prophylactic use of antibiotics is not indicated to prevent oral bacterial infections. Oral rinses, such as chlorhexidine or 2% hydrogen peroxide, can be used as local disinfectants.

Viral infections

The most frequent viral oral infection in cancer patients is caused by herpes simplex virus type 1 (HSV-1).[39] The asymptomatic presence of HSV-1 in the oral mucosa is detected in 70% of cancer patients by means of polymerase chain reaction.[40] A clinical diagnosis can normally be made, but, whenever feasible, exfoliative cytology is helpful for virus isolation.[41] Presentation may be as a first infection or as a reactivation. In the former, it usually develops as a gingivostomatitis, with mouth vesicles, pain, and sometimes locoregional lyphadenopathy and fever. Treatment with oral acyclovir, 400 mg five times a day for 5 days, helps reduce symptom duration.[42]

Infection recurrence (herpes labialis), typically occurs in one-third of patients who have had a prior infection, because of reactivation of the latent virus in the trigeminal ganglia. Both chemotherapy and radiotherapy can act as trigger for disease recurrence.

Herpes labialis typically begins with painful blisters involving the skin or mucous membranes of the mouth or lips. Acyclovir cream 5% can be applied topically every 4 h for 5–10 days. More rarely, severe oral herpes zoster infections may occur, requiring systemic drugs such as Acyclovir 800 mg 5 times a day for 7 days or valacyclovir 1000 mg every 8 h for 7 days.

Osteonecrosis of the jaw

Osteonecrosis of the jaw (ONJ) is a rare complication observed in cancer patients receiving bisphosphonate-based treatments, especially zoledronate and pamidronate.[43,44] Although their mechanism of action is not completely understood, bisphosphonates are known to inhibit osteoclast synthesis and migration, and promote tumour cell apoptosis,[45] resulting in impaired osteoclast-mediated bone resorption.[46] The inhibition of osteoblast-mediated osteoclastic reabsorption and the antiangiogenic properties may impair blood supply resulting in hypodynamic bone with reduced biomechanical properties and accumulation of micro-damage. The involvement of the jaw has an anatomic rationale since this region has thin mucosa and periosteum which separates bone from a trauma-intense and microbiologically diverse oral environment. The jaw is exposed to dental microtrauma and infections so that reparative mechanisms are more important than in other sites. Because of bone turnover inhibition and hypovascularity, the increased demand for bone repair cannot be satisfied, and bone remodelling is compromised, resulting in osteonecrosis.[47]

The most important risk factors are history of dental surgery or dental infections, type of bisphosphonates, and delivered doses. Other risk factors include diabetes, anaemia, coagulopathies, infections, alcohol consumption, smoking or concomitant cancer treatments (chemotherapy, radiotherapy, corticosteroids), as they contribute to an altered oral environment.[48,49]

The initial presentation may include oral pain, recurrent alveolar abscesses, paraesthesia, fistula, soft tissue swelling, or exposed bone, especially after dental extraction or traumatic injuries. A conservative approach would consist of symptom control and cycles of antibiotics, antimycotics and local disinfectants, together with standard oral health care.

Many studies demonstrate that the application of preventive measures can significantly reduce the incidence of ONJ in cancer patients receiving bisphosphonate-based therapies. Identification of patients at risk and co-management with dental team members can improve treatment outcomes and increase the number of ONJ-free patients.[50,51]

Xerostomia

Xerostomia is the subjective feeling of dryness of the mouth. The prevalence of xerostomia is about 29% in the primary care setting, 30–97% in palliative care patients[52–54] and varies between 94% and 100% after therapeutic doses of radiation for head and neck cancer.[55] The most frequent causes of xerostomia in cancer patients are listed in Box 13.2.[53]

Up to 90% of saliva is produced by the parotid, submandibular and sublingual glands. Saliva is composed of ions (fluid component) and proteins secreted respectively by parasympathetic and sympathetic stimulation. Saliva is composed of a serous part (α-amylase), devoted to starch digestion, and a mucous component which acts as a lubricant. It is saturated with calcium and phosphate

Box 13.2 Causes of xerostomia

Reduced salivary secretion caused by:

- radiotherapy and/or chemotherapy of the head and neck regions;
- surgery in the buccal and submandibular regions;
- drugs: anticholinergics, antidepressants, antipsychotics, anxiolytics, anticonvulsants, hypnotics, antihistamines, analgesics, diuretics, beta-blockers, antihypertensives, muscle relaxants;
- obstruction, infection, aplasia, malignant destruction of salivary glands;
- encephalitis, brain tumours, neurosurgical operations, autonomic pathway destruction;
- hypothyroidism;
- autoimmune diseases, sarcoidosis.

Widespread erosion of buccal mucosa caused by:

- progression of oral cancer, immunodeficiency, stomatitis.

Oral infections (viral, bacterial, and fungal)

Dehydration caused by:

- anorexia, diarrhoea, fever, O_2 therapy, large bedsores and/or ulcers, vomiting, polyuria, haemorrhage, diabetes insipidus, difficulty in swallowing.

Depression, anxiety

Modified from De Conno *et al.*[53]

and is necessary for maintaining healthy teeth, modulating oral microbial flora, and maintaining the mucosal immune system. The bicarbonate content of saliva enables it to buffer and produce the conditions necessary for the digestion of plaque.[53] Moreover, saliva helps with bolus formation during mastication and lubricates the throat for easy passage of food. The organic and inorganic components of salivary secretions protect the tissues and organs of the mouth. They act as a barrier to irritants and as a means of removing cellular and bacterial debris. Saliva contains various components involved in defence against bacterial and viral invasion, including mucins, lipids, secretory immunoglobulin, lysozymes, lactoferrin, salivary peroxidase, and myeloperoxidase.

Reduced saliva may lead to damage of both the hard and soft tissues of the oral cavity, an increase in ulcerations, candidiasis, dental decay, taste alterations and difficulty in speech. Moreover the amount of oral intake decreases as swallowing and chewing become difficult and painful.

During the course of RT to the head and neck region and for many months after the end of RT, there is a marked reduction in saliva production as a consequence of inflammation and degeneration of the acini, ducts, connective tissue and vascular components of the salivary glands.[56] The damage is generally proportional to the radiation dose delivered to the salivary glands and the volume of parenchyma exposed. Saliva production decreases and its composition becomes more sticky, viscous and acidic, with a loss of organic and inorganic components that modify electrolyte and immunoglobulin composition. The microbial flora is altered and as a consequence there is increased growth of *Streptococcus*, *Lactobacillus* and *Candida* spp.[57] Box 13.2 shows the many drugs involved in xerostomia.[53] Most of those drugs act on the central nervous system and many palliative care patients take more than one of these medications daily. In two different studies Ventafridda *et al.* found a significantly higher incidence of xerostomia in patients treated with morphine in oral solution compared to a randomized group treated with oral methadone or controlled release morphine tablets.[58,59] In another study,[60] xerostomia was present in 35% of cancer patients treated with an anti-inflammatory and/or adjuvant drugs, 36% of the time during treatment with weak opioids and/or adjuvants, and 51% of the time during treatment with strong opioids and/or adjuvants. The management of xerostomia includes local measures, general measures and pharmacological treatments. Pre-irradiation oral care by a dental team is useful to treat any dental or periodontal pathology. The first step in the management of xerostomia consists of frequent oral hygiene and air humidification in the patient's room. Topical comfort is provided by sucking ice cubes, rinsing with cold tonic water and chewing sugarless gum which stimulate the production of saliva. Bitter substances stimulate salivary secretion, while sweet substances can increase the sensation of dry mouth. Alcohol and mouth rinses containing alcohol should be avoided. Artificial saliva as a solution, spray or gel usually provides relief for a short period of time, and is useful immediately before bedtime or speaking. Mucin-rich artificial saliva provides more symptomatic relief to xerostomic patients than conventional, non-mucin substitutes.[61–63] The role of antioxidants and free-radicals in reducing the toxic effects of RT is under investigation.[64] The role of amifostine as a protector against xerostomia during RT has been established in a large multicentre randomized study.[65] A dose of 200 mg/m^2 reduced the severity and duration of xerostomia 2 years after RT in 315 patients with head and neck cancer.[66] Unfortunately the drug is expensive, produces adverse effects and has to be administered daily via intramuscular or subcutaneous routes. Pilocarpine and cevimeline (approved recently for Sjögren syndrome) are pharmacological sialogogues. Pilocarpine[67–69] acts primarily by stimulating minor salivary glands. Controlled studies show that pilocarpine produces benefits with acceptable adverse effects (in particular sweating) at higher doses of 10 mg three times a day. Best results are obtained with continuous treatment for more than 3 months after RT with doses of 5 mg three times a day.[70] Patients with asthma, severe chronic obstructive disease, glaucoma, and congestive heart disease are potentially at risk for adverse effects when using this drug.[71] Cevimeline appears to have less toxicity, but needs to be further investigated.

Taste alteration

Taste disturbance occurs as a result of a reduction in taste sensation (hypogeusia), an absence of taste sensation (ageusia), or a distortion of normal taste sensation (dysgeusia). Potential causes are listed in Box 13.3.

Box 13.3 Potential causes of taste alterations in cancer patients

- Cancer diagnosis
- Local disease of the mouth and tongue caused by cancer
- Surgery of the tongue (partial glossectomy), palate, oropharynx
- Tobacco usage
- Elimination of the olfactory component of taste after laryngectomy
- Radiotherapy for head and neck cancer
- Radiotherapy of the abdomen and/or pelvis
- Damage to the nervous system following surgery or cerebral lesions
- Lesions of cranial nerves V, VII, IX, or X
- Lesion and infection of chorda tympani
- Complicated intubation before surgery
- Alteration of the cell regenerating cycle
- Malnutrition
- Immune deficiency
- Administration of chemotherapy (carboplatin, cisplatin, cyclophosphamide, doxorubicin, 5-fluorouracil, levamisole, methotrexate, paclitaxel)
- Any other kind of drug affecting taste
- Metabolic alterations/disorders
- Severe xerostomia
- Stomatitis, oral infections (candidiasis), ulcers, necrosis
- Endocrine factors (thyroidectomy, hypophysectomy, adrenalectomy, adrenal insufficiency or Cushing disease)
- Neurological diseases known to influence taste and/or smell sensitivity
- Irritation of oral cavity and oropharynx from endoscopic tube
- Local disease in nose or ears
- Modification in the receptor cells due to alteration of saliva by metabolic agents, drugs, radiation
- Dental pathology
- Complete or full upper dentures
- Bad dental hygiene
- Low plasma and/or salivary levels of zinc

The sensation of taste is mediated by the taste buds. There are about 10 000 taste buds, situated within the mucosa of the tongue, soft palate, uvula, pharynx, upper third of the oesophagus, epiglottis, larynx, lips and cheeks.[72,73]

The taste buds are connected to the oral cavity via the taste pores.[72] A 'gatekeeper' protein regulates the passage of saliva/tastants from the oral cavity, through the taste pore, and into the taste bud. The taste buds consist of about 50 cells, including specialised gustatory cells which are continuously being replaced (gustatory cells survive for about 10 days). Gustatory cells have a microvillus (containing the taste receptor), which projects into the taste pore; gustatory cells also have a synapse, which connects to sensory nerve fibres.

Each taste bud is innervated by about 50 nerve fibres, while each nerve fibre receives input from about five taste buds.[72] Taste information is transmitted via the V, VII, IX, and X cranial nerves to the nucleus of the tractus solitaris in the medulla, then onwards to the ventral posterior medial nucleus of the thalamus, and finally to the post-central gyrus in the parietal lobe. There is genetic variation in taste within a population.

The prevalence of taste disturbance is reported to be 31–35% in mixed oncology patients,[74,75] and 44–50% in advanced oncology patients.[76,77] Taste changes occur in 68% of patients receiving chemotherapy,[78] are relatively common in patients with cancers of the head and neck region,[79] and extremely common in patients who have received radiotherapy to the head and neck region.[80] RT has a toxic effect on the cells of the tongue, taste buds and innervation. It also reduces and changes saliva production which alters taste sensation. In some cases, improvement in taste disturbance occurs within a few weeks or months of treatment, but in many cases, taste problems persist for a long time after treatment. For example, Maes *et al.* reported that 50% of patients had subjective taste disturbance 12 months post radiotherapy.[79] Similarly, Mossman *et al.* reported that some patients had objective taste disturbance 7 years post radiotherapy.[81]

Taste alteration can lead to food aversion, reduced food intake, nutritional deficits, and weight loss.[82,83] Patients may report that 'food is tasteless' or 'the food is bitter' or has 'a metallic aftertaste'.

The management of taste disturbance involves good oral hygiene, treatment to increase salivation, and the withdrawal of drugs that can induce or increase the symptoms. Dietary therapy includes enhancing taste (using salt, sugar and other flavourings) and addressing the presentation, smell, consistency and temperature of the food.[84,85]

The most studied treatment in patients with taste disturbance is zinc therapy. Studies in patients with radiotherapy-related taste disturbance have produced conflicting results (Table 13.2).[86–94] Two small studies in patients with established taste disturbance suggest a possible therapeutic role for oral zinc supplements. Similarly, two small studies in patients undergoing radiotherapy suggest an additional prophylactic role for oral zinc supplements. Small uncontrolled studies and a case series also suggest that zinc administration may be effective.[91–94] Unfortunately, a recent large North Central Cancer Treatment Group study found no significant prophylactic effect, or therapeutic effect, for oral zinc supplements.

Oral zinc supplements are generally well tolerated, although they can cause dyspepsia and abdominal pain. Zinc must be administered in the middle of a meal to reduce the symptoms. In conclusion, it would seem reasonable to offer patients with taste disturbance a trial of an oral zinc supplement (in the absence of other treatment options).[95]

Local complications

Abscesses, fistula

Infections such as cellulitis and orocutaneous fistula make up about 22% of febrile episodes in patients with head and neck cancers.[96]

Table 13.2 Studies and case reports of zinc administration in patients with cancer

Authors	Design	Regimen	Outcomes
Mossman *et al.*[86]	Case series (n = 7; patients with taste disturbance post head and neck radiotherapy)	Variable Zinc 25 or 100 mg/day for 2–6 months	Improvement in objective taste disturbance.
Silverman and Thompson[87]	Case series (n = 30; patients with taste disturbance post head and neck radiotherapy)	Variable Zinc 100–150 mg/day for at least 1 month	Improvement in subjective taste disturbance (37% patients).
Silverman *et al.*[88]	Randomized controlled trials vs placebo (n = 19; patients pre head and neck radiotherapy)	Zinc 18 mg four times/day for duration of radiotherapy	No difference in objective taste disturbance during radiotherapy between groups. Earlier recovery of subjective taste disturbance in treatment group (64% vs 22% patients at 3 weeks post treatment).
Ripamonti *et al.*[89]	Randomized controlled trials vs placebo (n = 18; patients with taste disturbance during head and neck radiotherapy)	Zinc sulphate 45 mg three times/day from onset of subjective taste disturbance until 1 month post radiotherapy	Less objective taste disturbance during radiotherapy in treatment group. Earlier recovery of objective taste disturbance in treatment group.
Hakyard *et al.*[90]	Randomized controlled trials vs placebo (n = 169; patients pre head and neck radiotherapy)	Zinc sulphate 45 mg three times/day from onset of radiotherapy (≤7 days) until 1 month post radiotherapy	No difference in subjective taste disturbance during radiotherapy between groups. No difference in recovery of subjective taste disturbance between groups.
Henkin and Bradley[91]	Case reports: 1 patient with multiple myeloma, 1 patient with cystinuria	$ZnCl_2$ 60 mg Zn^{2+}/day	Improvement in taste acuity
Schnarch and Markitziu[92]	Case report: 1 patient with cerebello-pontine angle meningioma	Dose not reported	Improvement in taste acuity
Mossman and Henkin[93]	Case reports: 7 patients; head and neck cancer treated with radiotherapy	2 patients 25 mg Zn^{2+}/day 5 patients 100 mg Zn^{2+}/day	Improvement in taste acuity
Henkin[94]	Case reports: patients with head and neck cancer treated with radiotherapy	Zn 25 mg three times/day	Development of less severe hypogeusia

Data from Ripamonti C and Fulfaro F. [95]

An orocutaneous fistula is an abnormal communication between the skin and the oral cavity (external fistula) and is preceded by a cutaneous abscess. In oncological patients, the most frequent causes of fistulas are related to local progression of the disease, relapse ONJ, or treatments such as surgery, radiotherapy, chemotherapy, and photodynamics, In advanced cancer patients with head and neck cancer, cutaneous fistulae are reported in 21%.[97] The onset of a fistula produces various complications: infections, electrolyte imbalance, dehydration, malnutrition, cutaneous lesions, bleeding, delay in oncological treatments, psychosocial problems (distortion of body image, isolation, social discomfort). In advanced cancer patients, treatment is conservative and includes surrounding skin care (barrier cream) and local disinfection with povidone-iodine solution, control of local itching and pain, control of odour, management of nutrition and electrolytes (possible use of nasogastric tube, percutaneous endoscopic gastrostomy, or total parenteral nutrition), control of infections, use of antibiotics against anaerobic bacteria (metronidazole), pouching of secretions, and therapy for psychosocial distress.[53,98]

Trismus

Trismus is a severe restriction of mouth opening that may occur in head–neck cancer patients. The prevalence is variable, with 5–38% of patients developing trismus after treatment for head–neck cancer.[99,100]

Trismus may result directly from tumour which can cause a reflex contraction or prevent relaxation of mouth-closing muscles. It may also be the consequence of head and neck cancer treatments, such as radiotherapy, which results in necrosis and fibrosis of the mandible, pterygoid or masseter muscle).[101] Surgery can produce scars that impair normal opening of the mouth. A mouth interincisal opening of 35 mm is the cut-off value used to define patient's quality of life as impaired.[102] A restricted mouth opening can arise at different times and may seriously limit patients' food intake, chewing, swallowing and oral hygiene. A mean decrease of 32% in initial interincisal distance at 4 years after radiotherapy has been reported, with a rapid rate of evolution 1–9 months after radiation therapy, then becoming slower and protracted over later years.[103]

Some tools are used to either enhance exercise compliance or to improve therapeutic effectiveness. These tools include rubber plugs, wooden tongue blades, the Thera-Bite® system and dynamic bite openers, with variable results.[10,104]

Intensity-modulated radiotherapy (IMRT) in nasopharyngeal carcinoma patients has successfully prevented trismus and achieved a normal maximal interincisal distance in the 5–12 months following IMRT.[105]

References

1. Bensinger W, Schubert M, Ang KK, *et al.* (2008) NCCN Task Force Report: prevention and management of mucositis in cancer care. *J Natl Compr Canc Netw*, **6**(Suppl 1), S1–21.
2. McGuire DB, Correa ME, Johnson J, Wienandts P (2006) The role of basic oral care and good clinical practice principles in the management of oral mucositis. *Support Care Cancer*, **14**, 541–7.
3. López-Galindo MP, Bagán JV, Jiménez-Soriano Y, Alpiste F, Camps C (2006) Clinical evaluation of dental and periodontal status in a group of oncological patients before chemotherapy. *Med Oral Patol Oral Cir Bucal*, **11**(1), 17–21.
4. Sadler GR, Stoudt A, Fullerton JT, Oberele-Edwards LK, Nguyen Q, Epstien JB (2003) Managing the oral sequelae of cancer therapy. *Medsurg Nursing*, **12**(1), 28–36.
5. Southern H (2007) Oral care in cancer nursing: nurses' knowledge and education. *J Adv Nurs*, **57**(6), 631–8.
6. Costa EMM, Fernandez MZ, Quindere LB, de Souza LB, Pinto LP (2003) Evaluation of an oral preventive protocol in children with acute lymphoblastic leukemia. *Pesqui Odontol Bras*, **17**(2),147–50.

7. Turhal NS, Erdal S, Karacay S (2000) Efficacy of treatment to relieve mucositis-induced discomfort. *Support Care Cancer*, **8**, 55–8.
8. Poggi P, Rodriguez y Baena R, Rizzo S, Rota MT (2003) Mouthrinses with alcohol: cytotoxic effects on human gingival fibroblasts in vitro. *J Periodontol*, **74**(5), 623–9.
9. Trotti A, Garden A, Warde P, *et al.* (2004) A multinational, randomized phase III trial of iseganan HCl oral solution for reducing the severity of oral mucositis in patients receiving radiotherapy for head-and-neck malignancy. *Int J Radiat Oncol Biol Phys*, **58**, 674–81.
10. Sciubba JJ, Goldenberg D (2006) Oral complications of radiotherapy *Lancet Oncol*, **7**(2), 175–83.
11. Sonis ST, Elting LS, Keefe D, *et al.* (2004) Perspectives on cancer therapy-induced mucosal injury: pathogenesis, measurement, epidemiology, and consequences for patients. *Cancer*, **100**(9 Suppl), 1995–2025.
12. Trotti A, Colevas AD, Setser A, *et al.* (2003) Common Terminology Criteria for Adverse Events version 3.0: development of a comprehensive grading system for the adverse effects of cancer treatment. *Semin Radiat Oncol*, **13**, 176–81.
13. Sutherland SE, Browman GP (2001) Prophylaxis of oral mucositis in irradiated head-and-neck cancer patients: a proposed classification scheme of interventions and meta-analysis of randomized controlled trials. *Int J Radiat Oncol Biol Phys*, **49**, 917–30.
14. Stokman MA, Spijkervet FK, Boezen HM, *et al.* (2006) Preventive intervention possibilities in radiotherapy- and chemotherapy-induced oral mucositis: results of meta-analyses. *J Dent Res*, **85**, 690–700.
15. Nasilowska-Adamska B, Rzepecki P, Manko J, *et al.* (2007) The influence of palifermin (Kepivance) on oral mucositis and acute graft versus host disease in patients with hematological diseases undergoing hematopoietic stem cell transplant. *Bone Marrow Transplant*, **40**, 983–8.
16. Spijkervet FK, van Saene HK, van Saene JJ, *et al.* (1991) Effect of selective elimination of the oral flora on mucositis in irradiated head and neck cancer patients. *J Surg Oncol*, **46**, 167–73.
17. Stokman MA, Spijkervet FKL, Burlage FR, *et al.* (2003) Oral mucositis and selective elimination of oral flora in head and neck cancer patients receiving radiotherapy: a double-blind randomised clinical trial. *Br J Cancer*, **88**, 1012–16.
18. Cerchietti LC, Navigante AH, Körte MW, *et al.* (2003) Potential utility of the peripheral analgesic properties of morphine in stomatitis-related pain: a pilot study. *Pain*, **105**, 265–73.
19. Keefe D, Schubert M, Elting L, *et al.* (2007) Updated clinical practice guidelines for the prevention and treatment of mucositis. *Cancer*, **109**(5), 820–31.
20. McGuire DB (2003) Barriers and strategies in implementation of oral care standards for cancer patients. *Support Care Cancer*, **11**, 435–41.
21. Epstein JB, Silverman S Jr, Paggiarino DA, *et al.* (2001) Benzydamine HCl for prophylaxis of radiation-induced oral mucositis: results from a multicenter, randomized, double-blind, placebo-controlled clinical trial. *Cancer*, **92**, 875–85.
22. Dodd MJ, Miaskowski C, Greenspan D, *et al.* (2003) Radiation induced mucositis: a randomized clinical trial of micronized sucralfate versus salt and soda mouthwashes. *Cancer Invest*, **21**, 21–33.
23. El-Sayed S, Nabid A, Shelley W, *et al.* (2002) Prophylaxis of radiation associated mucositis in conventionally treated patients with head and neck cancer: a double-blind, Phase III, randomized, controlled trial evaluating the clinical efficacy of an antimicrobial lozenge using a validated mucositis scoring system. *J Clin Oncol*, **20**, 3956–63.
24. Migliorati CA, Oberle-Edwards L, Schubert M (2006) The role of alternative and natural agents, cryotherapy, and/or laser for the management of alimentary mucositis. *Support Care Cancer*, **14**, 533–40.
25. Meropol NJ, Somer RA, Gutheil J, *et al.* (2003) Randomized Phase I trial of recombinant human keratinocyte growth factor plus chemotherapy: potential role as mucosal protectant. *J Clin Oncol*, **21**, 1452–8.

26. Dazzi C, Cariello A, Giovanis P, *et al.* (2003) Prophylaxis with GMCSF mouthwashes does not reduce frequency and duration of severe oral mucositis in patients with solid tumors undergoing high-dose chemotherapy with autologous peripheral blood stem cell transplantation rescue: a double blind, randomized, placebo-controlled study. *Ann Oncol*, **14**, 559–63.
27. Jobbins J, Bagg J, Parsons K, Finlay I, Addy M, Newcombe RG (1992) Oral carriage of yeasts, coliforms and staphylococci in patients with advanced malignant disease. *J Oral Pathol Med*, **21**(7), 305–8.
28. Yeo E, Alvarado T, Fainstein V, Bodey GP (1985) Prophylaxis of oropharyngeal candidiasis with clotrimazole. *J Clin Oncol*, **3**(12), 1668–71.
29. Davies AN, Brailsford SR, Beighton D, Shorthose K, Stevens VC (2008) Oral candidosis in community-based patients with advanced cancer. *J Pain Sympt Manag*, **35**(5), 508–14.
30. Davies AN, Brailsford S, Broadley K, Beighton D (2002) Oral yeast carriage in patients with advanced cancer. *Oral Microbiol Immunol*, **17**, 79–84.
31. Barret AP (1984) Evaluation of nystatin in prevention and elimination of oropharyngeal Candida in immunosuppressed patients. *Oral Surgery*, **58**, 148–51.
32. Barkvoll P, Attramadal A (1989) Effect of nystatin and chlorhexidine digluconate on *Candida albicans*. *Oral Surg Oral Med Oral Pathol*, **67**, 279–81.
33. Meunier F (1990) Fluconazole treatment of fungal infections in the immunocompromised host. *Semin Oncol*, **17** (Suppl 6), 19–23.
34. Goodman JL, Winston DJ, Greenfield RA, *et al.* (1992) A controlled trial of fluconazole to prevent fungal infections in patients undergoing bone marrow transplantation. *N Engl J Med*, **326**(13), 845–51.
35. Tarumi Y, Pereira J, Watanabe S (2002) Methadone and fluconazole: respiratory depression by drug interaction. *J Pain Sympt Manag*, **23**(2), 148–53.
36. Clarkson JE, Worthington HV, Eden OB (2007) Interventions for preventing oral candidiasis for patients with cancer receiving treatment. *Cochrane Database Syst Rev*, **24**(1).
37. Overholser CD Peterson DE, Williams LT, Schimpff SC (1982) Periodontal infections in patients with acute non lymphocytic leukemia: prevalence of acute exacerbations. *Arch Inter Med*, **142**, 551–4.
38. Peterson DE, Overholser CD (1981) Increased morbidity associated with oral infections in patients with non acute lymphocytic leukaemia. *Oral Surg Oral Med Oral Pathol*, **51**, 390–3.
39. Montgomery RT, Redding SW, Le Maistre CF (1986) The incidence of oral herpes simplex virus infection in patients undergoing cancer chemotherapy. *Oral Surg Oral Med Oral Pathol*, **61**, 238–42.
40. Djuric M, Pavlica D, Jankovic L, Milasin J, Jovanovic T (2007) Presence of herpes simplex virus on the oral mucosa in patients undergoing chemotherapy. *Scott Med J*, **52**(1), 28–31.
41. Barret AP, Buckley DJ, Greenberg ML, Earl MJ (1986) The value of exfoliative cytology in diagnosing of oral herpes infection in immunosuppressed patients. *Oral Surg Oral Med Oral Pathol*, **62**, 175–8.
42. Leflore S, Anderson PL, Fletcher CV (2000) A risk-benefit evaluation of acyclovir for the treatment and prophylaxis of herpes simplex virus infections. *Drug Saf*, **23**(2), 131–42.
43. Marx RE (2003) Pamidronate (Aredia) and zoledronate (Zometa) induced avascular necrosis of the jaws: a growing epidemic. *J Oral Maxillofac Surg*, **61**, 1115–7.
44. Ruggiero SL, Mehrotra B, Rosenberg TJ, Engroff SL (2004) Osteonecrosis of the jaws associated with the use of bisphosphonates: a review of 63 cases. *J Oral Maxillofac Surg*, **62**, 527–34.
45. Iguchi T, Miyakawa Y, Saito K, *et al.* (2007) Zoledronate-induced S phase arrest and apoptosis accompanied by DNA damage and activation of the ATM/Chk1/cdc25 pathway in human osteosarcoma cells. *Int J Oncol*, **31**(2), 285–91.
46. Rogers MJ (2003) New insights into the molecular mechanisms of action of bisphosphonates. *Curr Pharm Des*, **9**(32), 2643–58.
47. Hellstein JW, Marek CL (2005) Bisphosphonate osteochemonecrosis (bis-phossy jaw): is this phossy jaw of the 21st century? *J Oral Maxillofac Surg*, **63**(5), 682–9.

48. Bamias A, Kastritis E, Bamia C, *et al.* (2005) Osteonecrosis of the jaw in cancer after treatment with bisphosphonates: incidence and risk factors. *J Clin Oncol*, **23**, 8580–7.
49. Durie B, Katz M, Crowley J (2005) Osteonecrosis of the jaw and bisphosphonates. *N Engl J Med*, **351**, 99–102.
50. Ripamonti CI, Maniezzo M, Campa T, *et al.* (2009) Decreased occurrence of osteonecrosis of the jaw after implementation of dental preventive measures in solid tumour patients with bone metastases treated with bisphosphonates. The experience of the National Cancer Institute of Milan. *Ann Oncol*, **20**(1), 137–45.
51. La Verde N, Bareggi C, Garassino, *et al.* (2008) Osteonecrosis of the jaw (ONJ) in cancer patients treated with bisphosphonates: how the knowledge of a phenomenon can change its evolution. *Support Care Cancer*, **16**(11), 1311–5.
52. Ventafridda V, De Conno F, Ripamonti C, Gamba A, Tamburini M (1990) Quality-of-life assessment during a palliative care program. *Ann Oncol*, **1**, 415–20.
53. De Conno F, Sbanotto A, Ripamonti C, Ventafridda V (2004) Mouth care. In: Doyle D, Hanks GWC, MacDonald N (eds), *Oxford Textbook of Palliative Medicine*, 3rd edn, pp. 673–687. Oxford: Oxford University Press.
54. Fusco F (2006) Mouth care. In: Bruera E, Higginson IJ, Ripamonti C, von Gunten C (eds), *Textbook of Palliative Medicine*, pp. 774–9. London: Hodder Arnold.
55. Kies MS, Haraf DJ, Rosen F, *et al.* (2001) Concomitant infusional paclitaxel and fluorouracil, oral hydroxyurea, and hyperfractionated radiation for locally advanced squamous head and neck cancer. *J Clin Oncol*, **19**, 1961–9.
56. Makkonen TA, Tenovuo J, Vilja P, Heimdahl A (1986) Changes in the protein composition of whole saliva during radiotherapy in patients with oral or pharyngeal cancer. *Oral Surg*, **62**, 270–5.
57. Reddy SP, Leman CR, Marks JE, Emami B (2001) Parotid-sparing irradiation for cancer of the oral cavity: maintenance of oral nutrition and body weight by preserving parotid function. *Am J Clin Oncol*, **24**, 341–6.
58. Ventafridda V, Ripamonti C, Bianchi M, Sbanotto A, De Conno F (1986) A randomized study on oral morphine and methadone in the treatment of cancer pain. *J Pain Sympt Manag*, 1, 203–7.
59. Ventafridda V, Saita L, Barletta L, Sbanotto A, De Conno F (1989) Clinical observations on controlled-release morphine in cancer pain. *J Pain Sympt Manag*, **4**, 124–9.
60. Ventafridda V, Tamburini M, Caraceni A, De Conno F, Naldi F (1987) A validation study of the WHO method for cancer pain relief. *Cancer*, 59, 850–6.
61. Duxbury AJ, Thakker, NS, Wastell DG (1989) A double-blind cross-over trial of a mucin-containing artificial saliva. *Br Dent J*, 166, 115–20.
62. Vissink A, Schaub RM, van Rijn LJ, Gravenmade EJ, Panders AK, Vermey A (1987) The efficacy of mucin-containing artificial saliva in xerostomia. *Gerodontology*, 6, 95–101.
63. Visch L, Gravenmade EJ, Schaub RM, Van Putten WL, Vissink A (1986) A double-blind crossover trial of CMC- and mucin-containing saliva substitutes. *Int J Oral Maxfac Surg*, 15, 395–400.
64. Konings AW, Coppes RP, Vissink A (2005) On the mechanism of salivary gland radiosensitivity. *Int J Radiat Oncol Biol Phys*, **62**, 1187–94.
65. Brizel DM, Wasserman TH, Henke M, *et al.* (2000) Phase III randomized trial of amifostine as a radioprotector in head and neck cancer. *J Clin Oncol*, **18**, 3339–45.
66. Wasserman TH, Brizel DM, Henke M, *et al.* (2005) Influence of intravenous amifostine on xerostomia, tumor control and survival after radiotherapy for head and neck cancer: 2-year follow-up of a prospective, randomized, phase III trial. *Int J Radiat Oncol Biol Phys*, **63**, 985–90.
67. Johnson JT, Ferretti Ga, Nethery WJ, *et al.* (1993) Oral pilocarpine for post-irradiation xerostomia in patients with head and neck cancer. *N Engl J Med*, **329**, 390–5.
68. Warde P, O'Sullivan B, Aslanidis J, *et al.* (2002) A phase III placebo-controlled trial of oral pilocarpine in patients undergoing radiotherapy for head and neck cancer. *Int J Radiat Oncol Biol Phys*, **54**, 9–13.

69. Ship JA, Hu K (2004) Radiotherapy-induced salivary dysfunction. *Semin Oncol*, **31**(Suppl 18), 29–36.

70. Zimmerman RP, Mark RJ, Tran LM, Juillard GF (1997) Concomitant pilocarpine during head and neck irradiation is associated with decreased post-treatment xerostomia. *Int J Radiat Oncol Biol Phys*, **37**, 571–5.

71. Vivino FB, Al-Hashimi I, Khan Z, *et al.* (1999) Pilocarpine tablets for the treatment of dry mouth and dry eye symptoms in patients with Sjögren syndrome: a randomized, placebo-controlled, fixed-dose, multicenter trial. *Arch Intern Med*, **159**, 174–81.

72. Ganong WF (2003) *Review of Medical Physiology*, 21st edn, pp. 191–4. New York: Lange Medical Books.

73. Schiffman SS (1983) Taste and smell in disease (first of two parts). *New Engl J Med*, **308**(21), 1275–9.

74. Portenoy RK, Thaler HT, Kornblith AB, *et al.* (1994) Symptom prevalence, characteristics and distress in a cancer population. *Qual Life Res*, **3**(3), 183–9.

75. Chang VT, Hwang SS, Feuerman M, Kasimis BS, Thaler HT (2000) The Memorial Symptom Assessment Scale Short Form (MSAS-SF). *Cancer*, **89**(5), 1162–71.

76. Tranmer JE, Heyland D, Dudgeon D, Groll D, Squires-Graham M, Coulson K (2003) Measuring the symptom experience of seriously ill cancer and noncancer hospitalized patients near the end of life with the Memorial Symptom Assessment Scale. *J Pain Sympt Manag*, **25**(5), 420–9.

77. Shorthose K, Davies A (2003) Symptom prevalence in palliative care. *Palliat Med*, **17**(8), 723–4.

78. Wickham RS, Rehwaldt M, Kefer C, *et al.* (1999) Taste changes experienced by patients receiving chemotherapy. *Oncol Nurs Forum*, **26**, 697–706.

79. Maes A, Huygh I, Weltens C, *et al.* (2002) De Gustibus: time scale of loss and recovery of tastes caused by radiotherapy. *Radiother Oncol*, **63**(2), 195–201.

80. Ruo Redda MG, Allis S (2006) Radiotherapy-induced taste impairment. *Cancer Treat Rev*, **32**(7), 541–7.

81. Mossman KL, Shatzman AR, Chencharick JD (1982) Long-term effects of radiotherapy on taste and salivary function in man. *Int J Radiat Oncol Biol Phys*, **8**(6), 991–7.

82. Williams LR, Cohen MH (1978) Altered taste thresholds in lung cancer. *Am J Clin Nutr*, 31, 122–5.

83. DeWys WD, Walters, K (1975) Abnormalities of taste sensation in cancer patients. *Cancer*, 36, 1888–96.

84. Twycross RG, Lack SA (1986) *Control of Alimentary Symptoms in Far Advanced Cancer*. Edinburgh: Churchill Livingstone.

85. Komurcu S, Nelson KA, Walsh D (2001) The gastrointestinal symptoms of advanced cancer. *Support Care Cancer*, **9**(1), 32–9.

86. Mossman KL, Henkin RI (1978) Radiation-induced changes in taste acuity in cancer patients. *Int J Radiat Oncol Biol Phys*, **4**(7–8), 663–70.

87. Silverman S Jr, Thompson JS (1984) Serum zinc and copper in oral/oropharyngeal carcinoma. A study of seventy-five patients. *Oral Surg Oral Med Oral Pathol*, **57**(1), 34–6.

88. Silverman JE, Weber CW, Silverman S Jr, Coulthard SL, Manning MR (1983) Zinc supplementation and taste in head and neck cancer patients undergoing radiation therapy. *J Oral Med*, **38**(1), 14–6.

89. Ripamonti C, Zecca E, Brunelli C, *et al.* (1998) A randomized, controlled clinical trial to evaluate the effects of zinc sulfate on cancer patients with taste alterations caused by head and neck irradiation. *Cancer*, **82**(10), 1938–45.

90. Halyard MY, Jatoi A, Sloan JA, *et al.* (2007) Does zinc sulfate prevent therapy-induced taste alterations in head and neck cancer patients? Results of phase III double-blind, placebo-controlled trial from the North Central Cancer Treatment Group (N01C4). *Int J Radiat Oncol Biol Phys*, **67**(5), 1318–22.

91. Henkin RI, Bradley DF (1970) Hypogeusia corrected by Ni^{++} and ZN^{++}. *Life Sci*, **9**, 701–9.

92. Schnarch A, Markitziu A (1990) Dysgeusia, gustatory sweating, and crocodile tears syndrome induced by a cerebellopontine angle meningioma. *Oral Surg Oral Med Oral Pathol*, **70**, 711–14.

93. Mossman KL, Henkin RI (1978) Radiation-induced changes in taste acuity in cancer patients. *Int J Radiat Oncol Biol Phys* **4**(7/8), 663–70.

94. Henkin RI (1972) Prevention and treatment of hypogeusia due to head and neck irradiation. *J Am Med Assoc*, **220**, 870–1.
95. Ripamonti C, Fulfaro F (2008) Taste disturbance. In: Davies A, Epstein J (eds), *Oral Complications of Cancer and its Treatment*, chapter 22. Oxford: Oxford University Press.
96. Barret AP (1988) Metronidazole in the management of anaerobic neck infection on acute leukemia. *Oral Surg Oral Med Oral Pathol*, **66**, 287–9.
97. Forbes K (1997) Palliative care in patients with cancer of the head and neck. *Clin Otolaryngol*, **22**, 117–22.
98. Fulfaro F, Ripamonti C (2006) Fistulas. In: Bruera E, Higginson IJ, Ripamonti C, von Gunten C (eds), *Textbook of Palliative Medicine*, pp. 780–6. London: Hodder Arnold.
99. Thomas F, Ozanne F, Mamelle G, Wibault P, Eschwege F (2006) Radiotherapy alone for oropharyngeal carcinomas: the role of fraction size (2Gy vs 2·5Gy) on local control and early and late complications. *Int J Radiat Oncol Biol Phys*, **15**, 1097–102.
100. Steelman R, Sokol J (1986) Quantification of trismus following irradiation of the temporomandibular joint. *Mo Dent J*, **66**, 21–3.
101. Vissink A, Jansma J, Spijkervet FK, Burlage FR, Coppes RP (2004) Oral sequelae of head and neck radiotherapy. *Crit Rev Oral Biol Med*, **14**, 199–212.
102. Scott B, Butterworth C, Lowe D, Rogers SN (2008) Factors associated with restricted mouth opening and its relationship to health-related quality of life in patients attending a maxillofacial oncology clinic. *Oral Oncol*, **44**(5), 430–8.
103. Wang CJ, Huang EY, Hsu HC, Chen HC, Fang FM, Hsiung CY (2005) The degree and time-course assessment of radiation-induced trismus occurring after radiotherapy for nasopharyngeal cancer. *Laryngoscope*, **115**(8), 1458–60.
104. Dijkstra PU, Sterken MW, Pater R, Spijkervet FK, Roodenburg JL (2007) Exercise therapy for trismus in head and neck cancer. *Oral Oncol*, **43**(4), 389–94.
105. Hsiung CY, Huang EY, Ting HM, Huang HY (2008) Intensity-modulated radiotherapy for nasopharyngeal carcinoma: the reduction of radiation-induced trismus. *Br J Radiol*, **81**(970), 809–14.

Chapter 14

Nausea and vomiting in advanced cancer

Mellar P. Davis

Introduction

Nausea and vomiting after chemotherapy is a well-studied symptom cluster, which has been divided into acute, delayed and anticipatory. Evidence for treatment is quite established with serotonin receptor-3 antagonists ($5HT_3RA$), dexamethasone and tachykinin (NK_1) receptor antagonists. Treatment guidelines for nausea and vomiting in advanced cancer, unrelated to chemotherapy, are not well established. Only a rare randomized controlled trial (RCT) has been successfully completed in this population. This is tragic since the prevalence of nausea and vomiting in advanced cancer (40–70%) matches the prevalence nausea and vomiting after moderate chemotherapy.[1–6] Patients may complain of nausea alone, vomiting alone or both. The pattern and severity, as well as associated symptoms other than nausea or vomiting, can provide clues as to the aetiology of nausea and vomiting.[7] Nausea contributes to weight loss in advanced cancer, vomiting will worsen bone pain or lead to complications such as pathological fractures. Both accelerate the demise of the patient. In fact, many dread nausea worse than pain and will forgo analgesics if it is suspected that nausea is opioid-induced.[1]

Nausea is an unpleasant sensation of the need to vomit. It is accompanied by autonomic symptoms such as pallor, cold sweats, tachycardia and diarrhoea. Retching is the spasmodic movement of the diaphragm without retrograde propulsion or peristalsis and is non-productive of vomitus (and thus differs from vomiting). However, vomiting and retching are frequently classified together.[1,8]

Multiple anti-emetics are available and have been reported to benefit patients with nausea.[1] Choices are usually made either based on presumed aetiological mechanisms according to clinical evaluation (aetiological guidelines) or guided by empiric single or multiple drug trials, irrespective of the mechanisms generating nausea and vomiting.[2,3,7] Individuals unaware of the various studies in advanced cancer may irrationally treat individuals based on guidelines that do not pertain to the population (such as guidelines based on chemotherapy prophylaxis) or by anecdotal experience.

Advances in our understanding of the physiology and pharmacology of the emetogenic reflex has led to the development of new classes of anti-emetics such as $5HT_3$ antagonists and neurokinin-1 receptor (NK_1) antagonists, which are instrumental in compassionately preventing chemotherapy-induced nausea and vomiting (CINV). Also an understanding of the emetic reflex has been key to the prospective studies of aetiological guidelines in advanced cancer. Such guidelines utilize presumed mechanisms based on presumed neurotransmitters and receptors which generate nausea to choose anti-emetics in a treatment paradigm which has been relatively successful.[2]

Neurocircuitry to nausea and vomiting

Peripheral signals

The emetic reflex involves phases of: (1) oesophageal dilatation, (2) relaxation of the lower oesophageal sphincter, (3) gastric dilatation, (4) gastric emptying, (5) gastric reflux; and

(6) oesophageal collapse in a cyclic pattern.[9] There is a coordinated relaxation of crural muscle and contraction of somatic abdominal and intercostal muscles. The small bowel generates a large retroperistalsis resulting in the production of vomitus. Prior to and during emesis the glottis closes and the soft palate elevates to protect the airway.[10–12]

In addition, there is a burst of autonomic activity that leads to sweating, tachycardia, hypotension. Vasopressin and oxytocin are released before or at the onset of nausea.[11] Several of the gastrointestinal reflexes that occur with nausea and vomiting may be seen with other gastrointestinal symptoms. Inhibition of the crural occurs with belching, changes in gastric accommodation with early satiety and relaxation of the lower oesophageal sphincter and crural diaphragm with gastro-oesophageal reflux disease.[11]

The research on nausea and vomiting using animal models is hampered by several factors. Although the ferret is usually the animal model of choice used in anti-emetic drug development, subspecies of ferrets differ in their sensitivity to various emetogenic stimuli.[12] There is no animal model for nausea, which is the symptom patients dread more than vomiting. Emetogenic responses to various agents (apomorphine, cisplatin, morphine) differ based on route of administration.[12] Little is known about the mechanisms that generate vomiting prior to drug absorption (gastric phase), where much is known about the signal pathways that generate post-absorption nausea and vomiting and is centred on the dorsal vagus complex (DVC). Non-vomiting species, such as rats, develop rapid conditioned food aversions, nippling-type food intake and pica in lieu of vomiting, as a protective mechanism, behaviours that advanced cancer patients may have. Many of the receptors which block emesis in humans block learned food aversions and pica in rats (ondansetron, $5HT_3RA$, δ-9-tetrahydrocannabinol and cannabinol receptor agonists].[11] Vasopressin is elevated with nausea in humans and many treatments that produce nausea and vomiting will increase vasopressin levels high enough to cause antidiuresis.[11] Certain causes of vomiting and nausea, such as motion, do not cause vasopressin to increase. Other hormones are also increased in nausea (adrenaline, cortisol, growth hormone, prolactin adrenocorticotrophic hormone, pancreatic polypeptide), yet it is not known if this is cause or effect.[11] Nausea may be associated with other symptoms. Nausea is often associated with pain, and pain can produce nausea and vomiting. Postoperative pain and nausea occur together, and when pain is relieved, nausea resolves.[13,14] Nausea and visceral pain may share some neural pathways. The emetic response to staphylococcal enterotoxin induced experimentally is not reduced by vagotomy or splanchnic, whereas interrupting both pathways abolishes emesis.[14] As a general rule, afferent nerves that travel with the sympathic autonomic nerves in the gut produce visceral pain, whereas vagal afferents in humans are responsible for vomiting.[11] However, splanchnic afferents can be the alternative emetogenic circuit when the subdiaphragmatic vagus is sectioned.[15] Vomiting after subdiaphragmatic vagotomy may occur due to activation of cardiac vagal afferents; pulmonary vagal afferents do not cause nausea. Increased plasma levels of several hormones, previously mentioned, could potentially be the alternative afferent route.

Overall most would agree that upper gastrointestinal tract vagal afferents are the most important pathways for postabsorption nausea. On the other hand, the vagal afferents are not essential for nausea. Even those with bilateral abdominal vagotomy experience nausea.[11] Hence, like vomiting, the circuit that induces nausea is mainly through vagal afferents, but is not essential.[12]

Central circuits for nausea and vomiting

The autonomic, smooth and striated muscle contraction and relaxation that occurs with vomiting is coordinated at the level of the medulla oblongata. This region is located from the opening of the central canal into the fourth ventricle to the level of the nucleus ambiguous (Figures 14.1 and 14.2). An area deep to the DVC near the nucleus ambiguous and retrofacial nucleus is a non-discrete set of neurons termed the central pattern generator (CPG) which controls the timing and activation of voluntary and involuntary muscles involved in emesis.[10,16] Afferent vagal input synapse in the area postrema and nearby nucleus tractus solitarius (NTS) is an important input to the CPG. In close proximity is the dorsal motor nucleus (DMN) part of the DVC which is involved in governing gastric motility (Figure 14.1). Three structures make up the DVC: area postrema, NTS and DMN. Neurons within the DVC and CPG control swallowing, baroreceptor reflexes, respiration and tone/mobility of oesophagus and stomach.[10,16] Half of pre-ganglionic motor neurons in the DMN innervate the lower oesophageal sphincter and fundus of the stomach. The area in and around the nucleus ambiguous (area of the CPG) innervates larynx, pharynx, expiratory respiratory muscles, sympathetic outflow for blood pressure, and parasympathetic outflow to the heart.[10] Connections between the NTS to the mango-cellular hypothalamic neurons and catecholamine neurons in ventrolateral medulla to hypothalamus are responsible for releasing both vasopressin and oxytocin.[10] Efferent output from the nucleus ambiguous to the C5–7 spinal cord governs phrenic nerve output to the diaphragm.[10]

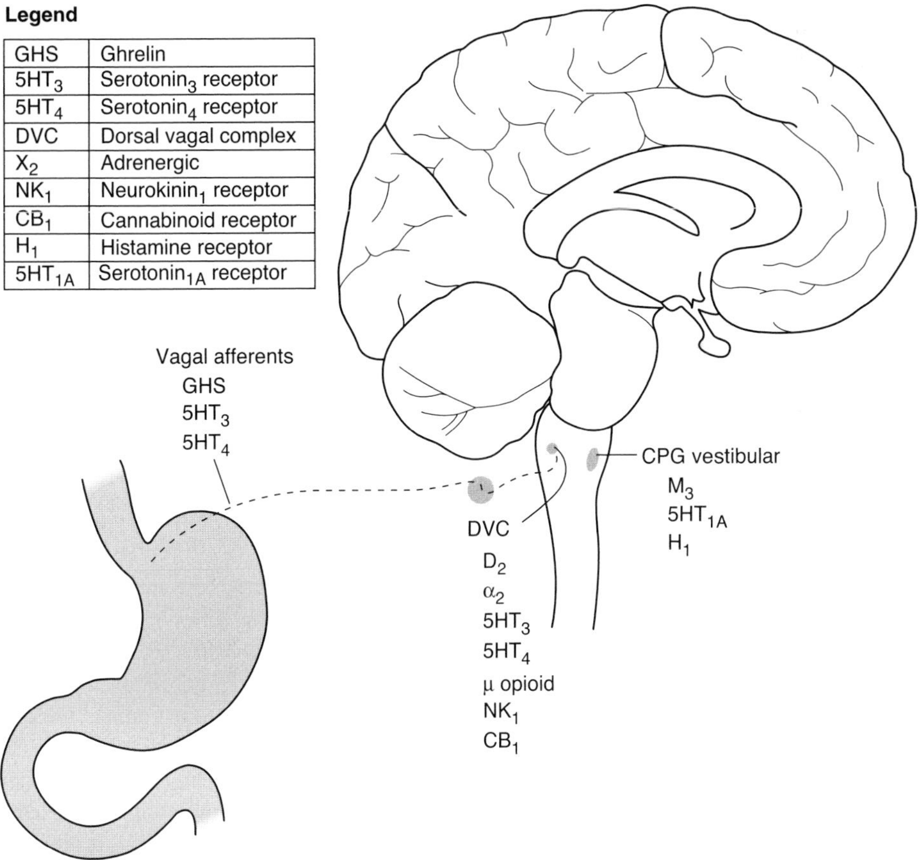

Fig. 14.1 Emetic neurotransmitters. GHS, ghrelin; $5HT_3$, serotonin$_3$ receptor; $5HT_4$, serotonin$_4$ receptor; DVC, dorsal vagal complex; α_2, adrenergic; NK_1, neurokinin$_1$ receptor; CB_1, cannabinoid receptor; CPG, central pattern generator; M_3, muscarinic; H_1, histamine receptor; $5HT_1A$, serotonin$_{1A}$ receptor.

Legend

NTS	Nuclues tractus solitarus
LES	Lower esophageal sphincter
DMN	Dorsal motor neuron
XII	12th cranial nerve
AP	Area postrema
Gel	Subnucleus gelatinosus
Int	Intermediate subnucleus
TS	Tractus solitarius
VL	Ventrolateral subnucleus
V4	4th ventricle
CPC	Central pattern generator

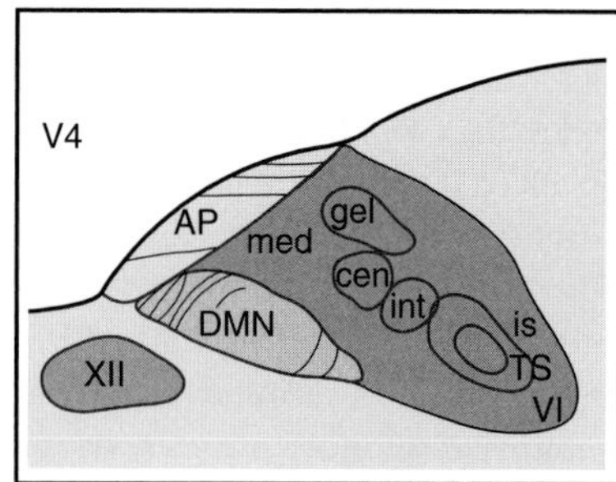

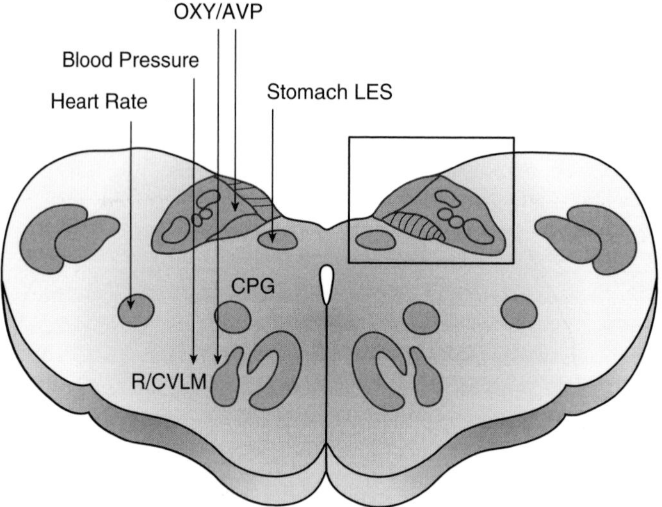

Fig. 14.2 Central neuroanatomy important to the emesis reflex. LES, lower oesophageal sphincter; CPG, central pattern generator; R/CVLM, right caudal ventrolateral medulla; OXY, oxytocin; AVP, arginine vasopressin; V4, 4th ventricle; AP, area postrema; DMN, dorsal motor neuron; XII, 12th cranial nerve; gel, subnucleus gelatinosus; med, medial subnucleus; cen, central subnucleus; int, intermediate subnucleus; is, interstitial subnucleus TS, tractus solitarius; vl, ventrolateral subnucleus.

Little is known about the neural circuits responsible for nausea, but these appear to be anatomically distinct from circuits which generate emesis.[11] The vomiting reflex is confined to the brainstem (decerebrate animals are capable of emesis). Autonomic activation, sepsis and motion will induce vomiting in decorticate individuals.[11] Conscious awareness, typical of nausea, is a cerebral function. If conditioned food aversion in rats is analogous to nausea in humans, then the forebrain region is involved in the perception of nausea.[11] Nausea and emesis also appear to be pharmacologically distinct. Serotonin receptor antagonists ($5HT_3RA$) such as ondansetron control acute emesis in chemotherapy quite well, but more than half of patients experience nausea.[17,18] Nausea is often more troublesome usually continuous and less responsive; emesis is episodic and more responsive to multiple anti-emetics. It is generally assumed that nausea is a low level stimulus that increases to climax in emesis. However, because nausea is more difficult to treat, has a greater aversive affective component and can be separately experienced, it is unlikely that nausea is a low grade affect of vomiting. Raised intracranial pressure will produce vomiting without nausea and so the two can be generated by distinctly different circuits. This may also occur with radiation therapy and during pregnancy.[11] Nausea originating from cerebral and vestibular sites might directly access higher centres responsible for nausea and bypass brainstem circuits that generate vomiting. AP lesions in experimental animals prevent vomiting with many emetogenic drugs but do not prevent vomiting with motion or by activation of vagal afferents.[19]

Drugs will initiate emesis from different sites within the DVC. Apomorphine, a dopamine D_2 receptor agonist, is a commonly used experimental emetic agent. Emesis is blocked by domperidone, metoclopramide and ablation of the AP.[12] $5HT_3$ receptors, which are blocked by ondansetron, are located presynaptically in the NTS and are effective in reducing cisplatin-induced emesis, whereas phenothiazines and low dose metoclopramide (D_2 receptor antagonists) are relatively ineffective.[12] Neurokinin-1 receptor antagonists are broad-spectrum antagonists relative to $5HT_3$RA and prevent delayed nausea from cisplatin, where ondansetron is fairly ineffective. Neurokinin-1 receptor expression is greatest in DMN, which is responsible for gastric fundus relaxation.[20,21] Gamma aminobutyric acid $(GABA)_A$ receptors are found also in the DMN. $GABA_A$ and $GABA_B$ receptor agonists block lower oesophageal sphincter relaxations and thus have anti-emetic activity. Gabapentin, which may interact with GABA receptors, reduces postoperative nausea and vomiting.[22–24] Midazolam reduces postoperative nausea and vomiting.[25] Nicotinic receptors are found in the DMN and NTS; three different nicotinic receptors are found in the dorsal medulla oblongata, which influence gastrointestinal function and, presumably, nausea. Each site where nicotinic cholinergic receptors are found appears to have an independent action.[26] It is unlikely that a 'universal' anti-emetic will be found due to the complex interactions of multiple receptors and neurotransmitters found between the DVC and CPG and within the DVC. In addition, combinations of anti-emetics may be needed or medications with broad receptor-binding profiles may be needed to control emesis (and perhaps nausea) in a significant number of individuals whose nausea and vomiting has failed to respond to a single anti-emetic.

Finally, there is plasticity in the organization of the emetic pathway and reflex. Ferrets, post bilateral vagotomy, become hypersensitive to copper sulphate. $5HT_3$RA does not reduce the emesis of abdominal radiation in vagotomized animals. This may be due to radiation-induced release of a peptide from the gastrointestinal wall which induces emesis via entrance into the AP.[12] As a result, responses to anti-emetics may be dependent on the clinical situation. Plasticity involving the emetic circuit can lead either to loss of control or failure to respond to anti-emetics.

Receptors and neurotransmitters

Nicotinic, muscarinic, dopaminergic NK_I GABA cannabinoid and histamine receptor antagonists have anti-emetic actions in a variety of clinical situations.[27]

Certain serotonin receptors are emetogenic ($5HT_3$) and others reduce emesis ($5HT_1$A and $5HT_4$). Muscarinic receptors are found in high density within the DVC, less so in the reticular formation of the central power generator and in a lesser density in the vestibular area.[28] Muscarinic receptors occur presynaptically on vagal afferent terminals. Expression is significantly reduced by vagotomy.[29,30] Cholinergic axons terminating on noradrenaline neurons within the AP induce emesis when activated. Some cholinergic terminals bypass the AP to synapse deeper in the DVC.[31]

Dopamine receptors are found predominately in the AP. Apomorphine, a D_2 receptor agonist, induces vomiting, which is completely prevented by AP ablation.[12] In the ferret, D_1-like receptors and D_4 receptors have no emetic effect; only D_2 and D_3 receptor agonists induce vomiting.[32]

Histamine receptors (H_1) are found throughout the DVC. Most histamine receptor antagonists block cholinergic receptors, which complicates our understanding of the contribution of H_1 receptor agonists' contribution to emesis and H_1 antagonists to anti-emesis.[27] The inhibitory constant (K_1) of diphenhydramine and promethazine at the H_1 receptor is only slightly lower than the K_1 for muscarinic receptors.[27] Therefore, most clinically available anticholinergic medications will also, to a certain extent, block histamine receptors.

More than 80% of 5HT in the body is located in enterochromaffin cells within the gastrointestinal mucosa.[33] 5HT is released from the intestinal mucosa upon exposure to many, but not all, chemotherapy agents and by radiation. Decarbazine and nitrogen mustard are exceptions. Urinary excretion of 5-hydroxyindoleacetic acid (5HIAA) and chromagranin A are markers of serotonin release from the gut.[33] Acetylcholine increases 5HT release (and anticholinergics reduce 5HT release, which may be a mechanism by which anticholinergics reduce nausea). Cisplatin-induced acute emesis correlates with 5HIAA levels. Serotonin binds to $5HT_3$ receptors on vagal afferents as the main mechanism of inducing emesis. $5HT_3$ receptors are also found in the DVC.[12,33–37] $5HT_3$RA do reduce DVC serotonin levels,[33] thus having a central effect on emesis. $5HT_3$RA have a relatively narrow spectrum of anti-emesis relative to NK_1 receptor antagonists. Experimentally, $5HT_3$ blockers do not reduce emesis from erythromycin, pilocarpine, apomorphine, loperamide, copper sulphate or motion.[12] $5HT_3$ receptors are a family of ligand-gated ion channels which are composed of subunits. As a result, several subtypes exist due to polymorphisms of heteromers ($5HT_3$B1, $5HT_3$A).[38] Different $5HT_3$RA may produce different responses due to polymorphisms and splice variants of the $5HT_3$ receptor. Hence, $5HT_3$RA switch may produce a response where the first receptor blocker failed to control emesis.[33,38]

Other 5HT receptors are involved in emetogenic pathways. $5HT_1$A receptor agonists may be more effective anti-emetics than $5HT_3$ receptor antagonists in certain animal species.[37,39] $5HT_1$A receptor agonists may work peripherally by preventing release of 5HT from enterochromaffin cells.[33] $5HT_4$ receptors are found in the gastrointestinal tract and mainly govern secretory function and motility. $5HT_4$ receptors are found within the mucosa (whereas $5HT_3$ receptors are found mainly in visceral neurons). $5HT_4$ receptor agonists block the release of serotonin from the gut.[33] Combinations of $5HT_3$RA and $5HT_1$A or $5HT_4$ receptor agonists may be more effective than either class of medication alone in reducing emesis but at the present time this is speculative. Neurokinin receptors (NK_1) are activated by substance P, which is found both on vagal afferents and within the DVC.[40] Substance P may activate $5HT_3$ receptors and NK_1 receptor activation may facilitate 5HT release.[33] In addition, NK_1 receptor antagonists are thought to work in the central nervous system (CNS), either within the area postrema or by blocking vagal motor neurons within the DMN.[10] NK_1 receptors are also found in certain animal species within the central pattern generator.[41] As a result, NK_1 receptor antagonists act synergistically with $5HT_3$RA to inhibit emesis and have a broader spectrum of activity than $5HT_3$RA.

Agonist anti-emetics

Both $5HT_1$A and $5HT_4$ receptor agonists are anti-emetics. Other receptor agonists that have anti-emetic activity are cannabinoid CB1 receptor agonists, opioid receptor agonists, $GABA_B$ receptor agonists and ghrelin.[27]

Cannabinoids have well-documented anti-emetic effects in a variety of species for a wide range of central- and peripheral-acting emetogenic agents (cisplatin, apomorphine, morphine, intragastric saline infusion). The anti-emetic effects occur at lower doses than those that cause psychotomimetic side-effects. The action appears to be mediated by CB_1 receptors in the DVC.[27] A second potential mechanism involves down-modulation or blockade of $5HT_3$ receptors which overlaps with $5HT_3$RA actions. CB_1 receptor agonists have well-established anti-emetic effects clinically, but the effects on nausea are not as well established.

Opioid receptor agonists such as morphine are well known for emetic effects, but at high doses this appears to be lost.[42] In animal studies, morphine and selective opioid receptor agonists have a broad spectrum of anti-emetic effects (apomorphine, copper sulphate, cyclophosphamide, cisplatin, and nicotine). This anti-emesis is reversed by naloxone.[27] Opioid receptors may interact with NK_1 receptor agonists and $5HT_1A$ receptor agonists to further inhibit emesis.[43]

Selective $GABA_B$ receptor agonists, such as baclofen, reduce emesis to a wide range of emetic initiators in the ferret. This includes cyclophosphamide, radiation, cisplatin and morphine. Clinically, baclofen has reduced emesis in neurologically impaired children with gastro-oesophageal reflux disease.[44]

Ghrelin binds to and activates the growth hormone secretogogue (GHS) receptor type Ia. GHS receptors are found in the hypothalamus, but the highest concentrates are found in the stomach.[45] GHS receptors have effects similar to motilin in the regulation of gastrointestinal mobility,[45] the beneficial effects on appetite and gastric motility, whereas deacylated ghrelin delays gastric emptying and diminishes appetite.[46] Ghrelin reduces cisplatin dyspepsia in rodents.[47] Individuals with functional dyspepsia benefit from ghrelin which reduces meal-related symptoms including nausea and enhances gastric emptying.[48] Ghrelin, a peripheral-acting anti-emetic, may act in synergy with central-acting anti-emetics.

Clinical relevance to understanding anti-emetic neurocircuitry

Research into anti-emetics involves identification of neurotransmitters and receptors that generate emesis in particular clinical situations. The goal of drug development is to find or synthesize agents which interfere with neurotransmission. This approach has identified D_2, H_1, M_3/M_5, $5HT_3$ and NK_1 receptors as major mediators of emesis. It has been assumed that a single neurotransmitter and/or receptor is involved in the generation of emesis from a particular stimulus. However, emesis may occur through several pathways simultaneously, or is amplified by interacting receptors. This may explain why $5HT_3RA$ and NK_1 receptor antagonists work synergistically to reduce cisplatin emesis and H_1 and M_3/M_5 receptor antagonists reduce motion sickness.[27] Adding non-overlapping anti-emetics which have different receptor-binding profiles has been successful in managing postoperative nausea and vomiting in addition to chemotherapy-induced nausea and vomiting.[49]

Identification of agents with anti-nausea activity is a challenge. There are no animal models. Physicians often prescribe anti-emetics for nausea, yet the pathways for nausea and emesis are distinctly different (though there may be some overlap in the brainstem). Nausea, which is a conscious awareness of the need to vomit, may bypass the brainstem DVC and CPG. The affective component of nausea which causes patients to suffer and complain is a cortical activity (perhaps prefrontal lobe area, similar to pain and food aversions in certain animals) of which we have little knowledge. If anticipatory nausea prior to chemotherapy is a clinical manifestation of a cortical-generated symptom, then anti-emetics for the most part fail to work or poorly control nausea.

Nausea and vomiting in advanced cancer: history, physical examination and diagnostic tests

Assessment and treatment of symptoms are based on an understanding of mechanisms. Pathophysiological mechanisms are inferred by a careful history, physical examination and diagnostic tests.[3] A key step to successful management involves combining the clinical picture with knowledge of emetic neuron-pharmacology in order to develop single or combination drug treatment regimens.

A pattern of infrequent large volume vomitus which relieves nausea suggests gastroparesis, gastric outlet obstruction or small bowel or colonic obstruction. Colic, constipation and abdominal pain are helpful additional clues.[1] On physical examination, abdominal distention and borborygami may be present in the case of a small bowel obstruction or colonic obstruction. The abdomen may not be distended in a high small bowel or gastric outlet obstruction, but a succession splash may be elicited. Periumbilical adenopathy (Sister Mary Joseph nodes) or a rim of tumour felt around the cul de sac on rectal examination (Blumer Shelf) are indications of extensive intra-abdominal and/or pelvic carcinomatosis, which would raise concerns about bowel obstruction. Ascites may produce nausea and vomiting unrelated to bowel obstruction. Nausea and vomiting will respond to a paracentesis in this case. A flat plate radiograph of the abdomen (commonly called kidney, ureter, bladder, or KUB X-ray) may demonstrate air-fluid levels in about 60–70% of those with a bowel obstruction.[1] Computed tomography and oral contrast studies may be necessary to determine the cause of obstruction and locate the area of obstruction(s) for those who are surgical candidates. If obstruction remains a concern after a plain abdominal film and endoscopy, a small bowel follow-through will reliably detect a partial high-grade obstruction, but will miss a subtle partial obstruction. Enteroclysis, which is a combination of barium and methylcellulose instilled into the proximal small bowel, should be considered if clinical suspicion for a symptomatic partial small bowel obstruction remains after standard studies, and despite a normal small bowel follow-through.[50] Gastric emptying studies (either with [^{99m}Tc] sulphur colloid in egg or ^{13}C breathe test) do not reliably help in the management of nausea and vomiting, nor influence decision-making or treatment options.

The clinical feature that most characterizes those suffering from drug, chemical or metabolic causes are persistent severe nausea unrelieved by vomiting.[7] Retching rather than vomiting may be present with intractable nausea. Reflux, hiccups, early satiety and headaches do not separate patients into clearly defined syndromes.[7] Serum electrolyte abnormalities may be the result rather than the cause of nausea and vomiting (hypokalaemia, azotaemia, and metabolic alkalosis).[51] Medications associated with nausea and vomiting are listed in Box 14.1.

Timing of the onset of nausea and/or vomiting with introduction of new medications is an important part of the history (Box 14.2).[51]

CNS metastases or leptomeningeal spread of cancer may produce nausea and vomiting, which is relatively refractory to first line anti-emetics (metoclopramide or haloperidol), but responsive to antihistaminic/anticholinergics or dexamethasone. Vomiting may occur without nausea. Posterior fossa metastases are most commonly associated with early morning nausea and vomiting.[2] New neurological deficits, delirium and/or papillo-oedema may be helpful associated signs.

Vertigo and nausea may occur with Ménière disease, labyrinthitis and leptomeningeal disease. Positional nausea and vomiting without vertigo occur with mesenteric traction.[1]

Metabolic causes of nausea and vomiting include uraemia, diabetic ketoacidosis, hyperparathyroidism, hypoparathyroidism, hyperthyroidism and Addison's disease. This is more commonly seen in the older patient and may be an associated comorbidity which should be considered in this population.[50] In addition, individuals with acute myocardial infarction and worsening heart failure may present with isolated nausea and vomiting unrelated to cancer.[50] This is also true for pancreatitis, hepatitis, cholecystitis and mesenteric ischaemia from vascular disease.[50]

Aetiological guidelines for managing nausea and vomiting in advanced cancer

A guideline for management of nausea and vomiting based on the clinical picture (syndrome) has been developed by three groups.[2,7,50] Two major steps are involved in these guidelines: (1) identify potentially reversible causes; (2) treat based on clinical features and presumed aetiology (Box 14.1, Table 14.1).

Box 14.1 Medications associated with nausea and vomiting

Aspirin

Non-steroidal anti-inflammatory drugs

Allopurinol

Anti-arrhythmic

Antihypertensives

Analgesics, particularly opioids

Anti-seizure medications

Antibiotics

- Erythromycin
- Tetracycline
- Sulphonamides
- Acyclovir

Anti-asthmatics, particularly theophylline

Beta-blockers

Calcium channel blockers

Diuretics

Unlike single drug studies, the entire guideline has been prospectively evaluated in the management of nausea and vomiting. These studies are basically 'single arm' studies testing a guideline rather than a drug. The effectiveness of single drugs across the spectrum of nausea and vomiting syndromes cannot be inferred from these studies. Haloperidol, for example, is recommended for chemical and metabolic causes of nausea and vomiting, yet there are no prospective studies which have shown if and how effective haloperidol is in this circumstance.[2,3,7,52] On the other hand, the $5HT_3RA$ tropisetron is not included in any of the aetiological guidelines (Table 14.2) yet has been shown to be effective as a single drug or in combination.[53,54] A number of the medications are limited to regional availability. For instance, cyclizine and levomepromazine are not available in the USA, so that substitutions would need to be made if guidelines were to be followed to the letter. In general, vomiting is usually more responsive than nausea by these guidelines.[2] Success rates range from 50% to 80% depending on criteria for response. Approximately 40% will need more than one drug to control nausea and vomiting.[2] Responses may take several days up to 1 week

Box 14.2 Presumed aetiology of nausea and vomiting in order of prevalence

1 Chemical/drug
2 Gastroparesis/gastric outlet obstruction
3 Visceral serosal/intestinal obstruction
4 Cranial/vestibular
5 Cortical/unclear causes

Table 14.1 Reversible causes of nausea and vomiting

Cause	Treatment
Drugs	Drug discontinuation/switch
Uraemia	Dialysis/hydration
Hypercalcaemia	Biphosphonates
Infection	Antibiotics
Anxiety	Psychotherapy, benzodiazepine
Constipation	Laxatives
Gastric irritation	Drug discontinuation/proton pump inhibitor
High (level) obstruction	Venting gastrostomy tube/stents

with the mean time to response of 3.4 days.[7] Nearly 60% will require parenteral administration of anti-emetics (Table 14.3).[7] The aetiology of emesis can be identified in 75% of circumstances, though physicians will change their opinion in 25% with repeat assessment.[2] Second-line medications are recommended if individuals with nausea and vomiting are unrelieved by first-line choices.[2,7,55] The population, as in single drug studies, is heterogeneous and each study size is relatively small with a fairly high chance of bias. It is not possible to compare treatment by aetiological guidelines with single drug studies.[3]

Empiric drug studies

Empiric trials of anti-emetics are patterned on designs used in oncological drug studies. These generally consist of single agent trials in a single arm. Randomized trials comparing two agents or one active drug and another placebo plus rescue anti-emetics or comparisons between single and

Table 14.2 Aetiological guidelines

Cause	First line	Second line
Chemical/metabolic	Haloperidol	Levomepromazine Cyclizine $5HT_3RA$
Gastroparesis/impaired gastric output/ obstruction	Metoclopramide Domperidone	Levomepromazine
Visceral, serosal Intestinal obstruction	Cyclizine Hyoscine butylbromide	Levomepromazine Domperidone Octreotide
Cranial	Cyclizine Corticosteroids	Levomepromazine Promethazine
Unclear/unknown	Haloperidol Cyclizine	Levomepromazine
Vestibular	Cyclizine Promethazine	Levomepromazine
Cortical/emotional	Benzodiazepine (lorazepam)	Levomepromazine

Table 14.3 Anti-emetics and dose

Anti-emetic	Oral	Parenteral
Haloperidol	1.5–10 mg/day	2.5–10 mg/day
Metoclopramide	30–80 mg/day	30–120 mg/day
Cyclizine	25–50 mg q 6–8/h	75–200 mg/day
Promethazine	10–25 mg q 6–8/h	25–100 mg/day
Hyoscine butylbromide	150–300 μg q 8/h	300–12 mg/day
Domperidone	10–20 mg q 6–8/h	–
Levomepromazine	6.25–25 mg/day	6.25–25 mg/day

multiple drug combination are rare. These trials may have a broad inclusion criterion or a narrower focus on a subset of patients with nausea and vomiting (most commonly bowel obstruction).

In a systematic review, Glare *et al.* found 21 trials through searching multiple databases and hand searches. Only seven were randomized controlled trials, two systematic reviews and 12 uncontrolled studies (case series, cohort studies). All RCTs had patient numbers <100. Confidence intervals, precision of estimates of effect size were not given for any study. Criterion for response was not uniform and meta-analysis was not possible due to heterogeneity of trials.[3]

The strength of recommendations for particular anti-emetics in RCTs and prospective single aim trials was graded by Glare *et al.* using the MERGE criteria (methods for evaluating research guideline evidence; 'A' criterion: has met most quality standards; 'B': most criteria fulfilled; 'C': criteria mostly unfulfilled; 'D': not fulfilled.[56–58] In addition, the US Department of Health and Human Services' Agency for Health Care Policy and Research grades of recommendations (A–C) was used. Box 14.3 lists recommendations based on grade of evidence.

In an audit of anti-emetic practices in a palliative care inpatient setting, the use of anti-emetics by physicians appeared to be a fusion of both aetiological and empirically derived recommendations. Serotonin receptor antagonists were frequently prescribed for reasons other than for chemotherapy or radiation prophylaxis. Aetiology was recognized by 90% and about 25% were prescribed two or more anti-emetics. Surprisingly, most prescriptions were given on an 'as-needed' basis rather than around-the-clock.[57] There is very little evidence in the literature to address dosing strategies (around-the-clock versus as-needed) and dose escalation. Implicitly, authors have suggested combining drugs with non-overlapping neurotransmitter receptor activity or switching a narrow-spectrum anti-emetic (haloperidol, metoclopramide) to a broad-spectrum anti-emetic (levomepromazine) when nausea and emesis fail to respond to initial choices.[2,54] Evidence for the use of combinations is level A, based on RCTs from a single group.[53,54,59]

Individual anti-emetics

Phenothiazines

Chlorpromazine was first used as an antipsychotic in 1951. Within 3–4 years of approval, three separate studies were published on the use of chlorpromazine for nausea and vomiting in cancer.[60–62] In one study, a subset of individuals underwent a double-blind comparison between chlorpromazine and placebo.[63] Patients had multiple causes for nausea and vomiting, including chemotherapy. Criteria for response included complete resolution of nausea and vomiting. Doses ranged from 10 to 50 mg and intervals from 4 to 6 h. Almost 400 patients were included in these three studies. Vomiting resolved in >60%, nausea resolved in <50%. In a subset with abdominal

Box 14.3

Level A evidence

- Metoclopramide is effective in the management of nausea and vomiting in advanced cancer.
- Serotonin receptor antagonists are more effective than metoclopramide and chlorpromazine.
- Corticosteroids are effective in reducing nausea, vomiting from bowel obstruction.

Level B evidence

- Aetiological guidelines based on neuropharmacology should be used to choose first-line anti-emetics.
- Cyclizine, corticosteroids and levomepromazine are effective in managing nausea and vomiting in advanced cancer.
- Olanzapine is effective in managing nausea and vomiting in advanced cancer.

Level C evidence

- Clinical practice guidelines are effective in managing nausea and vomiting in advanced cancer.
- Haloperidol is effective in the management of nausea and vomiting in advanced cancer.
- Cannabinoids (nabilone) are effective in managing nausea and vomiting in advanced cancer.

Level A: at least one good quality RCT as supportive evidence.

Level B: well-conducted clinical studies but no RCT evidence.

Level C: expert recommendations, no clinical evidence.

carcinomatosis, all responded with complete resolution of nausea and vomiting.[62] Patients receiving nitrogen mustard, a highly emetogenic agent, responded well, with 24 of 38 having complete resolution of nausea and vomiting.[60,62] Responses occurred regardless of aetiology. Debilitated patients had greater responses and side-effects. Chlorpromazine has been recently reported to improve nausea and vomiting in bowel obstruction when combined either with hyoscine butylbromide or octreotide.[64]

Side-effects to chlorpromazine in order of prevalence were sedation, dizziness, dry mouth and tachycardia.[61,63] Tolerance appeared to develop to sedation. Oral doses up to 100 mg every 4 h were not sedative as reported in one study.[63] Sedation appeared to be greater with parenteral administration.[63] Oral bioavailability of chlorpromazine is 20%, hence this may be due to a relative dose escalation when switching from oral to parenteral injection when using the same dose or due to hepatic metabolism and different metabolites derived from first pass clearance. One study from the same time period reported a reduction of postoperative nausea and vomiting with chlorpromazine in 100 patients. A dose of 12.5 mg i.m. was used and found to be safe.[65]

The chemical structure and receptor-binding spectrum of chlorpromazine and levomepromazine are quite similar.[66] Both have active metabolites which accumulate in the CNS.[67] Both are analgesic in addition to being anti-emetics.[68] The disadvantage to chlorpromazine is that it cannot be given subcutaneously. In countries where levomepromazine is not available, chlorpromazine may be a good, inexpensive substitution. In recent randomized studies, chlorpromazine responses were less marked than reported earlier. However, duration of control was the criterion of response, which was different from that in earlier studies, and a titration strategy was not utilized in the recent studies such that less than effective doses may have been used relative to the original studies.[53,59]

Levomepromazine

Levomepromazine reduces nausea and vomiting in advanced cancer, as demonstrated by case reports and single arm studies.[69–74] The total number of individuals treated in these trials was 281. Unlike chlorpromazine, most individuals had nausea and/or vomiting which was unresponsive to first-line anti-emetics. A group of 108 individuals received levomepromazine as prophylaxis for delayed nausea and emesis from cisplatin chemotherapy.[71,75] Doses in these studies ranged from 3.12 to 25 mg s.c./oral once daily to 15 mg twice daily. Responses were seen in the majority, ranging from 32% to 94% for complete response of nausea and from 32% to 94% for complete response of vomiting. A dose–response relationship could not be determined by these studies. The dose range utilized for refractory cancer-related nausea and vomiting was 6.25–12.5 mg/day with responses ranging from 32% to 94% (complete response) and for delayed nausea from cisplatin 25–30 mg per day, with complete responses (62–94%). In one study, no relationship was found between the dose of levomepromazine and response.[70] The patient population in these studies was heterogeneous and most, at least in one series, had multiple causes for their nausea and vomiting.[69] Approximately 25% had nausea and vomiting for unknown reasons.[69] Responses were seen within 1–2 days. The duration of control cannot be determined in these studies due in part to attrition, which can be significant in patients with advanced cancer.[69] Responses at day 5 were somewhat diminished in one study (54% vs 32%) but one-third of patients were no longer evaluable.[69] Side-benefits to levomepromazine may be reduction of pruritus and analgesia,[76,77] as well as reduction in delirium and anxiety.[77] The most common side-effects included sedation, hypotension and dry mouth.

Levomepromazine has greater receptor inhibitory activity for H_1, $5HT_2$ and D_2 receptors than chlorpromazine. $5HT_2$ receptor blockade reduces the risk for extrapyramidal reactions relative to pure D_2 receptor blockers such as haloperidol (Table 14.4). The brain:plasma ratio for levomepromazine is 10–30:1 (for haloperidol 22:1, as a comparison).[78] Brain elimination half-life is much longer than for serum.[78–80] Hence, small doses and long dosing intervals (12–24 h) between doses may be effective and serum concentrations will poorly reflect therapeutic levels.[66] The receptor binding spectrum of levomepromazine (and chlorpromazine) resembles that of atypical antipsychotics such as clozapine, due to the high binding affinity to $5HT_2$ receptors. Levomepromazine may have antidepression activity (similar to olanzapine) through blocking $5HT_2A$ receptor.[81] Levomepromazine is metabolized through the cytochrome CYP2D6 to *N*-desmethyl levomepromazine, which is as active as the parent drug. Both block α-adrenergic receptors to a greater degree than chlorpromazine, accounting for the side-effect of hypotension.[81] The half-life in serum is between 15 and 30 h and may depend on metabolizer status (CYP2D6 pharmacogenetics). Both levomepromazine and metabolites block multiple cytochromes (CYP1A2, CYP3A2, and CYP2D6), and hence drug interactions may potentially occur when switching to levomepromazine from other anti-emetics.[81,82]

Table 14.4 Receptor binding profile of chlorpromazine and levomepromazine[78] (KDNM)[1]

Drug	M_1	M_2	α_1	α_2	$5HT_1$	$5HT_2$	D_2
Levomeprazine	127	285	0.57	583	594	18.5	21.1
Chlorpromazine	134	570	4.4	980	752	41	32

Other phenothiazines

Thiethylperazine[83] perphenazine[84,85] and prochlorperazine[86,87] have been used to treat nausea and vomiting in advanced cancer reported in single aim studies. Thiethylperazine doses were 10 mg as needed (10 mg twice daily up to 20 mg 4 times daily), prochlorperazine 5 mg 3 times daily up to 80 mg daily in divided doses, and perphenazine 5–8 mg 2–4 times daily. The patient populations in these studies were heterogeneous. Some patients had nausea, which had not responded to other phenothiazines and responded by rotating the phenothiazines.[84] Phenothiazine switch from chlorpromazine or prochlorperazine to perphenazine resulted in control of nausea and vomiting.[65,84] Cancer patients generally made up only a portion of the study population; however, in the studies where patients with cancer were assessed separately, responses occurred in >50%.[83,84,86] One study added cyclizine or metoclopropramide to prochlorperazine for refractory nausea. This was required in 25% and was more commonly required for females.[87]

In summary, multiple studies have demonstrated significant benefits to phenothiazines in cancer-related nausea and vomiting. The most convincing evidence is for chlorpromazine and levomepromazine, both of which have pharmacological profiles which resemble atypical antipsychotics. The evidence for benefit is much greater than for haloperidol, yet haloperidol is more frequently used to treat cancer-related nausea and vomiting than phenothiazines in more recent studies. Most of the published experience dates to the 1950s and 1960s, yet the criterion for response included complete resolution of nausea and vomiting, which would match present-day standards for response. In countries where levomepromazine is not available, there is enough evidence that chlorpromazine may be substituted within aetiological guidelines. This would be relatively favourable in those regions with economic constraints relative to expensive atypical antipsychotics. This is particularly true in a capitated reimbursement system such as occurs with American hospices.

Haloperidol

Haloperidol has been available since 1958 and has been used as an anti-emetic for more than 10 years.[88] In animal models haloperidol prevents nausea from apomorphine. In a systematic review[59,88,89] 12 reports, 13 trials and 1994 patients were treated with haloperidol for nausea and vomiting. These studies involved patients experiencing postoperative nausea and vomiting, individuals with gastrointestinal diseases and nausea and those experiencing nausea and vomiting after chemotherapy and radiation.[88] There are no single-arm or RCTs for nausea and vomiting in advanced cancer. There are two trials using haloperidol in the management of bowel obstruction and three studies (previously cited) which included haloperidol as part of aetiological guidelines.[52] A single case report which used an '*n* of 1' method for evaluating responses found the combination of ondansetron and haloperidol effective in controlling refractory nausea and vomiting, whereas either drug alone was ineffective.[90] Doses used for bowel obstruction were 0.05 mg/kg/day s.c. or i.v. to 2–5 mg/day s.c. Reduction in vomiting was seen in the majority.[52,91–94]

Table 14.5 Comparisons of haloperidol and atypical antipsychotic receptor binding affinity (Ki) (NM)

Drug	D_1	D_2	$5HT_2A$	$5HT_3$	M_1	X_1	H_1
Haloperidol	25	1	78	>1000	>1000	46	>1000
Olanzapine	31	11	4	57	1.9	19	7

K (NM) inhibitory constant for receptor binding; low numbers reflect higher receptor binding.[95,96]

Haloperidol is a relative selective D_2 receptor blocker with mild affinity for D_1, $5HT_2A$ and H1 receptors (Table 14.5) , in contrast to the atypical antipsychotic olanzapine.[89] The lack of significant binding to H1 and M1 receptors suggests that haloperidol would be ineffective in reducing nausea and vomiting in motion sickness. There are no trials using haloperidol in this situation.[88] Despite its common use in managing nausea and vomiting in advanced cancer, there is little evidence as a single drug for its benefit, due to the lack of prospective trials, and although the three aetiological guideline studies used haloperidol for certain causes of nausea and vomiting, evidence of benefit as a single drug cannot be deciphered from these studies.[2,7,51]

Haloperidol metabolism is complex and consists of glucuronidation (50–60%), reduction and back oxidation through CYP2D6 and N-dealkylation to a toxic metabolite, presumably through CYP3A4. Poor metabolizers and those on medications which block CYP2D6 will have higher reduced haloperidol (which is an active metabolite).[89] The incidence of haloperidol-induced EPS is higher in slow metabolizers.[97] In addition, EPS is higher in frequency with oral administration (23%) compared to parenteral administration (7%), which may be related to haloperidol metabolites.[98] The half-life of haloperidol is 12–35 h (average 16 h) and oral bioavailability is 44–75% (average 60%).[89] Hence, haloperidol can be given twice daily. Conversion from parenteral to oral haloperidol is 1 to 2.

The popularity of haloperidol probably relates to its availability, versatility in routes and cost. Adverse effects include extrapyramidal reactions in 0.1% when doses per day range from 0.25 to 5 mg. Sedation increases with dose. When doses of 5 mg/day or more are used the risk of EPS and sedation increases, with the number needed to harm (NNH) for sedation 4.4 (1 out of 4 will experience sedation to the point of being clinically relevant).[88] Haloperidol will increase prolactin levels more than atypical antipsychotics which can lead to galactorrhoea and impotence.[99] However, hypotension (common with levomepromazine) is the same as placebo with haloperidol doses of ≤4 mg/day.[88] Extrapyramidal side-effects are responsive to benzodiazepines.[89,100,101] Extrapyramidal side-effects with haloperidol are dose-related and occur more frequently in younger individuals.[101] Extrapyramidal manifestations include akathisia and parkinsonism. Prolonged EPS side-effects may occur after haloperidol has been discontinued.[102]

Arrhythmias do not occur with haloperidol but at high doses prolongation of the QT_C interval can occur, which may be problematic if haloperidol is combined with other drugs that prolong the QT_C[103] such as methadone.[88] Fortunately, the doses needed to control nausea and vomiting are generally less than those required to treat psychosis.[88]

Haloperidol is equivalent to cannabinoids in managing post-chemotherapy nausea and vomiting.[104] Both would be considered inadequate by today's standards. Haloperidol has a long half-life, which allows for dosing every 12 h. This is convenient and increases compliance.

Olanzapine

Olanzapine has been documented by case report and small case series to be effective in the management of nausea and vomiting in advanced cancer.[105–108] Doses have ranged between 2.5 and 10 mg/day. Patients have usually received standard D_2 antagonists and then treated with olanzapine as a second-line anti-emetic. Doses are usually given once or twice daily because of the long half-life and the zydis form can be given under the tongue. It is not possible to determine any dose–response relationship from these small studies. Olanzapine comes in an injectable form, as an oral disintegrating tablet and standard tablets, and this offers route versatility. There is an impressive amount of evidence that olanzapine is quite effective when added to standard anti-emetics in preventing nausea and vomiting from highly emetogenic chemotherapy.[108–110] This includes delayed nausea and vomiting, which is usually poorly responsive to $5HT_3RA$, cannabinoids and haloperidol. An added benefit to olanzapine is its antipsychotic and antidepressive activity.[111,112] Olanzapine has been reported to reduce flushing and sweating from cancer,[113] and to reduce chronic pain and curtail opioid dose escalation in individuals with cancer pain.[114–117] Olanzapine would be preferred to haloperidol and metoclopramide in those with Parkinson disease.[118] Olanzapine will reduce nausea from selective serotonin reuptake inhibitor antidepressives[119] and reverses steroid psychosis.[120]

Olanzapine side-effects include the development of diabetes, which is not seen with other atypical antipsychotics such as risperidone,[121] quetiapine[122] or the butyrophenone haloperidol.[122] Olanzapine appears to produce insulin resistance without disturbing β-cell function.[123] Therefore, glucose intolerance and diabetes should resolve with discontinuation of olanzapine. Glucose should be monitored in individuals on olanzapine.[124] Antipsychotics prolong the QT_C interval by blocking repolarization via HERG-derived potassium channels. However, olanzapine appears to be one of the safest agents in this regard.[125,126] Individuals at risk for arrhythmias with a prolonged QT_C interval should be monitored closely or receive anti-emetics which will not further prolong the QT_C. Other side-effects are weight gain, dry mouth, sedation and nausea.[99,127]

Olanzapine binds to a multitude of receptors which are involved in initiating emesis (D_2, $5HT_2A$, $5HT_2C$, and $5HT_3$, M_1, α_1, and H_1). Olanzapine is a more potent inhibitor of $5HT_2$ receptors than D_2 receptors (Table 14.5), which differs from chlorpromazine and haloperidol. As a result, olanzapine has significantly fewer EPS effects and significantly greater antidepression activity.[128]

Olanzapine has a long half-life (27–38 h) and can be dosed once daily.[99] It is metabolized by multiple cytochromes (CYP1A2, CYP2D6) and is rapidly glucuronidated; hence there are few clinically significant drug interactions. All metabolites are less active than the parent drug.[127] Metabolism and drug pharmacokinetics are not influenced by renal failure or mild-to-moderate hepatic dysfunction. Food does not alter absorption.[99]

Another atypical antipsychotic, risperidone, in a retrospective study involving 20 patients using 1 mg per day resolved vomiting in 64% and nausea in 50%. Sedation was the major adverse effect.[129]

Metoclopramide

Metoclopramide has been studied retrospectively, in randomized trials, in comparison to levosulpride, sustained-release metoclopramide, placebo, ondansetron and in combination with dexamethasone and tropisetron.[53,59,130–134] Metoclopramide can be given orally, i.m. as a sustained release every 12 h or s.c. Doses ranged from 10 mg twice daily to as high as 3 mg/kg with multiple doses given (as for prophylaxes with highly emetogenic chemotherapy). Metoclopramide has been given as a rescue for chemotherapy-induced nausea and vomiting, for treatment of the cancer-associated dyspeptic syndrome (which includes nausea) and for relief of nausea associated with the opioid bowel syndrome.[130,133,135] From these studies, it appears that sustained-release metoclopramide is superior to immediate-release metoclopramide for the same daily dose, that levosulpride and tropisetron are superior to low dose metoclopramide and that the addition of dexamethasone to metoclopramide adds very little to anti-emetic activity.[52,131,132,134,136,137] In comparison studies, there is a suggestion of a dose–response relationship. In the study by Mystakidou *et al.*, responses with metoclopramide 10 mg by mouth 4 times daily (+ dexamethasone) were 16% (complete response); when 60–120 mg continuous s.c. infusion (plus dexamethasone) was used by Bruera *et al.*, all responded clinically without the need to change therapy. However, it is difficult to compare populations between studies and the measure of response differed between studies. The only direct comparison between metoclopramide doses found that 10 mg was as effective as 0.4 mg/kg as a single dose.[138] There are no studies which directly compare dose and response. In addition, the short half-life of metoclopramide is such that dosing intervals >4 h may be ineffective. This lends credence to the use of continuous infusion dosing strategies where 4 times daily schedules have failed to control vomiting.[132]

Metoclopramide, given preventively to individuals receiving morphine for acute pain, reduces nausea and vomiting (1.6% vs 3.7%). However, the incidence of nausea is quite low and does not justify the routine practice of prophylaxis.[139]

Metoclopramide has an oral bioavailability of 70–80%, which is not influenced by renal or liver disease, nor is it different in those >65 years of age.[140–142] Metoclopramide is metabolized to an N-dealkylated metabolite, monodeacetyl metoclopramide, by the cytochrome CYP2D6.[143] To a lesser extent, metoclopramide is metabolized by CYP1A2. Metoclopramide also inhibits CYP2D6 in a mechanism-based fashion, suggesting that drug interactions with medications metabolized through CYP2D6 are a concern. Metoclopramide clearance is likely to be slower in poor metabolizers.[143]

Metoclopramide also undergoes N-4 sulphate conjugation.[144] The elimination half-life of metoclopramide is dose dependent.[144] In diabetics and cancer patients receiving single 10 mg doses, the elimination half-life is 3.9–4 h.[145,146] Individuals receiving high dose metoclopramide as prophylaxis for cisplatin (doses ranging from 0.15 to 4.8 mg/kg over 15 min) have a terminal half-life ranging from 5.6–9.9 h.[142,147–150] This may be due to overwhelming CYP2D6 metabolism by high concentrations of substrate drug or to autoinhibition of CYP2D6 at high doses. Neonates, individuals with renal failure and hepatic failure will have delayed clearance of metoclopramide by 2–4-fold.[141,151–154] Dose intervals may need to be increased to 12 h or the dose reduced by half and intervals maintained. Metoclopropramide is a drug with route versatility and can be given by mouth, subcutaneously, per rectum and intravenously.

Metoclopramide is a D_2 receptor antagonist and $5HT_4$ receptor agonist, and hence is considered a gastrointestinal prokinetic drug.[155,156] At doses of >120 mg daily, metoclopramide blocks $5HT_3$ receptors. $5HT_4$ receptors require acetylcholine for prokinesis and anticholinergics will block metoclopramide prokinetic effects.[155] Side-effects include lethargy and in a subset, akathisia, which resembles psychological anxiety. The method of parenteral delivery may influence the risk of EPS effects. Metoclopramide given as a slow parenteral infusion over 15 min results in akathisia in 6% and if given rapidly over 2 min, 25% develop akathisia.[157] Unusual extrapyramidal reactions with metoclopramide include abdominal pain with rigidity, involuntary movements of limbs, trismus, torticollis and dystonic reactions which resemble tetanus.[158] Patients with a complete bowel obstruction may develop colic, nausea and vomiting when prescribed metoclopramide. Metoclopramide reduces renal plasma flow at high doses, which does not correlate with pretreatment creatinine clearance, age or gender. This may be clinically important in those individuals who are dehydrated or receiving nephrotoxic drugs.[159,160] Serum prolactin and aldosterone levels are also increased by low dose metoclopramide infusions, which may lead to gynaecomastia, menstrual abnormalities, impotence or fluid retention.[160]

Anticholinergic and antihistamine medications

Diphenhydramine was reported to reduce nausea and vomiting from radiation in 1946, and dimenhydrinate was reported to reduce nausea and vomiting from motion sickness in 1949.[161] Subsequent studies have demonstrated that anticholinergics reduce nausea and vomiting from air sickness, postoperative nausea and vomiting, nausea from morphine, cancer and pregnancy.[162–166] Most of the evidence is by case report, and a small case series except for morphine-induced nausea in which there is a randomized trial, and for motion sickness, for which there is a Cochrane review. Anticholinergics are also used frequently to manage bowel obstruction symptoms.

The only single drug trial of diphenhydramine in the management of nausea and vomiting in advanced cancer was published by McCawley *et al.* in 1951.[161] In this study, 150 patients received 50–300 mg day of diphenhydramine repeated every 3–4 h. Some had morphine or nitrogen mustard as a cause for nausea and vomiting. Diphenhydramine was ineffective at the 50 mg dose; some required 300 mg every 4 h for relief. Postoperative nausea and vomiting required 100 mg to be effective. Dimenhydrinate doses were effective at the 200 mg level in the study by McCawley *et al.*: 10–15% of individuals had failed to respond to diphenhydramine.[161] The population in this study was heterogeneous with mixed causes of nausea and vomiting. Sedation was the major side-effect. Diphenhydramine has been added to metoclopramide to reduce akathisia and improve metoclopramide tolerance.[167,168] A compounded formulation of lorazepam, diphenhydramine, haloperidol and metoclopramide has been used in hospice patients for refractory nausea and vomiting. Efficacy is unpublished, but the incidence of EPS is quite low (0.1%) despite combining metoclopramide and haloperidol together.[169] This is likely related to the addition of both a benzodiazepine and diphenhydramine, blocking extrapyramidal reactions. Diphenhydramine blocks CYP2D6 and probably delays metoclopramide clearance. The anticholinergic activity will prevent metoclopramide-induced prokinesis.[155,170]

A combination of metoclopramide 10 mg, plus diphenhydramine 25 mg and dexamethasone 4 mg has been given parenterally every 6 h for nausea and vomiting in an inpatient hospice unit. In this retrospective chart review, 57 of 63 (90%) had an objective reduction in vomiting and subjective improvement in nausea. Responses were usually seen within 2 days. Oral intake and improved activities were noted.[171] Vomiting was better controlled than nausea in this study. Individuals with nausea only partially controlled received a fourth drug, either a broad receptor-binding phenothiazine or a $5HT_3RA$.

Cyclizine has been included in aetiological guidelines[7,51] and in clinical practice recommendations for the management of bowel obstruction.[92] Recommended cyclizine doses are 100–150 mg daily or 50 mg every 8 h s.c. There are no single drug prospective studies of cyclizine in advanced cancer.[3] As s result, the effectiveness of cyclizine as a single drug cannot be determined by the available studies. Cyclizine may reduce nausea and vomiting associated with the use of morphine, but does not improve the control of postoperative nausea and vomiting when added to granisetron.[172,173] High dose chlorpheniramine (20–40 mg per day) and dimenhydrinate (50–100 mg s.c. as needed) have been substituted for cyclizine in countries where cyclizine is not available.[91,174] A two-case report illustrated the benefits to chlorpheniramine.[174]

Meclizine is commonly used for nausea and vomiting associated with vertigo. Meclizine reduces the incidence and severity of postoperative nausea and vomiting.[175] There are no single drug or combination drug trials in advanced cancer which have included meclizine as an anti-emetic.

Classic antihistamines are extensively metabolized with only a small amount of drug excreted unchanged. Most are metabolized through the cytochrome CYP2D6. Second generation antihistamines (astemizole and terfinadine) are metabolized through CYP3A4.[176] Antihistamines are well absorbed orally with effects lasting for 6 h. Diphenhydramine, cyclizine, chlorpheniramine and the antihistaminic phenothiazine, promethazine, are inhibitors of CYP2D6 at concentrations close to therapeutic plasma levels.[176–182] As a result, antihistamines will delay the clearance of commonly used anti-emetics such as metoclopramide and haloperidol, and will delay the clearance of cardiac medications such as metoprolol and other β-blockers and antidepressants such as venlafaxine. Antihistamines will boost the levels of metoclopramide and haloperidol (the active reduced metabolite) which may be the mechanism behind the benefits to combining the two medications.

Anticholinergics have almost exclusively been used to treat symptoms related to intestinal obstruction. Hyoscine butylbromide, hyoscine hydrobromide and glycopyrrolate are the most commonly reported anticholinergics.[64,91,93,183–186] In the original study by Ventafridda *et al.*, individuals were treated with morphine for pain, hyoscine butylbromide and haloperidol. All 22 patients had control of nausea and vomiting.[93] Since the original report, comparisons have been made between anticholinergics and octreotide in the management of obstruction. Octreotide was found to be highly effective in small case series.[187–189] In randomized studies, octreotide appears to be more effective than hyoscine butylbromide.[64,183,190] Octreotide reduced gastrointestinal secretions to a greater degree and allowed for removal of nasogastric tubes more often.[186] Recommendations by the European Association of Palliative Care (EAPC) are to use either an anticholinergic or octreotide with an anti-emetic (haloperidol, levomepromazine, chlorpromazine or prochlorperazine) or antihistamine drug (cyclizine or dimenhydrinate).[91] Patients who are not candidates for surgery and who continue to have nausea and vomiting despite optimal drug management should have a percutaneous venting gastrostomy placed.[91,191] Anticholinergic doses are hyoscine butylbromide 40–120 mg s.c./day, hyoscine hydrobromide 0.8–2.0 mg/day s.c. and glycopyrrolate 0.1–0.2 mg 3 or 4 times daily i.v. or s.c. Either glycopyrrolate or hyoscine butylbromide are preferred since these two medications do not cross into the CNS to a significant degree and do not cause cognitive failure or delirium.[192] Both hyoscine derivatives and glycopyrrolate are used to treat terminal secretions (death rattle) in addition to intestinal obstruction.[192]

Both hyoscine butylbromide and glycopyrrolate are quaternary ammonium anticholinergics, which do not penetrate into the CNS and thus have a low risk of inducing cognitive failure, unlike the tertiary ammonium anticholinergic hyoscine hydrobromide.[193–195] Glycopyrrolate levels in cerebrospinal fluid (CSF) are undetectable.[196] Either quaternary ammonium anticholinergic is the treatment of choice in the elderly. Oral absorption of glycopyrrolate and hyoscine butylbromide is poor and erratic and most drug effect will be limited to the bowel.[193,195] As a result, cardiac toxicity and bladder adverse effects will be less with oral administration. Hyoscine derivates are N-demethylated, presumably by CYP3A4, and glucuronidated. A significant proportion of the parent drug can be found in the urine (30%).[194] Grapefruit juice increases bioavailability by blocking gastrointestinal CYP3A4. Anticholinergics rapidly distribute to tissues.[196,197] Pharmacokinetics do change with age, as the elderly have higher sensitivity to anticholinergics.[197] Transdermal hyoscine hydrobromide has fewer side-effects than oral hyoscine hydrobromide and is superior to meclizine in reducing nausea and vomiting associated with motion sickness and equivalent to promethazine and dimenhydrinate.[198] Therapeutic levels are reached 8–12 h after applying the patch.

Side-effects include dry mouth (50–60%), reduced accommodation, and drowsiness (20%).[198] Blockade of central muscarinic receptors induces memory deficits and predisposes to delirium.[194,199]

Hyoscine derivatives at low concentration reduce heart rate and at high concentrations increase heart rate. Glycopyrrolate at usual doses appears to have fewer cardiac side-effects.[195,200] Dry mouth, urinary retention, mydriasis and cycloplegia are other side-effects.[194]

Anticholinergics will enhance the side-effects to tricyclic antidepressants, antihistamines and quinidine. Anticholinergics block the prokinetic activity of metoclopramide and the tachycardia of β-adrenoceptor agonists.[193]

$5HT_3$ receptor antagonists

$5HT_3$ receptor antagonists are effective in reducing postoperative nausea and vomiting and in preventing acute nausea and vomiting from cisplatin or other moderate to highly emetogenic chemotherapy drugs.[201–212] The combination of ondansetron and dexamethasone provides better prophylaxis for postoperative nausea and vomiting and chemotherapy-related nausea and vomiting than a $5HT_3RA$ alone.

Randomized trials have compared tropisetron, low doses of chlorpromazine or metoclopramide combined with dexamethasone, combinations of tropisetron plus chlorpromazine ± dexamethasone and tropisetron plus metoclopramide ± dexamethasone. Tropisetron alone was superior to low dose metoclopramide plus dexamethasone and low dose chlorpromazine plus dexamethasone in individuals who developed emesis on low doses of metoclopramide or chlorpromazine. Tropisetron complete responses in advanced cancer-related nausea and vomiting were 30–42.5%. The combination of chlorpromazine plus tropisetron produced complete responses in 42.5%. Combining chlorpromazine, tropisetron plus dexamethasone controlled nausea and vomiting in 35–65% and the three-drug combination with metoclopramide, tropisetron and dexamethasone, in 55–75%.[53,54,59] Doses of metoclopramide were 10 mg 4 times daily, and chlorpromazine doses were 25 mg twice daily. The low doses may account for the relatively low response rate with either drug. Dexamethasone added little to metoclopramide or chlorpromazine responses but did appear to add to responses with tropisetron–chlorpromazine or tropisetron–metoclopramide combinations.[53] Tropisetron is superior to alizapride in reducing nausea and vomiting related to high dose alkylating agent chemotherapy, in preparation for bone marrow transplantation.[213] Responses were inadequate to tropisetron, as patients still experienced five emetic episodes in the first 24 h. The addition of haloperidol to tropisetron in a second study done by the same group was superior to tropisetron alone.[214] Thus, a combination of a $5HT_3RA$ and D_2 receptor antagonist appears to be more effective in refractory nausea and vomiting in advanced cancer and nausea and vomiting associated with high dose chemotherapy. A RCT by Bruera *et al.* also found that dexamethasone did not improve metoclopramide responses in individuals.[136] The combination of dexamethasone plus a $5HT_3RA$ has not been reported in the management of nausea and vomiting in advanced cancer but would be of interest, in light of the benefits of this combination in postoperative and chemotherapy-related nausea and vomiting. Responses to the combination drug regimens increases over time. A greater number of complete responders were seen 7 days compared to day 1 or after 3 days of treatment.[53,54,59] Therefore, clinicians should give a combination of anti-emetics adequate time in order to gauge responses. Finally, it is impossible to determine if the proper strategy for treating nausea and vomiting in advanced cancer should be to titrate a single anti-emetic to maximum doses or to maintain the dose of a single anti-emetic and add on a second drug with a different receptor-binding profile (adding a $5HT_3RA$ to a D_2 receptor antagonist) or whether a combination of antiemetics should be started initially (a $5HT_3RA$, a D_2 receptor antagonist with or without dexamethasone). When metoclopramide is titrated to high doses (>120 mg), $5HT_3$ receptors are bound and blocked.[170] High dose metoclopramide becomes an expanded spectrum drug and acts like a D_2 receptor antagonist and $5HT_3$ RA.

$5HT_3RAs$ are rapidly absorbed and readily cross the blood–brain barrier.[36] Serum half-life is shorter for ondansetron (4 h) than for granisetron (9–11.6 h).[215] However, the biological effects of $5HT_3RAs$ are longer than the serum half-life and, hence, once-daily dosing will be effective in most circumstances.[35,216] The volume of distribution is quite large for $5HT_3RA$, indicating high tissue binding. Dolasetron is unique in that it is a pro-drug and requires activation to hydrodolasetron by CYP2D6 and CYP3A4 to be effective. $5HT_3RA$ are metabolized by various cytochromes;

ondansetron by CYP1A1, CYP1A2, CYP2D6, CYP3A3/4/5; tropisetron by CYP2D6, CYP3A43/4/5; granisetron by CYP3A3/4/5; and dolasetron by CYP2D6, CYP3A3/4/5.[217] $5HT_3$RAs do not inhibit cytochromes to a significant degree. Poor metabolizers have higher serum levels of ondansetron, tropisetron and poorly respond to dolasetron. Drugs which induce CYP3A4 will increase the clearance of ondansetron, tropisetron and granisetron.[218] In chemotherapy trials, there is comparative efficacy at therapeutic doses between $5HT_3$RAs, but there are significant inter-individual differences in pharmacokinetic–pharmacodynamic responses which suggest that in a particular individual, one $5HT_3$RA may be better than another and non-cross-tolerance occurs between $5HT_3$RAs.[219–221] Non-cross-tolerance may be due to: (1) differences in half-life (granisetron, tropisetron > ondansetron); (2) differences in metabolism; (3) nature of interacting with receptors (ondansetron is a competitive inhibitor, tropisetron and granisetron non-competitive inhibitors); (4) differences in inhibition of serotonin release from enterochromaffin cells (ondansetron does not inhibit release, granisetron and tropisetron do inhibit release); (5) interactions with other receptors (ondansetron with $5HT_1$B, $5HT_1$C, α_1 adrenergic and opioid receptors, tropisetron with $5HT_4$ receptors; (6) genetic differences in serotonin transporters which influence serotonin levels near receptors.[35,216,218,222–224] Switching from one $5HT_3$RA to another may produce an antiemetic response, as demonstrated in chemotherapy anti-emetic trials.[224] Therapeutic doses for $5HT_3$RA are listed in Table 14.6.

$5HT_3$RA causes an increase in the number and amplitude of non-propulsive intestinal contractions, increasing transit time and constipation. This may be of benefit in diarrhoea-predominant irritable bowel syndrome and advanced carcinoid. $5HT_3$RAs block cardiac potassium channels and repolarization, which can lead to mildly prolonged QT_C intervals. However, when combined with a butyrophenone (droperidol), QT_C intervals are not prolonged further relative to droperidol alone.[225] This is important when considering a combination of a D_2 receptor antagonist and $5HT_3$RA for refractory nausea. Tropisetron has anti-arrhythmic effects in those with ventricular arrhythmias. Dolasetron broadens the QRS complex. $5HT_3$RAs have a mild anxiolytic effect and antipsychotic effect and have been used to prevent relapse in alcohol or opioid abuse.[34] $5HT_3$RA are not associated with extrapyramidal side-effects and may improve memory performance in the elderly.[35] Other side-effects can include headache, sedation, fatigue and elevated transaminases and/or bilirubin.[216]

Dexamethasone

In RCTs, dexamethasone did not improve the anti-emetic benefits of metoclopramide nor chlorpromazine, either as initial treatment or in individuals who had not responded to low doses of metoclopramide or chlorpromazine.[53,54,59,136] Dexamethasone reduces nausea associated with radiation and in individuals with bilateral adrenal metastases and adrenal insufficiency.[226,227] Dexamethasone does improve the anti-emetic prophylaxis of $5HT_3$RAs ± metoclopramide in

Table 14.6 $5HT_3$RA therapeutic doses

Drug	Dose (day)
Ondansetron	8–32 mg
Tropisetron	5 mg
Granisetron	1–3 mg
Dolasetron	12.5–100 mg
Palonosetron	0.25 mg

individuals receiving emetogenic chemotherapy.[204,214,215] Dexamethasone 10 mg is equivalent to 20 mg in benefit as an anti-emetic. Both methylprednisone and dexamethasone given preoperatively reduce postoperative nausea and vomiting.[217,219] Vomiting is more responsive than nausea and 8 mg is better than 4 mg as a single dose in the preoperative setting.[201,219,220] Preoperative prophylaxis is improved when dexamethasone is combined with a $5HT_3$RA, gabapentin or mirtazapine.[201,221,228] There is a trend for bowel obstruction to resolve when individuals are treated with dexamethasone 6–16 mg daily. The number needed to treat for benefit is six.[229,230] Dexamethasone is frequently used to treat individuals with brain tumours or metastases who are experiencing nausea, vomiting and neurological deficits. There are no prospective studies which have demonstrated the effectiveness of corticosteroids in reducing nausea and vomiting in this situation. Dexamethasone has been used for pain, depression, fatigue and anorexia in advanced cancer.[231]

Single doses of dexamethasone, as frequently used as prophylaxis for chemotherapy and postoperative nausea and vomiting, have very little toxicity.[201] The clearance of dexamethasone is delayed by aprepitant, which is given to prevent delayed chemotherapy nausea and vomiting.[232] Dexamethasone is metabolized through CYP3A4 and may induce CYP3A4 expression if given over a period of time, leading to drug interactions.[233–235] Long-term corticosteroids have significant side-effects. The evidence for benefit in treating nausea and vomiting in advanced cancer do not justify routine or long-term use for this purpose. Individuals who appear to respond to corticosteroids should have doses tapered to the lowest effective dose.

Miscellaneous medications with anti-emetic activity

Cannabinoids

There are no prospective studies on the benefits of cannabinoids in the treatment of nausea and vomiting in advanced cancer.[3] There is a retrospective series treated for emesis which did demonstrate responses.[236] Cannabinoids, particularly nabilone, are superior to placebo, prochlorperazine, alizapride and domperidone, in managing acute chemotherapy-induced nausea and vomiting. Nabilone is equivalent to metoclopramide and chlorpromazine.[237] Combinations of cannabinoids and prochlorperazine or cannabinoids plus metoclopramide are better than either drug alone in controlling acute chemotherapy-induced nausea and vomiting.[237] Dexamethasone plus metoclopramide is superior to a cannabinoid plus prochlorperazine. Patients generally preferred cannabinoids over prochlorperazine, despite increasing side-effects from the cannabinoid.[238] Cannabinoids are equivalent to ondansetron in reducing delayed chemotherapy-induced nausea and vomiting and superior to placebo. The combination of a cannabinoid plus ondansetron was not superior to either drug alone.[239] This may be due to cannabinoid-induced $5HT_3$ receptor blockade (which may account for the anti-emetic activity of cannabinoids) rather than activation of CB1 receptors.[240,241] Cannabinoids have been recommended within reviews for chemotherapy-induced nausea and vomiting, but none of the recent guidelines has included cannabinoids.[242–244] Cannabinoids reduce nausea and vomiting in advanced acquired immune deficiency syndrome.[245,246] Additional benefits of cannabinoids are reported to be the relief of a central neuropathic pain syndrome, anorexia and cachexia.[238,247] However, the evidence for benefits in neuropathic pain is weak and predominately in those with multiple sclerosis.[237,248,249] A recent randomized study found that cannabinoids were as effective as placebo in the treatment of cancer-associated anorexia.[250] At the present time, there is little evidence to support the use of cannabinoids in the management of nausea and vomiting in advanced cancer.

Anti-seizure medications

Anti-seizure medications are not known to be anti-emetics. However, by case report, carbamazepine successfully resulted in complete cessation of nausea and vomiting in a patient with meningeal carcinomatosis.[251] Both zonisamide and levetiracetam controlled vomiting episodes in the adult cyclic vomiting syndrome.[252] Carbamazepine reduces nausea and vomiting in central demyelinating syndromes.[251] Preoperative gabapentin reduces pain, morphine requires and nausea and vomiting postoperative.[253,254–257] Combinations of gabapentin plus dexamethasone are superior to either drug alone. Gabapentin in a small case series reduced chemotherapy-induced nausea and vomiting in breast cancer.[258] By case report, gabapentin plus hyoscine hydrobromide reduced refractory nausea and vomiting from posterior fossa surgery.[259] Gabapentin also reduces hormone-related hot flashes and uraemic pruritus.[260,261] Anti-seizure medications may be helpful in those individuals with nausea and carcinomatosis meningitis, in treatment of paraneoplastic-related demyelination or as prophylaxis preoperatively to reduce postoperative nausea and vomiting.

Antidepressants

Antidepressants have been shown to reduce emesis in several clinical situations. However, there are no prospective studies of antidepressants in the management of nausea and vomiting in advanced cancer. Low doses of tricyclic antidepressants (amitriptyline, desipramine, nortriptyline, doxepin and imipramine) reduce nausea and vomiting from functional bowel syndrome.[262] Tricyclic antidepressants reduce nausea and vomiting in 88% of diabetics with delayed gastric emptying, whose nausea was unresponsive to prokinetic medications.[263] Mirtazapine completely controlled nausea and vomiting in an individual with severe gastroparesis unresponsive to multiple prokinetic drugs and pyloric injections of botulism toxin.[264] Low dose mirtazapine has been reported by case report to reduce primary (idiopathic) nausea and vomiting.[265] Responses were seen after nausea and vomiting failed to respond to multiple anti-emetics (metoclopramide, dimenhydrinate). Mirtazapine 30 mg preoperatively reduced postoperative nausea and vomiting.[228] Responses were further improved by the addition of dexamethasone to mirtazapine.[228]

The mechanism by which nausea and vomiting are improved by antidepressants is not known. However, serotonin modulates gastric motility and, in particular, fundic accommodation which is improved through activation of $5HT_1$ and $5HT_4$ receptors and through blocking acetylcholine receptors.[266] Tricyclics prevent serotonin reuptake, increase extracellular serotonin in the bowel, which binds to both receptors while tricyclics block acetylcholine receptors. Mirtazapine (like olanzapine) blocks $5HT_3$ and $5HT_2A$ receptors postsynaptically. The affinity for $5HT_3$ receptors is of the same magnitude as granisetron and ondansetron.[267] Mirtazapine facilitates activation of $5HT_1$ receptors, which would improve gastric accommodation. Mirtazapine also blocks H_1 receptors centrally, which may add to anti-emetic activity.[267]

Benzodiazepines

Anticipatory nausea and vomiting due to poorly controlled emesis from chemotherapy is relatively resistant to $5HT_3RA$, but may respond to benzodiazepines as a means of reducing anxiety-provoked emesis.[268] There are no prospective studies on the use of benzodiazepines in the management of nausea and vomiting in advanced cancer. Benzodiazepines, in particular midazolam, are widely used as a premedication to surgery, in part to reduce postoperative nausea and vomiting.[269–272] Lorazepam has been combined with haloperidol and diphenhydramine in a topical gel as a rescue combination in those experiencing chemotherapy-induced nausea and vomiting. Responses were reported in 70% of individuals treated with the gel.[273] Benzodiazepines reduce akathisia with metoclopramide, thus providing a rationale for the combination.[269] Benzodiazepines reduce dopamine in the DVC by activating GABA receptors. Dopaminergic neuron activity is diminished with GABA receptor activation.[274] In this sense, benzodiazepines act like a D_2 receptor antagonist.

Propofol

Propofol has been used for palliative sedation in benzodiazepine treatment refractory circumstances. In a cohort series of 13 cancer patients treated for intractable nausea and vomiting good to very good responses were seen in 69% treated with propofol. Doses ranged between 0.9 and 2.13 mg/kg/h.[275] Propofol also reduces postoperative nausea and vomiting.[276,277] The addition of dexamethasone to propofol improves responses in those experiencing postoperative nausea and vomiting.[278,279] Combinations of tropisetron plus propofol are more effective in reducing postoperative nausea and vomiting than tropisetron alone.[280] Propofol anti-emetic activity may be at least in part due to inhibition of 5-HT_3A receptors.[281]

Acupressure, acupuncture and gastric electrical stimulation

Acupressure of the P6 point has been reported to reduce post-chemotherapy nausea and vomiting in 70% (28/40) of individuals treated. These individuals failed to respond to standard anti-emetics.[282] Electro-acupuncture has been used to prevent nausea and vomiting in those receiving chemotherapy and to treat those whose nausea did not respond to a combination of a $5HT_3$RA and dexamethasone. Twenty-six of 27 (96%) individuals responded with a significant reduction in grade of nausea and episodes of vomiting when treated with electro-acupuncture.[283] In one RCT, wrist bands, which produced acupressure at the P6 point for 5 days, significantly reduced post-chemotherapy nausea and vomiting relative to controls.[284] Acupressure has been effective in reducing postoperative nausea and vomiting.[285] There are no prospective trials of acupressure or acupuncture in managing nausea and vomiting in advanced cancer. Stimulation may influence gastric myoelectrical activity, vagal neurotransmission and cerebellar vestibular activity, which in turn reduces emesis.[285]

High frequency gastric electrical stimulation has been used to treat refractory nausea and vomiting in those with gastroparesis.[286] Benefits may also be seen in those with normal gastric emptying and refractory nausea and vomiting.[286] Gastric electrical stimulation has also been effective in relieving vomiting in those with diabetic gastroparesis and chronic intestinal pseudo-obstruction.[287] There are no prospective studies using gastric electrostimulation in nausea and vomiting associated with advanced cancer.

The grading scale for evidence is provided on Box 14.3 and evidence for the use of anti-emetics and anti-emetic combinations to treat nausea and vomiting in advanced cancer is provided in Box 14.4.

Summary

The strength of the evidence is in favour of the use of metoclopramide $5HT_3$RAs or phenothiazines as initial management for nausea and vomiting. Dose response has not been established for most medications. There is both B2 level evidence and good reason for titrating metoclopramide or switching to a continuous infusion to improve response. In those individuals whose nausea and vomiting fails to respond to single anti-emetics, emesis may improve by either of the following: (1) drug rotation within class (to another phenothiazine); (2) switch to a $5HT_3$RA; (3) add a $5HT_3$RA to metoclopramide or a phenothiazine; (4) rotate to a broad receptor spectrum

Box 14.4 Level of evidence

Level A evidence

- Metoclopramide is effective in the management of nausea and vomiting in advanced cancer.[138]
- Dexamethasone does not significantly improve the anti-emetic activity of metoclopramide or chlorpromazine as initial treatment or as an add-on medication for those whose nausea and vomiting are not responding to low doses of chlorpromazine.[53,54,59,136]
- Tropisetron is effective in reducing nausea and vomiting which is not controlled by, or fails to respond to, low doses of metoclopramide or chlorpromazine.[53,54,59]
- The combination of low dose metoclopramide plus tropisetron or low dose chlorpromazine plus tropisetron is more effective in controlling nausea and vomiting than either drug alone.[53,54,59]
- The addition of dexamethasone to a chlorpromazine–tropisetron combination or a metoclopramide–tropisetron combination is more effective than the double-drug combination on refractory nausea and vomiting.[54,55]
- P6 acupressure does not improve emesis in advanced cancer.

Level B1 evidence

- Thiethylperazine is an effective anti-emetic in advanced cancer.[83]
- Perphenazine is an effective anti-emetic in advanced cancer.[85]
- Prochlorperazine is an effective anti-emetic in managing advanced cancer-related nausea and vomiting.[86,87]
- Diphenhydramine reduces nausea and vomiting in advanced cancer.[161]
- Switching from one phenothiazine to another in those whose nausea and vomiting has not responded to the first phenothiazines can improve response.[65,84]
- Levomepromazine will control nausea and vomiting which has not responded to first-line non-$5HT_3$RA anti-emetics and as first-line treatment.[69,70]

Level B2 evidence

- Haloperidol is effective in the management of nausea and vomiting in advanced cancer and bowel obstruction.[2,7,51]
- Cyclizine is an effective anti-emetic in the management of nausea and vomiting in advanced cancer.[7,51]
- Hyoscine butylbromide is an effective anti-emetic in the management of bowel obstruction.[64,93]
- Octreotide is more effective than hyoscine butylbromide in managing symptoms related to bowel obstruction, including nausea and vomiting.[64,91,183,186]
- Dexamethasone added to medical management of bowel obstruction may resolve bowel obstruction and nausea and vomiting.[229,230]
- Chlorpromazine and haloperidol are effective anti-emetics in managing nausea and vomiting associated with bowel obstruction.[64,93,183]

Level C evidence

- Olanzapine is an effective anti-emetic in advanced cancer and refractory nausea and vomiting.[105–108]

Box 14.4 Level of evidence *(continued)*

- Propofol is an effective anti-emetic in advanced cancer and refractory nausea and vomiting.[275]
- Titration of metoclopramide, and switching to a continuous subcutaneous infusion in individuals whose nausea and vomiting fails to respond to 10 mg every 4 h, improves responses.[132]
- Carbamazepine reduces nausea and vomiting associated with meningeal metastases.[251]
- Glycopyrrolate effectively reduces symptoms from bowel obstruction, including nausea and vomiting.[185]
- Cannabinoids improve nausea and vomiting in advanced cancer.[236]
- Ondansetron is an emetic antiemetic in advanced cancer.[288]

Level D evidence

- Benzodiazepines are effective anti-emetics in advanced cancer.
- Tricyclic antidepressants are effective anti-emetics in advanced cancer.
- Gabapentin is an effective anti-emetic in advanced cancer.
- Aetiological anti-emetic guidelines are superior to the use of rotating single agent anti-emetic dosing strategies.
- Adding anti-emetics at low doses is a more effective strategy than titrating single agent antiemetics to response or maximum therapeutic levels in the management of nausea and vomiting in advanced cancer.

A: Single drug benefits supported by at least one RCT.
B1: Single drug benefits supported by at least one prospective single arm study.
B2: Drug benefit demonstrated in a prospective RCT or single arm study in combination with other anti-emetics or as part of a prospective multiple anti-emetic guideline study, where single drug activity cannot be determined.
C: Single or multiple case reports, observational cohort series, retrospective review of clinical practice.
D: Expert opinion or by expert consensus.

phenothiazine (olanzapine, levomepromazine). Dexamethasone appears to add little anti-emetic activity to phenothiazines or metoclopramide, but may improve responses to a metoclopramide–$5HT_3RA$ or phenothiazine–$5HT_3RA$ combination. Alternatively, a strategy which adopts guidelines based on aetiology may be used. In individuals with refractory nausea and vomiting in whom palliative sedation is being considered, propofol is a reasonable choice.

The management of nausea and vomiting associated with a cancer-related bowel obstruction should consist of a combination of haloperidol plus a quaternary anticholinergic or phenothiazines plus a quaternary anticholinergic. In countries where octreotide is available, a substitution could be made for the anticholinergic; dexamethasone could be added in an attempt to resolve the intestinal obstruction.

Acknowledgement

The author would like to recognize the skills of Wendy L. Gatlin in preparing this manuscript.

References

1. Davis MP, Walsh D (2000) Treatment of nausea and vomiting in advanced cancer. *Support Care Cancer*, **8**(6), 444–52.

2. Stephenson J, Davies A (2006) An assessment of aetiology-based guidelines for the management of nausea and vomiting in patients with advanced cancer. *Support Care Cancer*, **14**(4), 348–53.
3. Glare P, Pereira G, Kristjanson LJ, Stockler M, Tattersall M (2004) Systematic review of the efficacy of antiemetics in the treatment of nausea in patients with far-advanced cancer. *Support Care Cancer*, **12**(6), 432–40.
4. Portenoy RK, Thaler HT, Kornblith AB, *et al.* (1994) Symptom prevalence, characteristics and distress in a cancer population. *Qual Life Res*, **3**(3), 183–9.
5. Reuben DB, Mor V (1986) Nausea and vomiting in terminal cancer patients. *Arch Intern Med*, **146**(10), 2021–3.
6. Mannix K (2006) Palliation of nausea and vomiting in malignancy. *Clin Med*, **6**(2), 144–7.
7. Bentley A, Boyd K (2001) Use of clinical pictures in the management of nausea and vomiting: a prospective audit. *Palliat Med*, **15**(3), 247–53.
8. Twycross RBI (1998) Nausea and vomiting in advanced cancer. *Eur J Pall Care*, **5**(2).
9. Brizzee KR (1990) Mechanics of vomiting: a mini-review. *Can J Physiol Pharmacol*, **68**(2), 221–9.
10. Hornby PJ (2001) Central neurocircuitry associated with emesis. *Am J Med*, **111**(Suppl 8A), 106S–12S.
11. Andrews PL, Horn CC (2006) Signals for nausea and emesis: implications for models of upper gastrointestinal diseases. *Auton Neurosci*, **125**(1–2), 100–15.
12. Andrews PL, Davis CJ, Bingham S, Davidson HI, Hawthorn J, Maskell L (1990) The abdominal visceral innervation and the emetic reflex: pathways, pharmacology, and plasticity. *Can J Physiol Pharmacol*, **68**(2), 325–45.
13. Andersen R, Krohg K (1976) Pain as a major cause of postoperative nausea. *Can Anaesth Soc J*, **23**(4), 366–9.
14. Sugiyama H, Hayama T (1965) Abdominal viscera as site of emetic action for staphylococcal enterotoxin in the monkey. *J Infect Dis*, **115**(4), 330–6.
15. Troncon LE, Thompson DG, Ahluwalia NK, Barlow J, Heggie L (1995) Relations between upper abdominal symptoms and gastric distension abnormalities in dysmotility like functional dyspepsia and after vagotomy. *Gut*, **37**(1), 17–22.
16. Saito R, Takano Y, Kamiya HO (2003) Roles of substance P and NK(1) receptor in the brainstem in the development of emesis. *J Pharmacol Sci*, **91**(2), 87–94.
17. Morrow GR, Andrews PL, Hickok JT, Stern R (2000) Vagal changes following cancer chemotherapy: implications for the development of nausea. *Psychophysiology*, **37**(3), 378–84.
18. Herrington JD, Kwan P, Young RR, Lagow E, Lagrone L, Riggs MW (2000) Randomized, multicenter comparison of oral granisetron and oral ondansetron for emetogenic chemotherapy. *Pharmacotherapy*, **20**(11), 1318–23.
19. Miller AD, Leslie RA (1994) The area postrema and vomiting. *Front Neuroendocrinol*, **15**(4), 301–20.
20. Dixon MK, Nathan NA, Hornby PJ (1998) Immunocytochemical distribution of neurokinin 1 receptor in rat dorsal vagal complex. *Peptides*, **19**(5), 913–23.
21. Krowicki ZK, Hornby PJ (2000) Substance P in the dorsal motor nucleus of the vagus evokes gastric motor inhibition via neurokinin 1 receptor in rat. *J Pharmacol Exp Ther*, **293**(1), 214–21.
22. Beaumont H, Jonsson-Rylander AC, Carlsson K, *et al.* (2008) The role of GABA(A) receptors in the control of transient lower oesophageal sphincter relaxations in the dog. *Br J Pharmacol*, **153**(6), 1195–202.
23. Kong VK, Irwin MG (2007) Gabapentin: a multimodal perioperative drug? *Br J Anaesth*, **99**(6), 775–86.
24. Sivarao DV, Krowicki ZK, Hornby PJ (1998) Role of $GABA_A$ receptors in rat hindbrain nuclei controlling gastric motor function. *Neurogastroenterol Motil*, **10**(4), 305–13.
25. Ho KM, Ismail H (2008) Use of intrathecal midazolam to improve perioperative analgesia: a meta-analysis. *Anaesth Intensive Care*, **36**(3), 365–73.
26. Ferreira M, Singh A, Dretchen KL, Kellar KJ, Gillis RA (2000) Brainstem nicotinic receptor subtypes that influence intragastric and arterial blood pressures. *J Pharmacol Exp Ther*, **294**(1), 230–8.

27. Sanger GJ, Andrews PL (2006) Treatment of nausea and vomiting: gaps in our knowledge. *Auton Neurosci*, **129**(1–2), 3–16.
28. Pedigo NW, Jr, Brizzee KR (1985) Muscarinic cholinergic receptors in area postrema and brainstem areas regulating emesis. *Brain Res Bull*, **14**(2), 169–77.
29. Leslie RA, Shah Y, Thejomayen M, Murphy KM, Robertson HA (1990) The neuropharmacology of emesis: the role of receptors in neuromodulation of nausea and vomiting. *Can J Physiol Pharmacol*, **68**(2), 279–88.
30. Reynolds DJ, Lowenstein PR, Moorman JM, Grahame-Smith DG, Leslie RA (1994) Evidence for cholinergic vagal afferents and vagal presynaptic M1 receptors in the ferret. *Neurochem Int*, **25**(5), 455–64.
31. Beleslin DB, Strbac M, Jovanovic-Micic D, Samardzic R, Nedelkovski V (1989) Area postrema: cholinergic and noradrenergic regulation of emesis. A new concept. *Arch Int Physiol Biochim*, **97**(1), 107–15.
32. Osinski MA, Uchic ME, Seifert T, *et al.* (2005) Dopamine D2, but not D4, receptor agonists are emetogenic in ferrets. *Pharmacol Biochem Behav*, **81**(1), 211–9.
33. Endo T, Minami M, Hirafuji M, *et al.* (2000) Neurochemistry and neuropharmacology of emesis—the role of serotonin. *Toxicology*, **153**(1–3), 189–201.
34. Tecott LH, Maricq AV, Julius D (1993) Nervous system distribution of the serotonin 5-HT3 receptor mRNA. *Proc Natl Acad Sci USA*, **90**(4), 1430–4.
35. Wolf H (2000) Preclinical and clinical pharmacology of the 5-HT3 receptor antagonists. *Scand J Rheumatol Suppl*, **113**, 37–45.
36. Waeber C, Dixon K, Hoyer D, Palacios JM (1988) Localisation by autoradiography of neuronal 5-HT3 receptors in the mouse CNS. *Eur J Pharmacol*, **151**(2), 351–2.
37. Gale JD (1995) Serotonergic mediation of vomiting. *J Pediatr Gastroenterol Nutr*, **21**(Suppl 1), S22–8.
38. Kaiser R, Tremblay PB, Sezer O, Possinger K, Roots I, Brockmoller J (2004) Investigation of the association between 5-HT3A receptor gene polymorphisms and efficiency of antiemetic treatment with 5-HT3 receptor antagonists. *Pharmacogenetics*, **14**(5), 271–8.
39. Wolff MC, Leander JD (1995) Comparison of the antiemetic effects of a 5-HT1A agonist, LY228729, and 5-HT3 antagonists in the pigeon. *Pharmacol Biochem Behav*, **52**(3), 571–5.
40. Diemunsch P, Grelot L (2000) Potential of substance P antagonists as antiemetics. *Drugs*, **60**(3), 533–46.
41. Onishi T, Mori T, Yanagihara M, Furukawa N, Fukuda H (2007) Similarities of the neuronal circuit for the induction of fictive vomiting between ferrets and dogs. *Auton Neurosci*, **136**(1–2), 20–30.
42. Thompson PI, Bingham S, Andrews PL, Patel N, Joel SP, Slevin ML (1992) Morphine 6-glucuronide: a metabolite of morphine with greater emetic potency than morphine in the ferret. *Br J Pharmacol*, **106**(1), 3–8.
43. Rudd JA, Cheng CH, Naylor RJ, Ngan MP, Wai MK (1999) Modulation of emesis by fentanyl and opioid receptor antagonists in *Suncus murinus* (house musk shrew). *Eur J Pharmacol*, **374**(1), 77–84.
44. Kawai M, Kawahara H, Hirayama S, Yoshimura N, Ida S (2004) Effect of baclofen on emesis and 24-hour esophageal pH in neurologically impaired children with gastroesophageal reflux disease. *J Pediatr Gastroenterol Nutr*, **38**(3), 317–23.
45. Inui A, Asakawa A, Bowers CY, *et al.* (2004) Ghrelin, appetite, and gastric motility: the emerging role of the stomach as an endocrine organ. *FASEB J*, **18**(3), 439–56.
46. Asakawa A, Inui A, Fujimiya M, *et al.* (2005) Stomach regulates energy balance via acylated ghrelin and desacyl ghrelin. *Gut*, **54**(1), 18–24.
47. Liu YL, Malik NM, Sanger GJ, Andrews PL (2006) Ghrelin alleviates cancer chemotherapy-associated dyspepsia in rodents. *Cancer Chemother Pharmacol*, **58**(3), 326–33.
48. Tack J, Depoortere I, Bisschops R, Verbeke K, Janssens J, Peeters T (2005) Influence of ghrelin on gastric emptying and meal-related symptoms in idiopathic gastroparesis. *Aliment Pharmacol Ther*, **22**(9), 847–53.

49. Apfel CC, Korttila K, Abdalla M, *et al.* (2004) A factorial trial of six interventions for the prevention of postoperative nausea and vomiting. *N Engl J Med*, **350**(24), 2441–51.
50. Lichter I (1993) Which antiemetic? *J Palliat Care*, **9**(1), 42–50.
51. Hasler WL, Chey WD (2003) Nausea and vomiting. *Gastroenterology*, **125**(6), 1860–7.
52. Critchley P, Plach N, Grantham M (2001) Efficacy of haloperidol in the treatment of nausea and vomiting in the palliative patient: a systematic review [Letter to Editor]. *J Pain Sympt Manag*, 631–4.
53. Mystakidou K, Befon S, Liossi C, Vlachos L (1998) Comparison of the efficacy and safety of tropisetron, metoclopramide, and chlorpromazine in the treatment of emesis associated with far advanced cancer. *Cancer*, **83**(6), 1214–23.
54. Mystakidou K, Befon S, Liossi C, Vlachos L (1998) Comparison of tropisetron and chlorpromazine combinations in the control of nausea and vomiting of patients with advanced cancer. *J Pain Sympt Manag*, **15**(3), 176–84.
55. Lichter I (1993) Results of antiemetic management in terminal illness. *J Palliat Care*, **9**(2), 19–21.
56. Tiddle J WM, Irwig L (1996) *Method of Evaluating Research and Guideline Evidence*. Sydney: NSW Health Department.
57. Burgess CL TP, Clifford RM (2007) Audit of nausea and vomiting management in palliative care hospital patients. *J Pharm Pract Res*, **37**(4), 306–9.
58. Glasziou PP, Irwig LM (1995) An evidence based approach to individualising treatment. *Br Med J*, **311**(7016), 1356–9.
59. Mystakidou K, Befon S, Trifyllis J, Liossi C, Papadimitriou J (1997) Tropisetron versus metoclopramide in the control of emesis in far-advanced cancer. *Oncologist*, **2**(5), 319–23.
60. Torres Del Toro JM, Albertson HA (1955) Chlorpromazine in the management of nausea and vomiting. *Va Med Mon* (1918), **82**(7), 306–8.
61. Homburger F, Smithy G (1954) Chlorpromazine in patients with nausea and vomiting due to advanced cancer. *N Engl J Med*, **251**(20), 820–2.
62. Moyer JH, Kent B, Knight RW, *et al.* (1954) Clinical studies of an anti-emetic agent, chlorpromazine. *Am J Med Sci*, **228**(2), 174–89.
63. Moyer JH, Kent B, Knight R, Morris G, Huggins R, Handley CA (1954) Laboratory and clinical observations on chlorpromazine (SKF-2601-A); hemodynamic and toxicological studies. *Am J Med Sci*, **227**(3), 283–90.
64. Mystakidou K, Tsilika E, Kalaidopoulou O, Chondros K, Georgaki S, Papadimitriou L (2002) Comparison of octreotide administration vs conservative treatment in the management of inoperable bowel obstruction in patients with far advanced cancer: a randomized, double- blind, controlled clinical trial. *Anticancer Res*, **22**(2B), 1187–92.
65. Stephen CR, Dent S, Bourgeois-Gavardin M (1955) Control of nausea and vomiting with chlorpromazine; incidence of side-effects. *Arch Intern Med*, **96**(6), 794–8.
66. Dahl SG, Hjorth M, Hough E (1982) Chlorpromazine, methotrimeprazine, and metabolites. Structural changes accompanying the loss of neuroleptic potency by ring sulfoxidation. *Molec Pharmacol*, **21**(2), 409–14.
67. Allgen LG, Hellstroem L, Santorp CJ (1963) On the metabolism and elimination of the psychotropic phenothiazine drug levomepromazine (Nozinan) in Man. *Acta Psychiatr Scand*, **39**(Suppl 169), 366.
68. Maxwell DR, Palmer HT, Ryall RW (1961) A comparison of the analgesic and some other central properties of methotrimeprazine and morphine. *Arch Int Pharmacodyn Ther*, **132**, 60–73.
69. Kennett A, Hardy J, Shah S, A'Hern R (2005) An open study of methotrimeprazine in the management of nausea and vomiting in patients with advanced cancer. *Support Care Cancer*, **13**(9), 715–21.
70. Eisenchlas JH, Garrigue N, Junin M, De Simone GG (2005) Low-dose levomepromazine in refractory emesis in advanced cancer patients: an open-label study. *Palliat Med*, **19**(1), 71–5.
71. McCabe HL, Maraveyas A (2003) Subcutaneous levomepromazine rescue (SLR) for high grade delayed chemotherapy-induced emesis (DCIE). *Anticancer Res*, **23**(6D), 5209–12.

72. Amesbury B, Alloway L, Hickmore E, Dewhurst G (2004) High-dose levomepromazine (methotrimeprazine) to control nausea in carcinoid syndrome. *J Palliat Care*, **20**(2), 117–8.
73. Higi M, Niederle N, Bierbaum W, Schmidt CG, Seeber S (1980) Pronounced antiemetic activity of the antipsychotic drug levomepromacine (L) in patients receiving cancer chemotherapy. *J Cancer Res Clin Oncol*, **97**(1), 81–6.
74. Krajnik M, Zylicz Z (2001) Understanding pruritus in systemic disease. *J Pain Sympt Manag*, **21**(2), 151–68.
75. Higi M, Niederle N, Schmidt CG, Seeber S (1980) [Improved antiemetic treatment with levomepromazine (author's translation)]. *Dtsch Med Wochenschr*, **105**(22), 794–5.
76. Bichel J, Brincker H (1965) Treatment of pruritus in Hodgkin's disease and in reticulum cell sarcoma. *Scand J Haematol*, **79**, 85–90.
77. Bronwell AW, Rutledge R, Dalton ML Jr (1966) Analgesic effect of methotrimeprazine and meperidine in postoperative patients. Double-blind study in 24 cases. *Am Surg*, **32**(9), 641–4.
78. Lal S, Nair NP, Cecyre D, Quirion R (1993) Levomepromazine receptor binding profile in human brain—implications for treatment-resistant schizophrenia. *Acta Psychiatr Scand*, **87**(6), 380–3.
79. Kornhuber J, Weigmann H, Rohrich J, *et al.* (2006) Region specific distribution of levomepromazine in the human brain. *J Neural Transm*, **113**(3), 387–97.
80. Kornhuber J, Wiltfang J, Riederer P, Bleich S (2006) Neuroleptic drugs in the human brain: clinical impact of persistence and region-specific distribution. *Eur Arch Psychiatry Clin Neurosci*, **256**(5), 274–80.
81. Green B, Pettit T, Faith L, Seaton K (2004) Focus on levomepromazine. *Curr Med Res Opin*, **20**(12), 1877–81.
82. Hals PA, Dahl SG (1995) Metabolism of levomepromazine in man. *Eur J Drug Metab Pharmacokinet*, **20**(1), 61–71.
83. Cox J, Collins JH (1962) Nausea and vomiting: control by thiethylperazine. *Curr Ther Res Clin Exp*, **4**, 178–81.
84. Homburger F (1958) Perphenazine as an antiemetic agent in cancer and other chronic diseases. *J Am Med Assoc*, **167**(10), 1240–1.
85. Ernst EM, Snyder AM (1958) Perphenazine in nausea and vomiting, and anxiety states. *Pennsylvania Med J*, **61**(3), 355–9.
86. Homburger F, Smithy G (1957) Proclorperazine for the treatment of nausea and vomiting in patients with advanced cancer and other chronic diseases. *N Engl J Med*, **256**(1), 27.
87. Walsh TD (1982) Antiemetic drug combinations in advanced cancer. *Lancet*, **1**(8279), 1018.
88. Buttner M, Walder B, von Elm E, Tramer MR (2004) Is low-dose haloperidol a useful. *Anesthesiology*, **101**(6), 1454–63.
89. Vella-Brincat J, Macleod AD (2004) Haloperidol in palliative care. *Palliat Med*, **18**(3), 195–201.
90. Cole RM, Robinson F, Harvey L, Trethowan K, Murdoch V (1994) Successful control of intractable nausea and vomiting requiring combined ondansetron and haloperidol in a patient with advanced cancer. *J Pain Sympt Manag*, **9**(1), 48–50.
91. Ripamonti CI, Easson AM, Gerdes H (2008) Management of malignant bowel obstruction. *Eur J Cancer*, **44**(8), 1105–15.
92. Ripamonti C, Twycross R, Baines M, *et al.* (2001) Clinical-practice recommendations for the management of bowel obstruction in patients with end-stage cancer. *Support Care Cancer*, **9**(4), 223–33.
93. Ventafridda V, Ripamonti C, Caraceni A, Spoldi E, Messina L, De Conno F (1990) The management of inoperable gastrointestinal obstruction in terminal cancer patients. *Tumori*, **76**(4), 389–93.
94. Mercadante S, Maddaloni S (1992) Octreotide in the management of inoperable gastrointestinal obstruction in terminal cancer patients. *J Pain Sympt Manag*, **7**(8), 496–8.

95. Bymaster FP, Nelson DL, DeLapp NW, *et al.* (1999) Antagonism by olanzapine of dopamine D1, serotonin2, muscarinic, histamine H1 and alpha 1-adrenergic receptors in vitro. *Schizophr Res*, **37**(1), 107–22.
96. Bymaster FP, Calligaro DO, Falcone JF, *et al.* (1996) Radioreceptor binding profile of the atypical antipsychotic olanzapine. *Neuropsychopharmacology*, **14**(2), 87–96.
97. Brockmoller J, Kirchheiner J, Schmider J, *et al.* (2002) The impact of the CYP2D6 polymorphism on haloperidol pharmacokinetics and on the outcome of haloperidol treatment. *Clin Pharmacol Ther*, **72**(4), 438–52.
98. Menza MA, Murray GB, Holmes VF, Rafuls WA (1987) Decreased extrapyramidal symptoms with intravenous haloperidol. *J Clin Psychiatry*, **48**(7), 278–80.
99. Stephenson CM, Pilowsky LS (1999) Psychopharmacology of olanzapine. A review. *Br J Psychiatry Suppl* **38**, 52–8.
100. Menza MA, Murray GB, Holmes VF, Rafuls WA (1988) Controlled study of extrapyramidal reactions in the management of delirious, medically ill patients: intravenous haloperidol versus intravenous haloperidol plus benzodiazepines. *Heart Lung*, **17**(3), 238–41.
101. Moleman P, Schmitz PJ, Ladee GA (1982) Extrapyramidal side effects and oral haloperidol: an analysis of explanatory patient and treatment characteristics. *J Clin Psychiatry*, **43**(12), 492–6.
102. White C, McPherson A, McCann MA, Sadler A, Fyvie J (2006) Prolonged extra-pyramidal side effects after discontinuation of haloperidol as an antiemetic. *Palliat Med*, **20**(3), 215–6.
103. Seneff MG, Mathews RA (1995) Use of haloperidol infusions to control delirium in critically ill adults. *Ann Pharmacother*, **29**(7–8), 690–3.
104. Neidhart JA, Gagen MM, Wilson HE, Young DC (1981) Comparative trial of the antiemetic effects of THC and haloperidol. *J Clin Pharmacol*, **21**(8–9 Suppl), 38S–42S.
105. Srivastava M, Brito-Dellan N, Davis MP, Leach M, Lagman R (2003) Olanzapine as an antiemetic in refractory nausea and vomiting in advanced cancer. *J Pain Sympt Manag*, **25**(6), 578–82.
106. Jackson WC, Tavernier L (2003) Olanzapine for intractable nausea in palliative care patients. *J Palliat Med*, **6**(2), 251–5.
107. Shinjo T, Okada M (2006) [Olanzapine use in cancer patients for refractory vomiting]. *Gan To Kagaku Ryoho*, **33**(3), 349–52.
108. Passik SD, Lundberg J, Kirsh KL, *et al.* (2002) A pilot exploration of the antiemetic activity of olanzapine for the relief of nausea in patients with advanced cancer and pain. *J Pain Sympt Manag*, **23**(6), 526–32.
109. Navari RM, Einhorn LH, Passik SD, *et al.* (2005) A phase II trial of olanzapine for the prevention of chemotherapy-induced nausea and vomiting: a Hoosier Oncology Group study. *Support Care Cancer*, **13**(7), 529–34.
110. Navari RM, Einhorn LH, Loehrer PJ, Sr, *et al.* (2007) A phase II trial of olanzapine, dexamethasone, and palonosetron for the prevention of chemotherapy-induced nausea and vomiting: a Hoosier oncology group study. *Support Care Cancer*, **15**(11), 1285–91.
111. Tohen M, Vieta E, Calabrese J, *et al.* (2003) Efficacy of olanzapine and olanzapine-fluoxetine combination in the treatment of bipolar I depression. *Arch Gen Psychiatry*, **60**(11), 1079–88.
112. Feldman PD, Kaiser CJ, Kennedy JS, *et al.* (2003) Comparison of risperidone and olanzapine in the control of negative symptoms of chronic schizophrenia and related psychotic disorders in patients aged 50 to 65 years. *J Clin Psychiatry*, **64**(9), 998–1004.
113. Zylicz Z, Krajnik M (2003) Flushing and sweating in an advanced breast cancer patient relieved by olanzapine. *J Pain Sympt Manag*, **25**(6), 494–5.
114. Bober DI, Star JE (2005) Olanzapine for the management of pain in an adolescent girl. *J Child Adolesc Psychopharmacol*, **15**(6), 842–3.
115. Freedenfeld RN, Murray M, Fuchs PN, Kiser RS (2006) Decreased pain and improved quality of life in fibromyalgia patients treated with olanzapine, an atypical neuroleptic. *Pain Pract*, **6**(2), 112–8.

116. Gorski ED, Willis KC (2003) Report of three case studies with olanzapine for chronic pain. *J Pain*, **4**(3), 166–8.

117. Khojainova N, Santiago-Palma J, Kornick C, Breitbart W, Gonzales GR (2002) Olanzapine in the management of cancer pain. *J Pain Sympt Manag*, **23**(4), 346–50.

118. Lertxundi U, Peral J, Mora O, Domingo-Echaburu S, Martinez-Bengoechea MJ, Garcia-Monco JC (2008) Antidopaminergic therapy for managing comorbidities in patients with Parkinson's disease. *Am J Health Syst Pharm*, **65**(5), 414–9.

119. Yoshida K, Higuchi H, Ozaki N (2007) Successful treatment of severe antidepressant-induced nausea with a combination of milnacipran and olanzapine. *Pharmacopsychiatry*, **40**(2), 84–5.

120. Budur K, Pozuelo L (2003) Olanzapine for corticosteroid-induced mood disorders. *Psychosomatics*, **44**(4), 353.

121. Fuller MA, Shermock KM, Secic M, Grogg AL (2003) Comparative study of the development of diabetes mellitus in patients taking risperidone and olanzapine. *Pharmacotherapy*, **23**(8), 1037–43.

122. Feldman PD, Hay LK, Deberdt W, *et al.* (2004) Retrospective cohort study of diabetes mellitus and antipsychotic treatment in a geriatric population in the United States. *J Am Med Dir Assoc*, **5**(1), 38–46.

123. Ebenbichler CF, Laimer M, Eder U, *et al.* (2003) Olanzapine induces insulin resistance: results from a prospective study. *J Clin Psychiatry*, **64**(12), 1436–9.

124. Beliard S, Valero R, Vialettes B (2003) Atypical neuroleptics and diabetes. *Diabetes Metab*, **29**(3), 296–9.

125. Crumb WJ, Jr, Ekins S, Sarazan RD, *et al.* (2006) Effects of antipsychotic drugs on I (to), I (Na), I (sus), I (K1), and hERG: QT prolongation, structure activity relationship, and network analysis. *Pharm Res*, **23**(6), 1133–43.

126. Kongsamut S, Kang J, Chen XL, Roehr J, Rampe D (2002) A comparison of the receptor binding and HERG channel affinities for a series of antipsychotic drugs. *Eur J Pharmacol*, **450**(1), 37–41.

127. Raggi MA, Mandrioli R, Sabbioni C, Pucci V (2004) Atypical antipsychotics: pharmacokinetics, therapeutic drug monitoring and pharmacological interactions. *Curr Med Chem*, **11**(3), 279–96.

128. Zhang W, Bymaster FP (1999) The in vivo effects of olanzapine and other antipsychotic agents on receptor occupancy and antagonism of dopamine D1, D2, D3, 5HT2A and muscarinic receptors. *Psychopharmacology (Berl)*, **141**(3), 267–78.

129. Okamoto Y, Tsuneto S, Matsuda Y, *et al.* (2007) A retrospective chart review of the antiemetic effectiveness of risperidone in refractory opioid-induced nausea and vomiting in advanced cancer patients. *J Pain Sympt Manag*, **34**(2), 217–22.

130. Bruera E, Michaud M, Partington J, Brenneis C, Paterson AH, MacDonald RN (1988) Continuous subcutaneous (CS) infusion of metoclopramide (MCP) using a plastic disposable infusor for the treatment of chemotherapy-induced emesis. *J Pain Sympt Manag*, **3**(2), 105–7.

131. Corli O, Cozzolino A, Battaiotto L (1995) Effectiveness of levosulpiride versus metoclopramide for nausea and vomiting in advanced cancer patients: a double-blind, randomized, crossover study. *J Pain Sympt Manag*, **10**(7), 521–6.

132. Bruera E, Seifert L, Watanabe S, *et al.* (1996) Chronic nausea in advanced cancer patients: a retrospective assessment of a metoclopramide-based antiemetic regimen. *J Pain Sympt Manag*, **11**(3), 147–53.

133. Bruera E, Brenneis C, Michaud M, MacDonald N (1987) Continuous Sc infusion of metoclopramide for treatment of narcotic bowel syndrome. *Cancer Treat Rep*, **71**(11), 1121–2.

134. Bruera E, Belzile M, Neumann C, Harsanyi Z, Babul N, Darke A (2000) A double-blind, crossover study of controlled-release metoclopramide and placebo for the chronic nausea and dyspepsia of advanced cancer. *J Pain Symptm Manag*, **19**(6), 427–35.

135. Nelson KA, Walsh TD (1993) Metoclopramide in anorexia caused by cancer-associated dyspepsia syndrome (CADS). *J Palliat Care*, **9**(2), 14–18.

136. Bruera E, Moyano JR, Sala R, *et al.* (2004) Dexamethasone in addition to metoclopramide for chronic nausea in patients with advanced cancer: a randomized controlled trial. *J Pain Sympt Manag*, **28**(4), 381–8.
137. Bruera ED, MacEachern TJ, Spachynski KA, *et al.* (1994) Comparison of the efficacy, safety, and pharmacokinetics of controlled release and immediate release metoclopramide for the management of chronic nausea in patients with advanced cancer. *Cancer*, **74**(12), 3204–11.
138. Cham S, Basire M, Kelly AM (2004) Intermediate dose metoclopramide is not more effective than standard dose metoclopramide for patients who present to the emergency department with nausea and vomiting: a pilot study. *Emerg Med Australas*, **16**(3), 208–11.
139. Bradshaw M, Sen A (2006) Use of a prophylactic antiemetic with morphine in acute pain: randomised controlled trial. *Emerg Med J*, **23**(3), 210–13.
140. O'Connell ME, Awni WM, Goodman M, *et al.* (1987) Bioavailability and disposition of metoclopramide after single- and multiple-dose administration in diabetic patients with gastroparesis. *J Clin Pharmacol*, **27**(8), 610–14.
141. Magueur E, Hagege H, Attali P, Singlas E, Etienne JP, Taburet AM (1991) Pharmacokinetics of metoclopramide in patients with liver cirrhosis. *Br J Clin Pharmacol*, **31**(2), 185–7.
142. Taylor WB, Bateman DN (1986) Oral bioavailability of high-dose metoclopramide. *Eur J Clin Pharmacol*, **31**(1), 41–4.
143. Desta Z, Wu GM, Morocho AM, Flockhart DA (2002) The gastroprokinetic and antiemetic drug metoclopramide is a substrate and inhibitor of cytochrome P450 2D6. *Drug Metab Dispos*, **30**(3), 336–43.
144. Bateman DN (1983) Clinical pharmacokinetics of metoclopramide. *Clin Pharmacokinet*, **8**(6), 523–9.
145. O'Connell ME, Awni WM, Goodman M, *et al.* (1987) Bioavailability and disposition of metoclopramide after single- and multiple-dose administration in diabetic patients with gastroparesis. *J Clin Pharmacol*, **27**(8), 610–14.
146. McGovern EM, Grevel J, Bryson SM (1986) Pharmacokinetics of high-dose metoclopramide in cancer patients. *Clin Pharmacokinet*, **11**(6), 415–24.
147. Havsteen H, Nielsen H, Kjaer M (1986) Antiemetic effect and pharmacokinetics of high dose metoclopramide in cancer patients treated with cisplatin-containing chemotherapy regimens. *Eur J Clin Pharmacol*, **31**(1), 33–40.
148. Bryson SM, McGovern EM, Kelman AW, White K, Addis GJ, Whiting B (1985) The disease. *Br J Clin Pharmacol*, **19**(6), 757–66.
149. Grevel J, Whiting B, Kelman AW, Taylor WB, Bateman DN (1988) Population analysis of the pharmacokinetic variability of high-dose metoclopramide in cancer patients. *Clin Pharmacokinet*, **14**(1), 52–63.
150. Taylor WB, Proctor SJ, Bateman DN (1984) Pharmacokinetics and efficacy of high-dose metoclopramide given by continuous infusion for the control of cytotoxic drug-induced vomiting. *Br J Clin Pharmacol*, **18**(5), 679–84.
151. Kearns GL, van den Anker JN, Reed MD, Blumer JL (1998) Pharmacokinetics of metoclopramide in neonates. *J Clin Pharmacol*, **38**(2), 122–8.
152. Wright MR, Axelson JE, Rurak DW, *et al.* (1988) Effect of haemodialysis on metoclopramide kinetics in patients with severe renal failure. *Br J Clin Pharmacol*, **26**(4), 474–7.
153. Albani F, Tame MR, De Palma R, Bernardi M (1991) Kinetics of intravenous metoclopramide in patients with hepatic cirrhosis. *Eur J Clin Pharmacol*, **40**(4), 423–5.
154. Kearns GL, Butler HL, Lane JK, Carchman SH, Wright GJ (1988) Metoclopramide pharmacokinetics and pharmacodynamics in infants with gastroesophageal reflux. *J Pediatr Gastroenterol Nutr*, **7**(6), 823–9.
155. Tonini M, Cipollina L, Poluzzi E, Crema F, Corazza GR, De Ponti F (2004) Review article: clinical implications of enteric and central D2 receptor blockade by antidopaminergic gastrointestinal prokinetics. *Aliment Pharmacol Ther*, **19**(4), 379–90.

156. Clarke DE, Craig DA, Fozard JR (1989) The 5-HT4 receptor: naughty, but nice. *Trends Pharmacol Sci*, **10**(10), 385–6.

157. Parlak I, Atilla R, Cicek M, *et al.* (2005) Rate of metoclopramide infusion affects the severity and incidence of akathisia. *Emerg Med J*, **22**(9), 621–4.

158. Khan NU, Razzak JA (2006) Abdominal pain with rigidity secondary to the anti-emetic drug metoclopramide. *J Emerg Med*, **30**(4), 411–3.

159. Israel R, O'Mara V, Austin B, Bellucci A, Meyer BR (1986) Metoclopramide decreases renal plasma flow. *Clin Pharmacol Ther*, **39**(3), 261–4.

160. Blumberg AL, Dubb JW, Allison NL, Aldins Z, Ramey K, Stote RM (1988) Selectivity of metoclopramide for endocrine versus renal effects of dopamine in normal humans. *J Cardiovasc Pharmacol*, **11**(2), 181–6.

161. McCawley CE, Kulasavage RJ, Warrington WR, Pasquesi TJ (1951) The intravenous use of diphenhydramine hydrochloride in the control of nausea and vomiting. *Portland Clin Bull*, **5**(3), 43–8.

162. Chinn HI, Strickland BA, Waltrip OH, Gainer SH (1951) Prevention of air sickness by benadryl-scopolamine mixtures. *US Armed Forces Med J*, **2**(3), 401–4.

163. Hume RH, Wilner WK, Jr (1952) The use of dramamine in control of postoperative nausea and vomiting. *Anesthesiology*, **13**(3), 302–5.

164. Warrington WR, Pasquesi TJ, Kulasavage RJ, McCawley EL (1953) Benadryl hydrochloride given intravenously to control postoperative nausea and vomiting. *Surgery*, **34**(5), 837–42.

165. Lin TF, Yeh YC, Yen YH, Wang YP, Lin CJ, Sun WZ (2005) Antiemetic and analgesic-sparing effects of diphenhydramine added to morphine intravenous patient-controlled analgesia. *Br J Anaesth*, **94**(6), 835–9.

166. Spinks AB, Wasiak J, Villanueva EV, Bernath V (2007) Scopolamine (hyoscine) for preventing and treating motion sickness. *Cochrane Database Syst Rev*, (3), CD002851.

167. Parlak I, Erdur B, Parlak M, *et al.* (2007) Midazolam vs diphenhydramine for the treatment of metoclopramide-induced akathisia: a randomized controlled trial. *Acad Emerg Med*, **14**(8), 715–21.

168. Grunberg SM, Ehler E, McDermed JE, Akerley WL (1988) Oral metoclopramide with or without diphenhydramine: potential for prevention of late nausea and vomiting induced by cisplatin. *J Natl Cancer Inst*, **80**(11), 864–8.

169. Weschules DJ (2005) Tolerability of the compound ABHR in hospice patients. *J Palliat Med*, **8**(6), 1135–43.

170. Briejer MR, Akkermans LM, Schuurkes JA (1995) Gastrointestinal prokinetic benzamides: the pharmacology underlying stimulation of motility. *Pharmacol Rev*, **47**(4), 631–51.

171. Kumar G, Hayes KA, Clark R (2008) Efficacy of a scheduled IV cocktail of antiemetics for the palliation of nausea and vomiting in a hospice population. *Am J Hosp Palliat Care*, **25**(3), 184–9.

172. Laffey JG, Boylan JF (2002) Cyclizine and droperidol have comparable efficacy and side effects during patient-controlled analgesia. *Ir J Med Sci*, **171**(3), 141–4.

173. Johns RA, Hanousek J, Montgomery JE (2006) A comparison of cyclizine and granisetron alone and in combination for the prevention of postoperative nausea and vomiting. *Anaesthesia*, **61**(11), 1053–7.

174. Morita M YT, Shishido H, Inoue S (2004) Chlorpheniramine maleate as an alternative to antiemetic cyclizine [Letter to Editor]. *J Pain Sympt Manag*, **27**(5), 388–90.

175. Forrester CM, Benfield DA, Jr, Matern CE, Kelly JA, Pellegrini JE (2007) Meclizine in combination with ondansetron for prevention of postoperative nausea and vomiting in a high-risk population. *Am Assoc Nurse Anesth J*, **75**(1), 27–33.

176. Sharma A, Hamelin BA (2003) Classic histamine H1 receptor antagonists: a critical review of their metabolic and pharmacokinetic fate from a bird's eye view. *Curr Drug Metab*, **4**(2), 105–29.

177. Akutsu T, Kobayashi K, Sakurada K, Ikegaya H, Furihata T, Chiba K (2007) Identification of human cytochrome p450 isozymes involved in diphenhydramine N-demethylation. *Drug Metab Dispos*, **35**(1), 72–8.

178. He N, Zhang WQ, Shockley D, Edeki T (2002) Inhibitory effects of H1-antihistamines on CYP2D6- and CYP2C9-mediated drug metabolic reactions in human liver microsomes. *Eur J Clin Pharmacol*, **57**(12), 847–51.

179. Hamelin BA, Bouayad A, Methot J, *et al.* (2000) Significant interaction between the nonprescription antihistamine diphenhydramine and the CYP2D6 substrate metoprolol in healthy men with high or low CYP2D6 activity. *Clin Pharmacol Ther*, **67**(5), 466–77.

180. Lessard E, Yessine MA, Hamelin BA, *et al.* (2001) Diphenhydramine alters the disposition of venlafaxine through inhibition of CYP2D6 activity in humans. *J Clin Psychopharmacol*, **21**(2), 175–84.

181. Hamelin BA, Bouayad A, Drolet B, Gravel A, Turgeon J (1998) In vitro characterization of cytochrome P450 2D6 inhibition by classic histamine H1 receptor antagonists. *Drug Metab Dispos*, **26**(6), 536–9.

182. Hiroi T, Ohishi N, Imaoka S, Yabusaki Y, Fukui H, Funae Y (1995) Mepyramine, a histamine H1 receptor antagonist, inhibits the metabolic activity of rat and human P450 2D forms. *J Pharmacol Exp Ther*, **272**(2), 939–44.

183. Mercadante S, Ripamonti C, Casuccio A, Zecca E, Groff L (2000) Comparison of octreotide and hyoscine butylbromide in controlling gastrointestinal symptoms due to malignant inoperable bowel obstruction. *Support Care Cancer*, **8**(3), 188–91.

184. De Conno F, Caraceni A, Zecca E, Spoldi E, Ventafridda V (1991) Continuous subcutaneous infusion of hyoscine butylbromide reduces secretions in patients with gastrointestinal obstruction. *J Pain Sympt Manag*, **6**(8), 484–6.

185. Davis MP, Furste A (1999) Glycopyrrolate: a useful drug in the palliation of mechanical bowel obstruction. *J Pain Sympt Manag*, **18**(3), 153–4.

186. Mercadante S, Casuccio A, Mangione S (2007) Medical treatment for inoperable malignant bowel obstruction: a qualitative systematic review. *J Pain Sympt Manag*, **33**(2), 217–23.

187. Mangili G, Franchi M, Mariani A, *et al.* (1996) Octreotide in the management of bowel obstruction in terminal ovarian cancer. *Gynecol Oncol*, **61**(3), 345–8.

188. Shima Y, Ohtsu A, Shirao K, Sasaki Y (2008) Clinical efficacy and safety of octreotide (SMS201-995) in terminally ill Japanese cancer patients with malignant bowel obstruction. *Jpn J Clin Oncol*, **38**(5), 354–9.

189. Massacesi C, Galeazzi G (2006) Sustained release octreotide may have a role in the treatment of malignant bowel obstruction. *Palliat Med*, **20**(7), 715–6.

190. Ripamonti C, Mercadante S, Groff L, Zecca E, De Conno F, Casuccio A (2000) Role of octreotide, scopolamine butylbromide, and hydration in symptom control of patients with inoperable bowel obstruction and nasogastric tubes: a prospective randomized trial. *J Pain Sympt Manag*, **19**(1), 23–34.

191. Gemlo B, Rayner AA, Lewis B, *et al.* (1986) Home support of patients with end-stage malignant bowel obstruction using hydration and venting gastrostomy. *Am J Surg*, **152**(1), 100–4.

192. Wee B, Hillier R (2008) Interventions for noisy breathing in patients near to death. *Cochrane Database Syst Rev*, (1)CD005177.

193. Tytgat GN (2007) Hyoscine butylbromide: a review of its use in the treatment of abdominal cramping and pain. *Drugs*, **67**(9), 1343–57.

194. Renner UD, Oertel R, Kirch W (2005) Pharmacokinetics and pharmacodynamics in clinical use of scopolamine. *Ther Drug Monit*, **27**(5), 655–65.

195. Ali-Melkkila T, Kanto J, Iisalo E (1993) Pharmacokinetics and related pharmacodynamics of anticholinergic drugs. *Acta Anaesthesiol Scand*, **37**(7), 633–42.

196. Kaila T, Ali-Melkkila T, Iisalo E, Kanto J (1990) Radioreceptor assay for pharmacokinetic studies of glycopyrrolate. *Pharmacol Toxicol*, **67**(4), 313–6.

197. Kanto J, Klotz U (1988) Pharmacokinetic implications for the clinical use of atropine, scopolamine and glycopyrrolate. *Acta Anaesthesiol Scand*, **32**(2), 69–78.

198. Nachum Z, Shupak A, Gordon CR (2006) Transdermal scopolamine for prevention of motion sickness: clinical pharmacokinetics and therapeutic applications. *Clin Pharmacokinet*, **45**(6), 543–66.

199. Wilden J, Rapeport D (2004) Presumed central anticholinergic syndrome from inadvertent intravenous hyoscine hydrobromide (scopolamine) injection. *Anaesth Intensive Care*, **32**(3), 419–22.

200. Diaz DM, Diaz SF, Marx GF (1980) Cardiovascular effects of glycopyrrolate and belladonna derivatives in obstetric patients. *Bull NY Acad Med*, **56**(2), 245–8.

201. Habib AS, Gan TJ (2004) Evidence-based management of postoperative nausea and vomiting: a review. *Can J Anaesth*, **51**(4), 326–41.

202. Bano F, Zafar S, Aftab S, Haider S (2008) Dexamethasone plus ondansetron for prevention of postoperative nausea and vomiting in patients undergoing laparoscopic cholecystectomy: a comparison with dexamethasone alone. *J Coll Physicians Surg Pak*, **18**(5), 265–9.

203. Warr DG (2008) Chemotherapy- and cancer-related nausea and vomiting. *Curr Oncol*, **15**(Suppl 1), S4–9.

204. Sarcev T, Secen N, Povazan D, *et al.* (2007) The influence of dexamethasone in the decrease of chemotherapy-induced nausea and vomiting. *J Balkan Union Ocol*, **12**(2), 245–52.

205. Sorbe BG (1994) Tropisetron (Navoban) alone and in combination with dexamethasone in the prevention of chemotherapy-induced emesis: the Nordic experience. *Semin Oncol*, **21**(5 Suppl 9), 20–6.

206. Smith DB, Newlands ES, Rustin GJ, *et al.* (1991) Comparison of ondansetron and ondansetron plus dexamethasone as antiemetic prophylaxis during cisplatin-containing chemotherapy. *Lancet*, **338**(8765), 487–90.

207. Olver I, Paska W, Depierre A, *et al.* (1996) A multicentre, double-blind study comparing placebo, ondansetron and ondansetron plus dexamethasone for the control of cisplatin-induced delayed emesis. Ondansetron Delayed Emesis Study Group. *Ann Oncol*, **7**(9), 945–52.

208. Ahn MJ, Lee JS, Lee KH, Suh C, Choi SS, Kim SH (1994) A randomized double-blind trial of ondansetron alone versus in combination with dexamethasone versus in combination with dexamethasone and lorazepam in the prevention of emesis due to cisplatin-based chemotherapy. *Am J Clin Oncol*, **17**(2), 150–6.

209. Malik I, Moid I, Khan Z, Hussain M (1999) Prospective randomized comparison of tropisetron with and without dexamethasone against high-dose metoclopramide in prophylaxis of acute and delayed cisplatin-induced nausea and vomiting. *Am J Clin Oncol*, **22**(2), 126–30.

210. Joss RA, Bacchi M, Buser K, *et al.* (1994) Ondansetron plus dexamethasone is superior to ondansetron alone in the prevention of emesis in chemotherapy-naive and previously treated patients. Swiss Group for Clinical Cancer Research (SAKK). *Ann Oncol*, **5**(3), 253–8.

211. Peterson C, Hursti TJ, Borjeson S, *et al.* (1996) Single high-dose dexamethasone improves the effect of ondansetron on acute chemotherapy-induced nausea and vomiting but impairs the control of delayed symptoms. *Support Care Cancer*, **4**(6), 440–6.

212. Bruntsch U, Drechsler S, Eggert J, *et al.* (1994) Prevention of chemotherapy-induced nausea and vomiting by tropisetron (Navoban) alone or in combination with other antiemetic agents. *Semin Oncol*, **21**(5 Suppl 9), 7–11.

213. Bregni M, Siena S, Di Nicola M, Bonadonna G, Gianni AM (1991) Tropisetron plus haloperidol to ameliorate nausea and vomiting associated with high-dose alkylating agent cancer chemotherapy. *Eur J Cancer*, **27**(5), 561–5.

214. Grunberg SM (2007) Antiemetic activity of corticosteroids in patients receiving cancer chemotherapy: dosing, efficacy, and tolerability analysis. *Ann Oncol*, **18**(2), 233–40.

215. Hamadani M, Chaudhary L, Awan FT, *et al.* (2007) Management of platinum-based chemotherapy-induced acute nausea and vomiting: is there a superior serotonin receptor antagonist? *J Oncol Pharm Pract*, **13**(2), 69–75.

216. Gregory RE, Ettinger DS (1998) 5-HT3 receptor antagonists for the prevention of chemotherapy-induced nausea and vomiting. A comparison of their pharmacology and clinical efficacy. *Drugs*, **55**(2), 173–89.

217. Weren M, Demeere JL (2008) Methylprednisolone vs dexamethasone in the prevention of postoperative nausea and vomiting: a prospective, randomised, double-blind, placebo-controlled trial. *Acta Anaesthesiol Belg*, **59**(1), 1–5.

218. Blower PR (2002) 5-HT3-receptor antagonists and the cytochrome P450 system: clinical implications. *Cancer J*, **8**(5), 405–14.

219. Warren A, King L (2008) A review of the efficacy of dexamethasone in the prevention of postoperative nausea and vomiting. *J Clin Nurs*, **17**(1), 58a–68.

220. Fujii Y, Nakayama M (2008) Dexamethasone for reduction of nausea, vomiting and analgesic use after gynecological laparoscopic surgery. *Int J Gynaecol Obstet*, **100**(1), 27–30.

221. Koc S, Memis D, Sut N (2007) The preoperative use of gabapentin, dexamethasone, and their combination in varicocele surgery: a randomized controlled trial. *Anesth Analg*, **105**(4), 1137–42.

222. McNulty R (2007) Are all 5-HT3 receptor antagonists the same? *J Natl Compr Canc Netw*, **5**(1), 35–43.

223. Cox EH, Veyrat-Follet C, Beal SL, Fuseau E, Kenkare S, Sheiner LB (1999) A population pharmacokinetic–pharmacodynamic analysis of repeated measures time-to-event pharmacodynamic responses: the antiemetic effect of ondansetron. *J Pharmacokinet Biopharm*, **27**(6), 625–44.

224. de Wit R AM, Blower PR (2005) Is there a pharmacological basis for differences in 5-HT3 receptor antagonist efficacy in refractory patients? *Cancer Chemother Pharmacol*, **56**, 231–8.

225. Charbit B, Alvarez JC, Dasque E, Abe E, Demolis JL, Funck-Brentano C (2008) Droperidol and ondansetron-induced QT interval prolongation: a clinical drug interaction study. *Anesthesiology*, **109**(2), 206–12.

226. Bausewein C, Kuhnbach R, Haberland B (2006) Adrenal insufficiency caused by bilateral adrenal metastases—a rare treatable cause for recurrent nausea and vomiting in metastatic breast cancer. *Onkologie*, **29**(5), 203–5.

227. Cole DR, Duffy DF (1974) Haloperidol for radiation sickness: control of associated nausea, vomiting, and anorexia. *NY State J Med*, **74**(9), 1558a–62.

228. Chen CC, Lin CS, Ko YP, Hung YC, Lao HC, Hsu YW (2008) Premedication with mirtazapine reduces preoperative anxiety and postoperative nausea and vomiting. *Anesth Analg*, **106**(1), 109–13, table of contents.

229. Feuer DJ, Broadley KE (2000) Corticosteroids for the resolution of malignant bowel obstruction in advanced gynaecological and gastrointestinal cancer. *Cochrane Database Syst Rev*, (2)CD001219.

230. Feuer DJ, Broadley KE (1999) Systematic review and meta-analysis of corticosteroids for the resolution of malignant bowel obstruction in advanced gynaecological and gastrointestinal cancers. Systematic Review Steering Committee. *Ann Oncol*, **10**(9), 1035–41.

231. Shih A, Jackson KC 2nd (2007) Role of corticosteroids in palliative care. *J Pain Palliat Care Pharmacother*, **21**(4), 69–76.

232. Nakade S, Ohno T, Kitagawa J, *et al.* (2008) Population pharmacokinetics of aprepitant and dexamethasone in the prevention of chemotherapy-induced nausea and vomiting. *Cancer Chemother Pharmacol*, **63**(1), 75–83.

233. El-Sankary W, Bombail V, Gibson GG, Plant N (2002) Glucocorticoid-mediated induction of CYP3A4 is decreased by disruption of a protein: DNA interaction distinct from the pregnane X receptor response element. *Drug Metab Dispos*, **30**(9), 1029–34.

234. Pascussi JM, Drocourt L, Gerbal-Chaloin S, Fabre JM, Maurel P, Vilarem MJ (2001) Dual effect of dexamethasone on CYP3A4 gene expression in human hepatocytes. Sequential role of glucocorticoid receptor and pregnane X receptor. *Eur J Biochem*, **268**(24), 6346–58a.

235. McCune JS, Hawke RL, LeCluyse EL, *et al.* (2000) In vivo and in vitro induction of human cytochrome P4503A4 by dexamethasone. *Clin Pharmacol Ther*, **68**(4), 356–66.

236. Maida V, Ennis M, Irani S, Corbo M, Dolzhykov M (2008) Adjunctive nabilone in cancer pain and symptom management: a prospective observational study using propensity scoring. *J Support Oncol*, **6**(3), 119–24.

237. Davis MP (2008) Oral nabilone capsules in the treatment of chemotherapy-induced nausea and vomiting and pain. *Expert Opin Invest Drugs*, **17**(1), 85–95.

238. Osei-Hyiaman D (2007) Endocannabinoid system in cancer cachexia. *Curr Opin Clin Nutr Metab Care*, **10**(4), 443–8.

239. Meiri E, Jhangiani H, Vredenburgh JJ, *et al.* (2007) Efficacy of dronabinol alone and in combination with ondansetron versus ondansetron alone for delayed chemotherapy-induced nausea and vomiting. *Curr Med Res Opin*, **23**(3), 533–43.

240. Oz M, Zhang L, Morales M (2002) Endogenous cannabinoid, anandamide, acts as a noncompetitive inhibitor on 5-HT3 receptor-mediated responses in *Xenopus* oocytes. *Synapse*, **46**(3), 150–6.

241. Fan P (1995) Cannabinoid agonists inhibit the activation of 5-HT3 receptors in rat nodose ganglion neurons. *J Neurophysiol*, **73**(2), 907–10.

242. Slatkin NE (2007) Cannabinoids in the treatment of chemotherapy-induced nausea and vomiting: beyond prevention of acute emesis. *J Support Oncol*, **5**(5 Suppl 3), 1–9.

243. Hesketh PJ (2008) Chemotherapy-induced nausea and vomiting. *N Engl J Med*, **358a**(23), 2482–94.

244. Sutton IR, Daeninck P (2006) Cannabinoids in the management of intractable chemotherapy-induced nausea and vomiting and cancer-related pain. *J Support Oncol*, **4**(10), 531–5.

245. Green ST, Nathwani D, Goldberg DJ, Kennedy DH (1989) Nabilone as effective therapy for intractable nausea and vomiting in AIDS. *Br J Clin Pharmacol*, **28**(4), 494–5.

246. Flynn J, Hanif N (1992) Nabilone for the management of intractable nausea and vomiting in terminally staged AIDS. *J Palliat Care*, **8**(2), 46–7.

247. Ashton JC, Milligan ED (2008) Cannabinoids for the treatment of neuropathic pain: clinical evidence. *Curr Opin Invest Drugs*, **9**(1), 65–75.

248. Martin Fontelles MI, Goicoechea Garcia C (2008) Role of cannabinoids in the management of neuropathic pain. *CNS Drugs*, **22**(8), 645–53.

249. Wilkins MR (2006) Cannabis and cannabis-based medicines: potential benefits and risks to health. *Clin Med*, **6**(1), 16–18.

250. Strasser F, Luftner D, Possinger K, *et al.* (2006) Comparison of orally administered cannabis extract and delta-9-tetrahydrocannabinol in treating patients with cancer-related anorexia–cachexia syndrome: a multicenter, phase III, randomized, double-blind, placebo-controlled clinical trial from the Cannabis-In-Cachexia-Study-Group. *J Clin Oncol*, **24**(21), 3394–400.

251. Strohscheer I, Borasio GD (2006) Carbamazepine-responsive paroxysmal nausea and vomiting in a patient with meningeal carcinomatosis. *Palliat Med*, **20**(5), 549–50.

252. Clouse RE, Sayuk GS, Lustman PJ, Prakash C (2007) Zonisamide or levetiracetam for adults with cyclic vomiting syndrome: a case series. *Clin Gastroenterol Hepatol*, **5**(1), 44–8.

253. Hurley RW, Cohen SP, Williams KA, Rowlingson AJ, Wu CL (2006) The analgesic effects of perioperative gabapentin on postoperative pain: a meta-analysis. *Reg Anesth Pain Med*, **31**(3), 237–47.

254. Pandey CK, Priye S, Ambesh SP, Singh S, Singh U, Singh PK (2006) Prophylactic gabapentin for prevention of postoperative nausea and vomiting in patients undergoing laparoscopic cholecystectomy: a randomized, double-blind, placebo-controlled study. *J Postgrad Med*, **52**(2), 97–100.

255. Tiippana EM, Hamunen K, Kontinen VK, Kalso E (2007) Do surgical patients benefit from perioperative gabapentin/pregabalin? A systematic review of efficacy and safety. *Anesth Analg*, **104**(6), 1545–56, table of contents.

256. Mathiesen O, Moiniche S, Dahl JB (2007) Gabapentin and postoperative pain: a qualitative and quantitative systematic review, with focus on procedure. *BMC Anesthesiol*, **7**, 6.

257. Dierking G, Duedahl TH, Rasmussen ML, *et al.* (2004) Effects of gabapentin on postoperative morphine consumption and pain after abdominal hysterectomy: a randomized, double-blind trial. *Acta Anaesthesiol Scand*, **48**(3), 322–7.

258. Guttuso T, Jr, Roscoe J, Griggs J (2003) Effect of gabapentin on nausea induced by chemotherapy in patients with breast cancer. *Lancet*, **361**(9370), 1703–5.

259. Guttuso T, Jr, Vitticore P, Holloway RG (2005) Responsiveness of life-threatening refractory emesis to gabapentin-scopolamine therapy following posterior fossa surgery. Case report. *J Neurosurg*, **102**(3), 547–9.

260. Pandya KJ, Thummala AR, Griggs JJ, *et al.* (2004) Pilot study using gabapentin for tamoxifen-induced hot flashes in women with breast cancer. *Breast Cancer Res Treat*, **83**(1), 87–9.

261. Vila T, Gommer J, Scates AC (2008) Role of gabapentin in the treatment of uremic pruritus. *Ann Pharmacother*, **42**(7), 1080–4.

262. Prakash C, Lustman PJ, Freedland KE, Clouse RE (1998) Tricyclic antidepressants for functional nausea and vomiting: clinical outcome in 37 patients. *Dig Dis Sci*, **43**(9), 1951–6.

263. Sawhney MS, Prakash C, Lustman PJ, Clouse RE (2007) Tricyclic antidepressants for chronic vomiting in diabetic patients. *Dig Dis Sci*, **52**(2), 418–24.

264. Kim SW, Shin IS, Kim JM, *et al.* (2006) Mirtazapine for severe gastroparesis unresponsive to conventional prokinetic treatment. *Psychosomatics*, **47**(5), 440–2.

265. Pae C-U (2006) Low-dose mritazapine may be successful treatment option for severe nausea and vomiting. *Prog Neuro-Psychopharm Biol Psychiat*, **30**, 1143–5.

266. Gershon MD, Tack J (2007) The serotonin signaling system: from basic understanding to drug development for functional GI disorders. *Gastroenterology*, **132**(1), 397–414.

267. Kast RE, Foley KF (2007) Cancer chemotherapy and cachexia: mirtazapine and olanzapine are 5-HT3 antagonists with good antinausea effects. *Eur J Cancer Care (Engl)*, **16**(4), 351–4.

268. Watson M, Meyer L, Thomson A, Osofsky S (1998) Psychological factors predicting nausea and vomiting in breast cancer patients on chemotherapy. *Eur J Cancer*, **34**(6), 831–7.

269. Rodola F (2006) Midazolam as an anti-emetic. *Eur Rev Med Pharmacol Sci*, **10**(3), 121–6.

270. Di Florio T, Goucke CR (1999) The effect of midazolam on persistent postoperative nausea and vomiting. *Anaesth Intensive Care*, **27**(1), 38–40.

271. Jung JS, Park JS, Kim SO, *et al.* (2007) Prophylactic antiemetic effect of midazolam after middle ear surgery. *Otolaryngol Head Neck Surg*, **137**(5), 753–6.

272. Lee Y, Wang JJ, Yang YL, Chen A, Lai HY (2007) Midazolam vs ondansetron for preventing postoperative nausea and vomiting: a randomised controlled trial. *Anaesthesia*, **62**(1), 18–22.

273. Bleicher J, Bhaskara A, Huyck T, *et al.* (2008) Lorazepam, diphenhydramine, and haloperidol transdermal gel for rescue from chemotherapy-induced nausea/vomiting: results of two pilot trials. *J Support Oncol*, **6**(1), 27–32.

274. Crowe S (2002) Midazolam—an anti-emetic? *Anaesthesia*, **57**(8), 830.

275. Lundstrom S, Zachrisson U, Furst CJ (2005) When nothing helps: propofol as sedative and antiemetic in palliative cancer care. *J Pain Sympt Manag*, **30**(6), 570–7.

276. Gauger PG, Shanks A, Morris M, Greenfield ML, Burney RE, O'Reilly M (2008) Propofol decreases early postoperative nausea and vomiting in patients undergoing thyroid and parathyroid operations. *World J Surg*, **32**(7), 1525–34.

277. Tarhan O, Canbay O, Celebi N, *et al.* (2007) Subhypnotic doses of midazolam prevent nausea and vomiting during spinal anesthesia for cesarean section. *Minerva Anestesiol*, **73**(12), 629–33.

278. Fujii Y, Nakayama M (2007) Prevention of postoperative nausea and vomiting with a small dose of propofol alone and combined with dexamethasone in patients undergoing laparoscopic cholecystectomy: a prospective, randomized, double-blind study. *Surg Endosc*, **22**(5), 1268–71.

279. Fujii Y, Nakayama M, Nakano M (2008) Propofol alone and combined with dexamethasone for the prevention of postoperative nausea and vomiting in adult Japanese patients having third molars extracted. *Br J Oral Maxillofac Surg*, **46**(3), 207–10.

280. Akin A, Esmaoglu A, Gunes I, Boyaci A (2006) The effects of the prophylactic tropisetron-propofol combination on postoperative nausea and vomiting in patients undergoing thyroidectomy under desflurane anesthesia. *Mt Sinai J Med*, **73**(2), 560–3.

281. Barann M, Linden I, Witten S, Urban BW (2008) Molecular actions of propofol on human 5-HT3A receptors: enhancement as well as inhibition by closely related phenol derivatives. *Anesth Analg*, **106**(3), 846–57, table of contents.

282. Gardani G, Cerrone R, Biella C, *et al.* (2006) Effect of acupressure on nausea and vomiting induced by chemotherapy in cancer patients. *Minerva Med*, **97**(5), 391–4.

283. Choo SP, Kong KH, Lim WT, Gao F, Chua K, Leong SS. Electroacupuncture for refractory acute emesis caused by chemotherapy (2006) *J Altern Complement Med*, **12**(10), 963–9.

284. Molassiotis A, Helin AM, Dabbour R, Hummerston S (2007) The effects of P6 acupressure in the prophylaxis of chemotherapy-related nausea and vomiting in breast cancer patients. *Complement Ther Med*, **15**(1), 3–12.

285. Streitberger K, Ezzo J, Schneider A (2006) Acupuncture for nausea and vomiting: an update of clinical and experimental studies. *Auton Neurosci*, **129**(1–2), 107–17.

286. Gourcerol G, Leblanc I, Leroi AM, Denis P, Ducrotte P (2007) Gastric electrical stimulation in medically refractory nausea and vomiting. *Eur J Gastroenterol Hepatol*, **19**(1), 29–35.

287. Andersson S, Lonroth H, Simren M, Ringstrom G, Elfvin A, Abrahamsson H (2006) Gastric electrical stimulation for intractable vomiting in patients with chronic intestinal pseudo-obstruction. *Neurogastroenterol Motil*, **18**(9), 823–30.

288. Currow DC, Coughlan M, Fardell B, Cooney NJ (1997) Use of ondansetron in palliative medicine. *J Pain Sympt Manag*, **13**(5), 302–7.

Chapter 15

Early satiety

Mellar P. Davis

Introduction

Early satiety is a sense of premature satiation during a meal, which limits food intake to small amounts.[1] More fundamentally, it is a feeling that the stomach is overfilled soon after starting to eat, out of proportion to the size of the meal, so that the meal cannot be finished.[2] Linguistically, the term should be early satiation rather than early satiety, however, the term early satiety has been associated with the symptom, hence the title of this chapter (Figure 15.1).[3]

Early satiety is common in the normal population. Functional dyspepsia occurs in 15–20% of the general population; 34% have some degree of early satiety.[4,5] A multitude of potential causes for early satiety have been cited; delayed gastric emptying, *Helicobacter pylori* infections, gastrointestinal hypersensitivity, impaired fundic accommodation, altered duodenal sensitivity, abnormal duodenal–jejunal motility and altered central nervous system signals.[4,6]

Most patients with cancer-related anrexia will not volunteer early satiety as a symptom.[7] Early satiety is one of the top 10 symptoms experienced by individuals with cancer and portends a poor survival,[1] yet is not included in most general symptom assessment tools.[8] Paradoxically, individuals with early satiety complain of loss of appetite, yet may be hungry when fasting. Early satiety is frequently considered with nausea and vomiting, but is associated more commonly with a symptom cluster that includes anorexia and fatigue and, therefore, appears to have a different mechanism than nausea and vomiting.[9,10] Early satiety is experienced more often by females irrespective of primary site, in those with advanced stages of cancer,[11–13] and along with dry mouth and anorexia is largely neglected and poorly managed by physicians.[14,15]

The physiology of satiety

Central signals

Central signals govern appetite, meal size and number and are probably the reason why early satiety clusters with anorexia in cancer.

Injections of neuropeptideY (NPY) into the caudal hypothalamus reduce gastric motility and increase sympathetic outflow, while injections into the paraventricular nucleus of the hypothalamus stimulate gastric motility and enhance vagal output by stimulating neurotransmission through the dorsal vagal motor nucleus near the nucleus tractus solitarius in the medulla. Coritcotropin-releasing factor (CRF) appears to block motility stimulated by NPY.[16] Pro-opiomelanocortin (POMC) neurons follow in parallel with NPY neurons from the arcuate nucleus,and when activated release CRF and thyrotropin-releasing hormone (TRH) which alters gastric motility and delays gastric output.[17] These neurons also project to the brainstem vagal dorsal motor nucleus, to influence gastric motility.[18]

IL_1 produces rapid relaxation of the gastric fundus in experimental animals and reduces gastric emptying by specific IL_1 receptors or through CRF_2 receptor activation.[19] IL-1 increases CRF

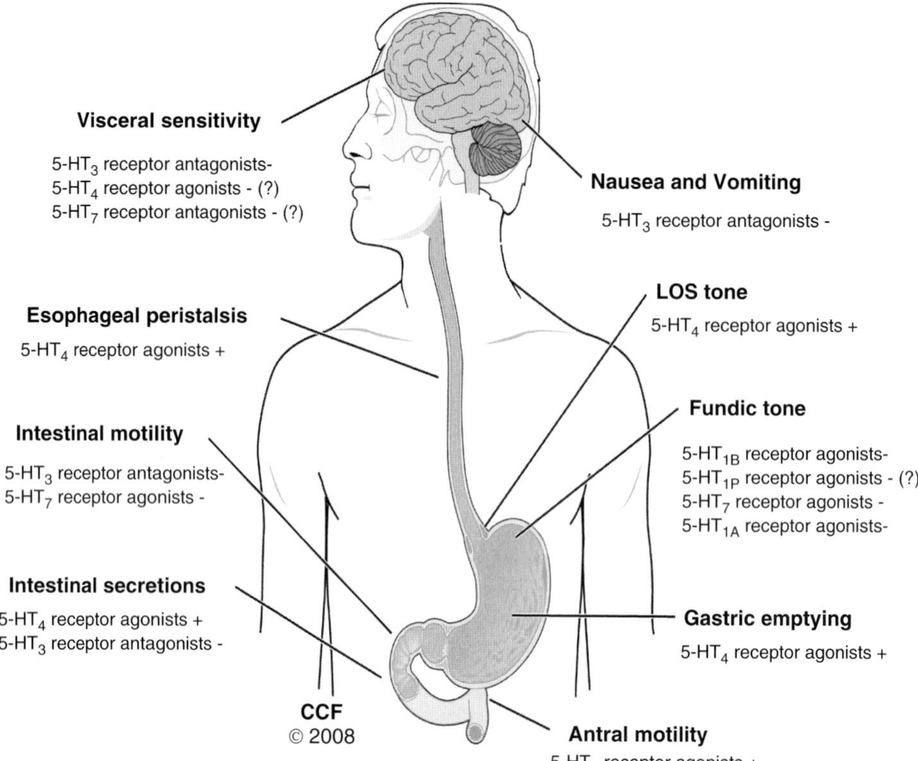

Fig. 15.1 Serotonin receptors and gastrointestinal function.

release via prostaglandin pathways, reduces gastric emptying, and slows gastrointestinal motility by decreasing acetylcholine release from enteric neurons.[20]

There is also a reciprocal relationship between the lateral hypothalamic area (LHA) and ventromedial hypothalamus (VMH) that regulates food intake and a direct relationship between dopamine levels in the LHA and meal size. Dopamine released from the LHA stimulates the dorsal motor nucleus of the vagus within the medullary dorsal vagus complex, to facilitate gastric accommodation.[21]

Peripheral signals

Satiety signals from the stomach are derived from food and liquid volume rather than nutritional content, whereas satiety signals from the small bowel are generated by nutritional content rather than volume.[22] Total vagotomy attenuates, but does not eliminate satiation from gastric distension and in at least one study, autonomic dysfunction in cancer did not appear to be associated with early satiety.[23] Normally, there is a positive relationship between satiety and gastric distension and an inverse relationship between distension and appetite.[24] Accommodation of the proximal stomach plays a role in satiety. Relaxation of the proximal stomach is induced by vago-vagal pathways and by non-vagal mechanisms via generation of nitric oxide.[25,26] Impaired accommodation forces food into the distal stomach, causing distension and activation of mechanoreceptors which cause early satiety.[27] Distention of the antrum produces more severe symptoms in response to the same volume, in the fundus.[28] Intraduodenal nutrients reduce antral motility, increase antral area and promote fundic relaxation. Duodenal lipids increase pyloric pressure, but reduce antral pressures and increase fundic accommodation to a greater degree than carbohydrate or protein.[29]

A number of medications are known to influence the neurotransmitters and receptors associated with gastric accomodation and motility. Serotonin acts as a paracrine messenger, and responses (nausea, motility, accommodation, visceral sensitivity) are dependent on the type of serotonin receptor (5HTR) which is activated (Figure 15.2). $5HT_3$Rs on vagus afferents generate vomiting and nausea when activated, while $5HT_4$Rs on enteric neurons and smooth muscle enhance acetylcholine release, which promotes gastrointestinal reflexes via excitatory post-synaptic currents, leading to increased peristalsis and amplified acetylcholine signals. Both $5HT_1$Rs and $5HT_4$Rs in the gastric fundus increase gastric accommodation.[30] As a result cisapride, a $5HT_4$R agonist, tegaserod, as well as metoclopromide enhance motility and improve gastric accommodation. Sumatriptan improves gastric accommodation through activation of $5HT_1$ARs.[31] Buspirone, a non-selective $5HT_1$AR agonist[32] and venlafaxine, a selective norepinephrine, serotonin reuptake inhibitor and mirtazapine also improve gastric accommodation.[33–35] 5HT1R agonists increase gastric accommodation by activating nitric oxide synthase, which increases nitric oxide, a smooth muscle relaxant. Sildenafil, a phosphodiestease inhibitor, prevents cyclic GMP breakdown, and amplifies nitric oxide effects in the gut. As a result, sildenafil increases gastric accommodation but not gastric emptying for solids (Table 15.1).[36]

Macrolides are motilin analogues which improve gastric emptying, but reduce gastric accommodation.[37]

Opioids are assumed to worsen gastrointestinal symptoms and delay gastric emptying, however, in healthy volunteers, blocking opioid receptors (via naloxone) reduces meal-related accommodation and the amount of food that could be ingested before satiety. Since naloxone does not alter gastric emptying,[38] it seems opioids (or endogenous opioid signalling) govern fundic accommodation more than gastric emptying.

Adrenergic neurotransmission within the gastrointestinal tract influences motility. $Alpha_2$ adrenergic receptors in presynaptic nerve terminals inhibit acetylcholine release from enteric neurons and increase gastric accommodation.[39] Short-term clonidine reduces meal-induced satiety in functional dyspepsia.[40]

Grehlin, a growth hormone secretogogue receptor agonist, increases appetite centrally, reduces pro-inflammatory (IL_1) expression, increases gastric acid secretion, motility and gastric emptying as a paracrine effector.[41–43]

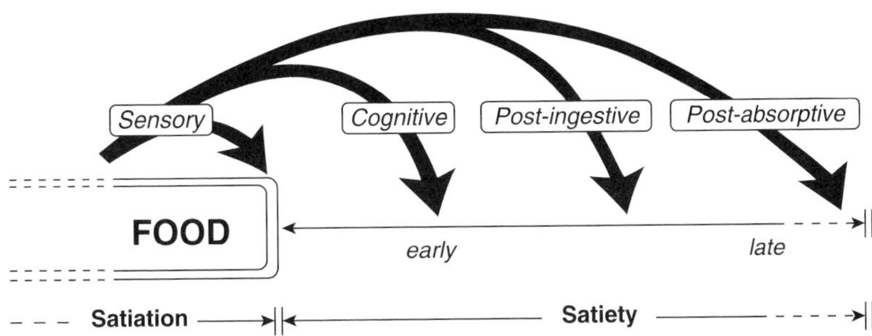

Fig. 15.2 Mediating processes.

Table 15.1 Medications and gastric motility and accomodation

Drug	Gastric emptying	Accommodation	Sensitivity
Cisapride	↑	a ↑	↑
Tegaserod		a ↑	–
SSRI	–	a ↑	+/–
Metoclopramide	↑	a →	N/A
Motilin analogue	↑	b ↓	N/A
Clonidine	→	a ↑	N/A
SRRI	→	a ↑	N/A
Sumatriptan	↓	a ↑	→
Buspirone	→	a ↑	N/A
$5HT_3$ antagonists	→	→	a ↓

SSRI, selective serotonin reuptake inhibitor. SRRI, serotonin receptor reuptake inhibitor.
[a]Reported to reduce early satiety in normals or in cancer-associated dyspepsia.
[b]Known to induce satiety in normals.

Pathophysiology of early satiety

Altered central signals

The proposed central mechanisms of early satiety include inhibition of NPY release, heightened melanocortin signals and a blunted ghrelin response. Elevated cytokines also induce the release of CCK and insulin, which act centrally as satiety signals.[44] IL_1 induces satiety and adversely influences meal size, meal duration and frequency in rats through activation of gluco-sensitive neurons in the VMH. In tumor-bearing rats, CSF IL_1 concentrations correlate inversely with food intake[45]. Brain serotonin and IL_1 are increased which may contribute to cancer-related early satiety.

Experimental tumors alter serotonin and cytokine levels within the hypothalamus, upregulate receptors to both and produce qualitative changes in NPY and quantitative changes in melanocortins. $5HT_1A$ agonists (mianserin), dopamine and IL_1 receptor blockers increase meal numbers when injected into the VMH of tumor-bearing rats.[46]

Peripheral signals: taking a cue from functional dyspepsia

In a hierarchal analysis of a 1000-patient dataset of symptoms, early satiety clustered with weight loss, anorexia and taste changes and to a lesser extent with easy fatigue, lack of energy, weakness and dry mouth.[9] Early satiety does not cluster with nausea, suggesting that the pathophysiology of early satiety in advanced cancer is distinct from nausea, vomiting, bloating and belching. Early satiety in cancer occurs in >40% and in a small study of 20 individuals with cancer, early satiety correlated with delayed gastric emptying.[47] Cytokines may play an important role by sensitizing vagal afferents in the gastrointestinal tract which mediate a sense of fullness and satiety.[48]

There is a vast amount of literature about early satiety in functional dyspepsia. Approximately 40% of those with functional dyspepsia have early satiety.[49] Objective evaluation of gastric mobility in functional dyspepsia reveals that gastric accommodation is abnormal in 40–50%, gastric emptying is impaired in 35-40% and 25% have abnormal gastric accommodation with normal (or even accelerated) gastric emptying.[50–52] Early satiety has been correlated with reduced gastric volumes, as measured by single-photon emission computed tomography (SPECT).[53,54]

On the other hand, early satiety did not correlate with delayed gastric emptying as measured by the ^{13}C octanoic acid breath test[55] or by the ^{99m}Tc sulphur colloid meal test.

In a group of individuals with severe functional dyspepsia and impaired gastric emptying, early satiety and weight loss correlated with impaired accommodation, in addition to delayed gastric emptying.[56] Objective improvement in gastric emptying by prokinetics poorly correlates with symptom response. Administration of motilin analogs like erythromycin improves gastric emptying, but increases meal-induced satiety and reduces caloric intake in normal individuals.[57]

Therefore, it appears that early satiety best correlates with impaired gastric fundus accommodation in individuals with functional dyspepsia. The exact mechanism behind the dysaccommodation (hormonal, neural or muscular) is not known.

Symptom assessment of early satiety

There are a few research instruments which assess early satiety in cancer patients including the Bristol Myers Anorexia/Cachexia Recovery Instrument,[58] and the Functional Assessment of Anorexia/Cachexia Therapy (FAACT) (Question 10).[59] The Gastroparesis Cardinal Symptom Index contains four items about early satiety, has a high test and retest reliability, internal consistency, and is responsive to changes over time.[60]

Objective assessment of fundic accommodation and gastric motility

A ^{13}C glycine or ^{13}C octanoic acid breath test has been used to determine motility effects and gastric emptying.[61] Nuclear scintigraphy after a ^{99m}Tc-radiolabelled egg meal is the standard for measuring gastric emptying. Scintigraphy images should be extended to 4 h to improve accuracy. [62] A 'poor man's gastric emptying study' involves swallowing radio-opaque markers, followed by repeat abdominal plain radiographs over 6 h.[63] Other ways of measuring gastric emptying include ultrasound, real-time paramagnetic resonance imaging, the H^+ breath test after lactulose, a radiolabelled CO_2 breath test and timed acetaminophen oral absorption.[64,65]

Measurements of gastric accommodation include intraluminal gastric barostats (which is the standard measure), ultrasound estimates of gastric volume pre- and during the meal, scintigraphy assessment of gastric volumes using ^{99m}Tc single photon emission computer tomography (SPECT), magnetic resonance scan volumes and the satiety drink test.[49] The satiety drink test is able to assess symptoms and objectify findings better than gastric emptying studies.[51] The satiety drink test involves two beakers with ingestion of a nutrient drink at a rate of 15 ml/min via a peristaltic pump which fills the beakers. Satiety is graded at 5 min intervals (0, none; 5, maximum satiety). Patients stop at maximum satiety (5 on the numerical scale) and the volume of ingested drink is measured. Individuals with early satiety generally stop at 500 ml, while normal individuals can ingest 1200–1500 ml before maximum satiety.[52] The satiety drink test has been validated against barostats and is more amenable to clinical use than gastric barostats.[66]

Clinical management of early satiety

There are a wide variety of potential causes for altered gastric motility and early satiety in cancer (Box 15.1).

Intra-abdominal cancer may cause autovagotomy from micrometastases or retroperitoneal nodes resulting in interruption of input to the enteric nervous system. An autoantibody

Box 15.1 Causes for altered gastric motility

- Tumor infiltration
- Paraneoplastic autoimmunity
- Chemotherapy-induced autonomic neuropathy
- Surgical interruption of vagus or enteric nervous system
- Radiation enteritis or neuropathy
- Co-morbidities
  - Pre-morbid functional dyspepsia
  - Hypothyroidism
  - Diabetes or collagen vascular diseases
- Medications
  - Anticholinergics
  - Opioids
- Infections
  - Helicobacter pylori
  - Cytomegalovirus
  - Herpes simplex

(anti-neuronal nuclear antibody type I or ANNA-1) is known to produce a visceral neuropathy.[67,68] Immune destruction of enteric pacemaker cells (interstitial cells of Cajal) will produce intestinal pseudo-obstruction and adversely influence gastric motility.

Whipple pancreatectomies and pylorus sparing pancreaticoduodenectomies cause gastroparesis and loss of motilin from the duodenum, resulting in impaired mobility. Recovery from surgically-induced gastroparesis is slow and may take six months.[69,70] Gastrectomy (partial) will produce gastroparesis in the remaining stomach in 5–15% depending on the procedure, if vagotomy was performed, the extent of nodal dissection and stage of cancer.

Gastroparesis is reported in 18% of those undergoing bone marrow transplantation which may be due to infections with cytomegalovirus (CMV), herpes simplex or as a result of graph versus host disease.[71,72] Gastroparesis may be the delayed sequelae from abdominal radiation.[73]

The approach to early satiety in cancer should include an assessment for mechanical outlet obstruction or an infiltrative process involving the gastric wall.[74] Also, small bowel obstruction not seen on upper gastrointestinal endoscopy may produce symptoms of early satiety. A negative upper endoscopy and CT scan of the abdomen will eliminate most mechanical causes for early satiety.[75] Treatment of *H. pylori* may be helpful, although infection correlates poorly with early satiety. Trials of prokinetics should follow if early satiety is present and obstruction is not an issue, even though objective improvement in gastric emptying by prokinetics correlates poorly with symptom response.[76,77] Individuals with gastrointestinal CMV, herpes simplex or *H. pylori* infections and early satiety should have their infections treated and re-evaluated for response (objective and subjective) before undergoing gastric motility studies.

Medication management of early satiety

Most studies have targeted anorexia and relief of anorexia as the main outcome and not assessed early satiety. A recent single arm study at the Cleveland Clinic using thalidomide for cancer anorexia found reduction in early satiety in the majority of those completing two weeks of treatment (D. Walsh, personal communication).

Within the published literature, there is very little evidence as to the management of early satiety in cancer. Radioisotope emptying studies were done in a 10-patient cohort with upper gastrointestinal cancers and gastroparesis. Metoclopramide improved symptoms, gastric emptying and individuals gained weight.[78] Nelson and colleagues reported the use of metoclopramide in 20 advanced cancer patients. Although appetite bloating, belching and nausea improved, only four of 18 individuals with early satiety improved.[47] The relationship between objective improvement of gastric emptying and subjective response of early satiety is not known

Metoclopramide and erythromycin are the only available prokinetics in the United States, as cisapride and tegeserod have been removed from the market. There is a difference among the prokinetics in effects on gastric accommodation. Tegeserod and cisapride improve gastric emptying and gastric accommodation, whereas erythromycin improves gastric emptying and impairs accommodation.[79,80] Some countries have domperidone, which increases gastric emptying and decreases bloating. A systematic review of prokinetics in the management of gastroparesis (36 studies, 514 patients mostly, if not exclusively, non-cancer patients) found that erythromycin and domperidone were superior to metoclopramide and cisapride in improving symptoms, though the influence on early satiety is not known.[81]

A multitude of studies have found that subjective responses to prokinetics do not correlate with objective response. Subcutaneous metoclopramide (10 mg every 6 h) improves nausea, vomiting, bloating and heartburn in individuals with gastroparesis, with no associated improvement in gastric emptying.[82] Erythromycin improves symptoms related to dyspepsia, but symptom response did not correlate with gastric emptying times.[83]

Initial treatment of early satiety in cancer involves metoclopramide with titration to response from 10 mg every 6 h or four times daily before meals and at bedtime, to a total of 100–120 mg daily. The evidence for this is based on a small study where responses occurred in a minority at low doses.[47] The addition of a proton pump inhibitor is unlikely to add to metoclopramide responses.[84]

There is evidence showing medications which improve gastric accommodation in functional dyspepsia also improve early satiety. These include octreotide[85] sumatriptan sidenafil,[86] ondansetron, anticholinergics,[87] venlafaxine or buspirone[32] and mirtazapine.[34] Many of these medications can be added to metoclopramide, although, anticholinergics will block metoclopramide prokinesis. A high placebo response to medications (up to 80%) is noted with gastrointestinal symptoms in functional dyspepsia.[88]

Diet and early satiety

A standard recommendation by expert opinion and not by clinical studies is to take five or six small meals throughout the day. No recommendations have been made for macronutrient content, which may be as important. Individuals with functional dyspepsia associate a certain eating habit and specific foods with symptoms. Many eat fewer than three meals per day. A prescription of low volume but high caloric dense foods to make up for caloric deficits may be difficult to tolerate in those with early satiety and associated anorexia.

Oronasal stimulation through eating stimulates dopamine release from the LHA, which increases fundus accommodation in preparation to receive the food volume.[89] There is greater feed intolerance to nasogastric tubing feeding in the critically ill,[90] and reduced accommodation in those who receive small bowel nutrition. If an individual has an elevated glucose, this should be treated since hyperglycemia adversely affects gastric motility and accommodation. Intraduodenal lipids delay gastric emptying, increase pyloric pressures, reduce antral pressures and increase both CCK and PYY, which increases gastric accommodation.. Therefore, dietary modification may be important in managing early satiety, if postgastric hormonal changes are considered important. This has not been explored clinically.

Paradoxically, high-fat diets may produce less satiety if satiety is delayed by better gastric accommodation and not induced by delays in gastric emptying. Flavors found in high-fat meals may better stimulate LHA and VMN dopamine and improve gastric accommodation. There is evidence that high-fat food produce weak effects on satiation and intra-meal satiety signals.[91] Joule for joule, fat is less satiating than carbohydrate and protein.[92] Satiety is governed by volume and weight rather than caloric density.[93] Studies examining volume, macronutrient content and meal frequency need to be done in cancer patients with distressing early satiety.

Summary

Early satiety is common, distressing, frequently accompanied by anorexia and is prognostically important. Assessment tools are available. Gastric outlet obstruction, small bowel obstruction, gastric wall infiltration and infection (*H. pylori*, CMV and herpes simplex) should be excluded clinically before an empiric trial of metoclopramide is started. Metoclopramide should be titrated to response. Individuals who fail to respond to metoclopramide could be investigated with gastric motility studies. Medications which improve gastric accommodation (triptans, sidenafil, venlafaxine, buspirone, ondansetron, octreotide) could be added to metoclopramide or used alone. Diet recommendations include small, frequent meals. Either a low or high fat content could be empirically tried, followed by reassessment for response.

Acknowledgement

The author would like to recognize the skills of Wendy L. Gatlin in preparing this manuscript.

References

1. Davis MP, Walsh D, Lagman R, Yavuzsen T (2006) Early satiety in cancer patients: a common and important but underrecognized symptom. *Support Care Cancer*, **14**(7), 693–8.
2. Talley NJ, Stanghellini V, Heading RC, Koch KL, Malagelada JR, Tytgat GN (1999) Functional gastroduodenal disorders. *Gut*, **45**(S2), 237–42.
3. Feinle-Bisset C, Andrews JM (2003) Treatment of functional dyspepsia. *Curr Treat Options Gastroenterol*, **6**(4), 289–97.
4. Tack J, Caenepeel P, Corsetti M, Janssens J (2004) Role of tension receptors in dyspeptic patients with hypersensitivity to gastric distention. *Gastroenterology*, **127**(4), 1058–66.
5. Geeraerts B, Vandenberghe J, Van Oudenhove L, *et al.* (2005) Influence of experimentally induced anxiety on gastric sensorimotor function in humans. *Gastroenterology*, **129**(5), 1437–44.
6. Walsh D, Donnelly S, Rybicki L (2000) The symptoms of advanced cancer: relationship to age, gender, and performance status in 1,000 patients. *Support Care Cancer*, **8**(3), 175–9.
7. Homsi J, Walsh D, Rivera N, *et al.* (2006) Symptom evaluation in palliative medicine: patient report vs. systematic assessment. *Support Care Cancer*, **14**(5), 444–53.
8. Donnelly S, Walsh D (1995) The symptoms of advanced cancer. *Semin Oncol*, **22** (S3), 67–72.
9. Walsh D, Rybicki L (2006) Symptom clustering in advanced cancer. *Support Care Cancer*, **14**(8), 831–6.

10. Armes PJ, Plant HJ, Allbright A, Silverstone T, Slevin ML (1992) A study to investigate the incidence of early satiety in patients with advanced cancer. *Br J Cancer*, **65**(3), 481–4.
11. Donnelly S, Walsh D, Rybicki L (1995) The symptoms of advanced cancer: identification of clinical and research priorities by assessment of prevalence and severity. *J Palliat Care*, **11**(1), 27–32.
12. Nielsen SS, Theologides A, Vickers ZM (1980) Influence of food odors on food aversions and preferences in patients with cancer. *Am J Clin Nutr*, **33**(11), 2253–61.
13. Theologides A (1976) Anorexia-producing intermediary metabolites. *Am J Clin Nutr*, **29**(5), 552–8.
14. Churm D, Andrew IM, Holden K, Hildreth AJ, Hawkins C (2008) A questionnaire study of the approach to the anorexia-cachexia syndrome in patients with cancer by staff in a district general hospital. *Support Care Cancer*, **17**(5), 503–7.
15. Andrew I, Kirkpatrick G, Holden K, Hawkins C (2008) Audit of symptoms and prescribing in patients with the anorexia-cachexia syndrome. *Pharm World Sci*, **2**, 489–96.
16 Monnikes H, Tebbe J, Bauer C, Grote C, Arnold R (2000) Neuropeptide Y in the paraventricular nucleus of the hypothalamus stimulates colonic transit by peripheral cholinergic and central CRF pathways. *Neurogastroenterol Motil*, **12**(4), 343–52.
17 Fujimiya M, Inui A (2000) Peptidergic regulation of gastrointestinal motility in rodents. *Peptides*, **21**(10), 1565–82.
18. Sim LJ, Joseph S (1991) Arcuate nucleus projections to brainstem regions which modulate nociception. *J Chem Neuroanat*, **4**(2), 97–109.
19. Montuschi P, Tringali G, Parente L, Preziosi P, Navarra P (1994) Interleukin-1 beta- and tumour-necrosis-factor-induced inhibition of rat gastric fundus motility in vitro. *Pharmacol Res*, **30**(1), 25–33.
20. Aube AC, Blottiere HM, Scarpignato C, Cherbut C, Roze C, Galmiche JP (1996) Inhibition of acetylcholine induced intestinal motility by interleukin 1 beta in the rat. *Gut*, **39**(3), 470–4.
21. Meguid MM, Fetissov SO, Varma M, *et al.* (2000) Hypothalamic dopamine and serotonin in the regulation of food intake. *Nutrition*, **16**(10), 843–57.
22. Powley TL, Phillips RJ (2004) Gastric satiation is volumetric, intestinal satiation is nutritive. *Physiol Behav*, **82**(1), 69–74.
23. Nelson K, Walsh D, Sheehan F (2002) Cancer and chemotherapy-related upper gastrointestinal symptoms: the role of abnormal gastric motor function and its evaluation in cancer patients. *Support Care Cancer*, **10**(6), 455–61.
24. de Graaf C, Blom WA, Smeets PA, Stafleu A, Hendriks HF (2004) Biomarkers of satiation and satiety. *Am J Clin Nutr*, **79**(6), 946–61.
25. Desai KM, Sessa WC, Vane JR (1991) Involvement of nitric oxide in the reflex relaxation of the stomach to accommodate food or fluid. *Nature*, **351**(6326), 477–9.
26. Tack J, Sarnelli G (2002) Serotonergic modulation of visceral sensation: upper gastrointestinal tract. *Gut*, **51**(S1), 77–80.
27. Caldarella MP, Azpiroz F, Malagelada JR (2004) Antro-fundic dysfunctions in functional dyspepsia. *Gastroenterology*, **124**(5), 1220–9.
28. Lee KJ, Vos R, Janssens J, Tack J (2004) Differences in the sensorimotor response to distension between the proximal and distal stomach in humans. *Gut*, **53**(7), 938–43.
29. Gershon MD, Tack J (2007) The serotonin signaling system: from basic understanding to drug development for functional GI disorders. *Gastroenterology*, **132**(1), 397–414.
30. Talley NJ, Camilleri M, Chitkara DK, *et al.* (2004) Effects of desipramine and escitalopram on postprandial symptoms induced by the nutrient drink test in healthy volunteers: a randomized, double-blind, placebo-controlled study. *Digestion*, **72**(3), 97–103.
31. Tack J, Broeckaert D, Coulie B, Janssens J (1998) The influence of cisapride on gastric tone and the perception of gastric distension. *Aliment Pharmacol Ther*, **12**(8), 761–6.

32. Tack JPH, Coulie B, Fischler B, De Gucht V, Janssens J (1999) A placebo-controlled trial of buspirone, a fundus relaxing drug in functional dyspepsia: effect on symptoms and gastric sensory motor function (abstract). *Gastroenterology*, **116**, A325.
33. Tack J, Broekaert D, Coulie B, Fischler B, Janssens J (2003) Influence of the selective serotonin re-uptake inhibitor, paroxetine, on gastric sensorimotor function in humans. *Aliment Pharmacol Ther*, **17**(4), 603–8.
34. Kim SW, Shin IS, Kim JM, *et al.* (2006) Mirtazapine for severe gastroparesis unresponsive to conventional prokinetic treatment. *Psychosomatics*, **47**(5), 440–2.
35. Moro E, Crema F, De Ponti F, Frigo G (2004) Triptans and gastric accommodation: pharmacological and therapeutic aspects. *Dig Liver Dis*, **36**(1), 85–92.
36. Sarnelli G, Sifrim D, Janssens J, Tack J (2004) Influence of sildenafil on gastric sensorimotor function in humans. *Am J Physiol Gastrointest Liver Physiol*, **287**(5), G988–92.
37. Tack J, Peeters T (2001) What comes after macrolides and other motilin stimulants? *Gut*, **49**(3), 317–8.
38. Geeraerts B, van Oudenhove L, Fischler B, *et al.* (2009) Influence of abuse history on gastric sensorimotor function in functional dyspepsia. *Neurogastroenterol Motil*, **21**(1), 33–41.
39. Thumshirn M, Camilleri M, Choi MG, Zinsmeister AR (1993) Modulation of gastric sensory and motor functions by nitrergic and alpha2-adrenergic agents in humans. *Gastroenterology*, **116**(3), 573–85.
40. Bisschops R, Tack J (2007) Dysaccommodation of the stomach: therapeutic nirvana? *Neurogastroenterol Motil*, **19**(2), 85–93.
41. Inui A, Asakawa A, Bowers CY, *et al.* (2004) Ghrelin, appetite, and gastric motility: the emerging role of the stomach as an endocrine organ. *FASEB J*, **18**(3), 439–56.
42. Liu YL, Malik NM, Sanger GJ, Andrews PL (2006) Ghrelin alleviates cancer chemotherapy-associated dyspepsia in rodents. *Cancer Chemother Pharmacol*, **58**(3), 326–33.
43. Dixit VD, Schaffer EM, Pyle RS, *et al.* (2004) Ghrelin inhibits leptin- and activation-induced proinflammatory cytokine expression by human monocytes and T cells. *J Clin Invest*, **114**(1), 57–66.
44. Perboni S, Inui A (2006) Anorexia in cancer: role of feeding-regulatory peptides. *Phil Trans R Soc Lond B Biol Sci*, **361**(1471), 1281–9.
45. Opara EI, Laviano A, Meguid MM, Yang ZJ (1995) Correlation between food intake and CSF IL-1 alpha in anorectic tumor bearing rats. *Neuroreport*, **6**(5), 750–2.
46. Laviano A, Gleason JR, Meguid MM, Yang ZJ, Cangiano C, Rossi Fanelli F (2000) Effects of intra-VMN mianserin and IL-1ra on meal number in anorectic tumor-bearing rats. *J Invest Med*, **48**(1), 40–8.
47. Nelson KA, Walsh TD (1993) Metoclopramide in anorexia caused by cancer-associated dyspepsia syndrome (CADS). *J Palliat Care*, **9**(2), 14–8.
48. Richards RD, Valenzuela GA, Davenport KG, Fisher KL, McCallum RW (1993) Objective and subjective results of a randomized, double-blind, placebo-controlled trial using cisapride to treat gastroparesis. *Dig Dis Sci*, **38**(5), 811–6.
49. Kim DY, Delgado-Aros S, Camilleri M, *et al.* (2001) Noninvasive measurement of gastric accommodation in patients with idiopathic nonulcer dyspepsia. *Am J Gastroenterol*, **96**(11), 3099–105.
50. Bisschops R, Karamanolis G, Arts J, *et al.* (2008) Relationship between symptoms and indigestion of a meal in dyspepsia. *Gut*, **57**(11), 1495–503.
51. Delgado-Aros S, Camilleri M, Cremonini F, Ferber I, Stephens D, Burton DD (2004) Contributions of gastric volumes and gastric emptying to meal size and postmeal symptoms in functional dyspepsia. *Gastroenterology*, **127**(6), 1685–94.
52. Tack J, Caenepeel P, Piessevaux H, Cuomo R, Janssens J (2003) Assessment of meal induced gastric accommodation by a satiety drinking test in health and in severe functional dyspepsia. *Gut*, **52**(9), 1271–7.
53. Piessevaux H, Tack J, Walrand S, Pauwels S, Geubel A (2003) Intragastric distribution of a standardized meal in health and functional dyspepsia: correlation with specific symptoms. *Neurogastroenterol Motil*, **15**(5), 447–55.

54. Kuiken SD, Samsom M, Camilleri M, *et al.* (1999) Development of a test to measure gastric accommodation in humans. *Am J Physiol*, **277**(6), G1217–21.
55. Talley NJ, Verlinden M, Jones M (2001) Can symptoms discriminate among those with delayed or normal gastric emptying in dysmotility-like dyspepsia? *Am J Gastroenterol*, **96**(5), 1422–8.
56. Karamanolis G Tack J (2006) Promotility medications-now and in the future. *Dig Dis*, **24**(4), 297–307.
57. Cuomo R, Vandaele P, Coulie B, *et al.* (2006) Influence of motilin on gastric fundus tone and on meal-induced satiety in man: role of cholinergic pathways. *Am J Gastroenterol*, **101**(4), 804–11.
58. Cella DF, VonRoenn J, Lloyd S, Browder HP (1995) The Bristol–Myers Anorexia/Cachexia Recovery Instrument (BACRI): a brief assessment of patients' subjective response to treatment for anorexia/cachexia. *Qual Life Res*, **4**(3), 221–31.
59. Ribaudo, JM, Cella D, Hahn EA, Lloyd SR, *et al.* (2001) Re-validation and Shortening of the Functional Assessment of Anorexia/Cachexia Therapy (FAACT) questionnaire. *Qual Life Res*, **9**, 1137–46.
60. Revicki DA, Rentz AM, Dubois D, *et al.* (2004) Gastroparesis Cardinal Symptom Index (GCSI): development and validation of a patient reported assessment of severity of gastroparesis symptoms. *Qual Life Res*, **13**(4), 833–44.
61. Arts J, Caenepeel P, Verbeke K, Tack J (2005) Influence of erythromycin on gastric emptying and meal related symptoms in functional dyspepsia with delayed gastric emptying. *Gut*, **54**(4), 455–60.
62. Guo JP, Maurer AH, Fisher RS, Parkman HP (2001) Extending gastric emptying scintigraphy from two to four hours detects more patients with gastroparesis. *Dig Dis Sci*, **46**(1), 24–9.
63. Feldman M, Smith HJ, Simon TR (2004) Gastric emptying of solid radiopaque markers: studies in healthy subjects and diabetic patients. *Gastroenterology*, **87**(4), 895–902.
64. Ghoos YF, Maes BD, Geypens BJ, *et al.* (1993) Measurement of gastric emptying rate of solids by means of a carbon-labeled octanoic acid breath test. *Gastroenterology*, **104**(6), 1640–7.
65. Hornbuckle K, Barnett JL (2000) The diagnosis and work-up of the patient with gastroparesis. *J Clin Gastroenterol*, **30**(2), 117–24.
66. Kindt S, Coulie B, Wajs E, Janssens J, Tack J (2008) Reproducibility and symptomatic predictors of a slow nutrient drinking test in health and in functional dyspepsia. *Neurogastroenterol Motil*, **20**(4), 320–9.
67. Donthireddy KR, Ailawadhi S, Nasser E, *et al.* (2007) Malignant gastroparesis: pathogenesis and management of an underrecognized disorder. *J Support Oncol*, **5**(8), 355–63.
68. Chinn JS, Schuffler MD (2005) Paraneoplastic visceral neuropathy as a cause of severe gastrointestinal motor dysfunction. *Gastroenterology*, **95**(5),1279–86.
69. Tanaka M (2005) Gastroparesis after a pylorus-preserving pancreatoduodenectomy. *Surg Today*, **35**(5), 345–50.
70. Dong K, Yu XJ, Li B, Wen EG, Xiong W, Guan QL (2006) Advances in mechanisms of postsurgical gastroparesis syndrome and its diagnosis and treatment. *Chin J Dig Dis*, **7**(2), 76–82.
71. Brand RE, DiBaise JK, Quigley EM, *et al.* (1985) Gastroparesis as a cause of nausea and vomiting after high-dose chemotherapy and haemopoietic stem-cell transplantation. *Lancet*, **352**(9145), 1985.
72. Bityutskiy LP, Soykan I, McCallum RW. Viral gastroparesis: a subgroup of idiopathic gastroparesis--clinical characteristics and long-term outcomes. *Am J Gastroenterol*, **92**(9), 1501–4.
73. Layer P, Demol P, Hotz J, Goebell H (1986) Gastroparesis after radiation. Successful treatment with carbachol. *Dig Dis Sci*, **31**(12), 1377–80.
74. Talley NJ (2007) How to manage the difficult-to-treat dyspeptic patient. Nat Clin *Pract Gastroenterol Hepatol*, **4**(1), 35–42.
75. Camilleri M, Malagelada JR (1984) Abnormal intestinal motility in diabetics with the gastroparesis syndrome. *Eur J Clin Invest*, **14**(6), 420–7.
76. Davis RH, Clench MH, Mathias JR (1985) Effects of domperidone in patients with chronic unexplained upper gastrointestinal symptoms: a double-blind, placebo-controlled study. *Dig Dis Sci*, **33**(12), 1505–11.
77. Park MI, Camilleri M (2006) Gastroparesis: clinical update. *Am J Gastroenterol*, **101**(5), 1129–39.

78. Shivshanker K, Bennett RW, Jr, Haynie TP (1983) Tumor-associated gastroparesis: correction with metoclopramide. *Am J Surg*, **145**(2),221–5.
79. Boivin MA, Carey MC, Levy H (2003) Erythromycin accelerates gastric emptying in a dose-response manner in healthy subjects. *Pharmacotherapy*, **23**(1), 5–8.
80. Veldhuyzen van Zanten SJ, Jones MJ, Verlinden M, Talley NJ. Efficacy of cisapride and domperidone in functional (nonulcer) dyspepsia: a meta-analysis. *Am J Gastroenterology*, **96**(3), 689–96.
81. Sturm A, Holtmann G, Goebell H, Gerken G (1999) Prokinetics in patients with gastroparesis: a systematic analysis. *Digestion*, **60**(5), 422–7.
82. McCallum RW, Valenzuela G, Polepalle S, Spyker D (1991) Subcutaneous metoclopramide in the treatment of symptomatic gastroparesis: clinical efficacy and pharmacokinetics. *J Pharmacol Exp Ther*, **258**(1), 136–42.
83. Dhir R, Richter JE (2004) Erythromycin in the short- and long-term control of dyspepsia symptoms in patients with gastroparesis. *J Clin Gastroenterol*, **38**(3), 237–42.
84. Grudell AB, Camilleri M, Burton DD, Stephens DA (2006) Effect of a proton pump inhibitor on postprandial gastric volume, emptying and symptoms in healthy human subjects: a pilot study. *Aliment Pharmacol Ther*, **24**(7), 1037–43.
85. Cremonini F, Camilleri M, Gonenne J, *et al.* (2005) Effect of somatostatin analog on postprandial satiation in obesity. *Obes Res*, **13**(9), 1572–9.
86. Bianco A, Pitocco D, Valenza V, *et al.* (2002) Effect of sildenafil on diabetic gastropathy. *Diabetes Care*, **25**(10), 1888–9.
87. Lunding JA, Gilja OH, Hausken T, Bayati A, Mattsson H, Berstad A (2007) Distension-induced gastric accommodation in functional dyspepsia: effect of autonomic manipulation. *Neurogastroenterol Motil*, **19**(5), 365–75.
88. Mearin F, Balboa A, Zarate N, Cucala M, Malagelada JR (1999)Placebo in functional dyspepsia: symptomatic, gastrointestinal motor and gastric sensorial responses. *Am J Gastroenterol*, **94**(1), 116–25.
89. Yang ZJ, Koseki M, Meguid MM, Laviano A (1996) Eating-related increase of dopamine concentration in the LHA with oronasal stimulation. *Am J Physiol*, **270**(2), R315–8.
90. Nguyen NQ, Chapman M, Fraser RJ, Bryant LK, Burgstad C, Holloway RH (2007) Prokinetic therapy for feed intolerance in critical illness: one drug or two? *Crit Care Med*, **35**(11), 2561–7.
91. Blundell JE, MacDiarmid JI (1997) Fat as a risk factor for overconsumption: satiation, satiety, and patterns of eating. *J Am Diet Assoc*, **97**(7S), S63–9.
92. Stubbs RJ (1999) Peripheral signals affecting food intake. *Nutrition*, **15**(7), 614–25.
93. Rolls BJ, Bell EA (1999) Intake of fat and carbohydrate: role of energy density. *Eur J Clin Nutr*, **53**(Suppl 1), S166–73.

Chapter 16

Disordered bowel function

David Blum and Florian Strasser

Introduction

Patients with cancer care often suffer from disordered bowel function. Constipation is much more common than diarrhoea in advanced cancer.[1] In palliative care diarrhoea and constipation may occur at the same time because severe constipation can cause paradoxical diarrhoea.[2]

Physiological bowel function

Normal bowel function depends on intestinal integrity and the ability to regulate intestinal fluids. The digestive system produces 8–9 l of fluid per day, of which three-quarters are absorbed in the small intestine. The colon is able to absorb up to 5 l per day. Normally only 100 ml fluids are excreted and a difference of 150 ml fluids per day distinguishes constipation from diarrhoea. Bile acids, prostaglandins and bacterial toxins stimulate secretion, whereas short-chain amino acids increase absorption. Gut fluid absorption is a process involving passive (co-transport of Na^+, glucose and amino acids) and active (basal Na^+K^+-ATPase, mucosal cyclic-AMP-dependent Cl^- secretion) mechanisms in the intestinal epithelium. These mechanisms are mainly regulated by the cholinergic system and mediated by intracellular calcium. In addition to electrolyte balance the parasympathetic nervous system plays a central role in intestinal muscle function. Peristalsis involves ascending contractions (mediated by acetylcholine) and descending relaxation, (mediated by vasoactive intestinal peptide) producing segmental, propulsive movements. Other receptors of particular importance in cancer are opioid μ-receptors, found mainly in the myenteric plexus, and opioid δ-receptors in the submucosal plexus. Endogenous opioids seem to influence bowel function on many levels including increased electrolyte (and therefore water) absorption, reduced peristalsis of the entire intestine, reduction of sensitivity to colon distension, and increased ileocaecal and internal anal sphincter tonus.

Constipation

Epidemiology and definition

Constipation is a frequent symptom that occurs in more than 10% of healthy persons. Its prevalence increases with age, disease, and among cancer patients more than half of patients suffer from symptoms of constipation.[3]

Overall both asymptomatic and symptomatic constipation are widely underestimated, even in specialized palliative care settings. The 'physiological frequency' of bowel movements shows large individual variation, ranging from three per day up to one every third day. It is important therefore to ask about patients' bowel habits prior to their cancer diagnosis.

Constipation is diagnosed by the use of the Rome III criteria[4] (must include two or more of the following):

- straining during at least 25% of defecations;
- lumpy or hard stools in at least 25% of defecations;
- sensation of incomplete evacuation for at least 25% of defecations;
- sensation of anorectal obstruction/blockage for at least 25% of defecations;
- manual manoeuvres to facilitate at least 25% of defecations (e.g. digital evacuation, support of the pelvic floor);
- fewer than three defecations per week.

The type and dose of the laxatives used during the preceding weeks provides additional information about the degree of constipation.

In clinical practice an estimation of stool retained in the colon using plain abdominal films can be helpful. For each abdominal quadrant the stool content is ranked from 0 to 3, resulting in total scores from 0 to 12, as reported by Bruera.[5]

Symptoms associated with constipation such as nausea, bloating, abdominal pain, flatulence, sensation of incomplete evacuation or rectal fullness, anorexia, early satiety, and halitosis, are not specific for the diagnosis of constipation. Sometimes constipation is manifested by other non-gastrointestinal symptoms such as urinary retention.

There are no established staging systems for the severity of constipation, such as for pain or depression. Severe constipation may progress to faecal impaction, which is almost always symptomatic and may be accompanied by abdominal pain, distension, colic, spasmodic rectal pain or vomiting. The clinical presentation may range from a change in stool quality/frequency to overflow diarrhoea and faecal incontinence.

Pathogenesis and causes

Advanced disease and age affects the performance of many organs including the intestine.

Reduced nutritional intake and decreased intestinal fluids can contribute to constipation. In the Nurses Health Study regular physical exercise and higher fibre intake were associated with a reduced risk of constipation. Advanced age is associated with slower colonic transit but also with increased laxative use, which may explain the inverse association between age and constipation in this study.[6,7] Despite these findings, elderly patients may have decreased reserve and comorbidities including cognitive impairment, depression, and medications such as diuretics which predispose to dehydration and constipation.

Tumours that compromise the anatomic integrity of the intestine by internal obstruction or external compression can affect the quality and frequency of bowel movements. Direct involvement of sphincters by tumour growth will also affect function.

Severe obstinate constipation (obstipation) can be precipitated by medications including opioids, calcium channel antagonists (nifedipine, verapamil), potassium-depleting diuretics, drugs with anticholinergic effects (tricyclic antidepressant, phenothiazines, hyoscine, antiparkinson drugs), serotonin ($5HT_3$) antagonists, sympathomimetics (clonidine), iron, and neurotoxic drugs (vinca alkaloids and thalidomide cause constipation in up to 30% of patients). Other conditions affecting nerves include diabetes mellitus, paraneoplastic pseudo-obstruction, and spinal cord involvement. Reversible metabolic causes of constipation include hypothyroidism and hypercalcaemia.[8,9]

Assessment/monitoring

The crucial step is to perform continuous reassessments in those patients identified at risk of constipation. After diagnosing constipation, the causes (Table 16.1) and potential laxative treatments should be considered.

The Victoria Bowel Performance Scale (BPS) was designed as an ordinal nine-point scale from −4 (severe constipation) to +4 (severe diarrhoea) and includes three parameters: visual stool characteristics, bowel pattern, and ability to control defecation.[10] This scale appears to be reliable but requires further prospective testing in clinical care to confirm the reliability and clinical utility of the BPS. A BPS management guideline has also been developed to assist with decision-making for each BPS score.

Management

The first step is to treat the underlying cause (Box 16.1). Identifying a single cause may be difficult since constipation in advanced cancer patients is usually a multifactorial problem. Many of the causes may not be reversible, and are usually best managed by a multidisciplinary team.[11]

Constipation is a frequent side-effect of any opioid therapy (both oral and parenteral) and unfortunately tolerance to opioid-induced constipation does not develop. By contrast, other side-effects such as drowsiness and nausea usually abate a few days after initiating opioid therapy. Constipation can occur on a lower dose than is required for adequate analgesia. Increasing doses of opioids have only a weak correlation with more severe constipation.[12]

An oral-only laxative regimen can achieve control in two-thirds of patients, whereas the other one-third will need additional rectal laxatives. Lubricants (liquid paraffin, mineral oil), salines (Mg, Na-phosphate, Na-sulphate), osmotic agents (lactulose, sorbitol, mannitol) and contact laxatives (docusate, ricinoleic acid, bile salt), polyphenolics (bisacodyl, Na-picosulphate), synthetic (danthrone) and natural anthracenes (senna, cascara, casanthranol) are widely used. Polyethylene glycol is also used, particularly in children. Due to the risk for constipation and dehydration in advanced cancer, bulk-forming drugs (fibre) are rarely used because they increase the risk of impaction.

Table 16. 1 Causes of constipation

Cause	Management
Immobility/inactivity/age	Mobilization, physical therapy
Opioids	Laxatives, opioid rotation
Other drugs[a]	Laxatives, change drugs
Hypercalcaemia or hypokalaemia	Correct electrolyte imbalance
Neural plexus/spinal cord invasion	Prokinetics, laxatives
Autonomic neuropathy/cachexia	Prokinetics, treat anorexia/cachexia
Tumour compression of bowel	Palliative surgery, stent
Severe depression	Counselling, antidepressants
Severe pain	Pain management
Hypothyroidism	Replace thyroid hormone

[a]Anticholinergics, diuretics, non-steroidal anti-inflammatory drugs, tricyclics, phenothiazines, antihistamines, iron, thalidomide, others.

Box 16.1 Treatment of constipation

- Treat the cause, if possible.
- Start with a peristaltic stimulant such as senna or a stool softener.
- Titrate towards effect.
- Add osmotic laxatives such as lactulose or sorbitol every 4–6 h, until bowel movement, but avoid long-term use (fluid and electrolyte imbalances).
- Treat distal constipation with suppositories or enemas
- After no bowel movement for 3 days, follow the 'rescue' enemas with an increase in oral laxatives.
- Distal faecal impaction (digital exam) may require digital disimpaction and oil-retention enema.
- Proximal faecal impaction (flat X-ray) may require magnesium citrate and oral lubricants (mineral oil).

Several pharmacological features have to be taken into account when choosing laxatives. The latency period from drug administration until the bowel movement, the intensity of its effects as well as typical adverse effects need to be known (Box 16.2). For mild and moderate constipation, as well as prophylaxis, a combination of two laxatives with stool softening as well as peristaltic stimulatory effects are used. They can be titrated until a daily bowel movement is reached.

Box 16.2 Pharmacological treatment of constipation

Bulk-forming agents

- Cellulose, psyllium seed, bran.
- They increase mass and water content of stool; intraluminal fluid increased after gut microflora breakdown.

Lubricants

- Liquid paraffin, mineral oil.
- Adverse effects include impaired absorption of fat-soluble vitamins, irritation of perianal area, risk of lipoid pneumonia when aspiration occurs.
- Short-term use for faecal impaction.

Osmotic laxatives

- Lactulose, sorbitol (30–70%), mannitol.
- Sorbitol is cheaper than lactulose and as effective.
- Polyethylene glycol: no effect in small intestine, slow onset of effect.
- Short-chain organic acids lower intestinal pH and stimulate peristalsis and increase stool bulk.
- Adverse effects include flatulence in 20%.

Box 16.2 Pharmacological treatment of constipation *(continued)*

Saline laxatives

- Mg-hydroxide, Mg-citrate; Na-phosphate, Na-sulphate.
- Mg: most potent; sulphate more potent than phosphate.
- Increases intestinal water secretion; directly stimulates peristalsis.
- Rapid onset throughout the gut, not only in the colon.
- Adverse effects include systemic electrolyte accumulation and volume overload.

  Severe cramping, bloating, dehydration, bowel perforation.
  Phosphates may cause hypocalcaemia.

Contact laxatives

- Docusate

  Increases mucosal secretion and peristalsis.
  Probably will develop tolerance.
  Detergent or surfactant effect allows water and fat to mix with faeces and stool softener.
- Castor oil

  Hydrolysed by gut microflora to ricinoleic acid.
  Adverse effects include cramping and diarrhoea, malabsorption.

Diphenylmethane derivates or polyphenolics

- Phenolphthalein, bisacodyl, Na-picosulphate.
- Effect mainly in the colon, slow onset (12–24 h).
- Adverse effects include abdominal cramps, hypokalaemia, allergies.

Anthracenes/anthraquinone derivates

- Synthetic (danthrone) or natural (senna)

  Senna, cascara, casanthranol. Senna in form of glycosides has to be converted to active form by colonic bacteria.
  Directly stimulate myenteric plexus; inhibition of NaK-ATPase; stimulation of cyclic AMP; mucosal electrolyte transport and motility.
  Effect mainly in the colon; slow onset (12–24 h).
  Pink urine can occur.

Prokinetics

- Metoclopramide

  Dopamine antagonist at both central and peripheral levels, in addition a cholinergic $5HT_4$ agonist and weak antagonist for $5HT_3$.
  Increases tone and strength of gastroduodenal contractions. Less prokinetic in jejunum, ileum and colon. No stimulation of gastric, pancreatic, enteric, biliary secretions.
  Combined action chemoreceptor-triggerzone and intestinal motility.
  Adverse effects include drowsiness, lassitude, anxiety, extrapyramidal side-efects.

(continued)

Box 16.2 Pharmacological treatment of constipation *(continued)*

- Domperidone

  Peripherally acting D_2-receptor antagonist, which does not cross blood–brain barrier.
  Effect limited to stomach.
  Adverse effects include dry skin, rash, pruritis, diarrhoea.
- Macrolide antibiotics, erythromycin

  Mimic effect of motilin, improve gastrointestinal motility in colonic pseudo-obstruction.
  Adverse effects include nausea and multiple drug interactions.

Enemas and suppositories

- Short latency of action
- Stimulation of anocolonic reflex
- Sodium phosphate suppository/sodium phosphate or citrate enema

  Releases bound water from faeces, may stimulate peristalsis in the lower bowel (rectal or colonic).
  May cause hypocalcaemia, hyperphosphataemia.
- Arachis oil, olive oil

  Softens hard, impacted stool.
- Glycerin suppository

  Softens stool by osmosis, as well as a lubricant.
  Can cause mechanical stimulation.
- Sorbitol enema

  Sodium docusate, sodium-lauryl sulphoacetate, sodium alkyl sulphacetate.
  Water influx and penetration of hard stool.
  Milk and molasses
  Stimulates lower bowel; sugar is an irritant; can produce gas which distends the bowel.
  Tap water: induces peristalsis.
  Soap suds: stimulates lower bowel, promotes evacuation.
  Saline: stimulates lower bowel, promotes evacuation.
  Polyphenol.
- Bisacodyl suppositories
  Induces colonic peristalis after 15–60 min. Bisacodyl is superior to glycerine.

Opioid antagonist

- Naloxone, or methylnaltrexate

  Modulates excitatory and inhibitory neurotransmission.
  Acts both on cholinergic and non-adrenergic/non-cholinergic neurons.
  Accelerates colon transit without increasing the number of bowel movements.
  Adverse effects include cramping.
  Alvimopan.

Methylnaltrexone is an opioid-antagonist of the μ-receptor approved by the US Food and Drug Administration (FDA) and the European Medicines Agency for opioid-induced constipation. The drug is administered subcutaneously, as frequently as 48 h. In a large placebo-controlled study, half of patients reported laxation within 4 h after the first study dose compared to 15% receiving the placebo. There was no reduction of analgesia, and withdrawal was not observed.[13] The most common side-effects included abdominal pain 17% (placebo: 13%) and flatulence 13% (placebo: 7%).

The chemical structure of an orally administered opioid antagonist, alvimopan, restricts gastrointestinal absorption and prevents the drug from crossing the blood–brain barrier. The FDA has approved alvimopan for the use of post-operative ileus. The drug is restricted to inpatients because of an association with increased myocardial infarction and there have been no trials in cancer patients.

Other peripheral opioid antagonists are being developed, including an oral candidate (NKTR-118) in patients with opioid-induced constipation.

Non-pharmacological measures can be equally important. Good location (intimacy, comfort) timing (patience, rhythm), mobility and activity, are all necessary components.

Prophylaxis

Measures to prevent constipation should start as soon as a decrease in stool frequency is observed, or when any opioid therapy is initiated.

General measures to mitigate constipation must be discussed with patients and families. They include encouragement of adequate fluid intake, activity, avoidance of excess dietary fibre (although fruit fibre may be beneficial), compliant use of laxatives and titration of bowel regimen to effect. The patient's medications should also be reviewed for possible contributory causes other than opioids, including $5HT_3$ receptor antagonists, calcium channel blockers, gabapentin and thalidomide. Occasionally, an alternative to these medications might be feasible.

Complications

Severe constipation can result in bowel obstruction, nausea and vomiting, abdominal pain; overflow diarrhoea, urinary retention, cognitive failure, dehydration, anorexia, haemorrhoids or anal fissures. Unfortunately, many of these conditions may not be recognized as complications of constipation. Patients with cancer are also prone to develop a rare disorder (Ogilvie syndrome) characterized by massive dilation of the caecum in the absence of mechanical obstruction. Neostigmine has been shown to be effective therapy; however, increased respiratory secretions and bradycardia may be serious side-effects of this cholinergic agent.

Conclusion

Constipation is underestimated in patients with advanced cancer. A better awareness and an appreciation of the need for continuous ongoing symptom assessment will improve the management of constipation. New agents (e.g. methynaltrexone) to reverse opioid-induced constipation appear to be effective, and do not compromise analgesia.

Diarrhoea

Epidemiology and definition

Diarrhoea is less common than constipation in palliative care, but can be debilitating and even life-threatening. In palliative care less than 10% of patients suffer from diarrhoea[2] but this increases considerably in patients undergoing abdominopelvic radiotherapy (20–50%), patients receiving certain chemotherapy regimes containing fluoropyrimidines and topoisomerase inhibitors (50%), and patients with carcinoid tumours (80%).

Patients may perceive small stools, loose stools or faecal incontinence as diarrhoea. These symptoms have to be further clarified and patients need to be asked about the number of stools per day. Diarrhoea is commonly defined as more than three or four unformed stools per day.

The impact of diarrhoea should not be underestimated since in addition to fluid loss, and electrolyte disturbances, diarrhoea can cause anxiety, embarrassment, and impair quality of life.

Pathogenesis and causes

The mechanisms causing diarrhoea are dependent on the trajectory of the illness, the tumour type, and the therapeutic agents used either for the cancer or for other symptoms.

Diarrhoea may be precipitated by conditions or factors which are unrelated to the diagnosis of cancer. Pre-existing lactose intolerance, dietary habits with excessive fibre, alcohol consumption or sorbitol use, could be the cause of diarrhoea. Comorbidities such as diabetes, hyperthyroidism, and inflammatory bowel disease are also potential contributors to diarrhoea.

Patients receiving anti-tumour therapy may suffer from diarrhoea caused by chemotherapy regimens containing 5-fluorouracil (5FU), capecitabine, irinotecan or tyrosine kinase inhibitors. Diarrhoea due to 5FU is usually the result of damage to the epithelium, producing an imbalance in intestinal fluid regulation.[14]

Capecitabine, a precursor of 5FU, is a fluoropyrimidine cytotoxic agent that can be administered orally. In both agents the prevalence of diarrhoea is 30–40%, and in up to 20% it can be severe.

Irinotecan can produce a cholinergic effect and acute diarrhoea which is antagonised by administration of subcutaneous atropine. Late diarrhoea, occurring more than 24 h after administration of irinotecan (usually at day 5), is prolonged and can be life-threatening, leading to dehydration and electrolyte imbalances. Toxicity is not solely dose dependent, and physiological as well as genetic factors are probably important in determining the severity, which can range from mild colitis to necrotizing enterocolits.

Novel targeted therapy agents such as epidermal growth factor receptors or tyrosine kinase inhibitors can cause diarrhoea, which may be more severe in combination with other chemotherapeutic agents. Tyrosine kinase inhibitors such as sorafenib, suninitib, imatinib or the proteasome inhibitor bortezomib are all associated with diarrhoea. Diarrhoea occurs in 30–50% of patients on these agents and can be severe in 5–10%.

Radiation therapy of the abdomen or pelvis can cause severe diarrhoea due to mucosal damage which may persist for some weeks after termination of the radiotherapy.

Infections should always be considered in the differential diagnosis since they can be easily treated with antimicrobial agents. *Clostridium difficile* flourishes when normal intestinal flora is altered due to antibiotic therapy. Two cytotoxic exotoxins (Toxins A and B) cause diarrhoea by increasing vascular permeability and inciting a proinflammatory response. Toxin B plays an important role once the gastrointestinal wall has been damaged by Toxin A. *C. difficile*-associated diarrhoea may complicate chemotherapy-related gastrotoxicity even in the absence of recent antimicrobial therapy. Rapid enzyme immunoassay tests are able to detect both toxins with good specificity (95–100%) but reduced sensitivity (65–85%).[15–17151] Metronidazole is the drug of choice even for an initial recurrence, while vancomycin and adjunctive probiotic agents can be effective for those patients with multiple relapses.

Other bacteria commonly causing enteritis with diarrhoea (campylobacter, salmonella) can also occur in cancer patients.

Enteral nutrition can cause diarrhoea due to rapid administration, cool temperature or high osmolarity of the nutrients.

Diarrhoea due to malabsorption occurs in several different cancer types including pancreatic carcinoma, cholangio-carcinoma, and tumours secreting active hormones such as vipomas and carcinoid. Resection of portions of the gastrointestinal tract such as stomach or ileum or colon may produce diarrhoea.[18–20] It is important to inform patients with colostomy that their output should be softer and looser than physiological stool.

In advanced cancer, especially for patients on any opioid therapy, severe constipation can manifest as paradoxical diarrhoea. An abdominal X-ray may be required to confirm the suspicion that obstipation is producing the 'overflow diarrhoea'.

Commonly used drugs might be the cause of diarrhoea, including laxatives, antacids or anti-emetics (see Box 16.3).

Box 16.3 Causes of diarrhoea

Diet

- Alcohol, milk, and dairy products (particularly in patients with lactose intolerance).
- Caffeine-containing products (coffee, tea, chocolate), specific fruit juices (prune juice, unfiltered apple juice, sauerkraut juice).
- High-fibre foods (raw fruits and vegetables, nuts, seeds, whole-grain products, dried legumes); high-fat foods (deep fat-fried foods, high-fat-containing foods).
- Lactose intolerance or food allergies.
- Sorbitol-containing foods (candy and chewing gum); hot and spicy foods; gas-forming foods and beverages (cruciferous vegetables, dried legumes, melons, carbonated beverages).

Drugs

- Laxatives, antacids, antibiotics, magnesium-containing antacids, colchicine, digoxin, lactulose, laxatives, methyldopa, metoclopramide, misoprostol, potassium supplements, propanolol, theophylline.

Anticancer Therapies

- Chemotherapy: 5FU, irinotecan, docetaxel, epidermal growth factor receptor and tyrosine kinase inhibitors capecitabine, cisplatin, cytosine arabinoside, cyclophosphamide, daunorubicin, docetaxel, doxorubicin, 5FU, interferon, irinotecan, leucovorin, methotrexate, oxaliplatin, paclitaxel, topotecan,bortezemib.
- Radiotherapy: abdomen, pelvis.

Interventional procedure for pain

- Coeliac plexus block.

Infection

- *Clostridium difficile*, other enteritis-causing bacteria and viruses *Clostridium perfringens*, *Bacillus cereus*, *Giardia lamblia*, *Cryptosporidium*, *Salmonella* spp., *Shigella* spp., *Campylobacter* spp., rotavirus, norovirus.

Box 16.3 Causes of diarrhoea *(continued)*

Cancer-related

- Colon cancer, bowel obstruction.
- Pancreatic insufficency.
- Biliary obstruction.
- Surgical, including gastrectomy, pancreaticoduodenectomy (Whipple procedure), short bowel syndrome cholecystectomy, oesophagogastrectomy.
- Fistula.
- Carcinoid syndrome.
- Lymphoma involving the gastrointestinal system.
- Phaeochromocytoma.
- Medullary carcinoma of the thyroid.
- Graft-versus-host disease.

Comorbidities

- Diabetes, hyperthyroidism, inflammatory bowel disease (Crohn disease, ulcerative colitis), diverticulitis, HIV/AIDS.

Assessment and monitoring

General symptom assessment tools for palliative care such as the Edmonton Symptom Assessment System usually do not include diarrhoea as a symptom, but different bowel scales are found in the literature. A patient-rated visual analogue scale has been validated. The Victoria BPS is designed for diarrhoea and constipation.[10]

A history that includes dietary habits and medication must be obtained. The frequency, consistency, timing (e.g. nocturnal diarrhoea) and colour of the stools are important. Symptoms such as fever and faecal incontinence may require further evaluation including laboratory tests and radiographic imaging. A rectal examination and assessment of sphincter tone is vital if spinal compression is suspected.

Clinical examination of the abdomen including auscultation and palpitation might provide useful information, whereas evidence of orthostasis will suggest dehydration. An expert panel recommended that symptoms of chemotherapy-induced diarrhoea (CIN) be classified as uncomplicated or complicated [equivalent to National Cancer Institute (NCI) grade ≥3]. Complicated diarrhoea should include one or more of the following symptoms and signs: moderate to severe cramping, grade ≥2 nausea and vomiting, decreased performance status, fever, sepsis, neutropenia, frank bleeding or dehydration. Because loperamide may be less effective in patients with severe diarrhoea (NCI grade ≥3) the panel recommends starting octreotide therapy (either subcutaneously or intravenously) along with antibiotics.

Evaluation with a complete blood count, electrolyte profile, and stool for blood, faecal leukocytes, *C. difficile*, *Salmonella* spp., *E. coli*, *Campylobacter* spp., would be appropriate.

Management

Dehydration and electrolyte imbalance should be treated either orally or by infusion therapy and all offending medications must be discontinued if possible.

Chemotherapy-induced diarrhoea can be treated initially with oral loperamide (2 mg every 2 h) until the diarrhoea resolves. Loperamide has minimal systemic side-effects, but can induce severe obstipation.[21,22] An oral fluoroquinolone should be added if there is no improvement after ≥24 h. If diarrhoea persists despite the use of loperamide for ≥48 h, patients should be hospitalized and intravenous fluids administered.

Tincture of opium is the second most commonly used anti-diarrhoeal agent. It contains 10 mg/ml morphine and other alkaloids such as codeine, etc. Starting doses are 5–10 drops, dissolved in a glass of water, three to five times daily.

Acute radiation injury results in mucosal damage and inflammation and up to 40% of patients with rectal cancer treated with postoperative therapy will develop chronic diarrhoea. Comorbidities such as diabetes, irritable bowel syndrome and smoking as well as therapy-related factors including radiation dose, volume of bowel irradiated, time–dose–fractionation parameters, and use of concomitant bio- or chemotherapy determine the predisposition to diarrhoea and complications.[23] The mechanisms contributing to chronic diarrhoea are unclear but could include bile salt malabsorption, bacterial overgrowth, and vitamin B_{12} deficiency.[24] Radiation therapy-induced diarrhoea responds well to oral opiates. Several clinical trials have focused on preventing radiation therapy-induced diarrhoea with pharmacological therapies including sucralfate, glutamine, misoprostol and octreotide. Despite initial promise, subsequent randomized clinical trials have not supported the use of these agents. There is strong evidence from placebo-controlled trials that depot octreotide is not effective for the prevention of diarrhoea during pelvic radiation therapy.[25] In a clinical trial, moderate or worse diarrhoea was observed in 53% of patients receiving sucralfate (versus 41% of those receiving placebo) and more sucralfate-treated patients reported faecal incontinence (34% vs 16%) and nausea.[26] Although well tolerated, 4 g of glutamine daily also demonstrated no benefit versus placebo.

Mixed results have been reported for placebo-controlled trials with 5-aminosalicylic acid derivatives. Sulphasalazine (2 g/day) was found to be effective[27] in decreasing the symptoms of radiation enteritis, meslazine showed no benefit,[28] and olsalazine increased the severity of diarrhea[29] in a placebo-controlled trial of patients who underwent adjuvant postoperative radiation therapy after surgery for sigmoid, rectal, or cervical cancer. Probiotic lactic acid-producing bacteria may prove to be an easy, safe, potentially effective prophylactic therapy.[30]

Antimicrobial treatment will be required for *Clostridium difficile* and other bacteria causing enteritis. Diarrhoea with malabsorption due to pancreas insufficiency or excess bile salts may occur after abdominal radiation. Pancreatic enzymes can be replaced and biliary salt malabsorption may respond to a bile binder such as colveselem or cholestyramine. Zollinger–Ellison syndrome patients with diarrhoea as a result of hypergastrinaemia will respond to high dose proton-pump inhibitors.

If diarrhoea cannot be controlled with loperamide, octreotide should be considered. Octreotide suppresses gastrointestinal hormones, reduces motility and increases absorption in the gastrointestinal tract. It can be started at a dose of 100 μg subcutaneously three times per day and increased up to 500 μg. Adverse effects may include mouth dryness[31,32] fluctuating blood sugars, altered absorption of dietary fats and enhanced QTc prolongation when combined with QTc-prolonging agents.

Two trials failed to show that glutamine prevents diarrhoea in patients receiving allogeneic or autologous transplantation. A new oral suspension formulation of L-glutamine reduced the incidence of severe mucositis in a phase III trial; however, independent confirmation is needed.[33–35]

Conclusion

Diarrhoea in advanced cancer can have devastating consequences. Severe diarrhoea can be fatal secondary to dehydration and electrolyte imbalance. Chronic diarrhoea can exacerbate malnutrition and impair the immune system. Better awareness and understanding of the different causes and more targeted treatments are necessary. Tailored prophylaxis strategies should emerge in the future.

References

1. Goodman M, Low J, Wilkinson S (2005) Constipation management in palliative care: a survey of practices in the United kingdom. *J Pain Sympt Manag*, **29**, 238–44.
2. Alderman J (2005) Diarrhea in palliative care. *J Palliat Med*, **8**, 449–50.
3. Potter J, Hami F, Bryan T, Quigley C (2004) Symptoms in 400 patients referred to palliative care services: prevalence and patterns. *Palliat Med*, **17**(4), 310–4.
4. Drossman DA (1999) The Rome criteria process: diagnosis and legitimization of irritable bowel syndrome. *Am J Gastroenterol*, **94**, 2803–7.
5. Bruera E, Suarez-Almazor M, Velasco A, Bertolino M, MacDonald SM, Hanson J (1994) The assessment of constipation in terminal cancer patients admitted to a palliative care unit: a retrospective review. *J Pain Sympt Manag*, **9**(8), 515–9.
6. Dukas L, Willett WC, Giovannucci EL (2003) Association between physical activity, fiber intake, and other lifestyle variables and constipation in a study of women. *Am J Gastroenterol*, **98**, 1790–6.
7. Leung FW (2007) Etiologic factors of chronic constipation: review of the scientific evidence. *Dig Dis Sci*, **52**(2), 313–6.
8. Staats PS, Markowitz J, Schein J (2004) Incidence of constipation associated with long-acting opioid therapy: a comparative study. *South Med J*, **97**, 129–34.
9. Pappagallo M (2001) Incidence, prevalence, and management of opioid bowel dysfunction. *Am J Surg*, **182**(5AS), 11S–18S.
10. Downing GM, Kuziemsky C, Lesperance M, Lau F, Syme A (2007) Development and reliability testing of the Victoria Bowel Performance Scale (BPS). *J Pain Sympt Manag*, **34**(5), 513–22.
11. Larkin PJ, Sykes NP, Centeno C, *et al.* (2008) The management of constipation in palliative care: clinical practice recommendations on Constipation in Palliative Care European Consensus Group. *Palliat Med*, **22**(7), 796–807.
12. Fallon MT, Hanks GW (1999) Morphine, constipation and performance status in advanced cancer patients. *Palliat Med*, **13**(2), 159–60.
13. Thomas J, Karver S, Cooney GA, *et al.* (2008) Methylnaltrexone for opioid induced constipation in advanced illness. *N Engl J Med*, **358**(22), 2332–43.
14. Arnold RJ, Gabrail N, Raut M, *et al.* (2005) Clinical implications ofchemotherapy-induced diarrhea in patients with cancer. *J Support Oncol*, **3**, 227–32.
15. Poutanen SM, Simor AE (2004) *Clostridium difficile*-associated diarrhea in adults. *Can Med Assoc J*, **171**, 51–8.
16. Jarvis B, Shevchuk YM (1997) Recurrent *Clostridium difficile* diarrhea-associated with mitoxantrone and etoposide: a case report and review. *Pharmacotherapy*, **17**, 606–11.
17. Yamazawa K, Kanno H, Seki K, *et al.* (2001) Life-threatening *Clostridium difficile*-associated diarrhea induced by paclitaxel-carboplatincombination chemotherapy. *Acta Obstet Gynecol Scand*, **80**, 768–9.
18. Wakasugi H, Hara Y, Abe M (1996) A study of malabsorption in pancreatic cancer. *J Gastroenterol*, **31**, 81–5.
19. King CE, Toskes PP (1976) Malabsorption following gastric resection. *Major Probl Clin Surg*, **20**, 129–46.
20. Hofmann AF (1972) Bile acid malabsorption caused by ileal resection. *Arch Intern Med*, **130**, 597–605.
21. Ruppin H (1987) Review: loperamide—a potent antidiarrhoeal drug with actions along the alimentary tract. *Aliment Pharmacol Ther*, **1**, 179–90.
22. Cascinu S, Bichisao E, Amadori D, *et al.* (2000) High-dose loperamide in the treatment of 5-fluorouracil-induced diarrhea in colorectal cancer patients. *Support Care Cancer*, **8**, 65.

23. Hauer-Jensen M, Wang J, Boerma M, Fu Q, Denham JW (2007) Radiation damage to the gastrointestinal tract: mechanisms, diagnosis, and management. *Curr Opin Support Palliat Care*, **1**(1), 23–9.
24. Andreyev HJ (2007) Gastrointestinal problems after pelvic radiotherapy: the past, the present and the future. *Clin Oncol (R Coll Radiol)*, **19**(10), 790–9.
25. Martenson JA, Halyard MY, Sloan JA, *et al.* (2008) Phase III, double-blind study of depot octreotide versus placebo in the prevention of acute diarrhea in patients receiving pelvic radiation therapy: results of North Central Cancer Treatment Group N00CA. *J Clin Oncol*, **26**(32), 5248–53.
26. Martenson JA, Bollinger JW, Sloan JA, *et al.* (2000) Sucralfate in the prevention of treatment-induced diarrhea in patients receiving pelvic radiation therapy: a North Central Cancer Treatment Group phase III double-blind placebo-controlled trial. *J Clin Oncol*, **18**(6), 1239–45.
27. Kiliç D, Egehan I, Ozenirler S, Dursun A (2000) Double-blinded, randomized, placebo-controlled study to evaluate the effectiveness of sulphasalazine in preventing acute gastrointestinal complications due to radiotherapy. *Radiother Oncol*, **57**(2), 125–9.
28. Resbeut M, Marteau P, Cowen D, *et al.* (1997) A randomized double blind placebo controlled multicenter study of mesalazine for the prevention of acute radiation enteritis. *Radiother Oncol*, **44**(1), 59–63.
29. Martenson JA Jr, Hyland G, Moertel, *et al.* (1996) Olsalazine is contraindicated during pelvic radiation therapy: results of a double-blind, randomized clinical trial. *Int J Radiat Oncol Biol Phys*, **35**(2), 299–303.
30. Delia P, Sansotta G, Donato V, *et al.* (2007) Use of probiotics for prevention of radiation-induced diarrhea. *World J Gastroenterol*, **13**(6), 912–5.
31. Szilagyi A, Shrier I (2001) Systematic review: the use of somatostatin or octreotide in refractory diarrhoea. *Aliment Pharmacol Ther*, **15**, 1889–97.
32. Rosenoff S (2004) Resolution of refractory chemotherapy-induced diarrhea (CID) with octreotide long-acting formulation in cancer patients: 11 case studies. *Support Care Cancer*, **12**, 561–70.
33. Anderson P, Ramsay N, Shu X, *et al.* (1998) Effect of low-dose oral glutamine on painful stomatitis during bone marrow transplantation. *Bone Marrow Transplant*, **22**, 339.
34. Schloerb PR, Skikne BS (1999) Oral and parenteral glutamine in bone marrow transplantation: a randomized, double-blind study. *J Parental Enteral Nutr*, **23**, 117.
35. Peterson DE, Jones JB, Petit RG (2006) Randomized, placebo-controlled trial of Saforis for prevention and treatment of oral mucositis in breast cancer patients receiving anthracycline-based chemotherapy. *Cancer*, **109**, 322.

Chapter 17

Depression and fatigue

Elizabeth Kvale, Casey Balentine Azuero, Eric Walker

Introduction

Depression may contribute to cachexia in advanced cancer patients through the generation of inflammatory mediators, or may occur as a component of the anorexia–cachexia syndrome in response to inflammatory signals. Depression is a comorbid disabling syndrome affecting about 15–25% of cancer patients. According to the World Health Organization (WHO),[1] depression can be reliably diagnosed and treated in primary care settings although fewer than 25% of those affected have access to effective treatment. An estimated 16% of non-institutionalized adults have a major depressive disorder (MDD), and in people with cancer, the rate of MDD increases to 10–25% (varying by cancer type and treatment stage).[2,3]

After a diagnosis of cancer, patients experience a full spectrum of depressive symptoms ranging from normal sadness, to adjustment disorder with depressed mood, to MDD. Other syndromes include dysthymia and subsyndromal depression. Dysthymia is a chronic mood disorder in which a depressed mood is present on more days than not for at least 2 years.[2] By contrast, subsyndromal depression is an acute mood disorder that is less severe than MDD.[4]

Epidemiological studies suggest that at least half of all people diagnosed with cancer successfully adapt. Markers of successful adaptation include maintaining an active involvement in daily life; minimizing the disruptions caused by the illness to one's life roles (e.g. spouse, parent, employee); regulating the normal emotional reactions to the illness; and managing feelings of hopelessness, helplessness, worthlessness and/or guilt.[5]

Diagnosing depression in cancer patients is challenging because the somatic complaints of a depressed patient often mirror those of a cancer patient. For example, fatigue and poor appetite are typically present in both groups.[6] A critical part of care is the recognition of depressive symptoms and determining the appropriate level of intervention. Treatment may range from brief counselling or support groups to medication and/or psychotherapy. Concurrent and proactive efforts to stabilize weight loss among cancer patients experiencing depression are essential to minimize the impact of depression on clinical outcomes.

Weight loss in depression

MDD may manifest as either weight loss or weight gain in otherwise healthy populations. This chapter will focus on issues associated with weight loss among depressed individuals. It is uncertain whether the weight changes that occur are the result of an energy imbalance linked aetiologically to depression.[7] Although associations between depression and weight loss are identified in a number of cancer populations,[8–10] the majority of these studies are cross-sectional and do not provide insight into whether weight loss precedes or follows the onset of a depressive disorder. Within clinically depressed populations, management of the underlying depression is noted to stabilize associated weight loss. No studies are identified which demonstrate similar effects during the treatment of depressed cancer patients.

Mechanisms of MDD

The pathophysiology that underlies MDD is not clearly defined, and prevalent theories in the past have focused on the neurotransmitters serotonin, norepinephrine, and dopamine. Recently there has been an increasing focus in the literature on the association of inflammation with depression, and a potential role for inflammatory processes in the pathogenesis of MDD and depressive symptoms.[11] Because of this potential mechanistic relationship between cachexia and depression, the remainder of this discussion will focus on current hypotheses related to inflammation and depression. A clear temporal relationship between inflammation and depression has not been established, and a causative role for inflammatory processes with regard to depression is not clear. A number of studies demonstrate an association between inflammatory markers and depression or depressive symptoms among cancer patients.[12–15] In addition, cancer patients who are administered interferon (IFN)-α report a behavioural syndrome that is very similar to MDD in both its clinical manifestations and its responsiveness to standard antidepressant therapies.[16–18] IFNα is a potent inducer of inflammatory cytokines and activates the hypothalamic–pituitary–adrenal axis via sensitization of corticotrophin-releasing factor pathways.

The behavioural syndrome associated with the experimental or therapeutic administration of cytokine-inducing substances is termed 'sickness behaviour', and in both animal and human models is characterized by depression, fatigue, listlessness, weakness, difficulty with concentration or cognitive challenges, and anorexia.[19,20] The symptom of fatigue is both highly prevalent and profoundly troubling to many cancer patients, and is believed to be multifactorial in aetiology. The association of cytokine administration with fatigue lends theoretical support to hypotheses suggesting that inflammatory pathways may be a common mechanism for cachexia, depression, and fatigue.[21–23] Certainly, studies suggest that depression and fatigue are strongly associated in populations of cancer patients.[24,25] Studies attempting to correlate such symptoms with circulating levels of cytokines are mixed, either supporting such an association[13,26] or failing to identify correlations.[27]

Diagnosis

Although the aetiology of depression and cancer-related fatigue is not fully understood, the biopsychosocial and stress–diathesis models of illness suggest that significant emotional, social and environmental antecedents—such as the diagnosis of cancer—are clearly involved in the evolution of depression. These models illustrate the importance of acquiring a patient's detailed psychological personal and family history to determine the risk of depression. Diagnosing depression in cancer patients is important because of the impact on quality of life and possible association with survival.

The diagnosis of depression in cancer can be difficult because of problems inherent in distinguishing biological and physical symptoms of depression from symptoms of illness or toxic side-effects of treatment. This is particularly true in patients receiving active treatment or those with advanced disease.

Practitioners should familiarize themselves with the risk factors associated with depression in cancer patients. Some risk factors for depression in cancer are outlined in Box 17.1. Given the high prevalence of depression among cancer patients and evidence that cancer clinicians do not identify depression in the majority of patients who are experiencing depressive symptoms,[28–30] routine screening for depression may be helpful. A number of brief screening instruments can be utilized to identify cancer patients experiencing depression. A single item question asking 'Are you depressed?' performs better than a number of more complicated approaches in the identification of depressed cancer patients.[31]

Box 17.1 Risk factors for depression in people with cancer[a]

Cancer-related risk factors

- Depression at the time of cancer diagnosis
- Poorly controlled pain
- Advanced stage of cancer
- Increased physical impairment or discomfort
- Pancreatic cancer
- Being unmarried and having head and neck cancer
- Treatment with certain chemotherapy agents:

  Corticosteroids
  Procarbazine
  L-Asparaginase
  Interferon-α
  Interleukin-2
  Amphotericin-B

Non-cancer-related risk factors

- History of depression

  Two or more episodes in a lifetime
  First episode early or late in life
- Lack of family support
- Additional concurrent life stressors
- Family history of depression or suicide
- Previous suicide attempts
- History of alcoholism or drug use
- Concurrent illnesses that produce depressive symptoms (i.e. stroke or myocaradial infarction)
- Past treatment for psychological problems

[a]National Cancer Institute (2008).

Using both the Hospital Anxiety and Depression Scale (HADS)[32] in conjunction with the Beck Depression Inventory (BDI)[33] has a 90% sensitivity and specificity rate for diagnosing depression compared to the gold-standard clinical psychiatric interview in an outpatient oncology setting.[34] In a different approach, Chochinov[35] and a panel of experts determined a diagnostic process based on the *Diagnostic and Statistical Manual of Mental Disorders IV* (DSM-IV)[36] criteria for major depressive disorder. Box 17.2 illustrates the diagnostic steps that should be followed by practitioners to determine the presence of MDD.

Cancer care teams should recognize that the suicide rate among cancer patients is nearly twice that of the general population, and routine screening for suicide risk is recommended. Utilizing the Surveillance, Epidemiology, and End Results (SEER) database, Misono *et al.* demonstrated

Box 17.2 Diagnosing depression in cancer patients[35]

Step 1. Core symptoms of depression (one of two must be present to continue to steps 2 and 3)

- Depressed mood
- Diminished interest and/or pleasure

Step 2. Additional symptoms of depression (total of five symptoms from steps 2 and 3 must be present)

- Weight loss or gain
- Insomnia or hyperinsomnia
- Psychomotor agitation or retardation
- Fatigue
- Feelings of worthlessness or inappropriate guilt
- Reduced ability to concentrate
- Recurrent thoughts of death or suicide

Step 3. Differentiating symptoms from depression and cancer

- Late insomnia: waking up in the middle of the night with difficulty falling back to sleep because of worry or concern
- Mood variation: the patient may not report being depressed all of the time, but may report consistent depressed mood in the morning or evening
- Anxiety
- Agitation
- Loss of sexual interest

a suicide rate of 31.4 per 100 000 person-years, compared to a suicide rate of 16.7 in the general US population.[37] Factors associated with higher risk included male gender, older age at diagnosis, white race, and cancers of the lung, stomach, and head and neck.[37]

Treatment

Whether to initiate therapy for depression depends on the probability that the patient will recover spontaneously in the next 2–4 weeks, the degree of functional impairment, and the severity and duration of the depressive symptoms. Studies show that pharmacotherapy, combined with psychotherapy or psychological support, remain the best primary interventions for MDD.

Pharmacological

According to Chochinov, some general considerations should be kept in mind when selecting an antidepressant. First, the choice of medication is largely dictated by the patient's clinical status. Most antidepressants take 4–6 weeks to achieve their therapeutic effect, so patients whose life

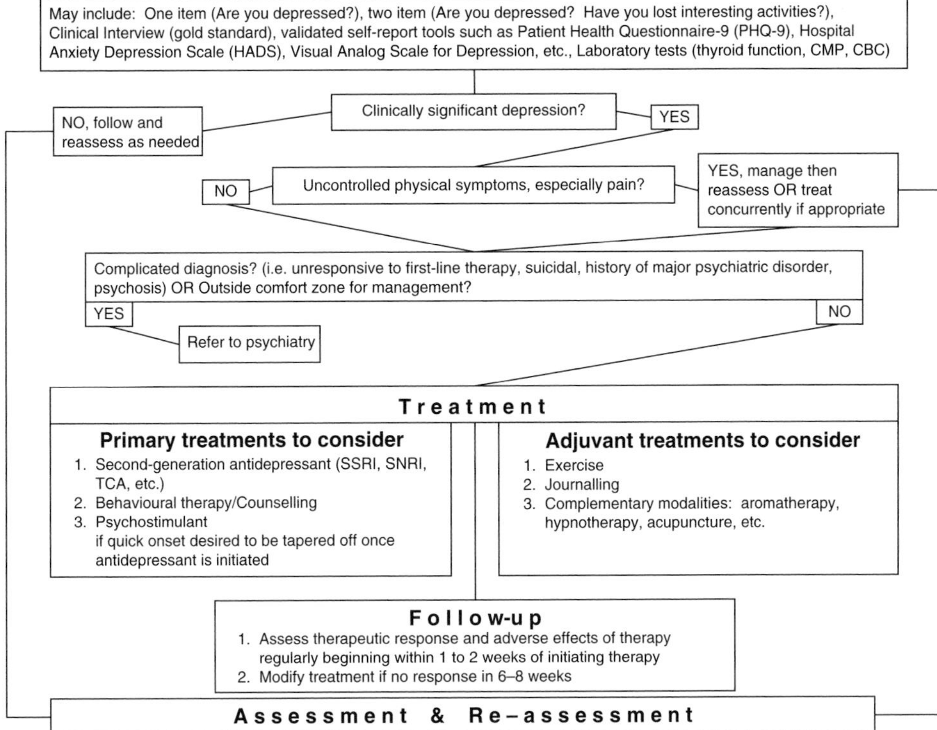

May include: One item (Are you depressed?), two item (Are you depressed? Have you lost interesting activities?), Clinical Interview (gold standard), validated self-report tools such as Patient Health Questionnaire-9 (PHQ-9), Hospital Anxiety Depression Scale (HADS), Visual Analog Scale for Depression, etc., Laboratory tests (thyroid function, CMP, CBC)
Clinically significant depression?
NO, follow and reassess as needed
YES
Uncontrolled physical symptoms, especially pain?
NO
YES, manage then reassess OR treat concurrently if appropriate
Complicated diagnosis? (i.e. unresponsive to first-line therapy, suicidal, history of major psychiatric disorder, psychosis) OR Outside comfort zone for management?
YES
NO
Refer to psychiatry
Treatment
Primary treatments to consider
1. Second-generation antidepressant (SSRI, SNRI, TCA, etc.)
2. Behavioural therapy/Counselling
3. Psychostimulant if quick onset desired to be tapered off once antidepressant is initiated
Adjuvant treatments to consider
1. Exercise
2. Journalling
3. Complementary modalities: aromatherapy, hypnotherapy, acupuncture, etc.
Follow-up
1. Assess therapeutic response and adverse effects of therapy regularly beginning within 1 to 2 weeks of initiating therapy
2. Modify treatment if no response in 6–8 weeks
Assessment & Re–assessment

Fig. 17.1 Algorithm for identification and management of depression in oncology supportive care settings. CMP, comprehensive metabolic panel; CBC, complete blood count; SSRI, selective serotonin reuptake inhibitor; SNRI, serotonin–norepinephrine reuptake inhibitor; TCA, tricyclic antidepressant.

expectancy is thought to be less will require a more rapidly acting drug (i.e. a psychostimulant). Other considerations for determining the best pharmacological therapy in an individual include a history of particular psychoactive medications that have been successful or unsuccessful in the past, or whether a first-degree relative has responded to a specific antidepressant. Depressed cancer patients are frequently taking several medications so possible drug interactions should also be considered.

Selective serotonin reuptake inhibitors (SSRIs) have become the preferred class of antidepressants for treating clinically depressed cancer patients,[35] although no antidepressant or class of antidepressants is shown to be superior in the management of the depressed cancer patient.[38] Mirtazapine may have a dual role in cancer patients who are experiencing anorexia since increased appetite is a common side-effect of this medication.[39] There is growing evidence supporting the use of methylphenidate for depression in cancer patients based on its quick response time and its effect on concomitant symptoms including fatigue, sedation and poor concentration.[3]

Early evidence suggests that psychotropic medications may have a role in the management of non-depressed individuals with primary cachexia. Mirtazapine has been tested in this setting, and early findings suggest benefit. Similarly, olanzapine may improve appetite in patients with cancer, without other indications for the medication. Utilization of psychotropic medications for the management of primary cachexia is off-label, and evidence is insufficient to support such a recommendation at this time.

According to the National Cancer Institute, antidepressant therapy should be continued for a minimum of 4–6 months after the depression resolves. When discontinuing treatment, the antidepressant agent should be gradually tapered.

Non-pharmacological management of depression and weight loss

As in non-cancer populations, psychotherapies appear to help depressed cancer patients. These therapies include psycho-educational interventions, cognitive behaviour therapy (CBT), interpersonal therapy, and problem-solving therapy. CBT is helpful in depressed cancer patients, particularly when combining behavioural activation with cognitive techniques.[40] These interventions focus on altering specific coping strategies aimed at improving overall adjustment and typically focus on specific thoughts and their relationship to emotions and behaviours. Some other goals of psychotherapy include enhancing coping skills, directly reducing distress, improving problem-solving techniques,[35–38] mobilizing support and developing a close relationship with a knowledgeable empathic health care provider.

Outside of behavioural and psychotherapies some people find meeting with a cleric or a member of a pastoral care unit to be beneficial. Also, cancer support groups are finding their way into many mediums such as face-to-face meetings, over the internet or chat rooms, making them increasingly accessible. These are instant support networks that may show the health benefits found in other forms of social support.

Complementary and alternative medicine (CAM) provides another approach to treating depression. CAM is a group of diverse medical and health care systems, practices, and products that are not generally considered part of conventional medicine (see Chapter 25). This overarching term includes therapies ranging from herbal supplements, movement therapy (i.e. yoga, tai chi), massage therapy, imagery and relation therapies, and acupuncture. Research into the safety and effectiveness of these therapies in cancer patients suffering from depression is limited. All patients interested in including CAM in their treatment should do so in collaboration with their medical practitioner. This is especially important when herbs and supplements are used, because of potential interactions with medications.

Physical activity in populations without illness increases appetite, enhances sensitivity to caloric needs, and modulates the immune system. Because proinflammatory cytokines play a role in the aetiology of depression, cachexia, fatigue and cancer treatment response, some researchers suggest an increase in physical activity and reduced fat intake could benefit symptoms and even prognosis.

Conclusion

Depression is a common comorbid disorder among cancer patients, presenting with depressed mood, loss of interest or pleasure, feelings of guilt or low self-worth, disturbed sleep or appetite, low energy and poor concentration. These problems can become chronic or recurrent and lead to substantial impairments in an individual's ability to take care of everyday responsibilities. Depression may be important in initiating or exacerbating unintentional weight loss among cancer patients, and both depression and associated fatigue should be addressed in the evaluation of cachectic cancer patients. Depression should be routinely screened for among cancer patients, especially those experiencing unintentional weight loss, and a low threshold should be maintained for initiating treatment.

References

1. World Health Organization (2009) Depression. Available from: http://www.who.int/mental_health/management/depression/definition/en/index.html (accessed 26 January 2009).

2. Dy SM, Lorenz KA, Naeim A, Sanati H, Walling A, Asch SM (2008) Evidence-based recommendations for cancer fatigue, anorexia, depression, and dyspnea. *J Clin Oncol*, **26**(23), 3886–95.
3. Pirl WF (2004) Evidence report on the occurrence, assessment, and treatment of depression in cancer patients. *J Natl Cancer Inst Monogr*, 32, 32–9.
4. Cancer Topics: Overview.; Available from: http://www.cancer.gov/cancertopics/pdq/supportivecare/depression/healthprofessional/page2 (accessed 2009 January 26).
5. Spencer S, Carver C, Price A (1998) Psychological and social factors in adaptation. In: Holland J (ed.), *Psycho-oncology*, pp. 211–22. New York: Oxford University Press.
6. Stoner S, Marken P, Sommi R (1998) Psychiatric comorbidity and medical illness. *Med Update Psychiatrists*, **3**(3), 64–70.
7. Payne M (2009) Nutrition and late-life depression. In: Bales CW, Ritchie CS (eds), *Handbook of Clinical Nutrition and Aging*, pp. 523–35. New York: Humana Press.
8. Tian J, Chen ZC, Hang LF (2007) Effects of nutritional and psychological status in gastrointestinal cancer patients on tolerance of treatment. *World J Gastroenterol*, **13**(30), 4136–40.
9. De Boer MF, McCormick LK, Pruyn JF, Ryckman RM, van den Borne BW (1999) Physical and psychosocial correlates of head and neck cancer: a review of the literature. *Otolaryngol Head Neck Surg*, **120**(3), 427–36.
10. O'Rourke RW, Diggs BS, Spight DH, *et al.* (2008) Psychiatric illness delays diagnosis of esophageal cancer. *Dis Esophagus*, **21**(5), 416–21.
11. Howren MB, Lamkin DM, Suls J (2009) Associations of depression with C-reactive protein, IL-1, and IL-6: a meta-analysis. *Psychosom Med*, **71**(2), 171–86.
12. Musselman DL, Miller AH, Porter MR, *et al.* (2001) Higher than normal plasma interleukin-6 concentrations in cancer patients with depression: preliminary findings. *Am J Psychiatry*, **158**(8), 1252–7.
13. Meyers CA, Albitar M, Estey E (2005) Cognitive impairment, fatigue, and cytokine levels in patients with acute myelogenous leukemia or myelodysplastic syndrome. *Cancer*, **104**(4), 788–93.
14. Bower JE, Ganz PA, Aziz N, Fahey JL (2001) Fatigue and proinflammatory cytokine activity in breast cancer survivors. *Psychosom Med*, **64**, 604–11.
15. Jacobson CM, Rosenfeld B, Pessin H, Breitbart W (2008) Depression and IL-6 blood plasma concentrations in advanced cancer patients. *Psychosomatics*, **49**(1), 64–6.
16. Capuron L, Gumnick JF, Musselman DL, *et al.* (2002) Neurobehavioral effects of interferon-alpha in cancer patients: phenomenology and paroxetine responsiveness of symptom dimensions. *Neuropsychopharmacology*, **26**(5), 643–52.
17. Capuron L, Neurauter G, Musselman DL, *et al.* (2003) Interferon-alpha-induced changes in tryptophan metabolism. Relationship to depression and paroxetine treatment. *Biol Psychiatry*, **54**(9), 906–14.
18. Capuron L, Raison CL, Musselman DL, Lawson DH, Nemeroff CB, Miller AH (2003) Association of exaggerated HPA axis response to the initial injection of interferon-alpha with development of depression during interferon-alpha therapy. *Am J Psychiatry*, **160**(7), 1342–5.
19. Dantzer R BR, Kent S, Goodall G (1993) Behavioral effects of cytokines: an insight into mechanisms of sickness behavior. *Methods Neurosci*, **17**,130–50.
20. Kelley KW, Bluthe RM, Dantzer R, *et al.* (2003) Cytokine-induced sickness behavior. *Brain Behav Immun*, **17**, S112–S8.
21. Cleeland CS, Bennett GJ, Dantzer R, *et al.* (2003) Are the symptoms of cancer and cancer treatment due to a shared biologic mechanism? A cytokine–immunologic model of cancer symptoms. *Cancer*, **97**(11), 2919–25.
22. Lee BN, Dantzer R, Langley KE, *et al.* (2004) A cytokine-based neuroimmunologic mechanism of cancer-related symptoms. *Neuroimmunomodulation*, **11**(5), 279–92.
23. Kurzrock R (2001) The role of cytokines in cancer-related fatigue. *Cancer*, **92**, 1684–8.

24. Stone P, Richardson A, Ream E, Smith AG, Kerr DJ, Kearney N (2001) Cancer-related fatigue: inevitable, unimportant and untreatable? Cancer Fatigue Forum. *Ann Oncol*, **11**(8), 971–5.
25. Chang VT, Hwang SS, Feuerman M, Kasimis BS (2000) Symptom and quality of life survey of medical oncology patients at a veterans affairs medical center: a role for symptom assessment. *Cancer*, **88**(5), 1175–83.
26. Rich T, Innominato PF, Boerner J, *et al.* (2005) Elevated serum cytokines correlated with altered behavior, serum cortisol rhythm, and dampened 24-hour rest–activity patterns in patients with metastatic colorectal cancer. *Clin Cancer Res*, **11**(5), 1757–64.
27. Ahlberg K, Ekman T, Gaston-Johansson F (2004) Levels of fatigue compared to levels of cytokines and hemoglobin during pelvic radiotherapy: a pilot study. *Biol Res Nurs*, **5**(3), 203–10.
28. Kirsh KL, Dugan C, Theobald DE, Passik SD (2003) A chart review, pilot study of two single-item screens to detect cancer patients at risk for cachexia. *Palliat Support Care*, **1**(4), 331–5.
29. Passik SD, Donaghy KB, Theobald DE, Lundberg JC, Holtsclaw E, Dugan WM (2000) Oncology staff recognition of depressive symptoms on videotaped interviews of depressed cancer patients: implications for designing a training program. *J Pain Sympt Manag*, **19**(5), 329–38.
30. Passik SD, Dugan W, McDonald MV, Rosenfeld B, Theobald DE, Edgerton S (1998) Oncologists' recognition of depression in their patients with cancer. *J Clin Oncol*, **16**(4), 1594–600.
31. Chochinov HM, Wilson KG, Enns M, Lander S (1997) "Are you depressed?" Screening for depression in the terminally ill. *Am J Psychiatry*, **154**(5), 674–6.
32. Zigmond AS, Snaith RP (1983) The hospital anxiety and depression scale. *Acta Psychiatr Scand*, **67**(6), 361–70.
33. Beck AT, Ward CH, Mendelson M, Mock J, Erbaugh J (1961) An inventory for measuring depression. *Arch Gen Psychiatry*, **4**, 561–71.
34. Berard RM, Boermeester F, Viljoen G (1998) Depressive disorders in an out-patient oncology setting: prevalence, assessment, and management. *Psychooncology*, **7**(2), 112–20.
35. Chochinov HM (2001) Depression in cancer patients. *Lancet Oncol*, **2**(8), 499–505.
36. American Psychiatric Association (1994) *Diagnostic and Statistical Manual of Mental Disorders*, 4th edn. Washington, DC: AMA.
37. Misono S, Weiss NS, Fann JR, Redman M, Yueh B (2008) Incidence of suicide in persons with cancer. *J Clin Oncol*, **26**(29), 4731–8.
38. Valentine AD (2003) Cancer pain and depression: management of the dual-diagnosed patient. *Curr Pain Headache Rep*, **7**(4), 262–9.
39. Davis MP, Dickerson ED, Pappagallo M, Benedetti C, Grauer PA, Lycan J (2001) Mirtazapine: heir apparent to amitriptyline? *Am J Hosp Palliat Care*, **18**(1), 42–6.
40. Weinberger MI, Roth AJ, Nelson CJ (2009) Untangling the complexities of depression diagnosis in older cancer patients. *Oncologist*, **14**(1), 60–6.

Part 5

Nutritional counselling

Chapter 18

Counselling by dietitians

Laura Elliott and Barbara Parry

Introduction

Nutrition plays a vital role in the care of a patient diagnosed with cancer. A third of all cancers diagnosed in 2009 were related to suboptimal diets, physical inactivity, and/or overweight and obesity.[1] Previous studies suggest that cancer patients are highly motivated to make positive changes in their health behaviours,[2] and oncology dietitians often are able to capitalize on such teachable moments to facilitate change.[3] In the USA, there is recognition of the importance of the dietitian in care of the patient with cancer; the 650 Association of Comprehensive Cancer Centers and 1435 programmes accredited by the Commission on Cancer include nutrition as an integral component of comprehensive cancer care.[4,5] A multidisciplinary approach is sought as the best way to assure the provision of quality care to the patient with cancer, and the dietitian is considered an important member of that team. Similarly, within the UK, the dietitian's role within a multidisciplinary care team is recognized, particularly where nutritional support needs are identified for a patient.[6,7]

The comprehensive education of a dietitian, not only in areas of diet, foods and nutrition, but also in counselling, psychosocial aspects of health, economics, physiology and chemistry, lends a unique blend of knowledge and expertise that can be communicated to both the patient and the patient's family members. This unique expertise both distinguishes and establishes the dietitian as a key member of the health care team.

Early nutrition assessment and intervention for improved outcomes

Recent studies evaluating nutrition interventions have shown improved outcomes with early nutrition screening, frequent monitoring, intervention as needed, and follow-up of cancer patients.[8–21] Both the National Institute for Health and Clinical Excellence in the UK[6] and the American Dietetic Association recognize the role of the dietitian and provide guidelines for nutritional care.[6,22] The Evidence Analysis Library of the American Dietetic Association currently includes 31 recommendations for eight specific cancer diagnoses.[22] Furthermore, these guidelines also include additional recommendations that highlight the importance of early and frequent contact by a dietitian for patients with head and neck, oesophageal, colon, and haematopoietic cancers (see Table 18.1).

To summarize, these studies found that compared to no intervention or to an intervention with only a medical food supplement, early screening in selected cancers and frequent intervention by a dietitian improved the preservation of weight and fat-free mass, and also increased treatment tolerance. Nutrition intervention provides positive outcomes in cancer patients including maintenance of an appropriate weight status, an adequate energy and protein intake, minimizing the symptoms of anorexia, nausea, vomiting and diarrhoea, and enhancing quality of life. Individualized dietary counselling has been acknowledged as the most effective nutrition intervention.[8]

Table 18.1 Summary of Oncology Nutrition, Medical Nutrition Therapy (MNT) recommendations from the Evidence Analysis Library, American Dietetic Association[22]

Type of cancer	Recommendation
Colorectal cancer, radiation therapy and MNT[8]	Dietitians should provide weekly MNT that includes an individualized nutrition prescription and counselling for patients with colorectal cancer undergoing pelvic radiation. Individualized counselling with a focus on the consumption of regular foods may improve calorie and protein intake, nutrition status, quality of life and reduce symptoms of anorexia, nausea, vomiting and diarrhoea. **Rating: Fair** Imperative
Oesophageal cancer, chemoradiation and MNT[9]	The dietitian should provide MNT consisting of a pre-treatment evaluation and weekly visits for six weeks during chemoradiation treatment for oesophageal cancer to improve outcomes. MNT may reduce the amount of weight loss, unplanned hospitalizations, length of stay, as well as improving tolerance to treatment and the likelihood of receiving prescribed radiation dose. **Rating: Weak** Imperative
Head and neck cancer, MNT and radiation therapy[10–13]	MNT that consists of nutrition assessment, intensive intervention, and ongoing monitoring and evaluation by a registered dietitian should be provided for patients with head/neck cancer being considered for radiation therapy. MNT has been shown to improve calorie and protein intake, maintain anthropometric measurements and improve quality of life. **Rating: Strong** Imperative
Head and neck cancer, pretreatment evaluation and radiation therapy[10–13]	The dietitian should provide MNT consisting of a pre-treatment evaluation and weekly visits during radiation treatment for head and neck cancer to improve outcomes. **Rating: Strong** Imperative
Haematological cancer, MNT and chemotherapy[14]	MNT that consists of nutrition assessment, intensive intervention, and ongoing monitoring and evaluation by a registered dietitian may be of benefit to patients with acute leukaemias undergoing chemotherapy. Daily monitoring of intake and incorporating patient preferences have been shown to increase nutrition intake which positively affects body weight and tumour therapy side-effects (e.g. fatigue and anorexia). **Rating: Weak** Imperative
Lung cancer, MNT and chemotherapy[15]	MNT that consists of nutrition assessment, intensive intervention, and ongoing monitoring and evaluation by a registered dietitian may be of benefit to patients with small cell lung cancer undergoing chemotherapy. Providing MNT may improve protein and calorie intake, which has been shown to improve weight status and quality of life. **Rating: Weak** Imperative

American Dietetics Association Evidence Analysis Library Oncology Recommendations, Executive Summary. http://www.adaevidencelibrary.com/default.cfm (accessed 16 November 2008). © American Dietetic Association. Reprinted with permission. Evidence-based Nutrition Practice Guideline on Oncology published on October 2007 at http://www.adaevidencelibrary.com/topic.cfm?cat=2819 and copyrighted by the American Dietetic Association. Evidence-based Nutrition Practice Guidelines are intended to serve as synthesis of the best evidence available to inform registered dietitians as they individualize nutrition care for their clients.Guidelines are provided with the express understanding that they do not establish or specific particular standards of care, whether legal, medical or other.

Cancer patients have a variety of nutritional needs which vary according to their diagnosis, stage of disease, treatment, and response to treatment. A dietitian's input to a patient's care plan is, therefore, individually tailored to the patient's needs, and engages the patient in the process of decision-making wherever possible. An assessment of current nutritional intake, current nutritional problems, the degree or likelihood of nutritional depletion, and the nutritional implications of specific cancer types form the basis of appropriate dietary counselling.[7]

The dietitian: education, training and certification

The British Dietetic Association (BDA) defines the role of the registered dietitian as follows:

> Registered Dietitians (RDs) are the only qualified health professionals that assess, diagnose and treat diet and nutrition problems at an individual and wider public health level. Uniquely, dietitians use the most up-to-date public health and scientific research on food, health and disease, which they translate into practical guidance to enable people to make appropriate lifestyle and food choices.[23]

The title 'dietitian' is protected by statute in the UK and a registered dietitian will most commonly have completed a Bachelor of Science Honours degree in dietetics or nutrition and dietetics from a training programme that has been accredited by the Health Professions Council to ensure subsequent eligibility for registration. Less commonly, holding a degree in a life science subject may allow a prospective dietitian to qualify by completing a two-year post-graduate course in dietetics.[24] The optimally trained oncology dietitian also is registered with a professional association, is a member of a specialist group of practising dietitians, and seeks out formal qualifications in their chosen field. In the UK, professional registration with the Dietitians' Board of the Health Professions Council (HPC) is mandatory for employment within the National Health Service. Specialist-level oncology expertise can be nurtured 'on the job', as a newly qualified dietitian develops professionally within a health service position. Further, opportunity exists for members of the BDA to join the oncology specialist group for support and continuing professional education. The Oncology Group was established in 1988 and was formally recognized as a specialist group of the BDA in 1998. The Oncology Group convenes regular meetings, publishes and distributes a periodic newsletter, and aims to be a resource for all dietitians working with cancer patients.[25]

Similarly, a registered dietitian in the USA must have completed undergraduate, and in many cases, graduate training within ADA certified academic programmes. Such training provides medically oriented coursework with an emphasis in human nutrition in health and disease, food composition, food science, adult education, counselling principles, critical thinking, statistics, world food issues and food law, as well as food production and food service systems management.[26] This coursework is then followed by an internship that provides educational opportunities for observation and experience in a myriad of settings within hospitals, clinics, food service operations, as well as various sites within the community, such as public health clinics and schools. This foundational experience provides exposure to evidence-based practice and also includes experience in professional communication, the development of collaborative relationships, and the management of food and human resources.[27] Registration examinations are offered to individuals who complete both an ADA-certified degree programme and internship; individuals who pass the examination earn the credentials of registered dietitian (RD). As in the UK, dietitians' knowledge specific to the field of oncology nutrition is gained from experience, as well as individual study. Aiding the practice of oncology dietitians within the USA is the Oncology Nutrition Dietetic Practice Group (ONDPG) of the ADA. This professional group is comprised of more than 1500 dietitians in 24 countries who practice or have interest in the broad field of oncology nutrition and applications in areas of prevention, treatment, recovery, palliative and hospice care, education, industry, and research. Special interest groups within the ONDPG include prevention, complementary and alternative medicine, survivorship, hospice and palliative care, research and pediatrics. The ONDPG has an active electronic mailing list with communication on emerging nutrition and oncology research, topics of interest or patient challenges and solutions, a website with news, resources and patient education resources;[28] a quarterly peer-reviewed newsletter; and an active publications team that develops resources for the membership. Affiliation with the ONDPG, and the support it provides in terms of interactions with other oncology nutrition professionals, as well as resources to guide current practice in an area which is constantly experiencing update, is vital to assuring quality practice of the oncology dietitian, who often is a sole oncology nutrition practitioner within an institution. The goal of this practice group is to develop and assure standards of practice and standards of professional performance in order to maintain best practice using evidence-based resources, including books, videos, toolkits, a website, and listserve.[29] In 2008, the ONDPG secured board certification in oncology nutrition for its membership. Certification enhances education and training of the oncology nutrition practitioner, promotes standards of practice and expertise, provides credibility and recognition of specialty experience, skills and expertise, as well as helping patients with cancer to navigate through the maze of cancer information and help them make informed decisions.[30] Dietitians who successfully complete the examination are able to use the credentials CSO (certified specialist in oncology) along with their RD credentials.[31]

Continuing education

In common with many other professions, a registered dietitian is required to undertake continuing professional education in order to maintain their fitness to practice. In the UK, the HPC requires a registrant to: (1) maintain a continuous, up-to-date and accurate record of their continuing professional development (CPD) activities; (2) demonstrate that their CPD activities are a mixture of learning activities relevant to current or future practice; (3) seek to ensure that their CPD has contributed to the quality of their practice and service delivery; (4) seek to ensure that their CPD benefits the service user; and (5) present a written profile containing evidence of their CPD on request.[32] In the USA, the RD must complete 75 h of continuing education credits every 5 years to maintain registration status.[33]

Guidance of practice

In the UK, the HPC defines standards of character, health, conduct, performance, ethics, proficiency, education and training and CPD.[32] Similarly, the ADA's code of ethics guides the practice of dietitians in the USA,[34] and provides guidance in sensitive situations that arise from conflicting patient goals, family wishes and medical practice.

The nutrition care process

The nutrition care process, as described by the ADA, is shown in Figure 18.1. It represents the complexity of qualifications, activities and decisions made by a dietitian as an active part of a multidisciplinary care team,[35] and summarizes nutrition screening, assessment, intervention, and evaluation.

Nutrition screening

Nutrition screening prepares a dietitian for the first consultation with a patient. It provides adequate and accurate background information, and defines the reason for the dietetic referral. Where there may be high demand for limited dietetic resources, the nutrition screening process also provides a basis for prioritizing patient contact. In certain instances, this may involve the use of a validated

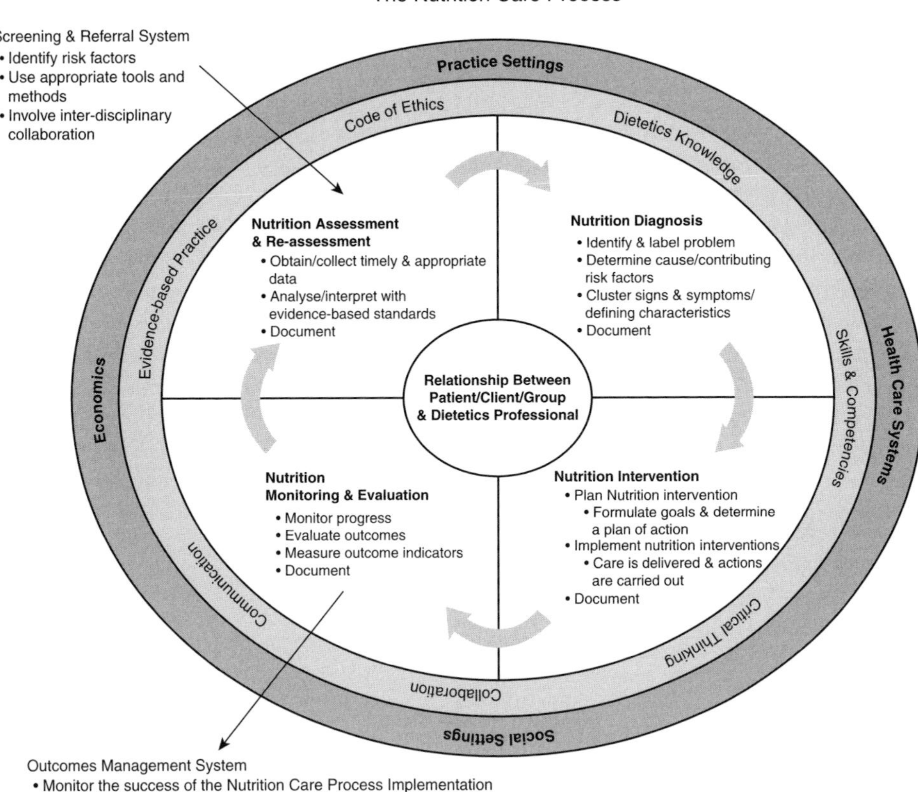

Fig. 18.1 Nutrition care process and model.
Reproduced from [29], with permission from Elsevier

screening tool to identify patients requiring nutrition intervention, and is aimed at preventing acute nutritional problems.[16] A number of nutrition screening tools are in use within health care. For example, the Patient-Generated Subjective Global Assessment (PG-SGA) is used in the USA and it includes an assessment of weight history, nutritional intake, patients' self-rated performance status and nutrition-related symptoms.[36] An equivalent tool used in the UK is the Malnutrition Universal Screening Tool (MUST), developed and validated by the British Association for Parenteral and Enteral Nutrition and its standing committee, the Malnutrition Advisory Group.[37]

Referral to a dietitian also may be triggered by clinical indicators such as weight loss of more than 5 pounds in one week; manifestation of symptoms affecting adequate nutrition such as nausea, vomiting or diarrhoea; manifestation of other symptoms that affect appetite including fatigue, pain and constipation; and/or the impact of various forms of treatment, including surgery, chemotherapy and/or radiation therapy. Multidisciplinary oncology teams that include the dietitian facilitate the nutrition care process.

In free-standing or tertiary cancer centres, this model may be routinely and formally used to assure optimal nutrition care. In smaller general hospitals, where cancer is treated in addition to many other diseases, a dietitian's regular ward visits may initiate referrals from both medical and allied health staff, as well as self-referrals from patients and their family members who have nutrition concerns or questions.

Nutrition assessment

Comprehensive assessment of the nutritional needs of a cancer patient considers the physical and psychosocial circumstances of the patient, as well as the effects of the disease and its treatment (see Figure 18.2).[7] Anxiety about cancer diagnosis, and feelings of depression following its confirmation, may adversely affect appetite. Food intake also may be impaired due to dysphagia, pain, vomiting and/or diarrhoea. Tumour growth itself may increase metabolic rate and increase energy needs.[38]

Consideration also should be given to the proposed treatment, past medical history including comorbidities, weight status prior to the onset of symptoms, current weight status, usual and current food intake, nutrition problems experienced, medications, and psychosocial factors including support systems available to the patient (see Chapter 3 for more information on nutrition assessment).

For many patients, the risk of undernutrition is high. Overall, Ravasco *et al.*[39] estimated that significant protein-energy malnutrition affects about 40% of advanced stage cancer patients.[39] For some cancer diagnoses up to 80% of patients may be malnourished at the time of diagnosis, e.g. cancers of the head and neck. Malnutrition can adversely affect not only treatment tolerance but also quality of life.

It also should be recognized that a cancer diagnosis does not automatically mean that nutrition intake deteriorates and that weight loss is inevitable. In breast cancer patients, more than 60% are likely to gain weight during the first year following diagnosis which, in itself, may impair prognosis

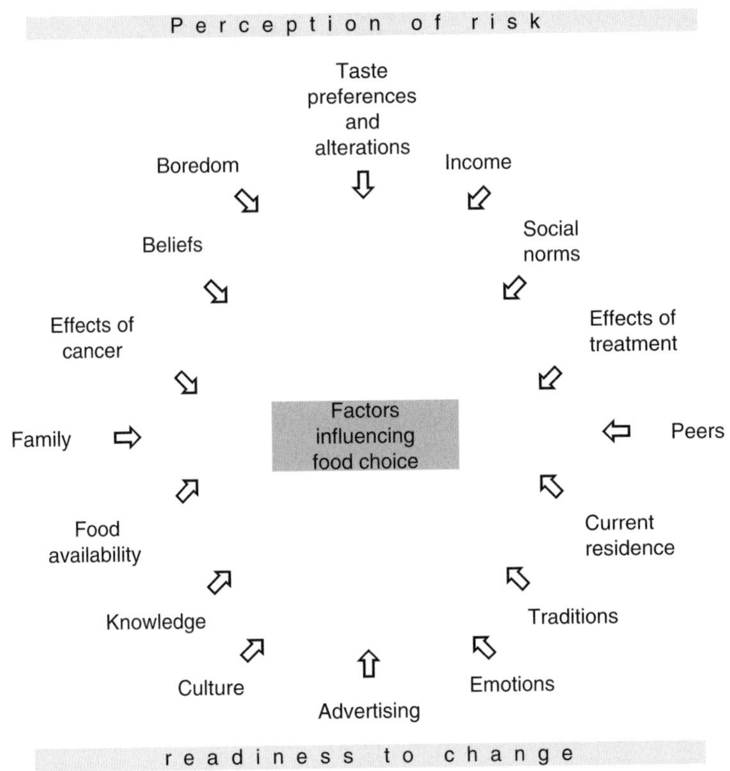

Fig. 18.2 Factors influencing food choice.

by increasing the risk of recurrence (see Chapter 27 regarding nutritional issues related to cancer survivorship).[40,41] While weight gain often is an unexpected consequence of cancer treatment, it provides yet another opportunity for a dietitian's expertise to be engaged in the promotion of the benefits of healthy eating and physical activity to such patients.

Nutrition intervention

Oncology interventions may range from providing simple symptom-related information to calculating involved plans with goals for calorie and protein intake or advising on the establishment of artificial feeding using enteral or parenteral nutrition. Communicating effectively with other members of the health care team regarding the potential need for feeding tubes and arranging for enteral formulae are essential to ensure that the patient's nutritional needs are met. Decisions should, wherever possible, be made jointly with the patients themselves and/or their family or caregivers. Dietitians will use their skills to provide appropriately targeted messages to all those involved in a patient's care and they also will intervene should problems arise which affect a patient's tolerance of the nutrition intervention recommended. Seeking a solution that is acceptable to the patient and their family members is essential if the intervention is to effectively meet nutritional needs throughout the course of the disease process (see Chapter 9 and 25 for detailed information on nutraceuticals and Chapters 13–17 for recommendations regarding nutrition-related symptom management).

Nutrition evaluation

Once a nutrition goal is established, evaluation should occur regularly and adjustments made as needed. If this is done in a timely fashion, patient care is enhanced and the probability of improved nutritional status is increased. Good practice dictates regular follow-up to evaluate the effectiveness of the interventions, and to provide responsive patient care.

Communication with other members of the multidisciplinary team is essential for good patient management and is an essential quality in a registered dietitian.[42,43] The ADA has created standardized language for use in charting patient visits that communicates, in clear and consistent language, a description of services the dietitian provides. The International Dietetics and Nutrition Terminology (IDNT) Reference Manual serves as a resource for the use of standardized language.[44] In the UK, effective communication is a recognised skill for all members of the health care team and communication skills training is recommended and supported by the Department of Health.[45]

Patient nutrition education

Good communication skills also underpin the effectiveness of nutrition education for patients and their families and/or caregivers. Changes in diet and other lifestyle factors, in the interest of improving prognosis or overall health and quality of life, may be facilitated by capitalizing on the 'teachable moment' that a cancer diagnosis may create.[46] A patients' perceived personal risk and level of worry and the challenges presented by a critical diagnosis may make patients more likely to implement change. Cancer patients also are motivated by their symptoms, and targeted messages that offer relief are often well received.

Good practice in patient communication and sharing of information is facilitated by:

- Seeking opportunities to meet the patient early in their treatment course in order to establish a comfortable relationship conducive to helpful communication throughout the course of cancer care.
- Taking account of a patient's history, treatment plan, goals for treatment, home situation, assistance available from the community and a patient's expressed well-being and degree of fatigue.

Reviewing relevant medical history information (both written and verbal from other members of the health care team) prior to a consultation can avoid overburdening the patient with excessive questions, and enhance rapport. This enables the dietitian to utilize their time with the patient more effectively and allows for more focused questioning and responses within a consultation.

- Meeting in as comfortable an environment as possible, providing advice in a calm, non-threatening manner to put the patient at ease during what may be a stressful time. Consideration of the wider factors influencing food choice such as a patient's social environment and socio-economic status is important for appropriately tailoring the intervention. Frequently the dietitian is asked to visit a patient to discuss a specific eating problem or symptom, which allows the dietitian to capitalize on teachable moments to provide this information.
- Involving family members or a caregiver can enhance the nutrition education process during a hospital stay, and can provide information in writing which may be of particular use once the patient is discharged. The provision of written guidance and an explanation of the goals of a nutrition intervention communicated through multiple channels enhances adherence and frees patients from being dependent on their memory, reducing patient burden and distress.
- Conducting interviews with the dietitian seated, if possible, to relax the patient while maintaining a respectful distance, and appropriate eye contact to establish good rapport. The dietitian should listen attentively and respectfully, asking questions in a way that is sensitive to the patient's clinical circumstances—for example, being mindful to keep the consultation as brief as possible should a patient be tired or emotionally distressed. Empathy is a key skill which is relevant to both effective communication and the ethos of a health care professional.
- Targeting nutrition messages to the problem at hand or, if the visit is made in advance of symptoms, providing information in a clear and concise way to avoid overwhelming the patient and their family members.[47–49] Sensitive recognition of a patient's level of literacy is an important factor in effectively communicating nutrition messages. Ideally, any written materials provided will have been assessed for readability (e.g. using the Flesch–Kinkade readability score or other index). In the UK, commercially published literature may be 'crystal marked' by the Plain English Campaign for clarity of content and readability.[50]
- Assisting a patient with understanding and processing the information given by other practitioners may enhance rapport in a dietetic consultation. Questions should be responded to, requesting additional assistance from colleagues within the health care team as necessary. The key lies in fostering good team communication and keeping the interests of the patient at the forefront of care.
- Providing a way in which the dietitian may be contacted following a consultation should the patient have further nutritional queries. Given the likelihood of changing nutritional needs during the course of cancer care, patients should be provided with the dietitian's contact information should their needs change or questions arise.
- Once a good relationship has been established, very brief, targeted interactions are possible that can achieve good outcomes in an efficient manner.

Oncology dietitians in practice

The oncology dietitian may practice in a variety of arenas. While many work as staff in hospitals and provide services to the oncology patient, some may work in other settings, including radiation centres, medical oncology physician practices and hospice and palliative care establishments. In addition, oncology specialist dietitians may contribute to the training of other dietitians, perform oncology-related research, or respond to the needs of cancer patients through consultancy roles within local or national cancer charities.

Registered dietitians in the hospital

The therapy provided in a hospital setting is, often, more acute in nature, and a patient may be too ill or fatigued to receive much in the way of dietary counselling. Under such circumstances, dietitians may be consulted to provide direct nutritional support without directly engaging the patient, but involving family members wherever possible. As a patient is prepared for discharge to home, or perhaps transfer to another health care establishment, the opportunity to provide dietary guidance and counselling may be more appropriate. A hospital stay may, however, provide many opportunities for brief interactions and messages that provide information and reinforcement.[47–49] Reducing the length of a patient's hospital stay to a minimum is recommended by government agencies to reduce risk of infection and overall health care costs.[51] Length of hospital stay may therefore be brief and restricted to intensive symptom management for oncology patients.[52]

A longer stay in hospital may allow for close monitoring of intake, perhaps using a food chart where food and drinks consumed by a patient are recorded and actual nutritional intake can be quantified. Although the patient's intake while in the hospital may not be an accurate reflection of intake at home, it provides a basis for discussing the types and amounts of foods needed to maintain weight and provide adequate nutrition.[19] In addition, the hospital dietitian may be called upon to calculate intake in the assessment of a patient who is to receive enteral nutrition (tube feeding) or parenteral nutrition (intravenous feeding) (see Part 6).

Registered dietitians in radiation centres or medical oncology outpatient departments

Outpatient clinic consultations allow for more anticipatory counselling, particularly when a nutrition screening tool is used that is sensitive enough to identify patients prior to the onset of symptoms. Because dietary issues can arise, increase in prevalence, and persist throughout all stages of cancer care, screening is important before, during and after treatment with referrals to a dietitian, if warranted.[53] The patient's care plan should reflect any changing needs. Similarly, clinical guidelines and oncology care pathways should alert the wider health care team towards appropriate referral to a dietitian at any stages of cancer care.[6]

An outpatient consultation may offer an opportunity for education prior to the placement of a feeding tube, discussion of food hygiene practices in the home or management of cancer-related symptoms. Should patients be identified as at increased risk of a future cancer diagnosis, an outpatient dietitian may lead or contribute to a programme of cancer prevention classes and demonstrations, and/or share information by constructing displays and contributing articles to newsletters. Further, an oncology dietitian also may be involved in cancer survivor education, providing information on healthy diet and health-directed behaviours to enhance quality of life and reduce the risk of a future cancer diagnosis.[54,55]

Registered dietitians in hospice and palliative care

Although patients in hospice or palliative care may have less interest in food and eating, the dietitian's responsibility to these patients and their families is no less important than in the acute health care setting. Hospice and palliative care work may offer a greater amount of time for the dietitian to discuss and address eating problems and feeding issues. Hydration and feeding are sensitive issues in end-of-life care. Achieving optimal nutritional solutions for both patients and their families may involve many hours of discussion with the wider health care team.

In the UK, the Liverpool Care Pathway[56] provides an example for best practice in end-of-life care. A hospice dietitian should have a sensitivity and understanding of the medico-legal aspects of feeding, be familiar with the landmark nutrition support cases, and have good communication and counselling skills in order to successfully contribute to the discussions that occur regarding end-of-life issues.

As part of the hospice team, the dietitian can help provide justification for admission, calculate total parenteral nutrition or tube feeding regimens, recommend weaning regimens when there is decreased need for enteral or parenteral nutrition, suggest texture and fluid consistency adjustments to prevent aspiration, discuss more palatable food choices, and help relax dietary restrictions as the patient's intake decreases.[57] There also is an opportunity, as in acute care, for collaboration with food service providers to facilitate the dietary interventions recommended, thus integrating the diagnosis, nutritional requirements and a patient's food preferences, to provide the best outcome for the patient at the end of life (see Chapter 30 for more information on palliative care).

Conclusion

The broad education and training that dietitians receive makes them a valuable health care team member. Their background in physiology, nutrition, food science, biochemistry and communications skills makes them uniquely qualified to communicate complicated information to patients and caregivers. Coupled with oncology-specific training, the specialist oncology dietitian is able to integrate detailed information from other health care team members, assess nutritional needs, identify interventions and effectively provide appropriate education to patients, enhancing further the dietitian's role in multidisciplinary care.

References

1. American Cancer Society (2009) *Cancer Facts and Figures, 2009*. Atlanta: American Cancer Society.
2. Griffiths M, Leek C (1995) Patient education needs: opinions of oncology nurses and their patients. *Oncol Nurs Forum*, **22**, 139–44.
3. Demark-Wahnefried W, Aziz NM, Rowland JH, Pinto BM (2005) Riding the crest of the teachable moment: promoting long-term health after the diagnosis of cancer. *J Clin Oncol*, **23**, 5184–830.
4. Association of Comprehensive Community Cancer Centers. *Cancer Program Guidelines*. Available at: http://accc-cancer.org/publications/publications_cpguidelines.asp (accessed 23 October 2008).
5. Commission on Cancer. *Cancer Program Approval*. Available at: http://www.facs.org/cancer/coc/whatis.html (accessed 23 October 2008).
6. National Institute for Clinical Excellence (NICE) (2004) *Improving Supportive and Palliative Care for Adults with Cancer: The Manual*. London: NICE.
7. Thomas B, Bishop J (eds) (2007) *Manual of Dietetic Practice*, 4th edn. Oxford: Blackwell.
8. Ravasco P, Montiero-Grillo I, Vidal P, Camilo M (2005) Dietary counseling improves patient outcomes: a prospective randomized, controlled trial in colorectal cancer patients undergoing radiotherapy. *J Clin Oncol*, **23**, 1431–8.
9. Odelli C, Burgess D, Bateman L, *et al.* (2005) Nutrition support improves patient outcomes, treatment tolerance and admission characteristics in oesophagel cancer. *Clin Oncol*, **17**, 639–45.
10. Gocalves Dias MC, deFatima NM, Nadalin W, Waitberg DL (2005) Nutrition intervention improves the caloric and protein ingestion of head and neck cancer patients under radiotherapy. *Nutr Hosp*, **20**, 320–5.
11. Isenring E, Capra S, Bauer J, Davies PS (2003) The impact of nutrition support on body composition in cancer outpatients receiving radiotherapy. *Acta Diabetol*, **40**(Suppl 1), S162–4.

12. Ravasco P, Montiero-Grillo I, Vidal P, Camilo M (2005) Impact of nutrition on outcome: a prospective randomized controlled trial in patients with head and neck cancer undergoing radiotherapy. *Head Neck*, **8**, 659–68.
13. Dawson ER, Morley SE, Robertson AG, Soutar DS (2001) Increasing dietary supervision can reduce weight loss in oral cancer patients. *Nutr Cancer*, **41**(1–2), 70–74.
14. Ollenschläger G, Thomas W, Konkol K, Diehl V, Roth E (1992) Nutritional behavior and quality of life during oncological polychemotherapy: results of a prospective study on the efficacy of oral nutrition therapy in patients with acute leukaemia. *Eur J Clin Invest*, **22**(8), 546–53.
15. Glimelius B, Birgegard G, Hoffman K, *et al.* (1992) Improved care of patients with small cell lung cancer. *Acta Oncol*, **31**(8), 823–32.
16. Capra S, Ferguson M, Reid K (2001) Cancer: impact of nutrition intervention outcomes—nutrition issues for patients. *Nutrition*, **17**, 769–72.
17. Hill D, Hart K (2001) A practical approach to nutritional support for patients with advanced cancer. *Int J Palliat Nurs*, **7**(7), 317–21.
18. Baldwin C, McGough C, Norman AR, Grost GS, Cunningham DC, Andreyev HJN (2006) Failure of dietetic referral in patients with gastrointestinal cancer and weight loss. *Eur J Cancer*, **42,** 2504–9.
19. Machin J, Shaw C (1998) A multidisciplinary approach to head and neck cancer. *Eur J Cancer Care*, **7**, 93–6.
20. Murphy PM, Modi P, Rahamim J, Wheatley T, Lewis SJ (2006) An investigation into the current peri-operative nutritional management of oesophageal carcinoma patients in major carcinoma centres in England. *Ann R Coll Surg Engl*, **88**, 358–62.
21. Tchekmedyian NS, Zahyna D, Halpert C, Heber D (1992) Clinical sspects of nutrition in advanced cancer. *Oncol* **49**(Suppl 2), 3–7.
22. American Dietetics Association. *Evidence Analysis Library Oncology Recommendations, Executive Summary*. Available at: http://www.adaevidencelibrary.com/default.cfm (accessed 16 November 2008).
23. British Dietetic Association. http://www.bda.uk.com (accessed 23 September 2009).
24. British Dietetic Association. *Want a Career as a Dietitian?* Available at: http://www.bda.uk.com/ced/CareersLeaflet.pdf (accessed 23 September 2009).
25. British Dietetic Association members' website. http://members.bda.uk.com/groups/oncology/index.html (accessed 23 September 2009).
26. Iowa State University. *Dietetics Coursework and Plans*. Available at: http://www.dietetics.iastate.edu/undergrad/program.php#courseworkRD (accessed 23 October 2008).
27. Foundation Knowledge and Competencies for Entry-Level Dietitians (2008) Available at: http://www.eatright.org/cps/rde/xchg/ada/hs.xsl/CADE_16200_ENU_HTML.htm
28. Oncology Nutrition Dietetic Practice Group website. Available at: http://www.oncologynutrition.org (accessed 23 October 2008).
29. American Dietetic Association (2006) Standards of practice and standards of professional performance for registered dietitians (generalist, specialty, and advanced) in oncology nutrition care. *J Am Diet Assoc*, **106**(6), 946–951.e21.
30. Grant B (2008) *Oncol Nutr Connection*, **16**, 5–10.
31. Commission on Dietetic Registration. Board Certified Specialist Eligibility Application and Fee. Available at: http://www.cdrnet.org/certifications/spec/eapplication%20onc.htmCSO (accessed 23 October 2008).
32. Health Professions Council UK. http://www.hpc-uk.org/index.asp (accessed 23 September 2009).
33. *Professional Portfolio Development Guide*. Available at: http://www.cdrnet.org/pdrcenter/portfolioTOC.htmPDP (accessed 23 Oct 2008).
34. Anonymous. Code of ethics (1999) *J Am Diet Assoc*, **99**(1), 109–13.
35. Anonymous. Nutrition care process and model part 1: the 2008 update (2008). *J Am Diet Assn* **108**(7), 1116.

36. Ottery F (1996) Supportive nutritional management of the patient with pancreatic cancer.*Oncology*, **10**(Suppl 9), 26–32.
37. British Association for Parenteral and Enteral Nutrition. *Malnutrition Universal Screening Tool.* Available at: http://www.bapen.org.uk/must_tool.html (accessed 24 September 2009).
38. Bozzetti F (2001) Nutrition support in cancer patients. In Payne-James J, Grimble G, Silk D (eds), *Artificial Nutrition Support in Clinical Practice*, Chapter 37, pp. 639–80. London: Greenwich Medical Media.
39. Ravasco P, Moneiro-Grillo I, Vidal PM, Camilo ME (2003) Nutritional deterioration in cancer: the role of disease and diet. *J Clin Oncol*, **15**, 443–50.
40. Harvie M, Howell A (2005) The need for lifestyle interventions amongst postmenopausal women with early breast cancer. *Women's Health*, **1**(2), 205–23.
41. Carmichael AR (2006) Obesity and prognosis of breast cancer, *Obesity Reviews*, **7**(4), 333–40.
42. Cant RP (2008) Exploring dietitians' verbal and nonverbal communication skills for effective dietitian–patient communication. *J Hum Nutr Diet*, **21**, 502–11.
43. Health Professions Council (2007) *Standards of Proficiency – Dietitians.* London: Health Professions Council.
44. American Dietetic Association (2008) *International Dietetics and Nutrition Terminology (IDNT) Reference Manual: Standardized Language for the Nutrition Care Process*, 1st edn. Chicago: ADA.
45. Department of Health (2003) *Statement of guiding principles relating to the commissioning and provision of communication skills training in pre-registration and undergraduate education for Healthcare Professionals.* Available at: http://www.dh.gov.uk/en/Publicationsandstatistics/Lettersandcirculars/Dearcolleagueletters/DH_4093504 (accessed 28 September 2009).
46. McBride CM, Puleo E, Pollak KI, Clipp EC, Woolford S, Emmons K (2007) Understanding the role of cancer worry in creating a "teachable moment" for multiple risk factor reduction. *Soc Sci Med*, **66**, 790–800.
47. Miller G (1994) The magic number seven, plus or minus two: some limits on our capacity for processing information. *Psychol Rev*, **101**(2), 343–52.
48. American Association fort the Advancement of Science (2008) *Communicating Science, Tools for Scientists and Engineers.* Available at: http://communicatingscience.aaas.org/Pages/newmain.aspx (accessed 16 November 2008).
49. Walker TJ. *Your Message. Media Training Worldwide.* Available at: http://www.mediatrainingworldwide.com (accessed 16 November 2008).
50. Plain English Campaign. http://www.plainenglish.co.uk/crystal_mark (accessed 29 September 2009).
51. Department of Health (2008) *High Quality Health for All – NHS Next Stage Review Final Report*, p. 47. London: Stationery Office.
52. Utilization and Volume. Available at: http://www.aha.org/aha/trendwatch/chartbook/2008/08appendix3.ppt (accessed 16 November 2008).
53. Gosselin TK, Gilliard L, Tinnen R (2008) Assessing the need for a dietitian in radiation oncology. *Clin J Oncol Nurs*, **12**(5), 781–7.
54. Institute of Medicine (2006) *From Cancer Patient to Cancer Survivor: Lost in Transition.* Available at: http://www.IOM.edu (accessed 23 October 2008).
55. World Cancer Research Fund/American Institute for Cancer Research (2007) *Food, Nutrition, Physical Activity and the Prevention of Cancer: a Global Perspective.* Washington DC: AICR.
56. *Liverpool Care Pathway for the Dying Patient.* http://www.endoflifecare.nhs.uk/eolc/lcp.htm (accessed 28 September 2009).
57. Wade E (1984) Nutrition support: enhancing the quality of life of the terminally ill patient with cancer. *J Am Diet Assoc*, **84**(9), 1044–5.

Chapter 19

Multidisciplinary approach to nutritional problems

Colette Hawkins, Inga Andrew, Tessa Aston, Trevelyan Beyer, Jacqueline Cairns, Bob Hansford, Jane Hopkinson, and Caroline Worsfold

Introduction

Living with cancer presents patients and their carers with a wide range of challenging experiences. It also brings them into contact with diverse groups of health care professionals, all bringing a particular perspective and various suggestions for managing problems. Working together, different professional groups can provide comprehensive care for the physical, psychosocial and practical problems the patient may experience. The challenge is to avoid overwhelming the patient with the sheer number of professionals and to avoid duplication of effort or, worse still, contradictory management plans. Role definition, clear to professionals as well as patients and carers, together with excellent communication, is necessary for effective team working.

Multidisciplinary team (MDT) working is central to the provision of effective palliative care. The aim is holistic care focused on the problems and objectives presented by the patient. Palliative Care MDT structures vary widely and still depend heavily on available resources. Nevertheless there is a continued drive to invest in better provision of specialist palliative care and teams are growing. Allied health professionals (AHPs) regularly working in MDTs with specialist nurses and doctors include dietitians, physiotherapists, pharmacists, social workers, occupational therapists, chaplains, and counsellors. Oncologists liaise closely with palliative care MDTs and volunteers offer an invaluable support service to MDTs in hospice units. The MDT approach to care applies to patients in any care setting, not just within specialist inpatient or day care services.

This chapter illustrates the potential benefit to patients and carers from MDT input. Specialists common to many UK cancer and palliative care MDTs present their unique perspective on a familiar clinical scenario relating to nutritional problems. The scenario described below, is fictitious.

> Mr Durham is a 64-year-old man with advanced adenocarcinoma of the pancreas. He has deteriorated despite Gemcitabine chemotherapy. He was admitted from home in to his local hospice because of abdominal pain. This responded quickly to an adjustment to his opioid medication. His family expressed concern about his appearance and poor appetite. He has lost 6 kg in weight over a 4-week period and his appearance has become wasted and gaunt. He has little energy to mobilize. The patient himself reports that he just 'doesn't feel like eating' and he is 'not bothered' by his weight. Family members however, report anxieties about his nutritional intake on a daily basis. They regularly attend the unit at mealtimes in order to encourage him to eat, bring in a range of foods to entice him and coerce him with the hope of him being 'built up' and gaining energy. When they see him continuing to decline, they request nutritional intervention.

Doctor

> 'He's not eating, doctor. He needs to be built up to keep fighting this. What are you going to do about it?' (Mr Durham's wife)

The scenario of carers approaching the doctor to express concern about the patient's poor nutritional intake is very common in the context of advanced cancer. On a human level, it is distressing to see someone unable to eat and lose weight. The sight of a severely cachectic patient can be upsetting to professionals as well as carers. Altered body image can have a profound effect on patients themselves although anxiety around anorexia often affects carers more than the patients themselves.[1]

Medical training tends to focus on a problem-solving approach. Consequently, doctors tend to be 'fixers'.

Approached by Mr Durham's anxious family, the doctor should consider appropriate intervention and this includes identification of treatable causes of difficulty eating. Assessment of patients with nutritional problems by medical staff is, however, variable and there are limited tools to support this.[2,3] This can mean that treatable contributory factors are missed. Appreciation of the symptoms commonly described by patients with anorexia–cachexia syndrome (ACS) is needed for appropriate assessment (Table 19.1). For example, early satiety (feeling full quickly), one of the most common symptoms described by patients with ACS,[4] is rarely considered by the professional's assessment.[2]

Standardised, simple tools to enable appropriate, comprehensive assessment of the symptoms seen in ACS are required. An abridged version of the Patient-Generated Subjective Global Assessment (PG-SGA)[5] has been used successfully to reveal a number of symptoms commonly associated with ACS (see Table 19.1.) and, with basic treatments, led to improved symptom profile.[6] This has been incorporated into a basic multiprofessional set of guidelines, the Macmillan Durham Cachexia Pack.[7] A thorough assessment for symptoms, many of which can be improved by simple strategies, is probably the most valuable intervention a doctor can provide in this situation and is the most likely to impact quickly on the patient's well-being.

The pathophysiology underlying ACS is complex and only partially understood. Treatments to reverse or retard the progression of ACS are the subject of considerable research effort.

Table 19.1 Symptoms listed on the PG-SGA tool and reported by 23 patients with anorexia–cachexia syndrome[4]

Symptom	Percentage of patients reporting symptom (n = 23)
Dry mouth	91
No appetite	74
Feel full quickly	70
Nausea or vomiting	61
Constipation	52
Altered taste	48
Problems swallowing	43
Mouth sores	39
Diarrhoea	22
Smells bother me	17

To date there is no effective treatment in advanced cancer. Anorexia as a symptom may be improved by some drug treatments, for example progestogens,[8] but these are not without side-effects and may be inappropriate for patients approaching the terminal phase. There is a risk-benefit judgement to be made with any intervention, particularly if the patient's prognosis is limited and likely benefits of the treatment are modest.

Mr Durham's family has requested 'tube feeding'. For many carers, and some patients, restoring or increasing nutritional intake equates to prolongation of life, increased energy and function and possibly further oncological treatment options. The basic problem can appear simple: the patient is not eating, thus the solution seems equally straightforward: the patient needs nutritional support. Decision-making by doctors is embedded within core ethical principles, for example the four principles of non-maleficence, beneficence, justice, and autonomy.[9] Within this framework, it is helpful to have awareness of additional elements which may contribute towards the decision-making process. To this end, it can be helpful to consider the following questions:

1) What is the aim of the proposed intervention (investigation/treatment)?
2) Is that aim a realistic one?
3) Who is being treated as a result of the proposed intervention?

In terms of the provision of intensive nutritional support (INS) for patients with advanced malignancy, these questions could be answered as follows:

1) INS is usually considered with the aim of weight gain/increased energy/being 'built-up' for further oncological treatments. This is appropriate in some patients, but not in others (see below). If INS is being considered by medical staff, the expectations of the treatment must be discussed clearly with the patient. It is surprising how often the patient and doctor approach nutritional intervention with different expectations of the outcome.
2) The likelihood of achieving the aims listed above in a patient with advanced cancer and established ACS is small. Evidence in the literature has demonstrated a general failure of INS to achieve any meaningful gain for the patient. Unfortunately the expectation of counteracting the nutritional deficit caused by ACS with intensive nutrition is both simplistic and unrealistic.[10] If the likelihood of success of any intervention is poor, the balance of risk and benefit to the patient must be considered very carefully.
3) Insight into the personal dynamics in the discussion around nutritional support in ACS is important. As a human being, a doctor is no less likely to be moved by the emotional connotations of anorexia and cachexia than anyone else. This, together with the discomfort of not intervening and the tendency to 'fix', puts doctors at risk of offering treatments with little or no gain, and potentially some burden, to patients. Similarly carers can be motivated by a deep desire to 'do something'. For many people, offering food to a sick loved one is such a central component to providing care that the presence of anorexia disempowers them unacceptably. It is fundamentally important that decisions around nutritional support are centrally motivated by the best interests of the patient. Awareness and some insight into the human factors affecting decision-making will facilitate this.

When Mr Durham's family are approached to ascertain their hopes and expectations of nutritional intervention, their comments include:

> 'He's so tired, it will give him energy.'
>
> 'He can't have more chemotherapy unless he's stronger.'
>
> 'He can't go on eating so little; he'll fade away.'

Awareness of anxieties held by carers and patients themselves is important, but not necessarily in order to define a medical treatment. Acknowledging concerns, explanation, and directing hope towards something achievable and comforting for the patient are hugely valuable interventions.

Armed with reasonably few medical options for treating the underlying problem, there is potential for the doctor to feel a sense of hopelessness and helplessness. And yet there is much that can be done to improve the experience of ACS for both the patient and the carers with a multi-professional approach. The key role of the doctor in supporting this is to provide appropriate comprehensive assessment of associated and contributory symptoms, manage these wherever possible and retain awareness of the factors driving treatment decisions.

Nurse

> 'I walked into the room and there they were, husband and wife, divided by a small dish of elegantly served pieces of strawberry and melon. They weren't just arguing, they were crying. He looks so wasted. It's easy to feel helpless in that sort of situation, but I knew what to do.' (Janet)

This is part of the story about Mr Durham, told by a clinical nurse specialist. The nurse had received training in the Macmillan Approach to Weight and Eating (MAWE), an approach that has been found effective in helping people live with cancer-induced ACS.[11] The training is available as an open access Learn Zone Module at http://www.macmillan.org.uk

Up to 80% of people with advanced cancer experience poor appetite.[12] Janet's account echoes how doctors can feel—helplessness when presented with anorexia in someone with ACS. Carers and family members can also feel helpless. The reasons are complex, but include the exposure of the limitations of medical science and that ultimately no amount of loving care will prevent the progression of advanced cancer. Silence can be a useful defence when nothing can be done to change a situation.[13] But breaking the silence, to explore the potential for intervention, can generate hope.

Nurses can generate hopefulness by helping patients and their carers manage eating-related distress.[14] In this way, they can add to the hope generated by doctors through the assessment and treatment of symptoms that contribute to eating problems.

Nurses and the management of eating-related distress

Nurses are core members of any MDT. They are typically the health care professional best placed to initiate the management of eating-related distress, because they spend most time with patients and their families. The role of the nurse can have different boundaries according to the make-up of the team. Some teams will include a specialist palliative care dietitian or psychologist, to whom nurses can refer the most complex eating-related problems. Other nurses may be in a position where they need to seek this expertise from outside the team.

The important nursing contribution to the management of eating-related distress is to: engage in discussion with patients and carers about eating; give information; and support the communication of love and care in ways that do not involve food.

Managing a personal sense of helplessness in order to break the silence

Being a member of a team is important for managing helplessness. Sharing feelings can mitigate a sense of isolation, but also facilitate a consensus on an appropriate team approach.[15] Some team members will have expertise in helping others manage emotions, such as social workers. It can be important to seek their support, either as a team or as an individual working with a challenging case.

Why break the silence?

Unless invited, patients and their carers are unlikely to volunteer eating-related distress: they have low expectation of help.[16] Misunderstandings about the cause of changing eating habits can contribute to distress. Examples include: a belief that emotional weakness is causing appetite loss and that increasing food intake will lead to improved strength. It is only possible to establish understandings of changing food intake by asking questions.

How to break the silence?

Questions that can help establish a patient's (or carer's) understanding of changing eating habits and associated distress can include:

- What did you have to eat yesterday?
- How is this different from what you used to eat before you were unwell?
- Why do you think your eating habits have changed?
- Are you troubled by the change in your eating habits?

Giving information

There is little to guide patients, carers or health care professionals in knowing what constitutes an appropriate diet for someone with advanced cancer.[17] A typical misunderstanding is that the diet promoted for the general population to reduce the risk of cancer can arrest the progression of advanced cancer. Simple advice on energy-and protein-dense foods that are easy to eat can mitigate distress.[17] These foods are appropriate for people who have lost weight and have a small appetite.[18] Thus the advice helps them to know how to optimize their nutritional intake within the confines of a small appetite.

Demonstrating feelings without feeding

Food can be a way of communicating feelings within a family.[19] The messages transmitted through the giving and receiving of food may not be obvious to family members: raising awareness of common meanings may be important to helping families manage distress. Encouraging expressions of care that do not involve food, such as the use of touch, can help people sustain relationships. Modelling caring behaviour, by acknowledging some of the difficulties imposed by changing eating habits for both patient and carer, can be another way of supporting relationships.

Back to the story

In order to help Mr and Mrs Durham manage their eating-related distress, Janet made a judgment that conflict was not typical of their relationship. She asked permission to speak to each of them on their own, to ask about the changes in Mr Durham's eating habits, why these changes had occurred and why they were troubling. This revealed that Mr Durham understood that cancer was suppressing his appetite, as his doctor had explained this. He had not shared this information with his wife, as he did not want to worry her. Meanwhile, his wife thought that he had given up and was not trying to eat. She felt inadequate as a carer because she could not motivate him to eat. Janet asked if they would each explain to the other why changing appetite was troubling and offered to facilitate this discussion. Mr and Mrs Durham listened to each other and spontaneously began to generate solutions to their conflict. For example, Mrs Durham suggested reading the local paper together rather than cookery books. Janet acknowledged that their experience was common for couples managing advanced cancer and shared examples, from her own experience, of how other couples had managed changing eating habits.

Dietitian

Dietitians, along with other AHPs, are increasingly working within specialist palliative care teams. Current evidence suggests that health professionals do not understand how to manage malnutrition adequately, lending weight to the value of a dietitian within the MDT. Barriers to better management include lack of awareness, knowledge, guidelines and time.[2,3,20]

The dietitian's role in supporting patients with cancer-induced ACS is to provide care based on the stage of disease (i.e. prognosis), individual needs and personal choice of the patient. With advancing disease it can be appropriate for principal objectives to become maximizing food enjoyment, if possible, and minimizing food-related discomfort.[21]

The identification of nutrition-related problems may come about in various ways—in this case, through Mr Durham's family expressing concern. However, there are also a number of screening tools available, including holistic measurement tools and nutritional screening tools such as the Distress Thermometer[22] and PG-SGA.[5,23] Active screening is important as it can assist health professionals in the timely identification of nutritional risk and eating-related concerns, and a symptom list can inform decisions about planning appropriate dietary and medical interventions. Use of a nutrition assessment tool may be undertaken by several MDT members, but good communication within the team will avoid unnecessary and unhelpful duplication.

Screening will stratify patients into categories of nutritional risk (high, medium and low) so that guided care plans can be used to assist staff in managing the level of risk identified. In patients needing to improve their oral intake, first-line advice should be to increase consumption of energy- and nutrient-dense foods combined with food fortification and frequency of foods and fluids. The objective is to capitalize on any remaining interest in food with small quantities of high-energy foods. High risk patients should be assessed by a suitably qualified health professional such as a dietitian or nutrition support team.[24]

In Mr Durham's case, screening may have already been carried out on his admission to the hospice. Initially hospice staff may have given first-line dietary advice. Subsequently, when Mr Durham has said that he just 'doesn't feel like eating' and he is 'not bothered' by his weight, the staff may have decided not to take any further dietary action so as to respect his wishes and avoid any further distress.

However, typically families will express concern over their loved ones' poor appetite, change in body image and weight loss. Some may specifically ask for a referral to the dietitian as they see this team member as providing the expertise to advise on nutritional intervention. Loss of appetite generates considerably more anxiety and distress among carers than patients.[1] Patients' anxiety is often due to frustration with their carer's preoccupation with food[25] and avoidance of social contact due to altered body image.[26]

In Mr Durham's case the dietitian should liaise with the MDT to clarify whether:

- Mr Durham consents to referral. In some cases talking about food can cause more patient distress;
- anyone has already discussed his concerns, if any, about not feeling like eating;
- anyone has discussed with Mr Durham the anxieties his family have about his weight loss and poor nutritional intake. This is important when considering talking with the family about potential conflict around eating;
- other team members have already counselled family members about nutritional issues;
- he has physical symptoms which could impact on his appetite or ability to eat;
- his prognosis can be estimated in order to plan realistic goals and a meaningful outcome.

As part of the assessment it is important to identify any nutrition-related problems or barriers to food and fluid intake and evaluate their impact (Box 19.1).

When assessing the patient's nutritional problems the dietitian should have good listening and counselling skills in order to create an empathic relationship with patients and their carers.[21] The dietitian should be able to discuss the changing role nutrition has, with the patient and carers, as the patient progresses towards the terminal phase of the disease.

If Mr Durham has expressed a wish that he could eat better and enjoy his food more, he may want direction or alternatively want to take control of any food and drink provision. He may have found his own solutions to his eating problems.

Simple strategies may include exploring food and drinks he fancies, eating when he wants, presenting small meals or snacks in a pleasing way and liaising with catering services to facilitate access to appropriate food provision. Any strategy should encompass careful discussion with Mr Durham and his family of realistic goals that may include promotion of self-management strategies.[27,28]

It is clear in this scenario that nutritional counselling should be directed to the family members in particular, as their efforts will undoubtedly add to the patient's psychological distress. It may help to meet the family separately so that they can 'air' their concerns without causing distress to the patient. They may feel a loss of control, anger or guilt. They may feel he should try harder or they may not understand his prognosis.

It is important to address the family concerns and to explain that coercing the patient to eat will not help to build him up and give him more energy. Feeling a sense of helplessness, the health professional may be tempted to recommend a prescription of oral nutritional supplements to help build Mr Durham up. However, this may lead to false hope by carers, giving unrealistic expectations and then anger when this is not successful. In addition, it may increase Mr Durham's distress by the pressure being diverted from getting him to eat to getting him the take the supplement drink.

Box 19.1 Identification of nutrition-related problems

- Oral problems: dry mouth (xerostomia), sore, painful mouth (mucositis). Fungal infection, taste changes. Poorly fitted dentures, physical swallowing problems.
- Posture and environment not conducive to eating/drinking.
- Cultural/spiritual issues: food restrictions, meal patterns, customs and beliefs.
- Gastric stasis (nausea/vomiting).
- Early satiety: may be related to tumour position/size/ascites/ACS.
- Altered bowel habit: diarrhoea/constipation/obstruction. Pancreatic enzyme replacement therapy may improve bowel habit in pancreatic cancers.
- Pain.
- Breathlessness/fatigue: practical difficulties of self-feeding as too weak.
- Other illness that may be contributing to general condition, e.g. poorly controlled diabetes mellitus.
- Depression/low mood: consider counselling, practical strategies to help improve self-confidence, and drug treatment.
- Fear of eating if the patient associates symptoms with food.

By giving information to the family on the mechanics of weight loss and cachexia, they can be helped to understand why their actions are not beneficial and that they could unwittingly have a negative impact on Mr Durham's quality of life. It is also important that the dietitian dispels any myths about diet in advanced disease.

Any action agreed with the patient and family should be communicated with the MDT members and generic staff involved with the patient's care to ensure consistency of information and consensus on management. It is important to clarify the dietitian's role in ongoing assessment. Repeated questioning about food-related issues may generate, or increase anxiety, and is a risk of the MDT approach. Review by the dietitian should be taken on where there is a clear role for this specialist.

The dietitian can input to discussions around ethical issues and role of drug treatments. Faced with such a challenging but commonly occurring clinical scenario, the role of the dietitian will be to help members of the MDT examine the nutritional problems and discuss the ethical dilemmas, if any, of nutritional and/or medication interventions. This requires members having an understanding of the complexity of nutritional problems in cancer and of the role food plays for the individual.[29] The dietitian will play a key role in the coordination of strategies for both the present situation and any future predictable changes.

Pharmacist

> 'He's hardly eating so trying to get him to swallow all those tablets at meal times is impossible.' (Mrs Durham)
>
> 'I mean what's the point ... all those tablets and I still feel awful?' (Mr Durham)

Pharmacists have long been seen as the experts in medicines[30] and it is this quality that gives them a unique and vital role in the MDT. Several other disciplines involved will have good pharmacological knowledge and in this respect overlap. However, the pharmacist's in-depth understanding of medicines and their use can add to, enhance and apply other members of the team's knowledge. Therefore pharmacists often have an advisory role within the team. Community pharmacists are part of the primary care MDT and an easily accessible resource for patients and generalist clinicians, shown to make valuable interventions with advanced cancer patients.[31]

The concerns expressed by Mr and Mrs Durham reveal information useful to the pharmacological management of the current symptoms. The following is a basic structure of how a specialist pharmacist working in advanced cancer might help Mr Durham.

Assessment

A careful assessment of the patient's current symptoms is an essential building block for any health care professional. The PG-SGA is a useful tool to assess patients with nutritional problems and has been discussed earlier in the chapter. The importance of not overwhelming the patient and avoiding duplication has also been discussed and would suggest that perhaps such a tool could be utilized by one team member and then referred to by others.

In Mr Durham's case, he has poor appetite and weight loss (although this does not bother him). An assessment would also probably reveal mouth problems (sore mouth, dry mouth, altered taste) given his recent history of chemotherapy.

Drug history

An accurate drug history can reveal a great deal about not only what the patient is currently taking but may also give explanation as to the cause of some symptoms. There are often differences between what a patient is taking and what has been prescribed. A three-fold approach ensures that any discrepancies are highlighted and can be resolved.

1 *Ask the patient*: what medications do you take?
2 Request to see all of the prescribed medication and *look*: what medications does the patient have and how are they labelled?
3 Seek information from the main prescriber and *ask the family doctor*: for a copy of the patient's most up-to-date repeat medication list.

A drug history will allow the pharmacist to review the known side-effects of the current medication and see if any of these could be contributing to symptoms. Mr Durham has had a recent increase in dose of opioid. Common side-effects of opioid medication include constipation, nausea and drowsiness. Unmanaged constipation can cause nausea, vomiting and anorexia. Nausea itself can certainly prevent patients from feeling like eating.

Tablet burden is something that both Mr and Mrs Durham describe, and this too can be assessed during the drug history process. Patients with advanced cancer are very often on large numbers of medications.[32] These can include medications initiated years ago, often by multiple prescribers, which are no longer being reviewed and monitored.[33] This can lead to the continuation of futile or inappropriate medicines. Examples of this might be anticholesterol medication such as 'statins' with proven long term benefits but futile prescriptions in this patient group.

Medicines use review

Having established what the patient's current medication regimen should be, it is important to find out whether this is being followed. The literature suggests that compliance is not always good in this patient group.[34] Practical aspects can also be addressed here, including route of delivery and form of drug most appropriate for the patient.

Mr Durham's comment conveys a sense of hopelessness on his part. It is quite likely that he is not conforming to the medication regimen set for him. The pharmacist is ideally placed to improve Mr Durham's concordance, to negotiate an acceptable regimen that would rationalize the current list of medicines and control the existing symptoms. More than 30 years of evidence suggests that knowledge improves concordance[35] and so the pharmacist would do well to spend time, listen, then educate and counsel Mr Durham about his medication.

Symptom control

Having gathered all the information described above, the pharmacist can suggest or prescribe (as many pharmacists are now supplementary or independent prescribers) medications that will improve the current symptoms. New medications need to be considered in terms of suitability for the individual patient, taking into account contraindications, cautions, side-effects and drug–drug interactions. The pharmacist will also consider non-pharmacological approaches to symptom management which may warrant a trial in advance of drug treatment.

Plan

Table 19.2 illustrates the outcome of the drug history, medicines use review and possible pharmacological approaches to symptom management for Mr Durham.

> 'I sort of see the point now, I mean there are still a good number of tablets to take but at least I feel better ... had a bit of an appetite for the first time in weeks.' (Mr Durham)

> 'It's much better now he can take some of the drugs as liquid medicines, he's even managing some small meals.' (Mrs Durham)

Table 19.2 Mr Durham: pharmacist assessment and management strategy

Medication assessment: medication currently prescribed	**Medication currently taken**
◆ Aspirin 75 mg mane ◆ Simvastatin 40 mg nocte ◆ Lansoprazole 30 mg mane ◆ Atenolol 25 mg mane ◆ Diclofenac 50 mg tds ◆ Creon® 25 000 units tds ◆ Morphine sulphate sustained release 120 mg bd ◆ Morphine sulphate immediate release 40 mg prn ◆ Paracetamol 1 g qds ◆ Lactulose 15 ml bd	◆ Morphine sulphate sustained release 120 mg bd ◆ Morphine sulphate immediate release 40 mg prn ◆ Aspirin 75 mg mane
Symptom assessment	**Suggested pharmacological management medications initiated**
1. No appetite 2. Feeling full quickly 3. Sore mouth (unknown cause) 4. Dry mouth 5. Nausea 6. Constipation (Weight loss was a symptom but the patient was not bothered by it and did not want it treated)	1. Dexamethasone 4 mg mane, 2-week course and review 2. Metoclopramide 10 mg tds and increase as needed, review after 1 week 3. Benzydamine mouthwash 15 ml up to hourly, review after 1 week 4. Artificial saliva spray/gel qds (e.g. AS Saliva Orthana® spray, Biotene Oralbalance® gel) 5. See 2. 6. Senna 15 mg nocte ± docusate 200 mg bd, or Movicol 1 sachet bd, review after 1 week (Use liquid medications where possible)
Suggested pharmacological management medications stopped (futile medication)	
◆ Aspirin 75 mg mane (preventative measure) ◆ Simvastatin 40 mg nocte (long term benefits) ◆ Atenolol 25 mg mane (BP 90/60) ◆ Lactulose 15 ml bd (not effective for opioid-induced constipation)	
Overall management: counselling points	
◆ Why removing the futile medicines is appropriate. ◆ Why more than one medication can work at the same time to manage pain in different ways, so the importance of taking the opioid, the NSAID and paracetamol. ◆ Why the Creon® capsules will help digest any food eaten. ◆ That there are various types of laxatives, used for different causes of constipation, and that continuous use of laxatives, if necessary, is safe. ◆ The benefits of all the new medications. ◆ That all the new medications are a trial and can be stopped at any time; negotiate 'giving them a go' for a week to see if symptoms improve. ◆ Leave a plan/information card with all the above documented.	

Physiotherapy and occupational therapy

'... I just can't see how we will manage at home now he is so weak ...'

Physiotherapists (PTs) and occupational therapists (OTs) in oncology and palliative care are familiar with close multidisciplinary working. This is apparent also in the context of nutritional problems in cancer. Within the wider team, PT and OT cooperate, communicate and work closely together towards rehabilitation and patient care. As well as assessing Mr Durham in the hospice setting, joint OT/PT domiciliary assessment (with or without Mr Durham) is likely to be appropriate. This was the time that Mrs Durham shared her fears and concerns about her husband's discharge and her own ability to cope if her husband does not eat to maintain his strength. Mrs Durham was reassured that there would be appropriate equipment, practical care assistance as required and therapy team follow-up once Mr Durham was home.

Fundamental to meaningful PT/OT intervention is collaborative goal-setting with patients. Goals must be realistic, specific and achievable. Though there is very close working, the PT and OT do have different focuses of assessment and use different skills.

Physiotherapy

Within the MDT, PT's specific role is defined as, '... a health care profession concerned with human function and movement and maximising potential'.[36] After full initial assessment Mr Durham revealed a strong desire to regain his premorbid level of functional ability. Skeletal muscle weakness and loss of muscle mass are characteristic of cancer-induced ACS.[37] These cause decreased mobility and other disabilities.

Conflict around rest

'... I keep pushing him to do more and to walk but he says he is too tired ...' (Mrs Durham)

Carers and families experience anxiety, fear and a sense of helplessness with regards to the consequences of ACS.[1,15] Reduced exercise/activity levels are also triggers of these feelings. The PT must educate carers on the need for balance between 'enabling' activity and 'allowing' rest. Tension and conflict arise between unrealistic expectations and actual physical ability.

The commonly held assumption, 'The harder I work the stronger I will get', is not valid in the presence of ACS in cancer. Metabolic pathways change in response to tumour factors leading to breakdown of skeletal muscle (proteolysis). Though inactivity does of course lead to de-conditioning,[38] it is the underlying disease that brings about the extreme wasted state. Helping Mrs Durham to understand this will undermine the notion that 'he is not helping himself'.

Activity and exercises

'I need some exercises to build up the strength in my legs again.' (Mr Durham)

There is no evidence that exercise can reverse the muscle-wasting effects of cancer-induced ACS. There is an indication that there may be some 'protective' effect and this view is shared by specialist PTs in palliative care/oncology. PTs are commonly asked for exercise programmes by patients.[39]

A simple, seated exercise programme (as published in the Durham Cachexia Pack[7] and summarized in Table 19.3) can contribute to well-being and, in this patient group, aims to:

- maintain muscle strength;
- maintain endurance of muscles;

Table 19.3 Seated exercise programme for patients with cancer-induced anorexia–cachexia syndrome[7]

Exercise	Repetitions	Frequency/day
Knee extension	3–10	1–3
Ankle dorsiflexion (bending up)	5–15	1–3
Sit to stand	1–5	1–3
Arm raises	3–10	1–3
Deep breaths	3	1–3

- increase oxidative capacity of muscles;
- improve self-reported quality of life markers;
- relieve symptoms of depression;
- be a positive focus for patients and carers.

Cancer-related fatigue management studies show benefits to increased activity levels including exercise programmes.[40] There are no studies involving cancer ACS sufferers but there is an assumption among professionals that exercise/activity is better than rest in controlling fatigue in this group.[39]

Occupational therapy (OT)

OTs use a variety of skills when working with a person who has cancer-induced ACS. These aim to assist with the fatigue and decreased energy levels associated with this condition as well as enabling independence.[7,41,42]

When dealing with Mr Durham's case the OT will work in both a holistic manner and adopt a client centred approach with an emphasis on patient choice.[43]

The initial interview with Mr Durham will allow the therapist to build a picture of what is important to him. This might include:

- leisure interests;
- personal activities of daily living;
- environmental issues;
- issues of spirituality;
- functional problems.[43]

The OT must understand the effect ACS is likely to have on Mr Durham if realistic goals are to be set. Mr Durham has generalised weakness due to muscle loss caused by ACS. The two core skills that an OT will use are activity analysis and the grading of activity.[44]

Mr Durham also identified the following problems:

- difficulty with feeding himself;
- maintaining personal activity of daily living;
- anxiety when family want him to eat.

Grading the activity

The OT will look at grading all aspects of the patient's daily activity and look towards scheduling high exertion activities for periods when the patient's energy levels are likely to be at their highest.

Activities would be prioritised so that those which a patient values most highly are given increased emphasis. Energy-consuming activities that are non-vital or peripheral would either be avoided or reduced in frequency.[44]

The OT will look at simplifying and enabling everyday tasks such as feeding. Mr Durham may benefit from repositioning while feeding, i.e. providing him with a higher chair or an adjustable height table reducing the energy required. Lightweight cutlery, lightweight cups, plate guards and careful timing of meals to try and coincide with periods of high energy levels are other examples of intervention here.[41]

Energy conservation

The OT must explain the benefits of avoiding exhaustion in activities and the need for regular rest breaks. To enable personal activities of daily living the OT may consider advising carers to assist, conserving energy for other valued activities. The OT will also look at providing adaptive equipment including perching stools, bath boards, 'long handle reachers', etc. It may be appropriate for Mr Durham to perch rather than stand while shaving or to place all lower garments over feet before standing up. The OT may play an educational/liaison role between the patient and the family in close working with the rest of the MDT.

Working together, PT and OT ensure that Mr Durham is achieving his potential in terms of independence and physical function. Together with the wider MDT, PT and OT will offer support, reassurance and education for both Mr and Mrs Durham as they face the disabling effects of ACS.

Chaplain

Listening to the personal story

The case study gives us some factual details but there is not much information as to who Mr Durham is. His spiritual and physical needs will become clearer once we have had time to listen to his story. Within this story we can discover perhaps the journey of illness as he sees it and learn a little more about the background to his statement that he is 'not bothered' by his weight loss.

Telling the story of our own life is a personal experience that demands attentiveness from the listener. Being well listened to may be nourishment for the soul, which at this stage may be more important than physical food.

Spiritual narratives

Personal stories are often the main sphere in which to work. The personal story may be the individual spiritual narrative of a person who tries to make sense of their illness through expression of their fears and hopes; their consideration of meaning and disillusionment and their discussion of close relationships. The consideration of food may also feature in this personal account of illness but it should be listened out for, and picked up on, rather than being directed to by the listener.

Religious narratives

A person with a religious background may have stories (and philosophies) from their own faith tradition around food that can be set alongside the individual's story. The significance of the cosmic religious stories may be discussed with the individual if that is appropriate.

Discussions might ensue as to what the patient needs in order to facilitate their religious observance; a respectful silence as a Hindu offers prayers before eating and the availability of water to bless the food, for example.

Insight

The religious stories may reveal something to professionals of an attitude to food that would be helpful in the care of Mr Durham. In the Jewish story, the Passover meal is central to God's redemption of the Israelites from slavery. Two aspects of the Passover meal are significant for people suffering anorexia. The first is that the preparation of food is paramount. The second is that the Passover meal was eaten in twilight and in haste.

People with cancer often live in a framework of time different from those who look after them. They want to eat when the moment of appetite comes upon them: there may be a sense of urgency, of eating when the time is right, a moment of haste. The time when the sickness has been momentarily suspended, and the possibility of eating has opened up, may not be the time when food or meals are available.

Does the hospice have the equipment to be able to store, prepare and cook food at any time? Are there staff who are available and able to prepare a light snack at any time? Will it be presented to patients in a manner that is acceptable to them?

If relatives are bringing in food for the patient, can this also be stored so that it is available when the patient wants it? It is helpful to encourage relatives to understand that waiting upon the moment of appetite may be more productive than the patient feeling pressured into eating at visiting time for the sake of the relatives. However, the family need to be assured that hospice staff will give the patient food that they have made, if he asks for it.

The availability of a refrigerator in each person's room may mean that the person has greater autonomy over the time of eating and the choice of food.

There is a meal at the heart of Christian worship too. The Eucharistic meal has now become symbolized by a tiny amount of bread and a small sip of wine. The quantity of the meal does not diminish the profound experience of eating this meal; for those who participate in this meal it is the opportunity to draw close to God. It also teaches us that a small amount may suffice. There is both the symbolic significance of taking a small amount of food to sustain the spiritual life of the person, and the physical reality that people with anorexia have small appetites and cannot ingest large amounts of food.

Memory and imagination

The partaking of meals in religious stories is often about remembering acts of salvation by God. Remembering may also be important for us in a physical sense in that it may enhance enjoyment of food.

One of our spirituality sessions in the hospice day care focuses upon taste. A plate of brightly coloured prepared fruits is laid out on a picnic cloth along with freshly baked bread and an array of childhood sweets. Participants are invited to share a memory of their favourite childhood sweets or an occasion when they have tasted strawberries or other fruit. The smell of the bread often conjures up baking days in their home as children. The opportunity to stimulate appetites through remembrance is one that can be shared within the relaxed atmosphere of other patients. It may be more difficult to share this exercise with the relatives present as this can sometimes provoke the response of buying in an excessive amount of a certain food that a patient has said he likes.

Using the imagination to stimulate appetite is another related tool that might be helpful. Conjuring up seaside holidays, with all the sights and sounds, may add to the delight of eating an ice lolly.

Anxiety

Given all of the above, it should be remembered that Mr Durham has no desire to eat and this does not cause him any distress. If *we* are distressed by his anorexia, perhaps the tension lies within our own psyche. For professionals working in palliative care, there is still a challenge when patients cannot have some quality of well-being: lack of food may challenge our ability to care. There are ethical discussions that need to take place within the team about artificial nutrition procedures that might be available in this situation. Some members of the team will find this a more difficult option than others. Combined with this, the team has to carry the anxieties of the family who believe that not eating means imminent death. Medical or nursing staff may be able to ease the anxieties of the relatives as they explain about the physiological changes that will happen when a person finds it difficult to eat. Helping the family to adjust their views may be as important as helping the team to honour the patient's experience. Perhaps this is the greatest challenge; to alter our notion of how we might nourish Mr Durham when he no longer desires to eat.

Volunteer

> 'He just sits and ignores his food. I try to encourage him, but he gets upset.' (Mr Durham's wife)
>
> 'I don't even want to try to eat. I know I won't eat very much and it just makes her more upset.' (Mr Durham)

The volunteer's role is interesting, challenging and rewarding.

Volunteers are fundamental to the workforce within UK hospices and take on a wide range of roles. They are often involved in meal preparation and presentation. They need to be mindful of the distinction between maximizing comfortable eating and drinking by the patient and coercing them. However, they have the opportunity to support the patient and their carers in the difficult problems around eating, and with patience, appropriate encouragement and sensitivity, it is often possible to improve the patient's intake. Ensuring the patient feels relaxed and not pressured is central to achieving this. Care of a patient outside their normal residence is unsettling in itself and this should be taken into consideration. There can be simple reasons other than the underlying cancer that makes someone not want to eat—for example, a change of mealtime or limited meal choice.

Mr Durham should be asked about the type of food and drink that he enjoys. If he normally has a glass of beer at home then this can be offered, or a small glass of sherry before a meal may help stimulate his appetite. Experience shows that presentation can help in encouraging the patient to want to try eating again. Investing effort in making the food look interesting and appetising often pays dividends. Meal trays can be set with a cloth, a glass with a napkin arranged in it and a small vase with a flower.

When serving the food it is important to serve small portions, often just a tablespoon of each vegetable and a very small piece of meat is all that the patient requires. If the plate is overfull with food this can discourage any attempt to eat. The patient is encouraged to eat little and often. Offer snacks and nibbles in between meals. Offer assistance where required by cutting food into small manageable pieces, and offer assistance with eating. Give the patient time to eat. It is both annoying and de-motivating to have dishes cleared away before one has finished eating. If the patient is not eating well, gently coax him. Be aware, however, of coercing the patient; the patient is the only effective judge of what he can and cannot manage. If the patient does start to eat, a positive comment can encourage the patient to continue to eat.

A change in surroundings can help encourage patients to eat, and many institutions can offer various places to eat. Giving a choice is often helpful to patients. Sitting at a table with others, rather than sitting in bed, facilitates social interaction; a fundamental part of eating in society. Family or carers visiting at meal times may, if they wish, assist the patient in eating; this can encourage the patient to eat, but be aware of the potential of carers to feel stressed about poor eating and respond by pressuring the patient. Good advice for the carers about how they can best help is empowering for them. To enable the patient time to eat meals without being disturbed, it is helpful to avoid clinical rounds at set meal times.

The volunteer role is often perceived as unthreatening by patients, separate from the medical and nursing staff involved. This can mean that the patient will divulge information to the volunteer in preference to anyone else; also that the volunteer can effectively communicate information relevant to the patient's nutritional care. This underpins the value of the volunteer within the MDT framework.

MDT coordination

The input of a range of health care professionals is of great value in the context of nutritional problems in patients with cancer. However, coordination of care is important, partly to avoid mixed messages and duplication of effort, but also to ensure clear ownership of patient care. Clinical responsibility usually rests with the senior doctor, and it is important that a lead is identified for ultimate decision-making. However, during the palliative stage of the patient's journey, it is often the case that a non-medical MDT member has greatest input and impact on the problems presented, so may be the most appropriate team member to lead decision-making. The development of a 'key worker' role is underway in the UK in recognition of this. The role is also intended to guard against the potential problem of ownership: multiple professionals involved but none taking responsibility for coordinating care.

Finally

The complexity of the experience generated by eating problems in patients with cancer demands an MDT approach. Individuals working within an MDT need to appreciate respective roles and responsibilities and be willing to communicate effectively. The consequence of this holistic approach is care that has far greater meaning and impact for patients and those around them.

References

1. Hawkins C (2000) Anorexia and anxiety in advanced malignancy; the relative problem. *J Hum Nutr Diet*, **13** (2), 113–17.
2. Churm D, Andrew I, Holden K, Hildreth A, Hawkins C (2009) A questionnaire study of the approach to the anorexia–cachexia syndrome in patients with cancer by staff in a district general hospital. *Support Care Cancer*, **17**(5), 503–7.
3. Spiro A, Baldwin C, Patterson A, Thomas J, Andreyev HJN (2006) The views and practice of oncologists towards nutritional support in patients receiving chemotherapy. *Br J Cancer*, **95**(4), 431–34.
4. Andrew I, Kirkpatrick G, Holden K, Hawkins C (2008) Audit of symptoms and prescribing in patients with the anorexia–cachexia syndrome. *Pharm World Sci*, **30**(5), 489–96.
5. Bauer J, Capra S, Ferguson M (2002) Use of the scored Patient Generated Subjective Global Assessment (PG-SGA) as a nutrition assessment tool in patients with cancer. *Eur J Clin Nutr*, **56**, 779–85.
6. Andrew I, Waterfield K, Hildreth A, Kirkpatrick G, Hawkins C (2009) Quantifying the impact of standardized assessment and symptom management tools on symptoms associated with cancer-induced anorexia cachexia syndrome. *Palliat Med* **23**(8), 680–8.
7. Macmillan Durham Cachexia Pack. Available at: http://learnzone.macmillan.org.uk (accessed 29 August 2008).
8. Berenstein EG, Ortiz Z (2005) Megestrol acetate for the treatment of anorexia–cachexia syndrome. *Cochrane Database Syst Rev*, (18)(2)CD004310.
9. Randall F, Downie RS (1999) Ethics and aims in palliative care. In: Randall F (ed.), *Palliative Care Ethics. A Companion for All Specialties*, 2nd edition, pp. 6–7. Oxford: Oxford University Press.

10. Skipworth RJ, Stewart GD, Dejong CHC, Preston T, Fearon KCH (2007) Pathophysiology of cancer cachexia: much more than host–tumour interaction? *Clin Nutr*, **26**, 667–76.
11. Hopkinson JB, Fenlon D, Nicholls P, *et al.* (2009) *Helping People Live with Advanced Cancer: An Exploratory Cluster Randomised Trial to Investigate the Effectiveness of the 'Macmillan Approach to Weight loss and Eating difficulties' (MAWE).* London: Macmillan Cancer Support.
12. Hopkinson JB, MacDonald J, Wright DNM, Corner JL (2006) The prevalence of concern about weight loss and change in eating habits in people with advanced cancer. *J Pain Sympt Manag*, **32**(4), 322–31.
13. Lazarus RS (1999) *Stress and Emotion: A New Synthesis.* London: Free Association Press.
14. Hopkinson JB (2008) Change in eating habits. In Corner JL and Bailey C (eds), *Cancer Nursing: Care in Context*, 2nd edn, pp. 525–32. London: Blackwell.
15. Speck P (2006) *Teamwork in Palliative Care: Fulfilling or Frustrating?* Oxford: Oxford University Press.
16. Hopkinson JB, Corner JL (2006) Helping patients with advanced cancer live with concerns about eating: a challenge for palliative care professionals. *J Pain Sympt Manag*, **31**(4), 293–305.
17. Hopkinson JB (2008) Carers' influence on diets of people with advanced cancer. *Nurs Times*, **104**(12), 28–9.
18. British Dietetic Association, Nutritional Advisory Group for the Elderly (2002) *Have You Got a Small Appetite? Your Guide to Eating Well.* Birmingham: NAGE.
19. Lupton D (1996) *Food, the Body and the Self.* London: SAGE.
20 Aston T (2006) Nutrition in palliative care: effective or ineffective? *J Commun Nurs*, **20**(7), 4–8.
21. Eldridge L (2007) Palliative care and terminal illness. In: Thomas B, Bishop J (eds), *The Manual of Dietetic Practice*, 4th edn, pp. 783–8. Oxford: Blackwell.
22. National Comprehensive Cancer Network (2007) *Clinical Practice Guidelines in Oncology. Distress Management. Version 1.2008.* Available at: http://www.nccn.org/professionals/physician_gls/PDF/distress.pdf (accessed 27 May 2008).
23. Ottery FD (1996) Definition of standardised nutritional assessment and interventional pathways in oncology. *Nutr Suppl*, **12**(1), S15–19.
24. National Institute of Health and Clinical Excellence (2006) *Nutrition Support in Adults: Oral Supplements, Enteral and Parenteral Feeding.* Available at: http://guidance.nice.org.uk/CG32/guidance/pdf/English (accessed 3 June 2008).
25. Poole K, Froggatt K (2002) Loss of weight and loss of appetite in advanced cancer: a problem for the patient, the carer, or the health professional? *Palliat Med*, **16**, 499–506.
26. Strasser F (2003) Eating-related disorders in patients with advanced cancer. *Support Care Cancer*, **11**, 11–20.
27. Hopkinson JB (2007) How people with advanced cancer manage changing eating habits. *J Adv Nurs*, **59**(5), 454–62.
28. Bauer JD, Ash S, Davidson WL, *et al.* (2006) Evidence based practice guidelines for the nutritional management of cancer cachexia. *Nutr Dietetics*, **63**(Suppl 2), S5–S32.
29. Souter J (2005) Loss of appetite: a poetic exploration of cancer patients' and their carers' experiences. *Int J Palliat Nurs*, **11**(10), 524–32.
30. NHS Choices: about NHS services: NHS pharmacists/chemists. Available at: http://www.nhs.uk/AboutNHSservices/pharmacists/Pages/PharmacistsFAQ.aspx (accessed 28 July 2008).
31. Needham DS, Wong ICK, Campion PD (2002) Evaluation of the effectiveness of UK community pharmacists' interventions in community palliative care. *Palliat Med*, **16**(3), 219–25.
32. Hanks G, Roberts CJC, Davies AN (2004) Principles of drug use in palliative medicine. In: Doyle D, Hanks G, Cherny N, Calman K (eds), *Oxford Textbook of Palliative Medicine*, 3rd edn, p. 213. Oxford: Oxford University Press.
33. Nicholson A, Andrew I, Etherington R, Gamlin R, Lovel T, Lloyd J (2001) Futile and inappropriate prescribing: an assessment of the issue in a series of patients admitted to a specialist palliative care unit. *Int J Pharm Pract*, R72.

34. Zeppetella G (1999) How do terminally ill patients at home take their medication? *Palliat Med*, **13**(6), 469–75.
35. Hulka BS, Cassel JC, Kupper LL, Burdette JA (1976) Communication, compliance and concordance between physicians and patients with prescribed medications. *Am J Public Health*, **66**(9), 847–53.
36. Chartered Society of Physiotherapy. *The Role of the Physiotherapist for People with Cancer—CSP Position Statement. July 2003*. Available at: http://www.csp.org.uk (accessed 29 August 2008).
37. Ardies CM (2002) Exercise, cachexia, and cancer therapy, a molecular rationale. *Nutr Cancer*, **42**, 143–57.
38. Kisner C, Colby L (1990) *Therapeutic Exercise: Foundations and Techniques*, 3rd edn. Philadelphia: FA Davis.
39. Beyer T (2007) Management of skeletal muscle wasting in cancer anorexia–cachexia syndrome (ACS)—the role of exercise prescription, in Macmillan Durham Cachexia Pack, Section 6. Available at: http://learnzone.macmillan.org.uk (accessed 29 August 2008).
40. Ingram C (2006) A home based, physical activity intervention increased physical activity, fitness, and vigour and reduced fatigue in sedentary women with early stage breast cancer. *Evid Based Nurs*, **9**(1), 19.
41. College of Occupational Therapists (2004) *Occupational Therapy Intervention in cancer. Guidance for Professionals, Managers and Decision-makers*. London: Simon Crompton for a working party of HOPE .
42. Lindsell G cited in, Cooper J (2006) *Occupational Therapy in Oncology and Palliative Care*, 2nd edn. New York: Wiley.
43. Law M, Baptiste S, Mills J (1995) Client centred practice: what does it mean and does it make a difference? *Can J Occup Ther*, **62**(5), 250–7.
44. Hagedorn R (2000) *Tools for Practice in Occupational Therapy: A Structured Approach to Core Skills and Processes*. London: Churchill Livingstone.

Part 6

Artificial nutritional support

Chapter 20

Nutritional support: an overview

Tim E. Bowling

As has been fully explored elsewhere, good nutrition is a key component to effective management for cancer patients, both for those who can be cured and for those who are to be palliated. However, such patients face a wide array of difficulties which will challenge their ability to maintain their nutritional status. These include somatic symptomatology either from the disease or its treatments, such as pain, nausea, vomiting, hiccoughs and diarrhoea/constipation; supratentorial influences, commonly depression; and cancer cachexia. Managing the patient nutritionally requires a holistic approach to consider all matters that will have a disadvantageous effect on a patient's ability to feed. Therefore, in addition to considering the need for nutritional support, effort should be directed at any concurrent symptomatology. Identification of treatable aetiologies, such as biochemical/metabolic disturbance (e.g. electrolyte imbalance, acid–base disturbance), dehydration and benign upper gastrointestinal tract disease (e.g. ulcers), can prove very effective. For those problems without obvious solutions, optimization of symptom control is paramount: analgesia anti-emetics (Chapter 14), anti-diarrhoeals, laxatives, chlorpromazine (for hiccoughs) and rationalization of drug therapy, where possible, are a brief list of areas that may need to be addressed. There are also some treatment options for appetite stimulation and cancer cachexia (see Part 3), and psychological help is often required, which most oncology centres can access.

Focusing specifically on nutritional support, counselling by dedicated teams is of tremendous value for cancer patients. Part 5 has dealt with nutritional assessment and counselling, and the roles of the various members of the multidisciplinary team in the management of the patient. This section will examine the role of artificial feeding for patients who are unable to meet their nutritional needs by normal dietary means.

As a general principle, feeding should be achieved by the simplest method possible. Therefore, if the gut works and the patient is able to feed orally, then dietary supplementation should be the first option to be explored. If oral feeding is not possible or inadequate, tube feeding can be considered. Intravenous feeding (parenteral nutrition) should only be resorted to (i) when the gastrointestinal tract is inaccessible or not working, or (ii) if an individual cannot meet requirements adequately with eating and/or enteral tube feeding.

For artificial nutritional support, there are two broad scenarios that are very different from each other. The first is patients who require short term nutritional support, for example to tide them over an acute intercurrent illness or short-lived complications of cancer therapy or surgery. The second is cancer patients needing nutritional support in the longer term to sustain adequate nutritional repletion, challenged either because of the effects of the illness and/or its treatment on their ability to meet nutritional needs by diet alone or because of irreversible intestinal failure. The approach to these two groups is different. The indications and practice of short term support is little different from any other patient group requiring artificial feeding. The issue of longer term feeding in cancer patients receiving palliative care to support life is an area of widely differing practice around the world. In home enteral and parenteral nutrition programmes in the USA and some European countries, cancer is the commonest indication. In other 'first world' countries, such as the UK, it is a minority activity. Whether this is due to clinical nihilism, indifference or resource allocation is a matter of ongoing debate and controversy. Nevertheless, enteral or parenteral feeding in terminally ill patients does have a role, but requires careful patient selection and, more importantly, good communication with the patient/carers, so that they are adequately informed of the benefits versus the burdens.

The following two chapters are designed to inform the reader about the basics of artificial nutritional support. They are not designed to be definitive texts.

Chapter 21

Oral and enteral nutrition

Jeremy Woodward

Introduction

Nutrition intake is impaired in malignant disease through a variety of mechanisms.[1,2] In many such situations weight loss is causally related to reduced caloric intake rather than solely to the catabolic effects of the underlying cancer, and is therefore potentially amenable to treatment.[3] Malnutrition is particularly prevalent for these reasons in patients with head and neck or gastrointestinal cancers.[4–7] Artificial nutrition support may allow for weight maintenance or even weight gain while treatment can be targeted at the cancer or the symptoms that cause reduced volitional oral intake and may be required in the longer term where such therapies are ineffective. However, it should not be seen as a substitute for detailed individual assessment of these symptoms and their relief. Artificial nutrition support is used in three principal settings in malignant disease—supplementing intake to meet requirements for weight maintenance or weight gain, for accessing the gastrointestinal tract where tumours result in obstruction or dysfunction, and for prevention of weight loss during therapy. This chapter outlines the options available for oral and enteral artificial nutrition support in malignant disease, the practicalities of providing such support in hospital and the community and the benefits that may be expected.

Oral nutrition support options

The ready availability of supplements designed to boost oral nutrient intake may lead to inappropriate overprescription. Following full nutritional and dietetic assessment and attempts to increase oral food intake by dietary counseling (see Part 5), oral nutrition supplements (ONS) may be employed. These are not, however, a substitute for increased food intake, which is preferable and more likely to be maintained in the longer term.[8]

Oral nutrition supplements taken by cancer patients include a wide variety of over-the-counter and non-formulary preparations of limited or questionable benefit and clinicians need to be alert to the likelihood that patients may not volunteer information about the use of such preparations.[9]

More conventional types of ONS available and utilized by healthcare professionals include formulations that are 'nutritionally complete' and provide all the essential macro and micronutrients in the appropriate proportions such that no other nutritional source is required if a sufficient quantity of the supplement is taken. ONS are milk-, soy-, yoghurt- or 'juice'-' based and are available in a variety of flavouurs, some of which have been tested on identified patient groups for palatability. Flavors may need to be specific to disease circumstances as taste preferences have been shown to be altered by cancer or cancer therapy.[10–12] Most are in a liquid form, but some are presented in different consistencies as 'puddings''. The majority of ONS contain 1–1.5 kcal/ml, but are available as 'concentrated' feeds up to 2 kcal/ml. Protein content varies from 4 to 10 g/100 ml. Modular ONS are also available as powders that can be added to food or drinks to provide additional carbohydrate calories or protein without vitamins and micronutrients, and high calorie flavoured liquid fat emulsions can boost calorie intake even in small quantities. The choice of the type of ONS depends on the proportion of the estimated energy requirement provided by diet and its nutritional value, the patient's ability to swallow different consistencies or tolerate fluid volume, as well as taste preference. The presentation of ONS in cartons allows the possibility of 'sip feeding' whereby adequate volumes can be taken in small amounts throughout the day and can overcome problems with early satiety or partially obstructing lesions of the gastrointestinal tract.

Newer formulations of ONS include preparations enriched with n-3 fatty acids or arginine[13–17] in an attempt to modulate inflammatory responses and cancer wasting (see Chapters 9 and 11).

To derive the optimal benefit from ONS, their use should be facilitated by appropriately trained professionals, such as dietitians. Unless specializing in clinical nutrition, clinicians may not be aware of the full range and variability as well as the relevant indications of the different products available.

Benefits of oral nutrition supplements

There is a possibility that the use of ONS might substitute for voluntary dietary intake and fail to augment, or even reduce total calorie or specific nutrient consumption. Properly conducted trials where attempts have been made to blind the subjects to the purpose of the study have established that ONS do not lead to a reduction in energy intake. However there is a suggestion that components of the diet may be altered to compensate for feed enrichment—for instance with the use of protein rich supplements.[18] Indeed, ONS may stimulate appetite,[19] presumably via a number of mechanisms including balanced nutrient intake and improved mood and energy levels. Over a wide range of clinical settings studied, the effect of ONS has been to increase total oral energy intake by 40–140% of the nutritional value of the supplement.[20] A greater augmentation of voluntary intake occurs in patients with a low starting body mass index. Studies in cancer patients are limited but suggest that it is possible to augment nutrient and protein intake with ONS in this setting.[8,21–24] However the increases may be short lived and overall nutrient intake can return to baseline over 1–2 months.[8,22]

Weight Gain

In most disease scenarios, the use of ONS also results in weight gain. However, in malignant disease, it has rarely been possible to demonstrate this despite increases in nutrient intake.[25,26] A review of 11 trials of nutritional supplementation in cancer revealed no benefit in terms of weight gain, body composition or functional outcomes.[27] Weight maintenance or a reduction of weight loss may be more achievable.[21,28] By way of illustration, a pilot study of 20 patients with pancreatic cancer demonstrated significant weight gain with the consumption of an n-3 fatty acid enriched feed [(eicosapentaenoic acid: (EPA).].[29] Unfortunately no additional benefit of EPA supplementation could be demonstrated in a subsequent randomized trial of this supplement against an isocaloric, isonitrogenous control supplement.[16] There was, however, a reduction in weight loss and a small increase in lean body mass after 4 and 8 weeks in both groups. A *post hoc* analysis showed a significant difference between patients who were compliant with a minimum of 1.5 cans per day (465 kcal and 24 g protein) compared to those who were not able to take this quantity, but this was independent of EPA supplementation.[30]

Improvement in function

Improvement in function has been even more difficult to demonstrate in patients with malignant disease taking ONS, and body composition has rarely been studied in trials of nutrition intervention in cancer patients.[16,28] However, those trials that have attempted to analyze tumour response rates, survival times[22,23,31] or toxicity and complications of therapy[32–34] have failed to highlight any significant differences in outcome with the use of ONS. One study has shown fewer treatment interruptions for head and neck cancer treated with radiotherapy and a non significant reduction in mucositis.[33]

Quality of Life

Despite the lack of beneficial functional outcome data for ONS in malignant disease, quality of life indices do appear to improve with nutritional supplementation.[8,15–16,26,28,35–38] This suggests that nutritional status or intake affects aspects of quality of life in cancer patients in ways that are not directly related to measurable changes in body mass or composition,[39] for example facilitating an increase in total energy expenditure and greater physical activity.[15]

The evidence supporting use of EPA-containing supplements is contentious but in the majority of studies there is no benefit demonstrated.[16,40] EPA in capsule form alone however, rather than as a component of ONS may improve physical activity scores in quality-of-life assessment despite no significant change in lean or whole body mass.[41]

Recommendations for use of ONS in cancer patients

There is a paucity of good quality studies of the use of ONS in cancer patients, with questionable demonstration of benefit. As a result, no meaningful cost:benefit analysis can be performed and it is difficult to provide firm advice on the use of ONS in cancer. Given that weight loss is inevitable where calorie intake does not meet requirements, and that supplementation will at least slow weight loss if not stop or reverse it, it is logical to aim to increase oral nutrient intake under these circumstances. If measures addressed at increasing volitional food intake fail to meet requirements, then ONS would be appropriately indicated. European Society for Clinical Nutrition and Metabolism (ESPEN) guidelines[42] recommend the institution of enteral nutrition support when the patient is malnourished or it is anticipated that the patient will be unable to eat for more than 7 days, or to meet more than 60% of estimated requirements for more than 10 days. In the case of terminal illness, where life expectancy is likely to be more than 2–3 months, then the use of ONS may improve quality of life. It is unlikely that ONS would significantly influence the dying phase of the illness and at this stage, their use would be inappropriate on grounds of futility as much as for the risk of prolonging suffering.

Enteral tube feeding options

If volitional intake of food or ONS does not meet requirements then enteral tube feeding (ETF) should be considered. The introduction of a tube to instill feed into the gastrointestinal tract carries additional risks and considerations which may influence the decision to proceed to ETF on failure of oral nutrition support.

Tube feeding acts as a bypass by delivering feed directly into the stomach where voluntary intake, ingestion, swallowing or oesophageal transit are impaired; or into the proximal small intestine to overcome gastric dysmotility or outlet obstruction. Tubes can be passed via the nose into the stomach or proximal small intestine, or through the abdominal wall into the stomach or intestine. These tubes can be placed surgically, endoscopically or radiologically.

Nasogastric/nasoenteral tubes

Passage of a feeding tube through the nose to access the upper gastrointestinal tract is the simplest form of ETF and the tube can be positioned at the bedside. Nasogastric (NG) tubes are made of polyurethane in order to optimize strength and flexibility while maintaining a high lumen to diameter ratio.[43] For feeding rather than drainage, bore sizes of 6–8F are preferred in children, and 8F in adults to balance comfort with risk of blockage.

Blind bedside NG tube insertion carries the risk of inadvertent malposition. Passage down the trachea and into the lung is the commonest misplacement;;[44] however, there are continued reports of accidental intracranial placement[45] (traversing the ethmoid sinus after surgery or trauma) or intrapleural or even pericardial location.[46] Following several reported deaths from NG tube misplacement, the UK National Patient Safety Authority issued guidance on confirming intragastric placement using pH of gastric aspirate as the bedside test of choice, resorting to X-ray in case of uncertainty.[47] Direct visualization at radiological or endoscopic placement may be required where bedside placement proves difficult—for instance in partially obstructing lesions of the pharynx or oesophagus. A review of more than 2000 endoscopy-facilitated feeding tube placements in patients with aero-digestive cancers reported a 96% success rate overall with one death recorded due to tumour perforation at NG tube placement.[48] Complications of nasogastric tubes that are unrelated to placement or inadvertent feeding into the wrong cavity are unusual but include local irritation and sinusitis.[49]

In situations where there is either gastric stasis or outflow obstruction, it will be necessary to position the tip of the feeding tube beyond the pylorus. This can be more challenging. It is usually achieved with fluoroscopic or endoscopic guidance, and these have equivalent success rates.[50] There are also a variety of alternative techniques for bedside placement, such as the use of prokinetic agents[51,52] or magnetic steering devices,[53,54] which have their protagonists but the success rates claimed are not always borne out in routine clinical practice. An electromagnetic imaging device has recently been developed that provides a three dimensional representation of the tube as it is being placed and allows observation of manipulation beyond the pylorus without recourse to invasive techniques.[55,56] Further studies are required to ascertain the effectiveness of this new technique.

Nasogastric or nasoenteral tubes are most practical for short term use in a hospital setting. Difficulties in securing the tube result in frequent displacement and trained staff are often required to reposition it. This can result in dramatic reduction of feed delivery—in one study as little as 55% of that prescribed.[57] The presence of the tube interferes with social functioning and can be irritant and is therefore not ideal for use in the community.[58] However, patients or carers can be trained to pass the tubes themselves and NG tube feeding is successfully employed in young children and in some adults with a tube inserted each night and removed the following morning.[59] NG feeding can be considered in the short term in the community where there is good nursing support, and the use of a taped 'bridle' looped around the nasal septum and attached to the tube can provide additional confidence.[60]

Gastrostomy/jejunostomy tubes

For longer term enteral tube feeding, a tube can be inserted through the abdominal wall into the stomach or proximal jejunum. The indications for gastric or post-pyloric feeding are the same as they are for nasoenteral tubes, for instance, if the stomach does not empty either because of dysmotility or mechanical outflow obstruction then post-pyloric access will be required. Intragastric feeding requires a gastrostomy, and post-pyloric feeding some kind of jejunostomy.

For a gastrostomy, the preferred method is to place the tube using endoscopic techniques—the percutaneous endoscopic gastrostomy (PEG)'. Typically the 'pull through' method of PEG placement is employed, where needle puncture is used to introduce a thread into the stomach that can be removed through the mouth and allow a feeding tube to be drawn back into place by traction.[61] This tube design permits a 'bumper' or retention disc to retain the tube in the stomach but also to oppose the visceral and parietal peritoneal surfaces and prevent leakage of gastric contents into the abdominal cavity (Figure 21.1). A 'push' technique can also be used (Figure 21.2) where the

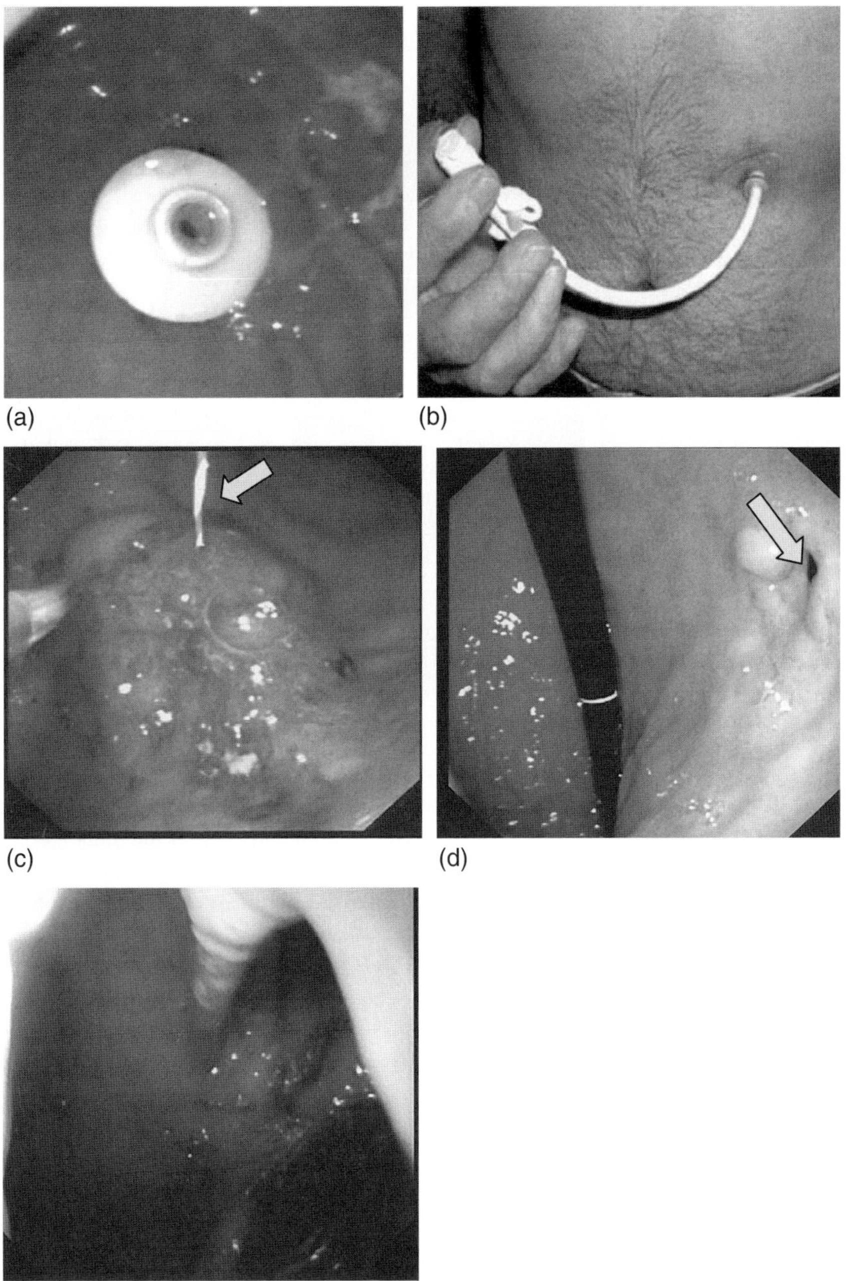

Fig. 21.1 The 'Pull' or bumper-retained percutaneous endoscopic gastrostomy (PEG) tube and complications. (a) Endoscopic view of the bumper disc retaining the PEG tube in the stomach and serving to oppose the gastric and abdominal walls by traction. (b) External view of the PEG in a typical location on the abdominal wall. (c) The 'buried bumper': too much tension on the PEG bumper has resulted in erosion of the underlying gastric mucosa and regrowth of the mucosa over the bumper. A wire has been inserted through the PEG from the external surface to demonstrate the lumen of the tube (arrow). (d) Erosion of the bumper through the gastric wall. In this case, initial inadvertent transcolonic placement of the PEG has only become apparent on attempted endoscopic exchange of a worn-out tube. The bumper has eroded through the gastric wall and into the transverse colon. The arrow demonstrates the opening of the gastrocolonic fistula. (e) View through the gastrocolonic fistula demonstrating the PEG tube in the transverse colon (arrow) [same case as in (c)].

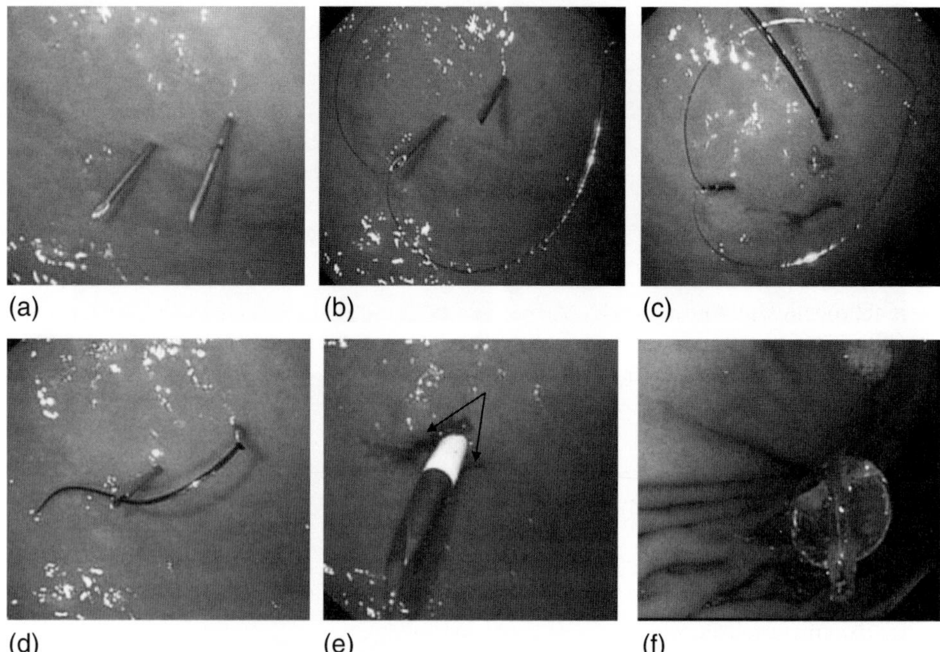

Fig. 21.2 Technique of placement of a 'push' balloon retained percutaneous endoscopic gastrostomy (PEG) in a patient with tonsillar carcinoma prior to commencement of chemoradiotherapy. (a) Twin-needle gastropexy device is inserted percutaneously into the stomach under direct gastroscopic visualization. (b) A preformed metal snare is opened and lies over the other needle. (c) A suture is passed through the needle and (d) The snare is closed, trapping the thread. The device is then removed from the patient and the suture tied on the exterior. This opposes the gastric and abdominal walls. (e) Following insertion of a second gastropexy suture (both arrows) a trocar is inserted inside a peel away sheath. The trocar is removed, the PEG tube placed through the sheath, balloon inflated and the sheath removed.

stomach is held up to the anterior abdominal wall with gastropexy sutures and a balloon-retained tube is placed through a track made using a trocar and pull-away sheath.[62] When endoscopic access to the stomach is not possible, for example obstructive pathology in the oropharynx or oesophagus, a radiologically inserted gastrostomy (RIG) can be placed, with similar rates of successful placement and complications.[63]

Complications of gastrostomy placement range from minor to major, and early to late. Early complications include localized pain, which typically lasts for a few days after the procedure and settles with simple analgesia. Occasionally leakage of gastric contents into the peritoneal cavity can result in a chemical peritonitis that normally settles with tightening of the tube and a short course of antibiotics, but may require laparotomy and surgical replacement of the tube. Other early complications relate to the procedure itself, such as cardiorespiratory compromise, aspiration pneumonia and haemorrhage at the site of insertion. Inadvertent placement of the tube across another viscus—including left lobe of the liver, colon or small intestine—is frequently reported but, surprisingly, associated with few immediate symptoms. The overall mortality within 30 days of insertion ranges from 5% to >more than 30% in the literature, but of course much of this relates to the underlying disease process rather than problems directly attributable to the gastrostomy itself. The commonest late complication is infection of the PEG site, which is usually localized and controlled easily by antibiotics, but can result in cellulitis or necrotizing fasciitis. There has been concern of tumour seeding in the stoma, especially in those with oropahryngeal or oesophageal cancer. However, such complications remain in the realms of case reports and small case series and are uncommon.

Percutaneous approaches to post-pyloric/jejunal placement include endoscopic placement of a PEG tube directly into the small intestine (:direct percutaneous endoscopic jejunostomy: DPEJ)[64] or transgastric placement of a fine bore 'extension" tube through a PEG directed into the intestine under direct (endoscopic or radiological) vision. This is known as a PEG-J or 'jejunal extension' PEG.[65,66] Placement of a DPEJ is technically much more difficult, and can be complicated by intestinal volvulus, perforation and leakage of irritant intestinal contents in up to 10% of cases.[64] The PEG-J is not associated with these complications, but is associated with a significant incidence of migration of the jejunal portion of the tube back into the stomach.[67] Where endoscopic or radiological placement is not possible, surgery may be required to position an enteral feeding tube. This may be performed laparoscopically or with a mini-laparotomy.

In addition to their use for feeding, large bore (up to 30F) gastrostomy tubes can be utilized for gastric drainage in those with intestinal obstruction further downstream—due, for example, to peritoneal malignancy, pseudomyxoma peritonei, metastatic ovarian, breast or colonic cancer.[68,69] More than 90% of patients treated in such series experience relief of nausea and vomiting and many thereafter manage to eat or drink small amounts for comfort. There is unfortunately a higher risk of complication with tubes used for this indication, including leakage of gastric contents.[69]

Feed types and administration

Blenderized home-prepared food can be given, but the risks of tube blockage, contamination and nutritional imbalance make it safer and easier to use proprietary self-contained brands of liquid feed. There are a number of different types of such feeds, which broadly speaking can be divided into the following groups:

- *Polymeric feeds.*. These contain whole protein, carbohydrate and fat and they can be used as a sole source of nutrition for those without any special nutrient requirements. The standard concentration is 1 kcal/ml, but they can be more or less energy dense (0.8–2.0 kcal/ml) and can also contain fibre, which can improve bowel function if this is problematic.
- *Elemental feeds.*. These diets contain protein in amino acid form and carbohydrate as glucose or maltodextrins. Fat content is very low. They are used primarily in situations of malabsorption, and have little indication in cancer scenarios.
- *Disease-specific feeds.* Certain clinical situations require alterations in diets. For example there are high energy/low electrolyte feeds designed for patients on dialysis, and low carbohydrate/high fat diets for patients with CO_2 retention, such as those on ventilators (carbohydrate has a higher respiratory quotient than fat or protein and leads to more CO_2 production). This may be of relevance in cancer patients with significant comorbidity
- *Immune-modulating feeds.*. These feeds contain extra substrates, which may alter the immune and inflammatory responses. The commonly used substrates are glutamine, arginine, RNA, ω-3 fatty acids and antioxidants. There is evidence gathering for the use of these products in certain surgical, trauma, critically ill and cancer patients. These are discussed in more detail in Chapter 9.

As with ONS, utilizing the right feed in the right patient requires healthcare professionals with appropriate knowledge, rather than a product randomly selected from the shelf.

The method of administering feed also has a number of options. It can be delivered by bolus or by continuous infusion using a pump or just gravity. There are benefits of both bolus and pump feeding that need considering and discussing with the patient. Bolus feeding is more physiological and appropriately satisfies appetite. It has the additional advantage of allowing the patient to be detached from giving sets for most of the day, thereby facilitating greater independence. However, there is the concern that it may lead the patient to feeling more bloated and uncomfortable. The theoretical fear of increased risk of pulmonary aspiration and chest infections over continuous feeding, however, is not supported in the literature. Continuous feeding can be spread over 12–24– h a day, dependent in part to how much feed the patient can tolerate. It would normally be over 12–16 h a day using a pump, to allow the patient some time free from equipment, with the patient semi-recumbent or upright (no less than 30°) to prevent aspiration. Night-time feeding allows daytime freedom, but sleep quality may be affected by the required patient positioning, noise from the pump and increased enuresis; daytime feeding will make activities difficult. On top of these considerations are more practical ones that will be determined by the accommodation of the patient, for instance, residential nursing homes may favour pump feeding because it is less time-consuming than bolus feeding several times a day. For optimizing quality of life, it should be the patients' wishes that are paramount in determining the method of feed delivery.

Complications of enteral feeding

On the whole enteral feeding is safe and complications are not usually serious. They can be divided into those due to the tubes and routes of feeding, which have been described already, and those due to the feeding itself. The latter group include:

Diarrhoea

This is the commonest complication, with rates quoted anywhere between 5% and 60%. It is most commonly associated with antibiotics, laxative use, contaminated feeds and hypoalbuminaemia. Management is: (i) to exclude other explanations, for example *Clostridium ddifficile*, colitis, malabsorption; (ii) to rationalize concomitant medication if possible, especially antibiotics. Treatment thereafter is usually successful with standard antidiarrhoeal medication (loperamide and/or codeine phosphate) and use of a fibre-containing diet.

Constipation

Usually due to a combination of inadequate fluid, dehydration, poor mobility and drugs (e.g. opiates). Management is to ensure that there is no other explanation such as colonic pathology, and then prudent use of laxatives and suppositories. Fibre feeds can also help and are usually worth trying.

Vomiting/aspiration/reflux

Both nasogastric and PEG feeding can increase the risk of aspiration. Both can interfere with gastro-oesophageal sphincter function, and wide-bore nasogastric tubes do so more than fine-bore tubes. Where possible, patients should be fed at 30–45°. Standard anti-emetics and prokinetic agents are usually effective. Alternative or additional management options include alteration of feed delivery (change from bolus to continuous feeding), or changing diet to a more energy-dense one, with smaller volumes delivering equivalent calories. Occasionally post-pyloric feeding is required.

Metabolic complications

Both under- and overhydration can be avoided by appropriate monitoring of fluid balance, and it should be remembered that enteral diets count as about 90% fluid, i.e. 1000 ml of feed = 900 ml fluid. Refeeding syndrome' is defined as severe fluid and electrolyte shifts and related metabolic implications in malnourished patients undergoing refeeding. In such patients administration of carbohydrate excess to their needs causes a surge of insulin secretion, which leads to massive cellular uptake of phosphate, magnesium and potassium and a consequent fall in their serum levels with disorder of glucose metabolism and fluid balance. This can all lead to dangerous arrhythmias and neurological events, and can be fatal. It is therefore vital that undernourished patients—and cancer sufferers will invariably fall into such a category—must not be fed excess to requirements however emaciated they may be.

Vitamin/trace element deficiencies

These are rare as most commercially available feeds are now nutritionally complete. Patients being enterally fed over a prolonged period of time may be at risk, but appropriate monitoring should avoid problems.

Indications for ETF in malignant disease

Unlike the use of ONS, ETF requires an invasive procedure that may be associated with significant complications and can impair the quality or duration of life. Although withdrawing and withholding nutrition support are considered ethically equivalent,[70] it may be difficult in practice to cease feeding through an existing gastrostomy and this may alter the manner of a patient's death and even unnecessarily prolong their suffering. Similarly, the placement of a feeding tube may alter the patient's domicile in view of nursing requirements and this could have a significant negative impact on their quality of life. The decision to place a feeding tube therefore needs to be taken with due consideration to all aspects of the patient's care and is best undertaken by a multidisciplinary team in consultation with the patient/family/carers.[71]

ETF prior to or during therapy

Prophylactic placement of an enteral feeding tube can be beneficial where mucositis or pain may limit the ability to swallow during or after treatment. This is most relevant for patients undergoing chemo-radiation therapy for head and neck cancer, but may also benefit patients with severe mucositis as a complication of chemotherapeutic regimens used for instance with bone marrow transplantation conditioning. In such cases, the discomfort of mucositis may be exacerbated by dysgeusia, xerostomia, nausea, vomiting and anorexia which can all be mitigated by tube feeding.

Head and neck ccancer

Patients undergoing therapy for head and neck cancer constitute a large proportion of all patients receiving ETF; however, there is considerable regional variation in the use of PEG tubes for this indication. In Germany and Spain, such patients constitute 60% of all patients fed at home by gastrostomy, whereas the proportion overall in the UK, Poland and Denmark is around 10%. There is however considerable regional variation in practice within countries—in Cambridge, UK 38% of all PEGs are placed for this indication.

Few studies have compared the use of tube feeding to dietary counselling and ONS in treatment for head and neck cancer. Two prospectively randomized trials compared 18 and 34 NG-fed patients respectively to oral feeding control groups, and demonstrated significant (7.3%, 9–12%) weight loss in the oral-fed group, which could be abolished entirely by nasogastric feeding.[72,73] However, despite the use of 40 kcal/kg in the tube-fed group, weight could only be stabilized and not regained.[72] The use of ONS may, however, reduce the requirement for tube feeding:—from 31% to 6% in one study of patients with oropharyngeal cancer treated by radiotherapy alone.[74]

Reports of ETF in head and neck cancer are largely anecdotal and retrospective. Patients generally prefer PEG tube placement rather than nasogastric tubes due to improved cosmesis and ease of use.[75,76] In addition, complication rates, including mechanical failure and aspiration pneumonia, have been reported to be lower with the use of gastrostomy tubes and this is reflected in quality-of-life scores.[77] The finding that PEG feeding is generally more prolonged than NG feeding in this setting is most likely to relate to the relative ease and desirability of removal of the NG tube following treatment completion.[76] The average duration of PEG feeding in this setting is more than 100 days.[76,80–82] compared to 8 weeks for NG feeding.[76] In the home setting, both NG and PEG tubes interfere significantly with social functioning, and psychological acceptance is low with up to one-third of tube-fed aero-digestive cancer patients uncomfortable about their body image.[78]

PEG placement can be undertaken prior to multimodality therapy, during surgery or, if significant feeding difficulties occur, subsequently. Placement prior to chemo-radiotherapy is associated with a reduction in weight loss during treatment compared to reactive tube feeding begun when feeding difficulties develop.[73,79] It is also associated with minimal complications[80,82] and reduced length of hospital stay.[73] Similarly, placement at the time of surgery is convenient and avoids complications of endoscopy under sedation.[83,84]

Seeding of tumour deposits into the gastrostomy track has been reported as a complication of the 'pull' technique of PEG placement in head and neck cancer patients. This occurs rarely—in less than 1% cases[85]—and there are only 44 instances reported in the literature.[86] Of these all but one are from squamous cell tumours. Mean survival after diagnosis of PEG site metastasis is around 4 months, but this is likely to reflect the high risk of seeding from already advanced tumouurs. This complication can be prevented by the use of a 'push' technique and is now the method of choice for such patients in many centres.[87] Furthermore, this technique can be employed in patients with severe trismus by the use of an ultrathin endoscope passed transnasally to guide PEG placement.[88]

Oesophagogastric cancer

Patients with oesophageal cancer are frequently malnourished at presentation due to obstructive dysphagia.

The use of chemoradiation for proximal squamous cell carcinoma may result in mucositis similar to that seen in patients with head and neck cancers. Nutrition support with dietary advice, ONS or ETF has been shown to reduce weight loss, increase radiotherapy completion rates and reduce hospital stays for such patients.[89] A previous study of patients undergoing chemoradiation therapy with curative intent showed that tube-fed dysphagic patients maintained their body weight better than non-dysphagic patients on standard oral diet.[90]

In the setting of oesophageal adenocarcinoma, the use of neo-adjuvant chemotherapy or chemoradiation may significantly prolong the time that patients are unable to feed orally. Nutrition support can be problematic for these patients due to the oesophageal obstruction impeding NG tube passage or endoscopy. Although NG tube feeding is preferable, PEG placement can be performed safely using endoscopic dilatation of the stricture[91,92] but carries significant risk of oesophageal perforation from the dilatation itself. An alternative is to site a 'push' PEG using an ultrathin endoscope to pass the tumour,[88] or ask a radiologist to site a RIG. A further consideration is that gastrostomy placement—either a PEG or a RIG—may prevent the use of the stomach as a conduit following oesophagectomy, although in practice this has only been reported in one case due to procedure-related thrombosis of the gastroepiploic artery.[93] Insertion of a feeding jejunostomy tube at the time of a staging laparoscopy may circumvent these concerns and its use can then be continued postoperatively.[94] It is now routine in most centres to place a feeding tube at the time of surgery for upper gastrointestinal malignancy, and although significant complications are reported they are outweighed by the nutritional benefits, with up to a quarter of patients requiring feeding via this route for more than 3 weeks and almost one in 10 continuing jejunostomy feeding at home after discharge.[95,96]

Recent guidelines recommend preoperative enteral feeding by ONS or ETF for 10–14 days in patients with gastrointestinal malignancy at severe risk of malnutrition-related complications,[97] even if this delays surgery. A systematic review recently demonstrated no overall benefit for EPA supplemented ETF in cancer patients undergoing surgery;;[24] however, the use of 'immune-enhancing' feeds is recommended by ESPEN for this indication—the evidence for this guidance is discussed in Chapter 9.

The combination of insufficient data and clinical variability preclude firm recommendations regarding the optimal route of ETF in oesophageal cancer, and much depends on the choice of therapy and the extent of obstruction.

Haemopoetic stem cell transplantation (HSCT)

The use of intensive conditioning regimens for allogeneic HSCT results in severe feeding difficulties due to mucositis or gastrointestinal intolerance from graft-versus-host disease. Patients experiencing severe symptoms rarely tolerate NG tube placement and parenteral nutrition is frequently required, and indeed recommended.[42] However, a small randomized controlled trial demonstrated no benefit of parenteral over enteral feeding, but a significant cost benefit for the latter.[98] A more recent observational study suggested a reduction in infectious mortality with ETF compared to parenteral nutrition and the optimal route of nutrition for HSCT requires more rigorous investigation.[99] There are no published data on the use of prophylactic PEG placement in patients undergoing HSCT. However, anecdotally this is associated with high complication rates that include severe PEG site infection as a result of neutropenia, and bleeding due to thrombocytopenia or massive splenomegaly. The challenges of nutritional support in HSCT are discussed in more detail in Chapter 28.

ETF in palliative care

Palliative nutrition support may be considered for patients with obstructing lesions of the upper gastrointestinal tract or with tumour-related anorexia.

The hazards and burden of tube insertion and maintenance need to be finely balanced with the predicted benefits of feeding in patients with advanced cancer. The priority necessarily shifts from that of longevity to quality-of-life issues. Geographical variability in the use of ETF demonstrates that cultural perspectives and patient expectations play a large part in this decision. In the UK, less than one-third of all home ETF patients have malignant disease[100] and it is rarely considered appropriate in the palliative care setting. On the other hand, in Italy and the USA, patients with advanced cancer make up more than 50% of the home enterally fed population.[101,102] Advocates of palliative home ETF would suggest that it improves quality of life, reduces readmission rates due to complications of malnutrition and allows patients more time at home and with their families in the later stage of their illness. However, the contrary view is that by prolonging life it may increase suffering, add to complications and concerns regarding the complexities of treatment. There is also a cost-benefit argument particularly with the requirement for increased healthcare provision in the community to manage patients at home. There are sadly few data available to inform the argument. The lack of positive outcomes in randomized controlled trials has led some to postulate that nutritional support should not be offered to patients in this setting.[103,104] However, this largely reflects the lack of evidence rather than a lack of demonstrated benefit.

Observational reports provide some information and suggest that the life expectancy for selected patients with malignant disease receiving ETF is comparable to that of patients with neurological dysphagia, for whom home ETF is an accepted and routine indication.[105,106] However, poor outcomes can be demonstrated with unselected patients[107] and a further report from Portugal of the use of PEG feeding in 154 palliative care patients over a 10-year period (mostly for head and neck and oesophageal cancer) demonstrated a median survival of 61 days, with 30% of patients dying within 1 month of PEG tube insertion.[108] Few centres would support the widespread use of ETF in this setting with such results. Patient selection is clearly vital and criteria have not yet been firmly established. Predicted survival for more than 6 weeks was considered by the Bologna group to be mandatory;;[109] however, prognostic estimates are notoriously unreliable in advanced cancer and no suitable tools exist that can provide any such accuracy. In this report, 30% of patients predicted to die within 6 weeks lived longer and a similar proportion of those who would have been eligible for home ETF by this criterion died prematurely. However, overall mean survival was 17 weeks for 135 enterally fed patients. Tube feeding was well accepted by the majority of patients who spent around 20% of their remaining life in hospital. A 4-year prospective follow-up study of patients in Kiel[3] could demonstrate no differences in survival or weight gain post-PEG insertion between patients with malignant disease or benign conditions (Figure 21.3). These outcomes would at least support a role for ETF at home with appropriate patient selection.

Studies of quality-of-life indices in palliative ETF for malignant disease are also extremely limited and generally of short duration.[78,110,111] It is currently not possible to state with any confidence that quality of life is significantly improved by ETF. Intuitively such an effect seems likely,

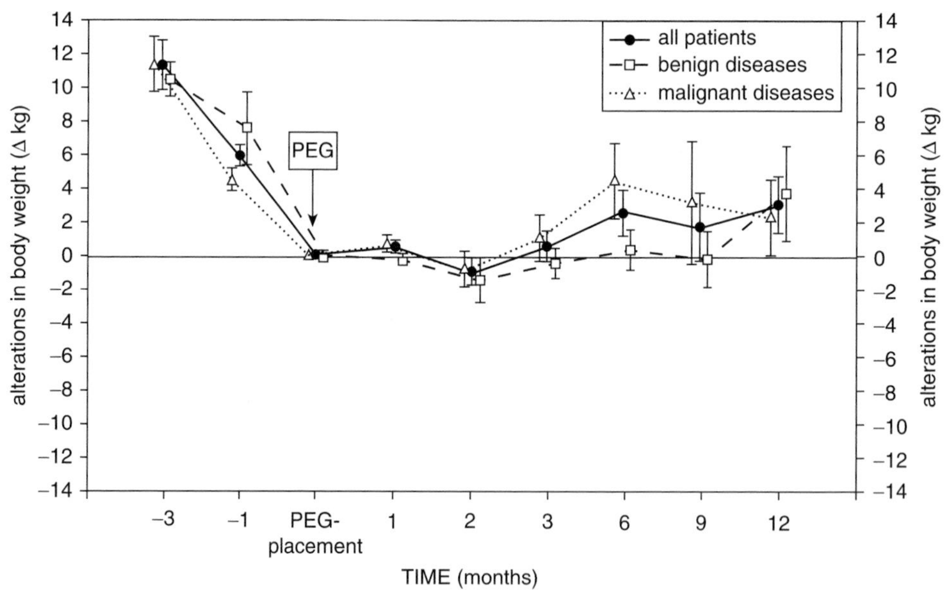

Fig. 21.3 Effect of percutaneous endoscopic gastrostomy (PEG) feeding on patients' weight from a 4-year prospective study in Kiel. All patients lost a considerable proportion of their weight prior to PEG feeding. Artificial nutrition abolished the weight loss and initially stabilized weight before gradually increasing but never returning to baseline. No differences could be detected between patients with benign or malignant diseases in this study. (From Loser *et al.*[3])

though others have argued that a 'symptom shift' may occur resulting in neutral or even negative quality-of-life experiences in this setting.[112]

Recommendations for the use of ETF in malignant disease

Despite the lack of objective data, it is still possible to make certain recommendations:

1. ETF should be considered when volitional oral intake is unlikely to meet requirements in the following settings:
   - During chemoradiotherapy for head and neck or oesophageal cancer. Preferred option: prior insertion of a 'push' PEG.
   - Preoperative nutritional optimization prior to definitive surgery. Preferred option: nasogastric tube feeding.
   - Postoperative feeding after surgery for upper gastrointestinal surgery. Preferred option: intraoperative jejunostomy tube placement.
2. ETF should only be considered in patients with advanced malignant disease who are unable to meet nutritional requirements orally where:
   - Projected life expectancy and quality of life justify the risks and complications of tube insertion.
   - The patient and carers are fully informed of the benefits and hazards of tube insertion, the issues relating to living with a feeding tube and managing feeding regimens at home.

Cultural, ethical and health economic considerations currently influence the decision to initiate ETF and it is hoped that future studies will help to clarify the role of ETF in advanced malignancy. However, due to the emotive nature of food and nutrition, and also of end-of-life issues, it is unlikely that such evidence will be forthcoming in the near future from prospective randomized controlled trials.

References

1. Rivadeneira DE, Evoy D, Fahey TJ, Lieberman MD, Daly JM (1998) Nutritional support of the cancer patient. *CA Cancer J Clin*, **48**, 69–80.
2. Ravasco P, Monteiro-Grillo I, Vidal PM, Camilo ME (2003) Nutritional deterioration in cancer: the role of disease and diet. *Clin Oncol*, **15**, 443–50.
3. Loser C, Wolters S, Folsch UR (1998) Enteral long term nutrition via percutaneous endoscopic gastrostomy (PEG) in 210 patients. A four year prospective study. *Dig Dis Sci*, **43**, 2549–57.
4. DeWys WD, Begg C, Lavin PT, *et al.* (1980) Prognostic effect of weight loss prior to chemotherapy in cancer patients. *Am J Med*, **69**, 491–7.
5. Wigmore SJ, Plester CE, Richardson RA, *et al.* (1997) Changes in nutritional status associated with unresectable pancreatic cancer. *Br J Cancer*, **75**, 106–9.
6. Brookes GB (1985) Nutritional status: a prognostic indicator in head and neck cancer. *Otolaryngol Head Neck Surg*, **93**, 69–74.
7. Sako K, Lore JM, Kaufman S, *et al.* (1981) Parenteral hyperalimentation in surgical patients with head and neck cancer: a randomized study. *J Surg Oncol*, **16**, 391–402.
8. Ravasco P, Monteiro-Grillo I, Vidal PM, Camilo ME (2005) Impact of nutrition on outcome: a prospective randomized controlled trial in patients with head and neck cancer undergoing radiotherapy. *Head and Neck*, **27**, 659–68.
9. Norman HA, Butrum RR, Feldman E, *et al.* (2003) The role of dietary supplements during cancer therapy. *J Nutr*, **133**, 3794–9S.

10. Gallagher P, Tweedle D (1983) Taste threshold and acceptability of commercial diets in cancer patients *J Paren Enteral Nutr*, **7**, 361–3.
11. Bolton J, Abbott R, Kiely M (1992) Comparison of three oral sip-feed supplements in patients with cancer. *J Hum Nutr Diet*, **5**, 79–84.
12. Wickham R, Rehwaldt M, Keter C (1999) Taste changes experienced by patients receiving chemotherapy. *Oncol NNurse FForum*, **26**, 697–706.
13. Senkal M, Haaker R, Linseisen J, *et al.* (2005) Preoperative oral supplementation with long chain omega-3 fatty acids beneficially alters phospholipids fatty acid patterns in liver, gut mucosa, and tumour tissue. *J Paren Enteral Nutr*, **29**, 236–40.
14. de Luis DA, Izaola O, Aller R, Cuellar L, Terroba MC (2005) A randomized trial with oral immunonutrition (omega-3 enhanced formula vs arginine enhanced formula) in ambulatory head and neck cancer patients *Ann Nutr Metab*, **49**, 95–9.
15. Moses AW, Slater C, Preston T, Barber MD, Fearon KC (2004) Reduced total energy expenditure and physical activity in cachectic patients with pancreatic cancer can be modulated by an energy and protein dense oral supplement enriched with n-3 fatty acids. *Br J Cancer*, **90**, 996–1002.
16. Fearon KCH, von Meyenfeldt MF, Moses AGW, *et al.* (2003) Effect of a protein and energy dense n-3 fatty acid enriched oral supplement on loss of weight and lean tissue in cancer cachexia: a randomised double blind trial. *Gut*, **52**, 1479–86.
17. Wigmore SJ, Barber MD, Ross JA, *et al.* (2000) Effect of oral eicosapentanoic acid on weight loss in patients with pancreatic cancer. *Nutr Cancer*, **36**, 177–84.
18. Stockley L, Jones FA, Broadhurst AJ, *et al.* (1984) The effect of moderate protein or energy supplements on subsequent nutrient intake in man. *Appetite*, **5**, 209–19.
19. Ovesen L (1992) The effect of a supplement which is nutrient dense compared to standard concentration on the total nutritional intake of anorectic patients. *Clin Nutrr*, **11**, 154–7.
20. Stratton RJ, Green CJ, Elia M (2003) *Disease-Related Malnutrition: An Evidence-Based Approach to Treatment.* : Wallingford, UK: CABI P.
21. Ovesen L, Allingstrup L (1992) Different quantities of two commercial liquid diets consumed by weight losing cancer patients *J Paren arent Enteral nteral Nutr,utr*, **16**, 275–8.
22. Arnold C, Richter M (1989) The effect of oral nutritional supplements on head and neck cancer *Int J Rad Oncol Biol Phys*, **16**, 1595–9.
23. Evans WK, Nixon DW, Daly JM, *et al.* (1987) A randomized study of oral nutritional support versus ad lib nutritional intake during chemotherapy for advanced colorectal and non-small cell lung .cancer... *J Clin Oncol*, **5**, 113–24.
24. Elia M, van Bokhorst-de Van de Schueren MA, Garvey J, *et al.* (2006) Enteral (oral or tube administration) nutritional support and eicosapentaenoic acid in patients with cancer: a systematic review. *Int J Oncol*, **28**, 5–23.
25. Ovesen L, Allingstrup L, Hannibal J, *et al.* (1993) Effect of dietary counseling on food intake, body weight, response rate, survival and quality of life in cancer patients undergoing chemotherapy: a prospective randomized study. *J Clin Oncol*, **11**, 2043–9.
26. Ravasco P, Monteiro-Grillo I, Vidal PM, *et al.* (2005) Dietary counseling improves patient outcomes: a prospective ra ndomized controlled trial in colorectal cancer patients undergoing radiotherapy. *J Clin Oncol*, **23**, 1431–8.
27. Stratton RJ, Elia M (1999) A critical, systematic analysis of the use of oral nutrition supplements in the community. *Clin Nutr*, **18**, S29–84.
28. Isenring EA, Capra S, Bauer JD (2004) Nutrition intervention is beneficial in oncology outpatients receiving radiotherapy to the gastrointestinal or head and neck area. *Brit J Cancer*, **91**, 447–52.
29. Barber MD, Ross JA, Preston T, Shenkin A, Fearon KCH (1999) Fish oil enriched nutritional supplement attenuates progression of the acute-phase response in weight losing patients with advanced pancreatic cancer. *J Nutr*, **129**, 1120–5.

30. Bauer J, Capra S, Battistuta D, *et al.* (2005) Compliance with nutrition prescription improves outcomes in patients with unresectable pancreatic cancer. *Clin Nutr*, **24**, 998–1004.
31. Elkort RJ, Baker FL, Vitale JJ, Cordano A (1981) Long term nutritional support as an adjunct to chemotherapy for breast cancer. *J Paren Enteral Nutr*, **5**, 385–90.
32. Bounous G, LeBel E, Shuster J, Gold P, Tahan WT, Bastin E (1975) Dietary protection during radiation therapy. *Strahlentherapie*, **149**, 476–83.
33. Nayel H, El-Ghoneimy E, El-Haddad S (1992) Impact of nutritional supplementation on treatment delay and morbidity in patients with head and neck tumours treated with irradiation. *Nutrition*, **8**, 13–18.
34. Flynn MB, Leighty FF (1987) Preoperative outpatient nutritional support of patients with squamous cancer of the upper aerodigestive tract. *Am J Surg*, **154**, 359–62.
35. Davidson W, Ash S, Capra S, *et al.* (2004) Weight stabilization is associated with improved survival duration and quality of life in unresectable pancreatic cancer. *Clin Nutfr*, **23**, 239–47.
36. Bauer JD, Capra S (2005) Nutrition intervention improves outcomes in patients with cancer cachexia receiving chemotherapy—a pilot study. *Support Care Cancer*, **13**, 270–4.
37. Marin Caro MM, Laviano A, Pichard C (2007) Nutritional intervention and quality of life in adult oncology patients. *Clin Nutr*, **26**, 289–301.
38. Marin Caro MM, Laviano A, Pichard C (2007) Impact of nutrition on quality of life during cancer. *Curr Opin Clin Nutr Metab Care*, **10**, 480—7.
39. Ravasco P, Monteiro-Grillo I, Vidal PM, *et al.* (2004) Cancer: disease and nutrition are key determinants of patients quality of life. *Support Care Cancer*, **12**, 246–52.
40. Jatoi A, Rowland K, Loprinzi CL, *et al.* (2004) An eicosapentaenoic acid supplement versus megestrol acetate versus both for cancer-associated wasting: a North Central Cancer treatment Group and National Cancer institute of Canada collaborative effort. *J Clin Oncol*, **22**, 2469–76.
41. Fearon KC, Barber MD, Moses AG, *et al.* (2006) Double-blind placebo controlled randomized study of eicosapentaenoic acid diester in patients with cancer cachexia. *J Clin Oncol*, **24**, 3401–7.
42. Arends J, Bodoky G, Bozzetti F, *et al.* (2006) ESPEN guidelines on enteral nutrition: non surgical oncology. *Clin Nutr*, **25**, 245—59.
43. Rees RG, Attrill H, Quinn D, *et al.* (1986) Improved design of nasogastric tubes. *Clin Nutr*, **5**, 203–7.
44. Sorokin R, Gottlieb JE (2006) Enhancing patient safety during feeding tube insertion: a review of more than 2000 insertions. *J Paren Enteral Nutr*, **30**, 440–5.
45. Hande A, Nagpal R (1991) Intracranial malposition of nasogatric tube following transnasal transphenoidal operation. *Br J Neurosurg*, **5**, 205–7.
46. Hanafy Eel-D, Ashebu SD, Naqeeb NA, *et al.* (2006) Pericardial sac perforation: a rare complication of neonatal nasogastric tube feeding. *Paediatr Radiol*, **36**, 1096–8.
47. National Patient Safety Authority. http://www.npsa.nhs.uk/patientsafety/alerts-and-directives/alerts/nasogastric-feeding-tubes/
48. Shastri YM, Shirodkar M, Mallath MK (2008) Endoscopic feeding tube placement in patients with cancer: a prospective clinical audit of 2055 procedures in 1866 patients. *Aliment Pharmacol Ther*, **27**, 649–58.
49. Desmond P, Raman R, Idikula J (1991) Effect of nasogastric tubes on the nose and maxillary sinus *Crit Care Med*, **19**, 509–11.
50. Thurley PD, Hopper MA, Jobling JC, *et al.* (2008) Fluoroscopic insertion of post-pyloric feeding tubes: success rates and complications. *Clin Radiol*, **63**, 543–8.
51. Kalliafas S, Choban PS, Ziegler D, *et al.* (1996) Erythromycin facilitates postpyloric placement of nasoduodenal feeding tubes in intensive care patients: randomized, double blinded, placebo controlled trial. *J Paren Enteral Nutr*, **20**, 385–8.

52. Silva CC, Saconato H, Atallah AN (2002) Metoclopramide for migration of naso-enteral tube. *Cochrane Database Syst Rev* CD003353.
53. Gabriel SA, McDaniel B, Ashley DW, *et al.* (2001) Magnetically guided nasoenteral feeding tubes: a new technique. *Am Surg*, **67**, 544–8.
54. Boivin M, Levy H, Hayes J (2000) A multicenter, prospective study of the placement of transpyloric feeding tubes with assistance of a magnetic device. The Magnetic-guided enteral feeding tube study group. *J Paren Enteral Nutr*, **24**, 304–7.
55. Young RJ, Chapman MJ, Fraser R, *et al.* (2005) A novel technique for post-pyloric feeding tube placement in critically ill patients: a pilot study. *Anaesth Intens Care*, **33**, 229–34.
56. Gray R, Tynan C, Reed L (2007) Bedside electro-magnetic guided feeding tube placement: an improvement over traditional placement technique? *Nutr Clin Pract*, **22**, 436–44.
57. Park RH, Allison MC, Lang J, *et al.* (1992) Randomised comparison of percutaneous endoscopic gastrostomy and nasogastric tube feeding in patients with persisting neurological dysphagia. *Br r Med ed J*, **304**, 1406–9.
58. Annoni JM, Vuagnat H, Frischknecht R, *et al.* (1998) Percutaneous endoscopic gastrostomy in neurological rehabilitation**: a report of six cases.** *DisabilRehab*, **20**, *308–14.*
59. *Delegge MH (2006) Enteral access in home care. J Paren Enteral Nutr*, **30**, *S13–S20.*
60. Anderson MR, O'Connor M, Mayer P, *et al.* (2004) The nasal loop provides an alternative to percutaneous endoscopic gastrostomy in high-risk dysphagic stroke patients. *Clin Nutr*, **23**, 501–6.
61. Gauderer MWL, Ponsky JL, Izant RJ (1980) Gastrostomy without laparotomy: a percutaneous endoscopic technique. *J Paediatr Surg*, **15**, 872–5.
62. Tucker AT, Gourin CG, Ghegan MD, *et al.* (2003) 'Push' versus 'Pull' percutaneous endoscopic gastrostomy tube placement in patients with advanced head and neck cancer. *Laryngoscope*, **113**, 1898–1902.
63. Silas AM, Pearce LF, Lestina LS, *et al.* (2005) Percutaneous radiologic gastrostomy versus percutaneous endoscopic gastrostomy: a comparison of indications, complications and outcomes in 370 patients. *Eur J Radiol*, **56**, *84–90.*
64. Maple JT, Petersen BT, Baron TH, *et al.* (2005) Direct percutaneous endoscopic jejunostomy: outcomes in 307 consecutive attempts. *Am J Gastroenterol*, **100**, 2681–8.
65. DeLegge MH, Duckworth PF Jr, McHenry L Jr (1995) Percutaneous endoscopic gastrojejunostomy: a dual center safety and efficacy trial. *J Paren Enteral Nutr*, **19**, 239–43.
66. Shike M, Latkany L, Gerdes H, *et al.* (1996) Direct percutaneous endoscopic jejunostomies for enteral feeding *Gastrointest Endosc*, **44**, 536–40.
67. Cameron E, Cottee S, Woodward J (2006) Long term PEG-J feeding: a single centre experience. *Gut*, **55**(Suppl 11), A103.
68. Brooksbank MA, Game PA, Ashby MA (2002) Palliative venting gastrostomy in malignant intestinal obstruction. *Palliat Med*, **16**, 520–6.
69. Pothuri B, Montemarano M, Gerardi M, *et al.* (2005) Percutaneous endoscopic gastrostomy tube placement in patients with malignant bowel obstruction due to ovarian carcinoma. *Gynecol Oncol*, **96**, 330–4.
70. House of Lords (1993) 48–58. *Report of Select Committee on Medical Ethics*, pp., London:: HMSO.
71. National Confidential Enquiry into Perioperative Deaths (2004) *Scoping our Practice.*: London: NCEPOD.
72. Hearne BE, Dunaj JM, Daly JM, *et al.* (1985) Enteral nutrition support in head and neck cancer: tube vs. oral feeding during radiation therapy. *J Am Diet Assoc*, **85**, 669–74.
73. Tyldesley S, Sheehan F, Munk P, *et al.* (1996) The use of radiologically placed gastrostomy tubes in head and neck cancer patients receiving radiotherapy. *Int J Radiat Biol Phys*, **36**, 1205–9.

74. Lee H, Havrila C, Bravo V, *et al.* (2008) Effect of oral nutritional supplementation on weight loss and percutaneous endoscopic gastrostomy tube rates in patients treated with radiotherapy for oropharyngeal carcinoma. *Support Care Cancer*, **16**, 285–9.
75. Lees J (1997) Nasogastric and percutaneous endoscopic gastrostomy feeding in head and neck patients receiving radiotherapy treatment at a regional oncology unit: a two year study. *Eur J Cancer Care*, **6**, 45–9.
76. Mekhail TM, Adelstein DJ, Rybicki LA, *et al.* (2001) Enteral nutrition during the treatment of head and neck carcinoma: is a percutaneous endoscopic gastrostomy tube preferable to a nasogastric tube? *Cancer*, **91**, 1785–90.
77. Magne N, Marcy PY, Foa, *et al.* (2001) Comparison between nasogastric tube feeding and percutaneous fluoroscopic gastrostomy in advanced head and neck cancer patients. *Eur Arch Otorhinolaryngol*, **258**, 89–92.
78. Roberge C, Tran M, Massoud C, *et al.* (2000) Quality of life and home enteral tube feeding: a french prospective study in patients with head and neck or oesophageal cancer. *Br J Cancer*, **82**, 263–9.
79. Pezner RD, Archambeau JO, Lipsett JA, *et al.* (1987) Tube feeding enteral nutritional support in patients receiving radiation therapy for advanced head and neck cancer. *Int J Radiol Biol Phys*, **13**, 935–9.
80. Wiggenraad RG, Flierman L, Goossens A, *et al.* (2007) Prophylactic gastrostomy placement and early feeding may limit loss of weight during chemotherapy for advanced head and neck cancer, a preliminary study. *Clin Otolaryngol*, **32**, 384–90.
81. Chandu A, Smith AC, Douglas M (2003) Percutaneous endoscopic gastrostomy in patients undergoing resection for oral tumours: a retrospective review of complications and outcomes. *J Oral Maxillofac Surg*, **61**, 1279–84.
82. Scolapio JS, Spangler PR, Romano MM, Mclaughlin MP, Salassa JR (2001) Prophylactic placement of gastrostomy feeding tubes before radiotherapy in patients with head and neck cancer: is it worthwhile? *J Clin Gastroenterol*, **33**, 215–17.
83. Cunliffe DR, Swanton C, White C, *et al.* (2000) Percutaneous endoscopic gastrostomy at the time of tumour resection in advanced oral cancer. *Oral Oncol*, **36**, 471–3.
84. Raynor EM, Williams MF, Martindale RG, Porubsky ES (1999) Timing of percutaneous endoscopic gastrostomy tube placement in head and neck cancer patients. *Otolaryngol Head Neck Surg*, **120**, 479–82.
85. Cruz I, Mamel JJ, Brady PG, Cass-Garcia M (2005) Incidence of abdominal wall metastasis complicating PEG tube placement in untreated head and neck cancer. *Gastrointest Endosc*, **62**, 708–11.
86. Capell MS (2007) Risk factors and risk reduction of malignant seeding of the percutaneous endoscopic gastrostomy track from pharyngo-oesophageal malignancy: a review of all 44 known reported cases. *Am J Gastroenterol*, **102**, 1307–11.
87. Foster JM, Filocamo P, Nava H, *et al.* (2007) The introducer technique is the optimal method for placing percutaneous endoscopic gastrostomy tubes in head and neck cancer. *Surg Endosc*, **21**, 897–901.
88. Lin CH, Liu NJ, Tang JH, *et al.* (2006) Nasogastric feeding tube placement in patients with oesophageal cancer: application of ultrathin transnasal endoscopy. *Gastrointest Endosc*, **64**, 104–7.
89. Odelli C, Burgess D, Bateman L, *et al.* (2005) Nutrition support improves patient outcomes, treatment tolerance and admission characteristics in oesophageal cancer. *Clin Oncol*, **17**, 639–45.
90. Bozzetti F, Cozzaglio L, Gavazzi C, *et al.* (1998) Nutritional support in patients with cancer of the oesophagus: impact on nutritional status, patient compliance to therapy and survival. *Tumori*, **84**, 681–6.
91. Stockeld D, Fagerberg J, Granstrom L, Backman L (2001) Percutaneous endoscopic gastrostomy for nutrition in patients with oesophageal cancer. *Eur J Surg*, **167**, 839–44.
92. Margolis M, Alexander P, Trachiotis GD, Gjharagozloo F, Lipman T (2003) Percutaneous endoscopic gastrostomy before multimodality therapy in patients with oesophageal cancer. *Ann Thorac Surg*, **76**, 1694–7.

93. Ohnmacht GA, Allen MS, Cassivi SD, *et al.* (2006) Percutaneous endoscopic gastrostomy risks rendering the gastric conduit unusable for oesophagectomy. *Dis Esophagus*, **19**, 311–12.
94. Jenkinson AD, Lim J, Agrawal N, Menzies D (2007) Laparoscopic feeding jejunostomy in oesophagogastric cancer. *Surg Endosc*, **21**, 299–302.
95. Yagi M, Hashimoto T, Nezuka H, *et al.* (1999) Complications associated with enteral nutrition using catheter jejunostomy after oesophagectomy. *Surg Today*, **29**, 214–18.
96. Ryan AM, Rowley SP, Healy LA (2006) Post-oesophagectomy early enteral nutrition via a needle catheter jejunostomy: 8-year experience at a specialist unit. *Clin Nutr*, **25**, 386–93.
97. Weimann A, Braga M, Harsanyi L, *et al.* (2006) ESPEN guidelines on enteral nutrition: surgery including transplantation. *Clin Nutr*, **25**, 224–44.
98. Szeluga DJ, Stuart RK, Brookmeyer R, Utermohlen V, Santos GW (1987) Nutritional support of bone marrow transplant recipients: a prospective, randomized clinical trial comparing total parenteral nutrition to an enteral feeding program. *Cancer Res*, **47**, 3309–16.
99. Seguy D, Berthon C, Micol JB (2006) Enteral feeding and early outcomes of patients undergoing allogeneic stem cell transplantation following myeloablative conditioning. *Transplantation*, **82**, 835–9.
100. Jones B, Holden C, Dalzell M, Micklewright A, Glencorse C (eds) (2006) *British Artificial Nutrition Survey (BANS)*. Available at: http://www.BAPEN.org.uk
101. Gaggiotti G, Orlandoni P, Ambrosi S, Catani M (2001) Italian Home Enteral Nutrition (IHEN) Register: data collection and aims. *Clin Nutrr*, **20**(S Suppl 2,), 69–72.
102. Howard L, Ament M, Fleming CR, Shike M, Steiger E (1995) Current use and clinical outcome of home parenteral and enteral nutrition therapies in the United States. *Gastroenterology*, **109**, 355–65.
103. Koretz RL (2007) Should patients with cancer be offered nutritional support: does the benefit outweigh the burden? *Eur J Gastroenterol Hepatol*, **19**, 379–82.
104. Koretz RL, Avenell A, Lipman TO, Braunschweig CL, Milne AC (2007) Does enteral nutrition affect clinical outcome? A systematic review of the randomized trials. *Am J Gastroenterol*, **102**, 412–29.
105. Sanders DS, Carter MJ, D' J, *et al.* (2000) Survival analysis in percutaneous endoscopic gastrostomy feeding: a worse outcome in patients with dementia. *Am J Gastroenterol*, **95**, 1472–5.
106. Schneider SM, Raina C, Pugliese P, Pouget I, Rampal P, Hebuterne X (2001) Outcome of patients treated with home enteral nutrition. *J Paren Enteral Nutr*, **25**, 203–9.
107. Cortez-Pinto H, Pinto Correia A, Camillo ME, Tavares L, Carneiro de Moura M (2002) Long term management of percutaneous gastrostomy by a nutritional support team. *Clin Nutr*, **21**, 27–31.
108. Goncalves F, Mozes M, Saraiva I, Ramos C (2006) Gastrostomies in palliative care. *Support Care Cancer*, **14**, 1147–51.
109. Pironi L, Ruggieri E, Tanneberger S, *et al.* (1997) Home artificial nutrition in advanced cancer. *J R Soc Med*, **90**, 597–603.
110. Fietkau R, Thiel HJ, Iro H, *et al.* (1989) Comparison between oral nutrition and enteral nutrition using a percutaneous endoscopically guided gastrostomy (PEG) in patients undergoing radiotherapy for head and neck tumors. *Strahlenther Onkol*, **165**, 844–51.
111. Marin Caro MM, Laviano A, Pichard C (2007) Nutritional intervention and quality of life in adult oncology patients. *Clin Nutr*, **26**, 289–301.
112. Jatoi A, Kumar S, Sloan JA, Nguyen PL (2003) On appetite and its loss. *J Clin Oncol*, **21**, 79–81.

Chapter 22

Nutrition in advanced malignancy: parenteral nutrition, palliative surgery and gastrointestinal stents

Pradeep F. Thomas and Dileep N. Lobo

Introduction

Oral with or without enteral nutrition is the intervention of choice for maintenance and/or repletion of adequate nutrition (Chapter 21). However, parenteral nutrition (PN) has a role to play in selected patients, and this chapter will discuss where it fits into the management algorithm of patients requiring nutritional support. Also discussed are the indications for surgical palliation and gastrointestinal stents in the management of patients with advanced or unresectable cancer to facilitate more effective nutritional intake.

Parenteral nutrition

The parenteral route is an invasive and relatively expensive form of nutrition support, and even in experienced hands is associated with risks from line placement, line infections, thrombosis and metabolic disturbance (and more so in inexperienced hands!). Careful consideration is therefore needed when deciding to whom, when and how this form of nutrition support should be given. Whenever possible, patients should be aware of why this form of nutrition support is needed and its potential risks and benefits.

Indications

Parenteral nutrition should only be used when oral or enteral nutrition is not feasible due either to lack of access to the gastrointestinal tract or to gastrointestinal failure or dysfunction.[1,2] It can also be used as a supplementary source of nutrition where oral/enteral intake is inadequate to meet requirements. Indications for PN can be broadly divided into two categories:

1 Short term to support the patient during/after treatment, e.g. chemoradiotherapy, bone marrow transplantation or surgery, and to cover any time-limited complications, e.g. severe mucositis, sepsis, enterocutaneous fistulae, intractable vomiting, radiation enteritis (see Chapter 31).

2 Long term because of unresolving/untreatable complication of the disease or its treatment, e.g. short bowel syndrome following extensive resection, intestinal obstruction, severe unresolving radiation enteritis, non-healing high output enterocutaneous fistulae. Its place in the palliated patient is discussed in more detail later in the chapter.

As a general principle the decision to start PN should be made by a multidisciplinary team, including those with expertise in nutrition support as well as the cancer team.

Access

Parenteral nutrition should be administered through a dedicated feeding line. The following routes are available for short term feeding (less than 28 days):[1]

A. Central line

- Central access is the ideal, with the proximal end of the catheter in the superior vena cava (or inferior vena cava for femoral lines). This allows standard PN feeds, which are hyperosmolar, to be introduced without complications.
- Greater complication rates for insertion.
- Ideally single lumen lines should be used exclusively for PN. Where venous access is required for other purposes, e.g. antibiotics and critical care management, multilumen lines will be required. However, even with meticulous line care, the exclusive use of one lumen in a multilumen line has a greater risk of line sepsis than a single lumen line used only for PN.
- The major complication is line sepsis (see Box 22.1).

Box 22.1 Line-related complications associated with parenteral nutrition (PN)

Infection (catheter-related sepsis CRS)[4]

- Common and potentially dangerous.
- Consider if pyrexia, leukocytosis and no other explanation (urine, chest).
- Stop PN and lock line with heparin.
- Swab exit site; peripheral and central blood cultures.
- If cultures indicate *Staphlococcus aureus* or *Candida albicans*, line must be removed, with insertion of a temporary line and treatment with systemic antibiotics. Other organisms: line may be salvageable—decision will depend in part on ease of alternative vascular access. If attempt at line salvage, lock with vancomycin, systemic antibiotics and observe closely. If sepsis persists, line will need removing; if sepsis settles, restart PN, but if pyrexia on infusion remove line.
- If cultures negative, reuse line and observe (and look for other sources). If in doubt, remove line.

Catheter occlusion

- Due to fibrin or lipid sludge.
- Lipid occlusion takes a while to build up. Therefore early occlusion (<7–14 days) is likely to be due to fibrin, and late occlusion (>14 days) more likely to be due to lipid.
- Fibrin can usually be dislodged with urokinase or concentrated alcohol, lipid with alcohol.

Catheter damage

- Can occur due to repeated clamping and unclamping.
- Repair kits available that can often avoid line replacement.

Catheter-related venous thrombosis

- When this causes failure of feed infusion, line needs to be removed and resited. Consider anticoagulation, especially if feeding intended for longer term.

Box 22.1 Line-related complications associated with parenteral nutrition (PN) *(continued)*

Thrombophlebitis (peripheral cannulae)

- Stop feed and remove line.
- Care of inflamed site with appropriate dressings and cleansing.

Extavasation of feed

- Occurs when line is displaced from vein and feed infiltrates into surrounding tissue.
- Remove line.

- The subclavian route is preferred to the jugular or femoral routes as the latter two have higher infection rates and it is more difficult to maintain sterile dressings.

B. Peripherally inserted central catheter (PICC)

- Inserted into the antecubital fossa and about 60 cm in length. The proximal end lies in the central veins thereby allowing hyperosmolar 'central' menus to be tolerated.
- Requires aseptic technique for insertion and should be done by trained personnel.
- Needs good size veins for placement.
- With good care these can last many months and are, therefore, a very good alternative to central lines. Indeed some authorities prefer this route.
- Major complications, other than failure to insert, are phlebitis (5–15%), malposition (8%) and catheter failure/leakage (4%).

C. Peripheral cannula

- Can be used, but its place is not as a route of first choice. The commonest complication is thrombophlebitis from the feed infusion, and to minimise this, hypo-osmolar/hypocaloric feeds are required which, by definition will be inadequate to meet a patient's needs. Therefore the use of peripheral cannulae should be reserved for patients who have unexpectedly lost cental venous access and need a temporary facility to administer PN.
- To optimize efficacy, the following are helpful.
  - Fine bore (22 or 24 french gauge polyurethane cannula).
  - Large forearm vein.
  - Hypocaloric, i.e. low osmolality, feed.
  - Glyceryl trinitrate patch distal to cannula.
  - Regular change of line (at least 48 hourly).

For long term feeding (>28 days) tunnelled central lines with a Dacron cuff (e.g. Hickman or Broviac catheters) or an implantable venous access disc will be required. These are more acceptable to patients, as well as minimizing risk of catheter sepsis.[1]

Whatever line is used, it must be inserted with meticulous aseptic technique, and subsequent care—dressings, handling and feed attachment—must adhere to strict and comprehensive protocol-led management. All healthcare facilities looking after patients on PN have a duty to have such protocols in place.

Prescribing and administering PN

The energy needs of patients are between 1 and 1.3 times the resting energy expenditure, and for most this amounts to 30–35 kcal/day, with equal amounts being contributed by fat and carbohydrate.[2]

Protein requirements are 1.0–1.5 g/kg/day and appropriate amounts of micronutrients (fat- and water-soluble vitamins), electrolytes (Na, K, Ca, Mg, PO_4) and minerals (Fe, Zn, Cu, Mn, Se) should be added.[2] There are many 'off the shelf' commercial preparations which are often entirely adequate to meet a patient's needs. Alternatively, individual components can be compounded under sterile conditions (laminar flow). A more detailed description of PN requirements and the wide variety and suitability of available PN products is beyond the remit of this text. The potential for complications (see below) as a result of inappropriate prescribing and inadequate monitoring is immense, and therefore PN prescribing should, although often does not, remain the responsibility of professionals with appropriate expertise and experience.

Parenteral nutrition is administered via an infusion pump either continuously over 24 h or cyclically over 12–16 h. Cyclical infusions can have physiological and psychological advantages. PN should be introduced at no more than 50% of estimated needs for the first 24–48 h and increased progressively till the patient's nutritional requirements are met.

Patients should be monitored closely, both clinically and biochemically. This should include basic bedside parameters, such as blood sugars, blood pressure and pulse; routine haematology and biochemistry, including renal and liver function, magnesium, phosphate, calcium and lipids (daily to start and twice weekly when stable); and more esoteric biochemistry for patients on longer term feeding, which would include the trace elements of manganese, zinc, copper and selenium (2–4 weekly).

There is no minimum length of time for the duration of parenteral nutrition, although an intended duration of less than a week is unlikely to lead to any (nutritional) benefit.[2] Discontinuation of PN should never be abrupt before alternative methods of feeding have been established, as rebound hypoglycaemia can occur. Once oral or enteral feeding has begun, PN can be weaned off gradually over 1–2 days. If PN needs to stop suddenly, e.g. line problems, a dextrose infusion should be administered.

PN lines can be removed at ward level as a sterile procedure and with the patient lying flat in bed. Hickman lines have to be dissected out by a doctor skilled in the procedure. All catheter tips should routinely be sent for culture to enable audit of infection rates to be done.

Complications of PN

Complications of PN can be divided into three groups:

1 (Line) insertion-related: These include pneumo- or haemothorax, air embolism, thoracic duct injury, cardiac arrhythmias and arterial puncture.

2 Line-related (see Box 22.1)

3 Feeding-related

   a) Metabolic

   Deficiencies/excesses of any electrolyte, trace element, vitamin or mineral are possible. Adequate monitoring should avoid such problems.

   Refeeding syndrome (see below).

   b) Hepatobiliary

   Direct complications from PN are unusual in short term feeding (<14 days). Thereafter cholestasis and hepatic steatosis can develop. Occasionally fibrosis and cirrhosis can occur, but this is unlikely to be a significant consideration for cancer patients.

Refeeding syndrome

This is an important but often underappreciated complication of feeding undernourished and/or cachectic patients, and is particularly relevant to the cancer population. It can occur after the institution of any form of feeding, be it oral, enteral or parenteral feeding.[3]

During starvation when there is excessive muscle breakdown and ketosis to generate energy, phosphate and potassium are lost from the cell in proportion to the breakdown of glycogen and protein (potassium being the main intracellular cation balancing the negative charges on proteins). There is, therefore, no clinical deficiency of these electrolytes until catabolism is abruptly reversed and resynthesis of glycogen and protein begins. This creates a sudden demand for inorganic phosphate for phosphorylation and ATP synthesis and for potassium to balance the negative charges on protein and glycogen. Magnesium, being involved in ATP synthesis, is also taken up by the cells. Upon the introduction of carbohydrate, insulin is released into the bloodstream and there is a shift of metabolism from fat to carbohydrate. Thiamine is a cofactor for glycolysis, and therefore this too can become deficient, with the risk of Wernicke's encephalopathy and cardiomyopathy. Excessive infusion of glucose may also cause hyperglycaemia leading to osmotic diuresis, dehydration and hyperosmolar non-ketotic coma. The production of fat from glucose due to lipogenesis can result in hypertriglyceridaemia and/or a fatty liver. Problems can be compounded by gut mucosal atrophy and impairment of pancreatic function due to prolonged undernutrition, which may predispose to severe diarrhoea following commencement of oral or enteral refeeding, and thereby further precipitate electrolyte and mineral imbalance.

The clinical features, therefore, of the refeeding syndrome can include an array of cardiac arrhythmias and myopathic deficiencies, heart failure and oedema secondary to the antidiuretic effect of hyperinsulinaemia, various central and peripheral neurological complications (fits, ataxia, encephalopathy, paraesthesia) and a miscellany of other system dysfunctions (gastrointestinal: abdominal pain, ileus, liver failure; renal: acute tubular necrosis; haematological: thrombocytopenia, haemolysis). There is, however, a spectrum or gradation in the features of the refeeding syndrome from asymptomatic cases with mild biochemical derangement to those with significant electrolyte abnormalities and resulting life-threatening symptoms. The cut-off point at which the 'refeeding syndrome' can be said to be present is, therefore, somewhat arbitrary. The full-blown syndrome should be defined by the presence of symptoms, but biochemical changes of sufficient degree to pose a potential risk should be acted upon without delay in order to prevent the clinical features developing.

Refeeding syndrome is effectively iatrogenic and can always be prevented, providing its possibility is considered. Strategies to prevent it include:

- awareness of the existence of refeeding syndrome and the circumstances in which it is likely to develop;
- refeed slowly—often no more than 10–15 kcal/kg/day to start with—and build up the macronutrient content of the feed over several days;
- monitor the patient clinically and biochemically frequently;
- anticipate the additional requirements, particularly of phosphate, potassium, magnesium and thiamine and provide proactively, rather than wait for deficiencies to develop;
- minimize salt intake, unless the patient is salt depleted.

Palliative treatment

Palliative oncological treatment (surgery/chemotherapy/radiotherapy) may be suitable for some patients in whom the disease is not amenable to curative treatment. Patients with a life expectancy of less than 1 month are considered to be in the terminal phase of disease and interventions should be kept to a minimum in these patients so as not to make the treatment worse than the disease (Chapter 33).[5,6]

The aim of palliative treatment is to achieve the best possible quality of life for patients and their families or carers, by maintaining or restoring the well-being and performance of the patient in everyday life.[5,7] Nutritional intervention in palliative care should focus primarily on controlling symptoms, maintaining an adequate hydration status and preserving body weight and composition (fat and lean tissues vs oedema and ascites) as far as possible.[8] The wishes of the patient and the family or carers should be considered[7] in conjunction with the risks and benefits related to nutritional intervention.[5,9]

Parenteral nutrition

Longer term PN needs to be considered when there is intestinal failure with no prospect of recovery, for example when advanced intra-abdominal cancers have caused intestinal obstruction and survival is dependent solely on nutritional support.[10,11] The survival of healthy individuals subject to total macronutrient starvation rarely exceeds 2 months, and is much less in patients with the burden of advanced cancer. Home parenteral nutrition (HPN) has been shown to maintain nutritional indices until death as well as stabilizing quality of life until 2–3 months before death.[12] Studies have demonstrated that 20–50% of patients with advanced cancer on HPN are alive at 6 months.[13,14] It also appears that patients and their families/carers relate HPN to benefits such as weight gain, higher energy, strength and activity levels, and security about the fulfilment of their nutritional needs.

The Northern Alberta HPN Program[11] has developed clinical practice guidelines for HPN and has suggested that the following criteria should be met before referring patients with advanced cancer for HPN:

- There should be a clear nutritional risk along with the diagnosis of cancer (e.g. intestinal obstruction or fistula).
- Patients should have an estimated life expectancy of at least 6–12 weeks.
- They should have a reasonable quality of life with a Karnofsky performance score of >50 (100 normal–10 moribund).
- They should be medically stable.
- Venous access should be available.
- Psychosocial factors should be considered to assess suitability.
- Patients and carers should have the opportunity to learn how to administer HPN.

The duration of HPN for the majority of these patients varies between a median of 2 and 4 months.[12,15,16] HPN is relatively safe, if facilitated by experienced centres, and the number of hospital readmissions is acceptable. Because there is little hard evidence demonstrating clear benefits of HPN in advanced cancer, the use of this form of palliative care is highly variable around the world, which probably says more about a country's culture and attitudes to palliation than about medical judgement. The dilemma remains whether to burden the patient/carer with complex technology with the risk of complications and readmittances to hospital to buy extra time and possibly a small improvement in quality of life, or let the patient die with dignity.[7]

This is, therefore, a management option with no clear indications, and which needs to be considered on an individualized basis, taking all factors into account, especially the patient's wishes.

Surgical palliation

Surgery has historically played a major role in palliation of symptoms from gastrointestinal cancers. The general principle is that removal or debulking of the tumour is the best possible palliation, although this is not always possible, particularly when tumour is either invading nearby essential organs or involving major vessels. The aim of palliative surgery for patients with advanced cancer is to ameliorate symptoms and improve quality of life. This is especially relevant for those who are unable to eat or receive enteral tube feeding due to intestinal obstruction. Palliative surgery is not indicated in asymptomatic patients, as it is not possible to improve their quality of life. Similarly, palliative surgery should not be contemplated in patients with a very short life expectancy or significant comorbidity, as the risks of surgery will outweigh the benefits.

If palliative surgery is being considered, the risks and benefits should be discussed thoroughly with the patient and family/carers so that an informed decision may be made. The patient should be under no illusions that the planned operation will be curative, and should understand that further palliative treatment in the form of chemotherapy or radiotherapy may be necessary thereafter. In most patients with advanced gastrointestinal cancer, palliative surgery is usually aimed at relieving luminal obstruction, which may be intrinsic or extrinsic. This may involve a non-curative resection of the obstructing cancer or a procedure that bypasses the obstruction. Relief of obstruction enables resumption of oral or enteral feeding. Rarely, surgery may be indicated for the placement of feeding tubes such as feeding gastrostomies and feeding jejunostomies, if endoscopic or radiological attempts at tube placement have been unsuccessful or are not possible. Surgical placement of a Hickman line may be necessary if long-term PN is envisaged. Palliative surgery in patients with advanced malignancy may also be indicated to treat enterocutaneous fistulae, haemorrhage or intra-abdominal sepsis.

Common sites of malignant obstruction to the gastrointestinal tract include the oesophagus, gastric antrum and pylorus, duodenum, small bowel and colon. It is relatively rare for rectal cancers to cause obstruction. Cancers of the pancreas and bile duct can cause obstructive jaundice, leading to malaise, loss of appetite and impaired digestion of fats.

Colonic interposition used to be a method of palliating oesophageal cancer and involved bypassing the obstructing lesion by anastomosing a pedicled segment of colon to the oesophagus and stomach. However, the morbidity of this procedure is high and it has largely been replaced by oesophageal stenting (see below).

Patients with gastric outlet obstruction secondary to malignancy may be suitable for a stent, and this is discussed below. Alternatively an anterior gastrojejunostomy is a relatively easy operation with good results. A loop of jejunum is brought up anterior to the colon and anastomosed in a side-to-side manner with the stomach either with staples or sutures (Figure 22.1). This is in contradistinction to the anastomosis being made on the posterior wall of stomach with a loop of jejunum brought through a window made in the transverse mesocolon in benign gastric outlet obstruction (retrocolic gastrojejunostomy). Prolonged obstruction to the gastric outlet may lead to gastric atony and recovery of gastric motility is often delayed after a gastrojejunostomy performed for obstruction. In this situation, placement of a large-bore nasogastric tube may be advisable for the first few postoperative days for drainage purposes. The other important complications of this surgery include anastomotic dehiscence, bile reflux gastritis, diarrhoea and the 'dumping syndrome'. Diarrhoea occurring after a gastroenterostomy is likely to be due to rapid gastric emptying with the creation of large volumes of liquid chyme and may necessitate the use of antidiarrhoeal drugs. The mechanisms leading to diarrhoea may cause dumping, which could

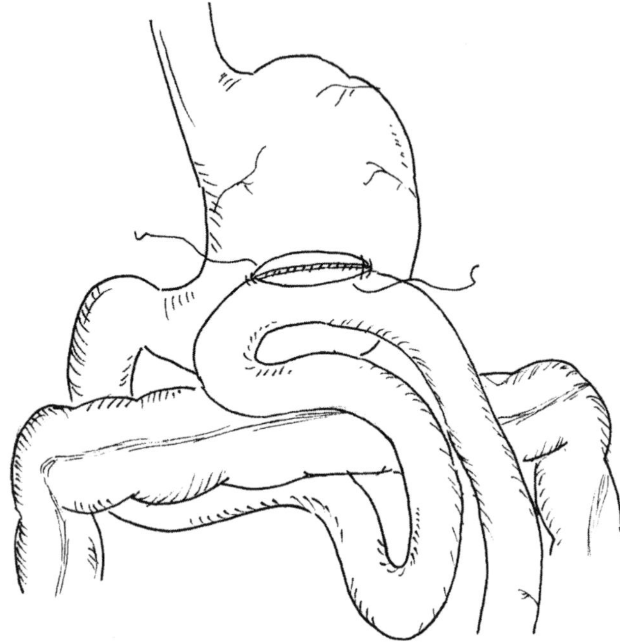

Fig. 22.1 An anterior, antecolic gastroenterostomy.

be early or late. Early dumping affects about 10% of patients, and leads to faintness, palpitations, sweating and abdominal discomfort almost immediately after eating. It is due to a high volume of osmotically active food moving rapidly into the small bowel, leading to the sequestration of circulating fluid into the gut. Patients tend to get some relief from lying down and they can be reassured that the situation usually improves with time. The somatostatin analogue octreotide can help ameliorate this. Late dumping is due to hypoglycaemia and patients experience similar symptoms as those with early dumping, but they tend to occur 30 min after eating. The rapid carbohydrate load leads to a rise in serum glucose, which leads to an increase in insulin secretion and hypoglycaemia. Patients can relieve the symptoms with a sugary drink or sweet, but octreotide can also be effective. Bile reflux gastritis and early dumping can be treated by converting the gastrojejunostomy into a Roux-en-Y reconstruction, but this sort of revisional surgery is rarely indicated in patients with advanced cancer.

Obstruction caused by small bowel tumours can be often resected and the ends reanastomosed. Resection may not be possible if the tumour is advanced and invading other vital structures. If the loop of small intestine cannot be freed, a side-to-side anastomosis is created in the adjoining small intestine to create a bypass. Sometimes multiple bypasses may be necessary. These bypasses can result in the formation of blind loops resulting in bacterial overgrowth.

In the case of unresectable obstruction to the right colon, a side-to-side anastamosis between the small intestine and transverse colon can be fashioned (Figure 22.2). This has the disadvantage of a blind end in the caecum which cannot be drained properly if the ileocaecal valve is competent, but can be remedied by adding a tube caecostomy to decompress the caecum. Some surgeons prefer to form a loop ileostomy in this situation.

Unresectable distal colonic or rectal tumours causing large bowel obstruction can be managed with formation of a loop colostomy (Figure 22.3). There are disadvantages with this procedure,

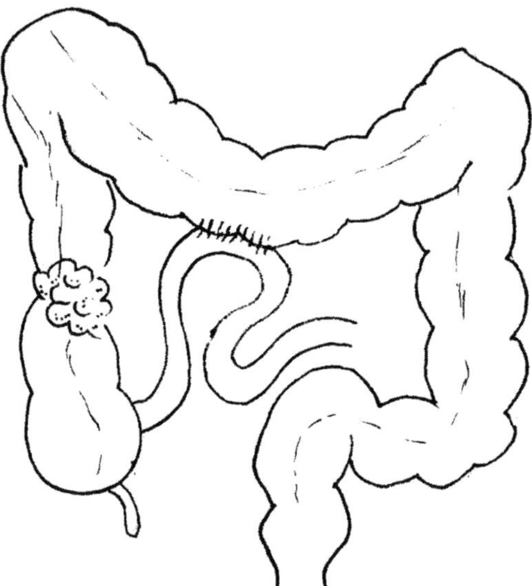

Fig. 22.2 A side-to-side ileocolic bypass for an obstructing tumour of the ascending colon.

including the psychological effects of having a stoma, difficulty educating patients/carers to manage their stoma, and the practical challenges of the various appliances required (Box 22.2). As the surgery is palliative and aimed at improving quality of remaining life, full and frank discussions need to be had before embarking on such a procedure.

Biliary obstruction secondary to cholangiocarcinomas or pancreatic cancers again may be amenable to endoscopic or percutaneous stenting, or alternatively will need a hepaticojejunostomy with or without a gastrojejunostomy. This is done after cholecystectomy and dissection of the

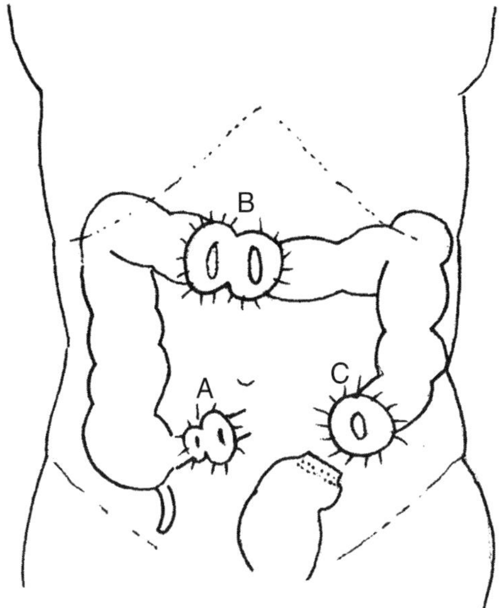

Fig. 22.3 Some types of intestinal stomas. (A) Loop ileostomy. (B) Loop transverse colostomy. (C) End descending colostomy.

Box 22.2 Complications of stomas

Early complications
- Ischaemia
- Retraction

Late complications
- Stenosis
- Prolapse
- Parastomal herniation
- Intestinal obstruction
- Haemorrhage
- Diversion colitis
- Dermatitis
- Psychological

common hepatic duct, which could be transected or opened partially and anastomosed with a loop of jejunum (Figure 22.4).

The increasing availability and expertise in laparoscopic surgery means that many of these bypass procedures can be done laparoscopically, reducing the morbidity and hospital stay.

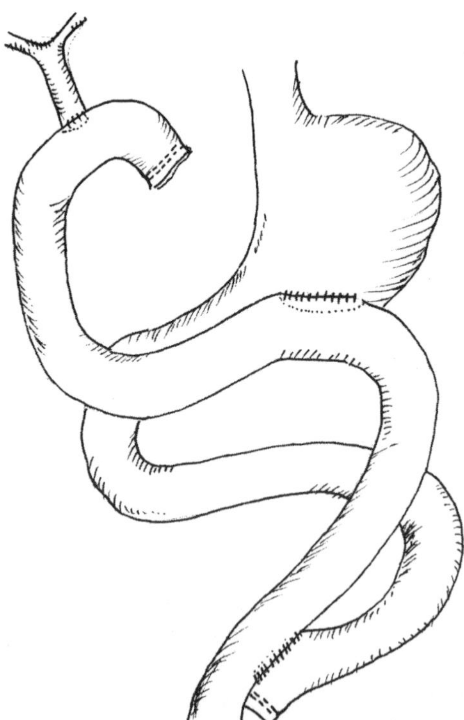

Fig. 22.4 A roux-en-Y hepaticojejunostomy and gastroenterostomy for a pancreatic tumour causing biliary and gastric outlet obstruction.

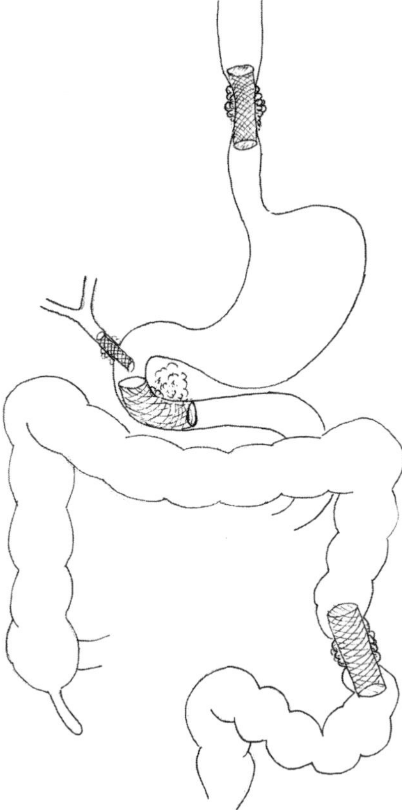

Fig. 22.5 Diagrammatic representation of oesophageal, biliary, duodenal and colonic stents.

There will be a few patients with multifocal gastrointestinal cancer or disseminated metastatic disease who are not amenable to resection or bypass. In this situation, life expectancy is usually very short, and although PN may be an appropriate palliative option, this is unlikely to influence the outcome. Compassionate care is probably the best option in such a situation.

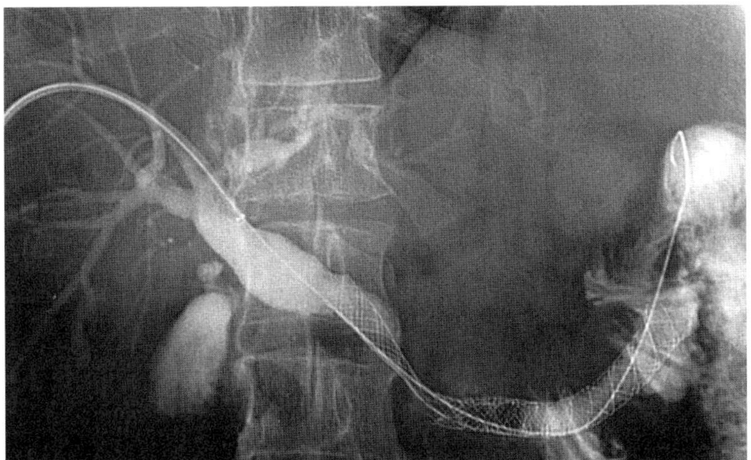

Fig. 22.6 X-Ray demonstrating insertion of a biliary and duodenal stent.

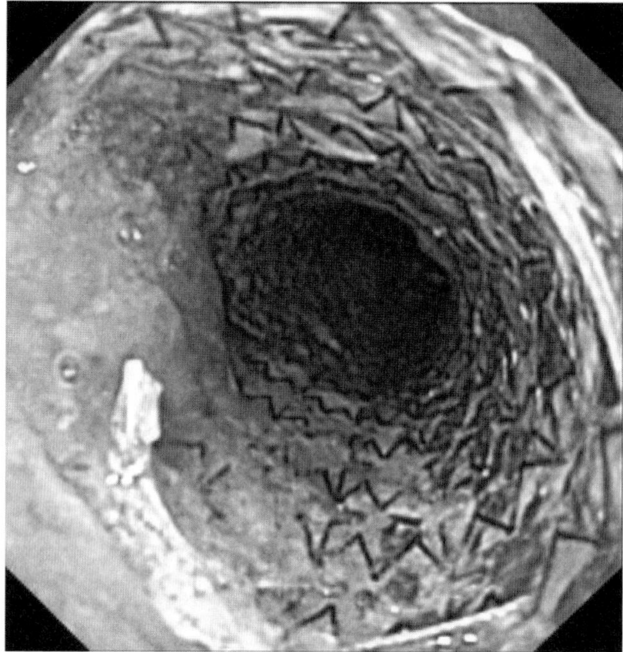

Fig. 22.7 Endoscopic view of a self-expanding oesophageal stent.

Stents

Not all patients are suitable for palliative surgery, and intraluminal stents (Figures 22.5–7) have significant advantages in patients in whom the risks of surgical intervention outweigh the benefits. General anaesthesia is not a prerequisite for the deployment of these stents and they are associated with less morbidity than surgery.

Patients with oesophageal carcinoma or post-oesophagectomy anastomotic strictures quite often present with severe dysphagia and odynophagia, and as a result are unable to maintain adequate oral intake. Oesophageal stents were the first stents available for the treatment of any gastrointestinal luminal obstruction or narrowing. Celestin introduced stents called 'Celestin tubes' which needed to be inserted during laparotomy. This was followed by the 'Atkinson tube' in the 1970s, which could be deployed endoscopically. These tubes were made of plastic and the material deteriorated over time. They also had a high risk of complications, including migration and oesophageal perforation. Current stents are self-expanding and are either made of steel, silicon or nitinol, which is an alloy of nickel and titanium and has the advantage of having 'shape-memory'.[17] There is a wide variety of products on the market, including covered and uncovered stents. Some of the more recent stents have a very soft flexible tube with a smaller diameter in the distal end which acts as a valve to prevent reflux; others have one or both ends flanged to avoid migration.

The primary purpose of a stent is to allow resumption of oral intake in patients where the oesophageal pathology was previously preventing this. It is, however, important for the patient to appreciate that even a successfully deployed stent may not allow a patient to have anything more than a diet of puréed food consistency. It will obviously allow a patient to maintain autonomy in feeding orally, but not with a 'normal' diet. It is also important to be aware that while some stents can be removed, most cannot and therefore once placed they will remain in situ. Therefore, stents should only be used as a last resort. Other than straightforward relief of dyshagia from obstructing neoplasms, covered stents are used in those with perforated tumours or tracheo-oesophageal fistulae, where they can effectively cover the perforation.

It is usually possible to manipulate a stent across the obstruction, either endoscopically or radiologically. When this is not possible, tumour tissue can be fulgurated by photodynamic therapy, laser beam therapy or alcohol injection. Intracavitary brachytherapy or external beam radiotherapy are other options. The usual choice of stent for oesophageal cancer is a covered stent, so as to avoid the tumour ingrowth which occurs through the mesh of uncovered stents. However, this benefit also gives the stent less purchase on the oesophageal wall, thereby making it more prone to migation. Even with a covered stent tumour, overgrowth can still occur at the top and bottom end of the stent. Management of tumour ingrowth/overgrowth is either by fulguration using the methods described above and/or deployment of a further stent to overlap with the original one. Other complications of stents include migration, oesophageal perforation, tracheo-oesophageal fistula, haemorrhage and stent fracture.

Self-expanding metal stents are becoming increasingly popular for management of malignant strictures elsewhere in the gastrointestinal tract such as the bile duct and duodenum (Table 22.1) and can be introduced under either endoscopic or radiological guidance.

Colonic stents (Table 22.2) are increasingly being used for the management of malignant strictures of the colon in patients where successful resection is not possible.[23] They are also used in patients who present with colonic obstruction with resectable tumours as a bridge to elective surgery, so that the patient can be stabilized and their general clinical status optimized prior to definitive elective surgery. These stents can be deployed in two ways. The stricture can be traversed by a guide wire passed through the endoscope; the stent is then passed over the guidewire, also through the endoscope, and deployed under direct endoscopic vision. The other system needs the endoscope to be removed after accurate placement of guidewire. The stent system is then passed over the guide wire and positioned and deployed under fluoroscopy guidance. Colonic stents have many advantages to operative management for advanced colonic tumours (Table 22.2). These include reduced mortality and morbidity, and shortened length of hospital stay.

Conclusions

The nutritional management of patients with advanced cancer often poses a clinical and ethical dilemma and decisions can only be made after careful consideration of the benefits versus the burdens and risks of further intervention, especially when these could be perceived as potentially dangerous and futile. Disease progress, performance status, projected life expectancy and the wishes of the patient, family and carers should all be taken into consideration in the decision-making process.

Table 22.1 Studies comparing surgical bypass with stents for duodenal obstruction

Wong *et al.*[18]	*n* = 17 gastojejunostomy vs 6 stents	In pancreatic cancer, stents result in early discharge and possibly improved survival.
Maetani *et al.*[19]	*n* = 20 stents vs 19 bypass	Stents provide better quality of life than bypass procedures.
Espinel *et al.*[20]	*n* = 24 stent vs 17 gastrojejunostomy	Less morbidity, earlier feeding and better quality of life with stents.
Jeurnink *et al.*[21] (systematic review)	*n* = 1045 stents vs 297 gastrojejunostomy	Better results with stent but bypass is probably better for patients with prolonged prognosis.
Kiely *et al.*[22]	*n* = 30 stents vs 21 bypass	Stents are safe and also useful for palliation for recurrent obstruction.

Table 22.2 Studies comparing stents to bypass surgery for colorectal cancers

Authors	Year	Patients	Outcome
Martinez-Santos *et al.*[24]	2002	n = 43 stents vs 29 bypass	Fewer complications and early discharge with stents.
Carne *et al.*[23]	2004	n = 22 stents vs 19 open surgery	Early discharge with stents. No difference in survival.
Johnson *et al.*[25]	2004	n = 18 stents vs 18 bypass	Can be available even to frail patients.
Ng *et al.*[26]	2006	n = 22 stent and resection vs 40 emergency colectomy	Bridging stent versus emergency resection. Better results in stented group.

Relatively simple interventions such as nutritional counselling, drug therapy and enteral nutrition should be considered before embarking on prolonged parenteral nutrition. Gastrointestinal stents and surgical bypass procedures are useful in the treatment of intestinal obstruction and can facilitate re-establishment of oral or enteral feeding.

References

1. ASPEN Board of Directors and the Clinical Guidelines Task Force (2002) Guidelines for the use of parenteral and enteral nutrition in adult and pediatric patients. *J Parenter Enteral Nutr*, **26**, 1SA–138SA.
2. National Collaborating Centre for Acute Care (2006) *Nutrition Support in Adults: Oral Nutrition Support, Enteral Tube Feeding and Parenteral Nutrition*. London: National Collaborating Centre for Acute Care.
3. Stanga Z, Brunner A, Leuenberger M, *et al.* (2008) Nutrition in clinical practice—the refeeding syndrome: illustrative cases and guidelines for prevention and treatment. *Eur J Clin Nutr*, **62**, 687–94.
4. O'Grady N P, Alexander M, Dellinger EP, *et al.* (2002) Guidelines for the prevention of intravascular catheter-related infections. *Am J Infect Control*, **30**, 476–89.
5. Bachmann P, Marti-Massoud C, Blanc-Vincent MP, *et al.* (2003) Summary version of the standards, options and recommendations for palliative or terminal nutrition in adults with progressive cancer. *Br J Cancer*, **89**(Suppl 1), S107–10.
6. Marin Caro MM, Laviano A, Pichard C (2007) Nutritional intervention and quality of life in adult oncology patients. *Clin Nutr*, **26**, 289–301.
7. McKinlay AW (2004) Nutritional support in patients with advanced cancer: permission to fall out? *Proc Nutr Soc*, **63**, 431–5.
8. Capra S, Ferguson M, Ried K (2001) Cancer: impact of nutrition intervention outcome—nutrition issues for patients. *Nutrition*, **17**, 769–72.
9. Nitenberg G, Raynard B (2000) Nutritional support of the cancer patient: issues and dilemmas. *Crit Rev Oncol Hematol*, **34**, 137–68.
10. Echenique M, Correia MI (2003) Nutrition in advanced digestive cancer. *Curr Opin Clin Nutr Metab Care*, **6**, 577–80.
11. Mackenzie ML, Gramlich L (2008) Home parenteral nutrition in advanced cancer: where are we? *Appl Physiol Nutr Metab*, **33**, 1–11.
12. Bozzetti F, Cozzaglio L, Biganzoli E, *et al.* (2002) Quality of life and length of survival in advanced cancer patients on home parenteral nutrition. *Clin Nutr*, **21**, 281–8.
13. Howard L (2000) A global perspective of home parenteral and enteral nutrition. *Nutrition*, **16**, 625–8.
14. Van Gossum A, Peeters I, Lievin V (1999) Home parenteral nutrition in adults: the current use of an experienced method. *Acta Gastroenterol Belg*, **62**, 201–9.

15. King LA, Carson LF, Konstantinides N, *et al.* (1993) Outcome assessment of home parenteral nutrition in patients with gynecologic malignancies: what have we learned in a decade of experience? *Gynecol Oncol*, **51**, 377–82.
16. Cozzaglio L, Balzola F, Cosentino F, *et al.* (1997) Outcome of cancer patients receiving home parenteral nutrition. Italian Society of Parenteral and Enteral Nutrition (S.I.N.P.E.). *J Parenter Enteral Nutr*, **21**, 339–42.
17. Martin R, Duvall R, Ellis S, Scoggins R (2009) The use of self-expanding silicone stents in esophageal cancer care: optimal pre-, peri-, and postoperative care. *Surg Endosc*, **23**, 615–21.
18. Wong YT, Brams DM, Munson L, *et al.* (2002) Gastric outlet obstruction secondary to pancreatic cancer: surgical vs endoscopic palliation. *Surg Endosc*, **16**, 310–12.
19. Maetani I, Tada T, Ukita T, Inoue H, Sakai Y, Nagao J (2004) Comparison of duodenal stent placement with surgical gastrojejunostomy for palliation in patients with duodenal obstructions caused by pancreaticobiliary malignancies. *Endoscopy*, **36**, 73–8.
20. Espinel J, Sanz O, Vivas S, *et al.* (2006) Malignant gastrointestinal obstruction: endoscopic stenting versus surgical palliation. *Surg Endosc*, **20**, 1083–7.
21. Jeurnink SM, van Eijck CHJ, Steyerberg EW, Kuipers EJ, Siersema PD (2007) Stent versus gastrojejunostomy for the palliation of gastric outlet obstruction: a systematic review. *BMC Gastroenterol*, **7**, 18–18.
22. Kiely JM, Dua KS, Graewin SJ, *et al.* (2007) Palliative stenting for late malignant gastric outlet obstruction. *J Gastrointest Surg*, **11**, 107–13.
23. Carne PWG, Frye JNR, Robertson GM, Frizelle FA (2004) Stents or open operation for palliation of colorectal cancer: a retrospective, cohort study of perioperative outcome and long-term survival. *Dis Colon Rectum*, **47**, 1455–61.
24. Martinez-Santos C, Lobato RF, Fradejas JM, Pinto I, Ortega-Deballón P, Moreno-Azcoita M (2002) Self-expandable stent before elective surgery vs. emergency surgery for the treatment of malignant colorectal obstructions: comparison of primary anastomosis and morbidity rates. *Dis Colon Rectum*, **45**, 401–06.
25. Johnson R, Marsh R, Corson J, Seymour K (2004) A comparison of two methods of palliation of large bowel obstruction due to irremovable colon cancer. *Ann R Coll Surg Engl*, **86**, 99–103.
26. Ng KC, Law WL, Lee YM, Choi HK, Seto CL, Ho JWC (2006) Self-expanding metallic stent as a bridge to surgery versus emergency resection for obstructing left-sided colorectal cancer: a case-matched study. *J Gastrointest Surg*, **10**, 798–803.

Part 7

Ethics, culture and spirituality

Chapter 23

Ethics and medically assisted nutrition and hydration

Paulina Taboada, Alejandra Palma, and Beatriz Shand

Introduction

Patients with advanced cancer decrease their oral intake as a result of various causes, including anorexia, nausea, vomiting, oral cavity lesions, odynophagia, dysphagia, delayed gastric emptying, bowel obstruction, cognitive impairment and mood disorders.[1,2] In preventing or treating the consequences of malnutrition in these patients, questions concerning the need for medically assisted nutrition and/or hydration (MANH) often arise.[3,4] This chapter focuses on the ethical dimension of decisions regarding MANH in advanced cancer patients. Attention shall be directed towards those situations in which advanced cancer patients are not able to eat or appear to be eating less than they should, losing weight, and/or becoming malnourished. Enteral nutrition (EN)—by means of oral nutritional supplements (ONS), tube feeding (TF)—or the implementation of parenteral nutrition (PN) may offer the possibility of increasing nutritional intake in these patients.

Since anorexia, undernutrition and cachexia occur frequently in cancer patients and are often indicators of poor prognosis,[1,2,5] decisions regarding the implementation of MANH in individual cases require an accurate evaluation and a sound foundation in order to avoid causing unnecessary suffering to patients at the end of life. Unfortunately, the available empirical evidence regarding the benefits and burdens of MANH in advanced cancer patients does not provide conclusive answers.[5–7] We contend (Box 23.1) that the eventual benefits and burdens of nutritional assistance need to be judged on a case-basis and that decisions regarding the use of MANH should be related to well-defined goals of care and solidly based on the ethical values/principles involved in the individual case.

Different authors and/or medical associations have proposed useful clinical guidelines for the use of artificial nutrition and/or hydration in cancer patients.[8–11] Some of these guidelines include a reference to the so-called 'principles of biomedical ethics', namely autonomy, non-maleficence, beneficence and justice.[6,12,13] The reference to these four principles corresponds to the principalistic trend of contemporary medical ethics.[14] For this complicated and controversial issue, we argue that the mere reference to formal principles is not enough to provide useful insights and concrete content for difficult decision-making in individual cases. In this chapter we briefly review the content of some traditional ethical values and principles that might be helpful in orienting decision-making for MANH in advanced cancer patients.

Decisions on the use of MANH in advanced cancer patients need to be related to well-defined goals of care and grounded simultaneously in a careful clinical assessment and ethical values and principles. Moreover, we maintain that the mere reference to formal ethical principles is not sufficient to guarantee good medical practice in relation to MANH, and that moral attitudes and virtues are of outmost importance in caring for advanced cancer patients. We emphasize that a periodic re-evaluation of decisions regarding the use of MANH is required to assess the attainability of pre-established goals of care and to consider eventual changes in the patient's condition, including quantity and quality of life.

Box 23.1 Key learning points on medically assisted nutrition and/or hydration (MANH)

1. Decisions regarding MANH in advanced cancer patients should be grounded simultaneously on careful clinical assessment and on ethical values/principles.
2. Empirical evidence regarding the benefits and burdens of MANH in advanced cancer patients does not provide conclusive results and so benefits and burdens need to be judged on a case basis.
3. Decisions on the use of MANH in advanced cancer patients need to be related to well-defined goals of care and solidly based on ethical values and principles.
4. Besides the formal ethical principles there are some traditional ethical values/principles that can provide content and guidance in difficult decision-making regarding the use of MANH in advanced cancer patients (see Box 23.2).
5. A periodic re-evaluation of the patient's condition is necessary to assess the attainability of the pre-established goals of care and to take into account eventual changes in the patient's condition, including the quantity and quality of life.

The ethical dimension of decisions about MANH in advanced cancer patients

In 1996, an expert committee, under the auspice of the European Association for Palliative Care (EAPC), proposed clinical guidelines on the use of artificial nutrition and hydration in advanced cancer patients.[11] These guidelines recommend a three-step approach (Box 23.2):

- Step I. Define the eight key elements necessary to reach a decision.
- Step II. Make the decision.
- Step III. Re-evaluate the patient and therapy at specified intervals.

This approach stresses the importance of a careful analysis of both the clinical status and the empirical evidence regarding benefits and burdens of MANH in advanced cancer patients. In 2006 the European Society for Clinical Nutrition and Metabolism (ESPEN) also proposed clinical guidelines on enteral nutrition for oncological patients[8] which provide evidence-based recommendations for the use of oral nutritional supplements (ONS) and tube feeding (TF) in cancer patients. Interestingly, the ESPEN complemented these recommendations with a reflection on the ethical and legal aspects related to enteral nutrition.[12] It becomes evident that empirical evidence alone is not sufficient to settle complex questions regarding the use of MANH in advanced cancer patients.

Decisions about the suitability of MANH in individual patients—especially at the end of life—require a broadened scope which includes the ethical, psychological, legal, cultural, spiritual and religious dimensions of medical care. Some examples of ethical questions related to decisions about MANH in advanced cancer patients include the following:

- Is MANH part of the 'basic care' we ought to provide to everyone or is it rather a form of 'medical treatment' that can be withheld or withdrawn?
- Which are the main ethical values and principles related to the use of MANH in advanced cancer patients?
- What is the role of patient autonomy in decision-making regarding nutrition and hydration? Are there any limits to a patient's right to refuse (or to demand) MANH?

Box 23.2 Guidelines on artificial nutrition/hydration in terminal cancer patients[a]

Step I. Define the eight key elements necessary to reach a decision

1. Oncological/clinical status.
2. Symptoms.
3. Expected length of survival.
4. Hydration and nutritional status.
5. Spontaneous or voluntary intake.
6. Psychological attitude.
7. Gut function and route of administration.
8. Need of special services (based on type of nutritional support prescribed).

Step II. Make the decision

1. Assessment of pros and cons to establish a well-defined goal of therapy.
2. Reference to ethical values and principles:[b]
   - Respect for life, heath and the dignity of the dying.
   - Pursue of proportionate medical care ('ethically adequate' medical care).
   - Exercise of responsible freedom (autonomy).
   - Respect for the symbolic, cultural, spiritual and/or religious meanings of care.
3. Explain the procedure to the patient and relatives.

Step III. Re-evaluate the patient and therapy at specified intervals

1. Periodic reevaluation of the decision in light of the attainability of expected goals.
2. Take into account changes in patient's conditions, including quality of life.

[a]Cf. Bozzetti *et al.*[11]
[b]Not included in the European Association for Palliative Care guidelines and intentionally included here.

Adapted from Cf. Experts Committee (1996): European Association for Palliative Care, *Nutrition*, **12**(3), 163 – 167, with permission

- Should health care professionals always respect advanced directives regarding MANH at the end of life?
- To what extent should health care professionals take into account the symbolic, cultural, spiritual and/or religious meaning attributed to acts of providing food and liquid to vulnerable people?

This chapter deals specifically with some of the ethical values and principles that underlie these questions.

MANH: 'basic care' or 'medical treatment'?

Ethical questions concerning MANH are sometimes framed as a problem of defining whether the use of intravenous fluids or feeding tubes corresponds to 'basic care' (and therefore always ethically obligatory) or to 'medical treatments' (and therefore required only under certain circumstances).[15,16] Ethicists usually agree that 'medical treatments' are not always morally obligatory, and the use of therapies that are not proportionate (or adequate) might be morally optional or even wrong.[14,17,18–22] Instead, 'basic care' is said to be always morally obligatory because without it the patient would probably do worse and eventually die. These basic measures assume a symbolic meaning in the context of health care and are regarded as a concrete expression of respect for human life and dignity. To deny someone's basic needs is not only to deny these particular needs, but necessarily undermines—and ultimately denies—human solidarity.[23]

A number of ethicists suggest that MANH should be regarded as 'medical treatments' that can be withheld or withdrawn, at least under certain circumstances.[16,24–29] There are also a number of authors that hold otherwise, considering these measures as part of the 'basic care' due to all human beings.[30–36] Among the main reasons supporting the latter position are statements that nutrition and hydration aim directly at preserving an organism's life and, as long as MANH preserves an individual's life and is relatively easy to implement, it should be regarded as morally obligatory (at least in principle). According to this perspective, to consider these rather simple measures as too burdensome—and therefore morally optional—might reflect a lack of sensibility for the value of human life.[36] There is a broad ongoing debate among ethicists, moral theologians and health care professionals on this particular issue.[37–41]

Regardless of whether one conceives MANH as 'basic care' or as 'medical treatment', it seems that framing the debate on the moral obligation of MANH on this distinction alone might be misleading in particular cases. The question regarding the ethics of MANH in individual cases (obligatory versus optional) cannot be definitively settled just by defining the category of acts under which MANH falls ('basic care' or 'medical treatment'). For instance, one may claim that some forms of MANH (e.g. intravenous hydration) correspond to basic medical assistance when individuals have an inadequate intake of oral fluids, but still regard its implementation as morally non-obligatory or even wrong under specific circumstances. To the contrary, some health care professionals may affirm that MANH should be formally included among the category of 'medical treatments', but still regard the intervention—in principle—as 'proportionate' and therefore morally obligatory, because it aims at preserving an individual's life and does not usually impose significant burdens.

The key ethical question regarding MANH is whether its implementation is morally obligatory in a particular case. In order to answer this ethical question, we need to identify the moral values and principles involved in that particular situation.

Main ethical values/principles related to MANH in advanced cancer patients

A reference to the principles of autonomy, non-maleficence, beneficence and justice is usually advocated to deal with ethical issues in health care.[6,12,13,42] In this chapter we briefly review the content of some traditional moral values and principles that might be helpful in decision-making regarding the implementation of MANH in advanced cancer patients. Some of the main values and principles related to this particular issue are listed in Box 23.3.

Respect for life, health and the dignity of the dying

Life is a basic human good and the foundation of a person's ability to fulfil other human goods and vital goals.[43] Life is an ethically relevant good that deserves an adequate value-answer, which is usually expressed as the moral obligation to respect and preserve life. Health, as an instrumental human good, also demands a value-response, commonly acknowledged as a moral duty to preserve health and to pursue medical care.[45,46] The moral obligation to preserve life and health has been acknowledged since ancient times, but it is equally evident that nobody is obliged to

Box 23.3 Main ethical values/principles related to medically assisted nutrition and/or hydration in advanced cancer patients

Some traditional principles of medical ethics:

1. Respect for life, heath and the dignity of the dying.
2. Duty to pursue of proportionate medical care ('ethically adequate' medical care).
3. Exercise of responsible freedom (autonomy).
4. Respect for the symbolic, cultural, spiritual and/or religious meanings of care.

So-called 'principles of biomedical ethics':

1. Autonomy.
2. Non-maleficence.
3. Beneficence.
4. Justice.

pursue all available means to preserve life and health. Greek physicians learned to distinguish situations in which a disease presents an obstacle to an otherwise healthy nature from situations in which disease leads human existence to its natural end.[47] Hippocratic physicians learned to acknowledge those medical efforts that would most probably fail:

> Whenever therefore a man suffers from an ill, which is too strong for the means at disposal of medicine, he surely must not even expect that it can be overcome by medicine.[47]

Consequently, Greek medicine did not consider death as a failure of medicine, but as the natural end of human life. The same idea was stressed centuries later by St Basil, who praised medicine as a divine gift, but condemned 'whatever requires an undue amount of thought or trouble or involves a large expenditure of effort and causes our whole life to revolve, as it were, around the solicitude for the flesh.'[48] St Basil's statement is perhaps one of the earliest contributions on the limits of our moral obligation to preserve life and to pursue health care. To accept that there are legitimate limits to our moral obligation to preserve life and to pursue health care implies the recognition of a moral duty to accept death as a constitutive part of human life.

Respect for the dignity of the dying person

We ought to respect the dignity of the dying person precisely because we respect human life and dignity in all its different stages and circumstances. In other words, the same ethical principle that urges us to respect human life and dignity demands from us a respect for a person's dying process. An important task of palliative care is to provide competent, active and concrete answers to these ethical demands. Defining the principles of palliative care, the World Health Organization (WHO) states that this discipline affirms life and regards dying as a normal process, neither hastening nor postponing death. [49] This definition corresponds to a concept of the so-called 'right to die with dignity'[50] not simply as a 'right to die',[51,52] but rather as a 'right to live one's life to the end'. The difference is important, because it points to the concrete ethical challenges that arise when caring for the terminally ill.

Once the diagnosis of a terminal status is established, there seems to be general agreement that the main goals of care should be relief of symptoms, the pursuit of the best possible quality of life and the patient's/family's preparation for death, including the psychological, spiritual, familial, and social dimensions of the dying process. Artificially prolonging a patient's distress would be contrary to the dignity of the dying person. The definition of 'terminally ill' therefore has practical implications for ethical decision-making regarding care, including MANH.[53,54]

Identifying the 'terminally ill'

Different definitions of 'terminally ill' are proposed in the literature.[55–57] In spite of the differences, some common features can be identified. A working definition, that summarizes the main elements to identify a patient as 'terminally ill', includes:

- the well-established diagnosis of an incurable, active and progressive disease that causes death;
- a lack of therapeutic interventions to cure the individual patient.

This is when there is no known medical intervention that can change the progression of the disease to death (at least according to the present state of medical art), or the available therapies have not been effective (or are no longer effective).

These elements that define a patient's status as 'terminal' have significant implications for ethical decision-making regarding medical care, including MANH. In this setting, some forms of MANH might be inadequate, especially if the goals of preserving life and relieving suffering through nutrition and/or hydration are no longer realistic. This idea leads us to the specific question about the foundation of our moral responsibility to preserve life and health through nutrition and hydration.

The moral obligation to preserve life and health through nutrition and hydration

Questions concerning the existence of a moral obligation towards nutrition and hydration have a long history. In the sixteenth century, moralists undertook a systematic analysis of this issue. In his famous *Relectiones Theologiae,* Francisco de Vitoria addressed the moral obligation to conserve life by means of food. He argued for a moral obligation regarding nutrition according to the natural inclination to self-preservation, the love a person owes to self, and the wrongness of suicide. In spite of arguing for the existence of a moral obligation for self-conservation by means of food, de Vitoria stated that a sick person who can take food 'only with the greatest of effort and as though by means of a certain torture' can be excused from this obligation based on 'a certain impossibility … especially where there is little hope for life, or none at all.'

In other words, de Vitoria thought that the moral obligation to take food might be suspended when a patient's life cannot be preserved any longer. He concluded that 'man is not held to employ all the possible means of conserving his life, but the means which are *per se* intended for that purpose' if they offer a reasonable hope for benefit, understood as the preservation of life and health.

These statements confront us with central questions concerning both the specific purposes for implementing MANH in advanced cancer patients and the legitimate limits of our moral obligation to preserve life and health through assisted nutrition and hydration.

Legitimate limits to the moral obligation to preserve life and health

The point of departure for a systematic reflection on the limits of our moral obligation to preserve life and health was Aquinas' tract on suicide. Following Aquinas, moralists usually introduce a distinction between 'positive' and 'negative' moral precepts. This distinction is relevant, as 'negative precepts' are said to oblige always (*semper*) and in every circumstance (*pro semper*), whereas 'positive precepts' oblige always (*semper*) but not in all circumstances (not *pro semper*). In other words, 'negative precepts' are always binding since they forbid what is intrinsically evil. On the contrary, one is not always bound to do something positively good, as *physical or moral impossibility* can excuse one from the fulfilment of affirmative precepts.

Applying this moral distinction to the question whether it is always obligatory to take food and/or liquids, de Vitoria proposed that unlike the 'absolute' moral obligation not to take innocent human life intentionally by depriving someone of nutrition and hydration, the extent of the 'positive' obligation to provide food and liquid rests on the possibility of obtaining benefit, which he understood as the preservation of life and health. His insights gave origin to the traditional moral distinction between 'ordinary' and 'extraordinary' (O/E) means for conserving life and health. This distinction, followed and further unfolded by subsequent moralists to this day,[19–21] is at the foundation of the current recognition of a moral obligation to pursue 'proportionate' (or 'ethically adequate') medical care.

If one accepts the premise that nutrition and hydration—even artificially administered—might be morally obligatory provided that its implementation can actually preserve an individual's life and health, then answering the question whether MANH does in fact preserve life and health in advanced cancer patients has important ethical implications (Box 23.4).

Does MANH preserve life and health in advanced cancer patients?

Does the omission of MANH cause death in advanced cancer patients?

Available empirical evidence is far from providing conclusive results to answer these questions.[58–62] Nevertheless, there are empirical data that provide helpful insights in this regard. If one takes into account the regular fluid losses of an organism, it is not hard to imagine that the expected survival of patients who do not receive the normal daily requirements would be affected.[63] A retrospective study of oncological patients who voluntarily refused food and fluids to hasten death observed a survival of 10 ± 7 days, with 85% of these patients dying within a period of 15 days.[64] Another retrospective survey, describing the experience of Dutch physicians who participated in cases of continuous deep terminal sedation, showed that almost three-quarters of the patients were not hydrated after inducing sedation and that 95% died within 7 days.[65]

Box 23.4 Some ethically relevant questions related to medically assisted nutrition and/or hydration (MANH) in advanced cancer patients

1. Which are the benefits and burdens related to MANH in advanced cancer patients?
2. How do health care professionals define clinical 'benefit' (medical utility/futility)?
3. How do health care professionals conceive the 'burdens' related to medical care?
4. Does MANH preserve life and health in advanced cancer patients?
5. Does the omission of MANH cause death in advanced cancer patients?
6. Does MANH relieve suffering in advanced cancer patients?
7. Can MANH contribute to improve a patient's responsible exercise of freedom (autonomy) at the end of life?
8. How do health care professionals respect the symbolic, cultural, spiritual and/or religious dimensions of MANH?

The situation is different in cases where the capacity to receive adequate fluid intake is spontaneously and irreversibly lost as a consequence of progression of the underlying disease. In such cases, the prognosis is intrinsically limited and the decreased liquid intake is considered to be part of the dying process. A systematic review showed that there is insufficient evidence to estimate the impact of artificial hydration in palliative care patients.

There is no convincing evidence that artificial hydration significantly changes the survival of those advanced cancer patients who are already in the dying process and for whom life expectancy is already severely reduced, although some authors suggest that particular groups of patients may benefit from artificial hydration at the end of life, especially if signs of dehydration or neurotoxicity are present.[61–72]

With regards to the effects of omitting nutritional support in advanced cancer patients, the available evidence is also not conclusive. Undernutrition and cachexia are very frequent phenomena and have been described as indicators of poor quality of life and limited prognosis in oncological patients.[5,8] Cancer cachexia is a syndrome characterized by progressive and involuntary weight loss, often associated with anorexia, anergy, fatigue, anaemia, hypoalbuminaemia and changes in the host cytokine and hormonal milieu. In the case of patients with obstructive head and neck cancers for whom aphagia is a consequence of anatomical factors and the main cause of nutritional deterioration is the lack of oral intake, nutritional support may significantly improve survival.[7,73] In those cases in which hypercatabolism and systemic inflammation predominate, artificial nutritional support has not been demonstrated either to recover or to prevent the progression of the patient's nutritional deterioration;[8] however, a positive effect of nutritional support in selected groups of patients, especially those with a relatively good prognosis, cannot be excluded.[74,75]

The ESPEN guidelines recommend that enteral nutritional support be started in advanced cancer patients if undernutrition already exists or if food intake is expected to be markedly reduced for more than 7 days because 'in patients who are losing weight due to insufficient nutritional intake, enteral nutrition should be provided to improve or maintain nutritional status and this may also contribute to the maintenance of quality of life.'[8] Independently of whether the main cause of nutritional deterioration is a difficulty in oral intake or the anorexia–cachexia syndrome, each oncological patient with a severely reduced oral intake who has an estimated survival of more than 3 months should be considered for MANH. A normal adult completely deprived of nutrients does not survive inanition for more than 2–3 months and, as a consequence, a key ethical question in decision-making regarding the use of MANH in a particular case is whether its omission may cause a patient's death.

Based on this kind of evidence, the French Fédération Nationale des Centres de Lutte Contre le Cancer recommends not implementing MANH in advanced cancer patients whose prognosis is less than 3 months and/or who have a severe and permanent deterioration of functional status, i.e. a Karnofsky index ≤50%.[76]

The ESPEN guidelines for cancer patients comment that palliative use of nutritional support in terminally ill cancer patients is rarely indicated and that those patients with a life expectancy of less than 40 days may be palliated with home intravenous fluid therapy. Consistently, the ESPEN recommendations are that

> … close to the end of life, guidelines for preserving nutritional state are no longer relevant and intensive nutritional therapy may worsen the condition of dying cancer patients. When the end of life is very close, most patients require only minimal amount of food and little water to reduce thirst and hunger. Small amounts of fluid may also help to avoid states of confusion induced by dehydration. Subcutaneous infused fluids in hospital or at home may be helpful and also provide a vehicle for the administration of drugs.'[8]

In summary, with regards to MANH in advanced cancer patients, the ethical principle of respect for life, health and the dignity of the dying demands that the prognosis of an oncological patient should be determined by the unavoidable progression of the cancer, rather than dehydration and or inanition because MANH support is omitted.[77] It also becomes evident that an accurate estimation of the patient's prognosis assumes a key role in individual decision-making regarding MANH. Unfortunately, our capacity to predict prognosis in individual patients is limited[78] so that ethically adequate decisions to implement or to withhold MANH in individual cancer patients have to be based not on a 'statistical certainty', but rather on the 'moral certainty' that our actions respect life, health and the dignity of the dying.

The pursuit of 'proportionate' or 'ethically adequate' medical care

A traditional principle of medical ethics states that the moral obligation to provide patients medical care should be adequately proportioned between the means to be employed and the expected results.[15,35] Medical interventions for which this adequacy of proportion does not hold are considered 'disproportionate' (or 'extraordinary') and therefore morally non-obligatory (or wrong). To the contrary, the implementation of means judged as 'proportionate' (or 'ordinary') is—in principle—morally obligatory. It is interesting to note that this traditional moral distinction is widely incorporated into contemporary medical ethics, in one way or another.[14,79–82]

According to the traditional moral distinction between 'ordinary' and 'extraordinary' (O/E) means of care, medical interventions are morally obligatory if they offer a reasonable *hope of benefit* (understood as the preservation of life and/or health) and do not impose *excessive burdens* on individual patients. Both conditions have to be fulfilled simultaneously. In other words, we can say that it is morally legitimate to withhold or withdraw medical interventions that are futile and too burdensome. It is important to note that both of these judgments have to be made in relation to a patient's individual condition at a particular point in time[83] and that in this context, the need for a clear understanding of the concepts of clinical 'benefit' and 'burden' becomes evident.

Which concept of 'benefit'?

Defining clinical benefit is not an easy task. The concepts of clinical 'benefit' or 'utility/futility' are widely explored in the medical literature.[84–87] Traditionally, clinical 'benefit' is understood as the capacity of a given medical intervention to offer a reasonable chance of preserving life and/or of maintaining/restoring health.[88] The development of evidence-based medicine seeks to provide statistical criteria in clinical practice, resulting in new attempts to demarcate the concepts of 'utility' and 'futility'. Christensen, for instance, introduces a helpful distinction between *absolute*, *statistical* and *disproportionate* futility.[89] According to this author, *absolute futility* refers to those completely ineffective interventions in physiological terms. Since there is a general agreement that a physician is not obliged to implement absolute futile measures, the limitation of this kind of measure does not pose difficult moral dilemmas. *Statistical futility* expresses a low probability of a specific measure to achieve a given goal, although the statistical information does not say very much about the moral obligation to implement the measure in a particular case. It certainly presents morally relevant clinical information that needs to be carefully considered in decision-making. The expression *disproportionate futility* qualifies a value-laden decision to abstain from a certain medical intervention—in spite of its low statistical probability of achieving a beneficial effect—because in a given situation it causes suffering and increases risks or costs to the patient and/or the family. A similar concept is proposed by Caplan, who states that 'medical utility must be understood as referring to both the probability and the desirability of attaining a particular diagnostic, therapeutic, or palliative goal'.[90]

A distinction can be made between those dimensions of clinical benefit/futility that are limited to the evidence-based probability of attaining a given goal and other dimensions related to the value-laden judgement about the desirability of attaining that specific goal. We might say that the statistical component of benefit/futility judgments belongs primarily to the domain of technical expertise while the value-laden component refers to the moral values involved in achieving—or failing to achieve—that given goal and/or to the risks and burdens associated with a specific medical intervention.

Which concept of 'burden'?

When applied to health care, the notion of 'burden' should not be too narrowly defined. In fact, one may regard as 'burdens' all the different sources of physical, psychological, spiritual, humane, familial, social, and financial distress associated with medical interventions.[21] Traditionally, judging a medical intervention as 'too burdensome' allows us to characterize it as morally non-obligatory.

The identification of a physical or moral 'impossibility' in using a given medical intervention is the classical criterion to define its ethically 'non-obligatory character'. Classical writers used a variety of expressions to describe different causes of *physical* or *moral impossibility* of medical care:

- an excessive effort (*summus labor, media nimis dura*);
- an unbearable pain (*quidam cruciatus, ingens dolor*);
- excessive expenses (*sumptus extraordinarius, media exquisita*);
- an intense fear or a very strong repugnance (*vehemens horror*).

The existence of at least one of these different causes of *physical* or *moral impossibility* allows for the definition of the 'extraordinary character' of care, thereby providing criteria for assessing the morally non-obligatory character of a given measure in individual cases.

According to the ethical principle of therapeutic proportionality, and in order to identify the moral character (obligatory, optional, illicit) of medical care—including MANH—a careful assessment of the potential benefits, risks and burdens is needed.

Comparative assessment of benefits, risks and burdens

Clinicians usually base their medical management on evidence of the possible benefits and risks/burdens of a given intervention. For instance, available medical guidelines on the use of MANH in advanced cancer patients categorize the patients into a series of groups, such as the type of cancer, the extent, the functional status, the likelihood of response to treatment, and the presence of malnutrition. The EAPC's guidelines propose a list of eight key clinical elements (Box 23.3) that include the oncological/clinical status, symptoms, expected length of survival, hydration and nutritional status, spontaneous or voluntary intake, psychological attitude, gut function, route of administration, and the need for special services based on the type of nutritional support prescribed.[11]

Based on these criteria, patients are classified according to the functional impact of the cancer and their prognosis and proximity to death. For example, one group consists of those who are undergoing therapy with a reasonable expectation of response or who are expected to live more than six months. Another group consists of malnourished cancer patients for whom treatments have been unsuccessful or whose disease is advanced and associated with a significant deterioration in functional status. These patients are bed-bound and unable to perform various tasks of self-care such as dressing and washing. Another group consists of individuals in the final phase of an irreversible decline, severe malnutrition and a life expectancy of less than 1–2 months.

It is evident that the possible benefits, risks and burdens associated with MANH for these three categories of patients are different. Consequently, the moral obligation to implement MANH will also vary, and if one accepts the premise that nutrition and hydration—even artificially administered—may be morally obligatory provided they preserve an individual's life/health and do not impose excessive burdens, then available empirical data regarding the actual benefits and burdens associated with MANH in the different groups of advanced cancer patients becomes ethically relevant for decision-making in individual cases. What does available medical evidence say regarding potential benefits and burdens of MANH in oncological patients?

Potential benefits of MANH in advanced cancer patients

Malnutrition and cachexia in advanced cancer patients are predictors of poor prognosis. Clinical evidence suggests that they can also have a great impact on quality of life, functionality and the adverse effects of oncological therapies in selected groups of patients.[5,8] It is argued that among the possible benefits of MANH in advanced cancer patients is the potential to improve nutritional status, to improve functional status, to reduce the risk of infections and pressure sores (due to poor nutritional status and immobility), to relieve symptoms (when these are experienced), prevent aspiration pneumonia, provide comfort, maintain human community, and respect the symbolic value of providing food and liquids.

Does MANH relieve suffering in terminally ill cancer patients?

It has been suggested that MANH may help prevent or treat unpleasant symptoms at the end of life. There are actually very few randomized controlled trials evaluating the efficacy of MANH in advanced cancer patients although there is evidence from less rigorously controlled studies indicating that MANH may have benefits in selected groups of patients and/or in relation to specific symptoms.

Functionality and quality of life

Head and neck cancer patients, who are losing weight as a consequence of a severely diminished oral intake, can improve their nutritional status, function and quality of life through MANH[7,73] Some studies show that tube feeding can improve the quality of life of patients with head and neck cancers and impaired nutrition when undergoing radiotherapy, as compared to oral feeding alone.[7] In patients with cancers of the head and neck, a feeding tube could be used to allow adequate intake around times of major surgery, chemo- and radiation therapy, when the ability to chew, swallow, retain and absorb food is impaired.[73]

Thirst and fluid balance

Terminally ill patients frequently complain of thirst and often lose the ability to consume an adequate amount of liquids.[91] The traditional approach of dealing with thirst in the terminally ill is to administer sips of water and to moisten the lips. Numerous studies have failed to show a positive correlation between the frequency and intensity of thirst and the presence of biochemical markers for dehydration, although there are clinical studies suggesting that, in cases where thirst is associated with hyperosmolarity, artificial hydration may be of help in relieving this symptom.[92,93] Artificial hydration is discussed further in Chapter 30.

Neurological symptoms

Neurological dysfunction, such as confusion or delirium, is a frequent source of distress for both patients and relatives at the end of life.[94] Several clinical studies suggest that dehydration may be a reversible cause of delirium in advanced cancer patients,[95,96] and it is possible that artificial hydration at the end of life may prevent or reverse delirium.[97–99]

Potential risks and burdens associated with MANH in advanced cancer patients

Some authors suggest that studies have consistently failed to demonstrate a meaningful clinical benefit of MANH in advanced cancer patients and that nutritional support is associated with risks and uncomfortable side-effects, including:

- Simple hydration administered subcutaneously or intravenously may cause irritation, infection, perforation of vessels, oedema and fluid accumulation.[66]
- Nasogastric tubes may cause irritation and discomfort, epistaxis, sinusitis and the need for restraint when patients are confused and repeatedly pull at the tube. Restraints can, in turn, lead to further complications such as pressure sores or agitation.
- Percutaneous endoscopic gastrostomy tubes can cause complications such as infection, perforation of the bowel, diarrhoea, cramping, nausea and vomiting.

Moral relevance of well-defined goals of care

If one accepts the premise that nutrition and hydration—even artificially administered—may be morally obligatory provided a reasonable hope of benefit (understood as the preservation of life/health) is offered and no excessive burdens are imposed, then available empirical data regarding the actual benefits, risks and burdens associated with MANH become ethically relevant for decision-making in individual cases. It is important to keep in mind that the moral character (i.e. obligatory, optional, illicit) of MANH cannot be derived exclusively from a comparative assessment of empirical data regarding its potential benefits, risks and burdens. In fact, according to the ethical principle of proportionality, to identify the moral character (obligatory, optional, illicit) of medical care, the empirical evidence needs to be analysed in light of well-defined goals of care and the moral relevance of pursuing these goals.

So in order to identify what constitutes an 'ethically adequate' use of MANH in oncological patients, it is important to establish well-defined goals of care that are both valuable and realistically attainable in the individual case. To make such a judgment assumes that the dimensions of medical decision-making limited to the evidence-based probability of attaining a given goal can be distinguished from other dimensions related to value-judgments regarding the desirability of attaining that goal in the individual case. In other words, defining both realistically attainable and morally relevant goals of care is central for ethical decision-making regarding MANH in oncological patients.

For example, if the cancer is curable and MANH appears to play a role in supporting the patient's hydration/nutritional status, functional status and/or quality of life, then judgements about the moral character of implementing MANH do not pose serious difficulties to clinicians. When the cancer cannot be cured, and particularly if the patient is approaching the terminal stage of the disease, clinicians seem to experience increasing difficulty in identifying the moral character of implementing MANH. In this context, it might be helpful to keep in mind that once the diagnosis/prognosis of a terminal condition has been established, there seems to be general agreement that the main goals of care should be the relief of symptoms, the pursuit of the best possible quality of life and the patient's/family's preparation for death, including the psychological, spiritual, familial, social, legal, etc. dimensions of the dying process.

In summary, according to the ethical principle of proportionality in medical care, judging the moral character (i.e. obligatory, optional, illicit) of medical interventions requires a comparative assessment of various clinical aspects connected with the actual benefits, risks and burdens, the establishment of well-defined goals of care, and the identification of the ethical values and principles involved in pursuing these goals. Although the moral character of implementing MANH in a particular case cannot be derived exclusively from a comparative assessment of data regarding its actual benefits and burdens, an accurate assessment of the clinical aspects is a necessary step of the ethical analysis.

Exercise of responsible freedom (autonomy)

A growing concern for patient's autonomy has characterized contemporary medicine and includes a respect for the choice to say 'no' to being overtreated (now or in the future) and even to refuse being treated at all. The importance of fostering a responsible exercise of freedom with regard to health care has obvious implications for the practice of medicine. It is interesting to note that although freedom and autonomy are highly valued in contemporary societies, the very concept of 'autonomy' is far from unambiguously understood and has become a 'Pandora's box' in contemporary bioethics. The word 'autonomy' derives from the Greek *autos* ('self') and *nomos* ('rule', 'governance' or 'law'). Beauchamp and Childress[14] remark that the expression 'autonomy' has been 'extended to individuals and has acquired meanings as diverse as self-governance, liberty rights, privacy, individual choice, freedom of the will, causing one's own behaviour, and being one's own person. Clearly, autonomy is not a univocal concept in either ordinary English or contemporary philosophy.' Before arguing for the existence of a moral value in respecting patients' and caregivers' exercise of responsible freedom and analysing its implications for decision-making regarding MANH in advanced cancer patients, it is important to make an attempt to clarify the concept of freedom and autonomy.

Fisher argues that 'in the classical tradition, at least up to Kant, *rational autonomy* might be said to be the capacity to make reasoned decisions for oneself—which implies not simply choosing and acting as we desire to, or even as we have reason to, but choosing and acting by reasons we endorse.'[100] He reminds us that 'for Kant autonomy was the state of will of one who recognizes that the demands of moral law are neither externally legislated nor subjectively constructed but are objective norms of reason clear to anyone with well-functioning mind and a will to apply them.' 'But for most of the sons of 'Enlightenment' (e.g. Hume and Mill) autonomy was not grasping the norms of reason but approving a course of action and experiencing the freedom to pursue it.'

Many twentieth century thinkers disconnected freedom from an objective rationality and tended to reduce autonomy to the pursuit of preferences, subjectively experienced as 'authenticity' in one's own decisions. So, for instance, libertarians conceive autonomy as the highest ethical principle and understand respect for autonomy as synonymous with allowing everyone to the make their own decisions, as long these decisions do not trespass another person's autonomy.[18,101,102] From this perspective, the decisive point is the fact *that* someone has chosen something without experiencing external constraints. The particular content of the decision does not matter very much, as long as it does not deprive others from their possibility to exercise autonomy.

Such a concept of autonomy has had enormous influence in shaping contemporary health care throughout the world. Its danger to the relationship between patients and health care professionals is not always sufficiently recognized and the current trend to overemphasize autonomous decisions may expose patients (and surrogate decision-makers) to a sort of 'medical abandonment'. Health care professionals may also fear to openly express their opinions regarding what constitutes 'best care', in order to avoid being accused of 'intruding' on patient autonomy. What used to be a participative relationship, in which health care professionals were personally engaged in effective communication and decision-making to pursue the 'best care' for their patients (solidarity), is at risk of becoming an 'aseptic' provision of information to allow individual decision-making (individualism).

It might be necessary to re-define the concept of 'autonomy' not merely as the capacity to decide for oneself (without experiencing external coercions), but as the 'responsible exercise of freedom'.[100] Such a concept stresses the moral value not only of permitting people to make free decisions, but also of fostering people's capacity to make *good* decisions. In other words, what matters is not only *that* people decide, but also the *content* of their decision, and it is according to the content of our free decisions that we form our 'moral personhood'. With regards to health care, we may act in a responsible or an irresponsible manner depending on the means we apply (or fail to apply) to preserve or restore health. For health care providers, such a concept of 'responsible freedom' implies the moral responsibility of becoming personally involved in a participative decision-making process that searches for what is objectively good for the individual patient, according to the circumstances ('best care').

Fostering a 'responsible exercise of freedom' involves each member of the triad of patient–family–health care professionals. It demands from each a serious effort to access accurate information with regards to the options in health care and requires implementing concrete strategies to preserve the patient's capacity to use their mental capacities, as long as it is possible. Therefore, an ethically relevant dimension of decisions about MANH in terminally ill patients is the question whether it may help preserve or restore a patient's mental faculties.

Can MANH contribute to improving patients' exercise of freedom at the end of life?

Neurological dysfunctions—such as confusion or delirium—are frequent at the end of life[94] and impede attention and communication, thereby affecting patients' exercise of freedom.[103] Delirium occurs in 88% of patients, often not in the final stages of the dying process, but some 16 days before death. Delirium is an independent predictor of poor survival and reversible in about 50% of cases. The causes of delirium are multifactorial, and its reversal influenced by minimally invasive measures such as discontinuing or reducing the dose of certain medications and hydrating patients.

One interesting study has a bearing on this issue. A comparison of patient and physician differences on factors considered important at the end of life showed that patients consistently consider 'being mentally aware' at the end of life important more often than physicians (92–65% of those surveyed). This suggests that patients are more likely than physicians to support the enhancement of cognitive functioning at the end of life over efforts to control symptoms if the two are in conflict.[104]

Responsible exercise of freedom and the role of advanced directives regarding MANH

Among substitute decision-makers who chose MANH for relatives with cognitive impairment, less than half would also choose MANH for themselves if they were in similar circumstances.[105] The reasons for providing MANH are usually connected with the respect for life and the symbolic meaning of providing nutrition and hydration to loved ones. On the other hand, when it comes to personal decisions, the arguments for withholding MANH are usually linked to the fear of becoming a burden to others and the rejection of a poor quality of life.

In the context of substitute decision-making, it is interesting to note that cultural and religious perceptions carry an important weight in substitute decision-making with regards to MANH. For instance, Orthodox Jews consider the provision of MANH for a family member with progressive dementia to be the standard of care. Although several prominent Catholic thinkers do not regard the provision of MANH to patients with advanced dementia as morally obligatory, others do. Keown is an example within the Catholic tradition who argues that the criteria for withholding or withdrawing MANH for any patient should depend on the worth of an intervention for a given patient. It should not be a judgement about the worth of the life of the individual, whether he or she has terminal cancer or advanced dementia. Keown argues that decisions to withhold or withdraw MANH based on the worth or quality of life of the patient cannot avoid being instances of intentional killing, and that it is an omission of an intervention with the intent to bring about the death of the patient.[106]

These findings have important implications for substitute decision-making regarding MANH. They point to the role that advanced directives can play in helping relatives know what their loved ones would have chosen in a given situation. They also suggest the idea that an individual's wishes are not *absolute* with regards to medical decision-making, including MANH at the end of life, and that there are moral and legal limits that ought to be respected. A responsible exercise of freedom demands that an individual or substitute medical decision-maker respect the moral values and principles that may be involved in a given situation, such as the duty to respect life, health and the dignity of the dying person, that he or she respect the obligation to pursue proportionate medical care, and respect cultural, spiritual and/or religious perceptions.

In summary, fostering a 'responsible exercise of freedom' in health care implies a participative decision-making process that involves all members of the triad 'patient–relatives–health care team' in the identification of what is objectively good for an individual patient (i.e. the 'best care', the 'proportionate care'), according to the circumstances, the moral values at stake and cultural and religious convictions.

Respect for the symbolic, cultural, spiritual and/or religious meanings

Caring for the sick includes the responsibility to seek the correct diagnoses and appropriate treatments, but also to provide the patient with the basic necessities of life, including shelter, nourishment, fluids, sanitary needs, toilet, etc. The idea of caring for someone is closely linked to the provision of food and liquids and is stronger when the sick are not able to personally take care of these needs. These measures assume a symbolic meaning in the context of health care and are regarded as a concrete expression of respect for human life and dignity.[107]

For most cultures, nutrition and hydration are tightly connected to ethical and symbolic values; however, the symbolic value attributed to nutritional assistance varies among different cultures. Empirical knowledge of the clinical benefits, risks and burdens associated with MANH may not be enough to clearly ground individual decisions, since emotional and cultural aspects heavily influence the decision-making process. Identifying cultural attitudes and personal beliefs regarding nutrition and hydration is both necessary and morally relevant in the context of MANH decisions.

Personal beliefs and cultural attitudes influence decision-making regarding MANH not only for patients and relatives, but also for different members of the health care team. It is interesting to note that clinical studies suggest the symbolic perception of MANH in patients, families and members of the health care team do not always coincide. For example, family members are often more concerned about anorexia than the patients themselves,[108–113] whereas, health care staff often underestimate the anxiety and distress that patients and relatives experience with anorexia.[114,115] A number of clinical surveys have explored the emotional,[116–121] cultural[122–126] and religious[127] dimensions of decisions regarding MANH.

Symbolic perceptions and cultural attitudes of patients/ families towards MANH

Some surveys suggest that the main concerns of patients and families regarding MANH are related to questions regarding effective feeding, survival and quality of life.[116] Among patients and families, the main factors favouring MANH were: preserving life, the palliation of symptoms, not abandoning the struggle against illness, and the presence of anxiety.[113,125] By contrast, the main reasons against initiating MANH were: preference for a natural death, not prolonging suffering, fear of dependence, and fear of abandonment.[116,128]

Reduced oral intake at the end of life is an important source of anxiety for relatives involved in patient care.[114,128–132] Canadian studies suggest that a reduced interest in eating, a limited capacity to digest food, fatigue and altered body image are all highly correlated with serious psychological distress in a terminally ill patient.[133] Moreover, from a spouse's perspective, the quantity and specificity of oral intake by the patient often functions as a barometer of the patient's overall condition.[108] Spouses may insist on maintaining what they regard as normal eating habits in the belief that not eating will rapidly lead to death. This trend in spouses' belief has been confirmed in different studies.[133,134]

The notion that reduced food and fluid intake accelerates death is prevalent in most western cultures. By contrast, the Hindu culture regards reduced oral intake as a sign of the proximity of death, rather than a cause.[134] The prevalent belief in Hindu culture is that a terminally ill person voluntarily gives up eating to prepare for an expected death, in a self-controlled and dignified process. Likewise, many Asian cultures recognize reduced oral intake as a normal part of the dying process, and a way of preparing for what is considered a good death. There are, however, regional differences among Asian cultures about what is considered a good death. For instance, many Taiwanese believe that if a person dies hungry the soul becomes restless and hungry, leading to a preference in Taiwan for MANH at the end of life, despite the physical discomfort that these measures can cause.[112]

It becomes evident that cultural, moral, spiritual and religious views of death shape what is considered to be appropriate behaviour toward the dying.[135] Since health care brings together people from different cultural and religious backgrounds, patients and their relatives may be surrounded by people that have different conceptions of a 'good life' and a 'good death'. Moreover, the emphasis on cure that characterizes contemporary medicine may encourage aggressive treatment—even if not clinically appropriate and/or contrary to patient's wishes—in order to avoid any perception of undertreatment.[21] Such a cultural trend, as well as the growing acceptance of euthanasia and physician-assisted suicide, may impose grave moral dilemmas on dying persons. Clinical surveys suggest that health care workers often fall into the temptation of using all available technology to avoid imminent death.[115]

How do health care professionals deal with the cultural and symbolic aspects of MANH?

Among medical professionals, the belief that MANH may prevent a patient's death from inanition and improve physical energy and overall well-being is reported in several studies.[130,134] Opinions regarding MANH vary in different countries and also according to the medical specialty. A study of Israeli doctors suggests that they positively value the administration of intravenous fluids to terminal patients.[125] Similarly, the majority of nurses in a Taiwanese study supported providing MANH to terminal patients and considered MANH as basic care, believing it helpful in preserving mental status, preventing delirium, and reducing anxiety or feelings of abandonment in both patients and families.[126] A Japanese study reported that the majority of doctors believed artificial hydration (AH) relieved feelings of thirst, though they were not able to cite conclusive clinical evidence to substantiate this belief.[123]

The same survey suggested that doctors who were more likely to recommend AH were typically less involved in the care of terminal patients and viewed AH as part of basic care. By contrast, doctors with expertise in palliative care believed that withholding hydration improved patients' overall well-being at the end of life, and considered AH a form of active medical treatment. Another study by the same group demonstrated that nurses were more informed of the clinical effects of AH than doctors.[136] An Australian study of palliative care doctors and nurses found differences in perception[137] between health care professionals and families. These professionals believed that MANH at the end of life was rarely beneficial to the patient, and instead asserted that mouth care was an effective relief of discomfort.

This perception of the moral character of MANH may be also related to the influence of cultural and religious factors. A transnational European study[138] reported that the withdrawal of support at the end of life was more frequently associated with doctors from Catholic, Protestant or no religious background. These physicians (Catholic, Protestant, no religion) were also more likely to discuss their decisions with families than were physicians from other religious groups.

A conclusion drawn from the various studies is that the different perceptions and beliefs regarding the use of MANH in terminal patients could be related to the professional background, the specialty and the cultural/religious views. Interdisciplinary palliative care teams must therefore promote good communication, not only between doctors and patients/relatives, but also among the diverse health care professionals themselves. They must be acutely aware of the high symbolic value of nourishment and the emotional impact of artificial hydration and nutrition on patients, families and other health care members.

Food and water as symbols of life and human community

Providing food and drink is usually understood as a concrete manifestation of an interpersonal bond that can be both expressed and cemented by sharing goods. Family members frequently consider nutrition and hydration—even when artificially administered—as a practical expression of love and care. MANH may seem analogous to basic care that expresses human community and solidarity so that decisions to withhold or to withdraw MANH might be regarded by family members as a form of abandonment. In individual decision-making about MANH, health care professionals should be attentive not only to the physiological utility/futility of the intervention, but also to the symbolic and cultural values linked to nutrition and hydration.

The position statement of the American Medical Association on tube feeding at the end of life may well express the difficulties many physicians have with the attempt to extend the symbolism of basic care to include MANH technologies.[139] It is far from evident that providing intravenous liquid or nutrition through nasogastric tubes is comparable to the typical way of feeding those who are hungry.[9] Moreover, it can be argued that patients may be abandoned to MANH and other technologies without being cared for humanely. Facing this sort of argument, some ethicists, such as Callahan, contend that there is a social significance attached to nourishing the vulnerable and dependent in our care that makes these acts substantially different from other medical acts involving life-sustaining technologies.[140] For Callahan, the norm of caring for another by providing food and water loses its meaning if the provision of MANH to some individuals is made optional. Fisher also maintains that 'food and water are not only sources but symbols of life and community. To deny these things which are so basic to someone is not only to deny them a need but necessarily undermines and ultimately denies all solidarity with them. Refusing food or water to someone is a powerful symbol of exclusion from the circle of the community, of humanity: but to do this when someone is weak or dying is especially revealing.'[24]

Conclusion

Ethical decision-making regarding MANH in advanced cancer patients demands an accurate assessment of the empirical evidence related to possible benefits, risks and burdens in light of both:

- the moral relevance of the goals of care pursued in the individual case;
- the ethical values and principles at stake in the situation.

When deciding whether to provide/withhold MANH in individuals with advanced cancer, we ought to attentively consider the moral values and principles that are actually pursued/trespassed when acting in one way or the other. Among the main moral values and principles that may be at stake are the value of respecting life/preserving health; the disvalue of intentionally causing a patient's death by omitting care; the value of relieving avoidable suffering, the disvalue of causing unnecessary suffering; the value of improving comfort and quality of life; the value of allowing a responsible exercise of freedom; the value of respecting the symbolic meanings of nutrition and hydration as manifestations of basic human solidarity.

These values guide judgements regarding MANH in advanced cancer, and medical care for these patients should be shaped by respect for vulnerable human life and the dignity of the dying. Care for these cancer patients demands a periodic re-evaluation of the patients' condition to assess the attainability of the pre-established goals of care and to take into account changes in the patients' circumstances, including the moral values that are at stake.

In concluding, we need to reflect on our understanding of decision-making in health care and whether we foster responsible exercise of freedom in medical decision-making. Are the individual's wishes absolute, and in what circumstances do we concede to substitute decision-making? Challenging questions also remain regarding spiritual considerations about goals of life, their related goals of health care, and whether these need to be part of judgements about MANH. We also need to be aware of and appreciate the symbolic, cultural and/or religious meanings attributed to the act of providing food and water to the vulnerable.

Funding source

This work was supported by a grant received from the Vicerrectoría Adjunta de Investigación y Doctorado and the Dirección General de Pastoral y Cultura Cristiana of the Pontificia Universidad Católica de Chile (Project N° DGP07-PBC017, entitled: 'Controversia actual sobre la noción de cuidados básicos en medicina. Análisis del concepto, las aplicaciones prácticas y las implicancias éticas').

References

1. Jaskowiak N, Alexander R (1998) The pathophysiology of cancer cachexia. In: Doyle D, Hanks G, MacDonald N (eds), *Oxford Textbook of Palliative Medicine*, 2nd edn, pp. 534–48. Oxford: Oxford University Press.
2. Del Fabbro E, Bruera E (2006) Pathophysiology of cachexia/anorexia syndrome. In: Bruera E, Higginson I, Ripamonti, vonGunten C (eds), *Textbook of Palliative Medicine*, pp. 527–37. London: Hodder Arnold.
3. Bruera E, MacDonald N (2000) To hydrate or not to hydrate: how should it be? *J Clin Oncol* **18**, 1156–8.
4. Winter S (2000) Terminal nutrition: framing the debate for the withdrawal of nutritional support in terminally ill patients. *Am J Med*, **109**, 723–6.
5. Dy S (2008) Enteral and parenteral nutrition in terminally ill cancer patients: a review of the literature. *Am J Hosp Pall Med*, **23**(5), 369–377.
6. Ganzini, L (2006) Artificial nutrition and hydration at the end of life: ethics and evidence. *Palliative Supportive Care*, **4**, 135–43.

7. Senft M, Fietkau R, Iro H, Sailer D, Sauer R (1993) The influence of supportive nutritional therapy via percutaneous endoscopically guided gastrostomy on the quality of life of cancer patients. *Supportive Care Cancer*, **1**, 272–5.
8. Arends J, Bodoky F, Bozzeti F, *et al.* (2006) ESPEN guidelines on enteral nutrition: non-surgical oncology. *Clin Nutr*, **25**, 245–59.
9. American Dietetic Association Report (2002) *J Am Dietet Assoc*, **102**(5), 716–722.
10. Federation National des Centres de Lutte Contre la Cancer (2001) *Standards, Options et Recommandations 2001 pour la Nutrition Artificielle a Domicile du Malade Cancereux Adulte (Rapport Integral).* Paris: FNCLCC.
11. Bozzetti F, Amadori D, Bruera E, *et al.* (1996) Guidelines on artificial nutrition versus hydration in terminal cancer patients. *Nutrition*, **12**(3), 163–7.
12. Körner U, Bondolfi A, Bühler E, *et al.* (2006) Ethical and legal aspects of enteral nutrition. *Clin Nutr*, **25**, 196–202.
13. Goldstein MK (1994) Intensity of treatment in malnutrition. The ethical considerations. *Primary Care*, **21**(1), 191–206.
14. Beauchamp T, Childress J (2001) *Principles of Biomedical Ethics*, 5th edn, chap. 1. Oxford: Oxford University Press.
15. Tollefsen C (2008) *Artificial Nutrition and Hydration. The New Catholic Debate.* Dordrecht: Spinger.
16. Goldstein MK, Fuller JD (1994) Intensity of treatment in malnutrition. The ethical considerations. *Primary Care*, **21**(1), 191–206.
17. Taboada, P (2006) Principles of bioethics in palliative care. In: Bruera E, Higginson I, Ripamonti, vonGunten C (eds), *Textbook of Palliative Medicine*, pp. 85–91. London: Hodder Arnold.
18. Cronin D (1989) Conserving human life. In: Smith R (ed.), *Conserving Human Life*, pp. 1–145. Braintree, MA: Pope John Center.
19. Kelly G (1951) The duty to preserve life. *Theol Stud*, **12**, 550–6.
20. Wildes K (1995) Conserving life and conserving means: lead us not into temptation. In: *Philosophy and Medicine 51*. Dordrecht: Kluwer.
21. Calipari M (2004) The principle of proportionality in therapy: foundations and applications criteria. *NeuroRehabilitation*, **19**(4), 391–7.
22. Sullivan S (2007) The development and nature of the ordinary/extraordinary means distinction in the Roman Catholic tradition. *Bioethics*, **21**(7), 386–97.
23. Fisher A (2008) Why do unresponsive patients still matter? In: Tollefsen C (ed.), *Artificial Nutrition and Hydration. The New Catholic Debate*, pp. 3–37. Dordrecht: Spinger.
24. Beauchamp T, Childress J (2001) *Principles of Biomedical Ethics*, 5th edn, chap. 3. Oxford: Oxford University Press.
25. Wildes K (1996) Ordinary and extraordinary means and the quality of life. *Theol Stud*, **57**(3), 500–12.
26. Clark P (2006) Tube feedings and persistent vegetative state patients: ordinary or extraordinary means? *Christ Bioeth*, **12**(1), 43–64.
27. Welie J (2005) When medical treatment is no longer in order: toward a new interpretation of the ordinary–extraordinary distinction. *Natl Cathol Bioeth Q*, **5**(3), 517–36.
28. Torchia J (2003) Artificial hydration and nutrition for the PVS patient: ordinary care or extraordinary intervention? *Natl Cathol Bioeth Q*, **3**(4), 719–30.
29. Devun M (1982) Extraordinary means in prolonging life. *J Am Med Assoc*, **248**(17), 2180.
30. Dolan JM (1991) Death by deliberate dehydration and starvation: silent echoes of the Hunger-Häuser. *Issues Law Med*, **7**, 173–97.
31. Heaney S (1994) "You can't be any poorer than dead": difficulties in recognizing artificial nutrition and hydrations as medical treatments. *Linacre Q*, 77–87.
32. Panicota M (2001) Catholic teaching on prolonging life: setting the record straight. *Hastings Center Rep*, **31**(6), 14–25.

33. Sulmasy D (2007) Double-effect reasoning and care at the end of life: some clarifications and distinctions. In: Monsour HD, Sullivan WF, Heng J (eds), *Dignity in Illness, Disability, and Dying*, pp. 49–109. Toronto: International Association of Catholic Bioethicists.
34. Pontifical Council *Cor Unum* (1981) *Dans le Cadre*. Vatican City: Editrice Vaticana, n. 2, 4, 4.
35. Pontifical Council for Pastoral Assistance to Health Care Workers (1995) *Charter for Health Workers*. Vatican City: Editrice Vaticana, n. 120.
36. Markwell H (2005) End-of-life: a Catholic view. *Lancet*, **366**, 1132–5.
37. Craig G (1994) On withholding nutrition and hydration in the terminally ill: has palliative medicine gone too far? *J Med Eth*, **20**, 139–43.
38. Dunlop RJ, Ellershaw JE, Baines MJ, Sykes N, Saunders CM (1995) On withholding nutrition and hydration in the terminally ill: has palliative medicine gone too far? A Reply. *J Med Eth*, **21**, 141–3.
39. Craig G (1996) On withholding artificial hydrating and nutrition from terminally ill sedated patients. The debate continues. *J Med Eth*, **22**, 147–53.
40. Shannon T (2006) Nutrition and hydration: an analysis of the recent papal statement in the light of the Roman Catholic bioethical tradition. *Christ Bioeth*, **12**(1), 29–41.
41. Mullooly J (1987) Ordinary/extraordinary means and euthanasia. *Wis Med J*, **86**(3), 4–8.
42. Day L, Drought T, Davis J (1995) Principle-based ethics and nurses' attitudes towards artificial feeding. *J Adv Nurs*, **21**(2), 295–8.
43. Gómez-Lobo A (2002) *Morality and the Human Goods. An Introduction to Natural Law Ethics*. Washington, DC: Georgetown University Press.
44. Seifert J (2004) The philosophical diseases of medicine and their cure. *Philosophy and Ethics of Medicine*, Vol. 1. *Foundations*. Dordrecht: Springer.
45. Nordenfeldt L (1987) *On the Nature of Health*. Dordrecht: Reidel.
46. Nordenfeldt L (1993) Concepts of health and their consequences for health care. *Theoretical Medicine*, **14**(4).
47. Hippocratic Corpus (1977) In: Reiser SJ, Dick AJ, Curran WJ (eds), *Ethics in Medicine: Historical Perspectives and Contemporary Concerns*, pp. 6–7. Cambridge, MA: MIT Press.
48. Engelhardt T, Smith A (2005) End-of-life: the traditional Christian view. *Lancet*, **366**, 1045–9.
49. World Health Organization (1990) Cancer pain relief and palliative care. Report of a WHO expert committee. *WHO Technical Report Series*, No. 804. Geneva: WHO.
50. Humphry D (1992) *Dying with Dignity. Understanding Euthanasia*. New York: Birch Lane Press.
51. Thomasma D (1996) An analysis of arguments for and against euthanasia and assisted suicide: Part one. *Cambr Q Healthcare Eth*, **5**, 62–76.
52. Thomasma D (1998) Assessing the arguments for and against euthanasia and assisted suicide: Part two. *Cambr Q Healthcare Eth*, 7, 388–401.
53. Goic A, Florenzano R, Piñera B, Valdés S, Armas-Merino R (1997) El cuidado del enfermo terminal (Mesa redonda). *Rev Med Chile*, **125**, 1517–25.
54. Serani A, Lavados M (1993) Regulación ética de la acción médica y limitación de tratamiento. In: Lavados M, Serani A (eds), *Ética Clínica. Fundamentos y aplicaciones*, pp. 129–39. Universidad Católica de Chile, Santiago de Chile.
55. Empire Medicare Services (1998) Hospice determining terminal status in non-cancer diagnosis—pulmonary disease. Policy number: (YPF # 169) (Ymed # 26). *Medicare News Brief*, 97–8.
56. Grupo de Estudios de Ética Clínica de la Sociedad Médica de Chile (2000) El enfermo terminal. *Rev Med Chile*, **128**, 547–52.
57. Monge MA (1991) El enfermo terminal. In: *Ética, Salud, Enfermedad*, pp. 119–129. Madrid: Ediciones Palabra.
58. Lynn J, Childress J (1983) Must patients always be given food and water? *Hastings Center Rep*, **13**(5)17–21.

59. Rabeneck L, Wray N, Petersen N (1996) Long-term outcomes of patients receiving percutaneous endoscopic gastrostomy tubes. *J Gen Intern Med*, **11**, 287–93.

60. McCann R, Hall W, Groth-Juncker (1994) Comfort care for terminally ill patients. The appropriate use of nutrition and hydration. *J Am Med Assoc*, **272**, 1263–6.

61. Finucane T, Christmas C (2000) More caution about tube feeding. *JAGS* **48**(9), 1167–8.

62. Lin A, Jabbari S, Worden F, *et al.* (2005) Metabolic abnormalities associated with weight loss during chemoirradiation of head-and-neck cancer. *Int J Radiat Oncol Biol Phys*, **63**(5), 1413–18.

63. Miller F, Meier D (1998) Voluntary death: a comparison of terminal dehydration and physician-assisted suicide. *Ann Intern Med*, **128**(7), 559–62.

64. Ganzini L, Goy ER, Miller LL, Harvath TA, Jackson A, Delorit MA (2003) Nurses' experiences with hospice patients who refuse food and fluids to hasten death. *N Engl J Med*, **4**(349), 359–65.

65. Hasselaar JG, Reuzel RP, Van den Muijsenbergh ME, *et al.* (2008) Dealing with delicate issues in continuous deep sedation: varying practices among Dutch medical specialists, general practitioners, and nursing home physicians. *Arch Intern Med*, **168**, 537–43.

66. Fainsinger R, Bruera E (1997) When to treat dehydration in a terminally ill patient? *Support Care Center*, **5**(3), 205–11.

67. Morita T, Tsunoda J, Inoue S, Chihara S (1999) Perceptions and decision-making on rehydration of terminally ill cancer patients and family members. *Am J Hospice Palliative Care*, **16**(3), 509–16.

68. Bruera E, Sala R, Rico M, Moyano J, Centeno C, Willey J, Palmer JL (2005) Effects of parenteral hydration in terminally ill cancer patients: a preliminary study. *J Clin Oncol*, **23**(10), 2366–71.

69. McCann R, Hall W, Groth-Juncker A (1994) Comfort care for terminally ill patients. The appropriate use of nutrition and hydration. *J Am Med Assoc*, **272**, 1263–6.

70. Lanuke K, Fainsinger R, DeMoissac D (2004) Hydration management at the end of life. *J Palliative Med*, **7**(2), 257–63.

71. Dalal S, Bruera E (2004) Dehydration in cancer patients: to treat or not to treat. *J Supportive Oncol*, **2**(6), 467–87.

72. Valero M, Álvarez R, García P, Sánchez R, Moreno JM, Léon M (2006) ¿Se considera la hidratación y la nutrición artificial como un cuidado paliativo? *Nutr Hosp*, **21**(6), 680–5.

73. Skelly R (2002) Are we using percutaneous endoscopy gastrostomy appropriately in the elderly? *Curr Opin Clin Nutr Metab Care*, **5**, 35–42.

74. Mirhosseini N, Fainsinger R, Baracos V (2005) Parenteral nutrition in advanced cancer: indications and clinical practice guidelines. *J Palliative Med*, **8**(5), 914–18.

75. Huhmann M, August D (2008) Review of American Society for Parenteral and Enteral Nutrition (A.S.P.E.N.) clinical guidelines for nutrition support in cancer patients: nutrition screening and assessment. *Nutr Clin Pract*, **23**, 182–8.

76. Bachmann P, *Marti-Massoud C, Blanc-Vincent MP, et al.* (2003) Summary version of the standards, options and recommendations for palliative or terminal nutrition in adults with progressive cancer. *Br J Cancer*, **89**(Suppl 1), S107–10.

77. Bozzeti F (2003) Home total parenteral nutrition in incurable cancer patients: a therapy, a basic humane care or something in between? *Clin Nutr*, **22**(2), 109–11.

78. Mirhosseini N, Fainsinger R, Baracos V (2005) Parenteral nutrition in advanced cancer: indications and clinical practice guidelines. *J Palliative Med*, **8**(5), 914–18.

79. Schotsmans P (2002) Equal care as the best care: a personalist approach. In: Engelhardt HT, Cherry M (eds), *Allocating Scarce Medical Resources: Roman Catholic Perspectives*, pp. 125–39. Washington, DC: Georgetown University Press.

80. Honnefelder L (2002) Quality of life and human dignity: meaning and limits of prolongation of life. In: Engelhardt HT, Cherry M (eds), *Allocating Scarce Medical Resources: Roman Catholic Perspectives*, pp. 140–53. Washington, DC: Georgetown University Press.

81. Taboada P (1998) El principio de proporcionalidad terapéutica en las decisiones de limitar tratamientos. *Boletín Escuela de Medicina*, **27**(1), 17–23.
82. Taboada P (2002) What is appropriate intensive care? A Roman Catholic perspective. In: Engelhardt HT, Cherry M (eds), *Allocating Scarce Medical Resources: Roman Catholic Perspectives*, pp. 53–73. Washington, DC: Georgetown University Press.
83. Meilaender G (1997) Questio disputata. Ordinary and extraordinary treatments: when does quality count? *Theol Stud*, **58**(3), 527–31.
84. Schneiderman L, Jecker N, Jonsen A (1990) Medical futility: its meaning and ethical implications. *Ann Intern Med*, **112**, 949–54.
85. Schneiderman L, Faber-Langendoen K, Jecker N (1994) Beyond futility to an ethical care. *Am J Med*, 96, 110–14.
86. Schneiderman L, Jecker N, *et al.* (1996) Medical futility: response to critiques. *Ann Intern Med*, **125**, 669–74.
87. Schneiderman L (1998) Commentary. Bringing clarity to the futility debate: are the cases wrong? *Cambr Q Healthcare Eth*, **7**, 269–78.
88. Taboada P (2009) Ordinary and extraordinary means of preserving life: the teaching of the moral tradition. In: Sgreccia E, Laffitte J (eds), *Alongside the Incurably Sick and the Dying Person: Ethical and Practical Aspects*, pp. 117–42. Vatican City: Libreria Editrice Vaticana.
89. Christensen K (1992) Applying the concept of futility at the bedside. *Cambr Q Healthcare Eth*, **1**, 239–48.
90. Caplan A (1996) Odds and ends: trust and the debate over medical futility. *Ann Intern Med*, **125**, 688–9.
91. McCann RM, Hall WJ, Groth-Juncker A (1994) Comfort care for terminally ill patients. The appropriate use of nutrition and hydration. *J Am Med Assoc*, **272**, 1263–6.
92. Ellershaw JE, Sutcliffe JM, Saunders CM (1995) Dehydration and the dying patient. *J Pain Sympt Manag*, **10**, 192–7.
93. Burge FI (1993) Dehydration symptoms of palliative care cancer patients. *J Pain Sympt Manag*, **8**, 454–64.
94. Bruera E, Higginson I, Gunten CV, Ripamonti C (eds) (2006) *Textbook of Palliative Medicine*. Oxford: Oxford University Press.
95. Lawlor PG (2002) Delirium and dehydration: some fluid for thought? *Support Care Cancer*, **10**, 445–54.
96. Waller A, Hershkowitz M, Adunsky A (1994) The effect of intravenous fluid infusion on blood and urine parameters of hydration and on state of consciousness in terminal cancer patients. *Am J Hosp Palliat Care*, **11**(6), 22–7.
97. Good P, Cavenaghi J, Mather M, Ravenscroft P (2008) Medically assisted hydration for palliative care patients. *Cochrane Database Syst Rev*, **16**(2).
98. Cerchietti L, Navigante A, Sauri A, Palazzo F (2000) Hypodermoclysis for control of dehydration in terminal-stage cancer. *Int J Palliat Nurs*, **6**(8), 370–4.
99. Faisinger R (2006) Dehydration and rehydration. In: Bruera E, Higginson I, Gunten CV, Ripamonti C (eds), *Textbook of Palliative Medicine*, pp. 727–35. Oxford: Oxford University Press.
100. *Steinhauser K,* Christakis NA, Clipp EC, McNeilly M, McIntyre L, Tulsky JA (2000) Patient/physician differences on factors considered important at the end of life. *J Assoc Med Assoc*, **284**, 2476–82.
101. Engelhardt HT (1986) *The Foundations of Bioethics*. New York: Oxford University Press.
102. Engelhardt HT (2000) *The Foundations of Christian Bioethics*. Lisse: Swets & Zeitlinger.
103. Gómez-Lobo A (2002) *Morality and the Human Goods. An Introduction to Natural Law Ethics*. Washington, DC: Georgetown University Press.
104. Lawlor P, Gagnon B, Mancini IL, *et al.* (2000) Occurrence, causes, and outcomes of delirium in patients with advanced cancer. *Arch Intern Med*, **160**, 786–94.

105. Mitchell S, Lawson F (1999) Decision-making for long-term tube-feeding in cognitively impaired elderly people. *Can Med Assoc J* **160**, 1705–9.

106. Keown J (2003) Medical murder by omission? *Clin Med*, **3**, 460–63.

107. Lynn J, Childress J (1983) Must patients always be given food and water? *Hastings Center Rep*, **12**, 17–21.

108. Holden CM (1991) Anorexia in the terminally ill cancer patient: the emotional impact on the patient and the family. *Hospice J*, **7**, 73–84.

109. Oi-Ling K, Man-Wah D, Kam-Hung D (2005) Symptom distress as rated by advanced cancer patients, caregivers and physicians in the last week of life. *Palliat Med*, **19**, 228–33.

110. Strasser F, Binswanger J, Cerny T (2007) Fighting a losing battle: eating-related distress of men with advanced cancer and their female partners. A mixed-methods study. *Palliat Med*, **21**, 129–37.

111. McClement S (2005) Cancer anorexia–cachexia syndrome: psychological effect on the patient and family. *J Wound Ostomy Continence Nurs*, **32**(4), 264–8.

112. Chiu TY, Hu WY, Chuang RB, *et al.* (2004) Terminal cancer patients' wishes and influencing factors toward the provision of artificial nutrition and hydration in Taiwan. *J Pain Sympt Manag*, **27**(3), 206–14.

113. Meares CJ (1997) Primary caregiver perceptions of intake cessation in patients who are terminally ill. *Oncol Nurs Forum*, **24**, 1751–7.

114. Strasser F, Binswanger J, Cerny T (2007) Fighting a losing battle: eating-related distress of men with advanced cancer and their female partners. A mixed-methods study. *Palliat Med*, **21**, 129–37.

115. SUPPORT Principal Investigators (1995) A controlled trial to improve care for seriously ill hospitalized patients. The study to understand prognoses and preferences for outcomes and risks of treatments (SUPPORT). *J Am Med Assoc* **274**(20), 1591–8.

116. Parkash R, Burge F (1997) The family's perspective on issues of hydration in terminal care. *J Palliat Care*, **13**(4), 23–7.

117. Morita T, Tsunoda J, Satoshi N, Satoshi C (1999) Perceptions and decision-making on rehydration of terminally ill cancer patients and family members. *Am J Hosp Palliat Care*, **16**(3), 509–16.

118. Steinhauser K, Christakis N, Clipp E, McNeilly M, McIntyre L, Tulsky J (2000) Factors considered important at the end of life by patients, family, physicians, and other care providers. *J Am Med Assoc*, **284**(19), 2476–82.

119. Mercadante S, Ferrera P, Girelli D, Casuccio A (2005) Patients' and relatives' perceptions about intravenous and subcutaneous hydration. *J Pain Sympt Manag*, **30**(4) 354–8.

120. Hughes N, Neal R (2000) Adults with terminal illness: a literature review of their needs and wishes for food. *J Adv Nurs*, **32**(5), 1101–7.

121. Orreval Y, Tishelman C, Herrington M, Permert J (2004) The path from oral nutrition to home parenteral nutrition: a qualitative interview study of the experiences of advanced cancer patients and their families. *Clin Nutr*, **23**, 1280–7.

122. Buiting H, Van Delden J, Rietjens J, *et al.* (2007) Forgoing artificial nutrition or hydration in patients nearing death in six European countries. *J Pain Sympt Manag*, **34**(3), 305–14.

123. Morita T, Shima Y, Adachi I (2002) Attitudes of Japanese physicians toward terminal dehydration. *J Clin Oncol*, **20**(24), 4699–704.

124. Miyashita M, Morita T, Shima Y, Kimura R, Takahashi M, Adachi I (2007) Physician and nurse attitudes toward artificial hydration for terminally ill cancer patients in Japan: results of 2 nationwide surveys. *Am J Hosp Palliat Care*, **24**(5), 383–9.

125. Musgrave C, Bartal N, Opstad J (1996) Intravenous hydration for terminal patients: what are the attitudes of Israeli terminal patients, their families and their health professionals? *J Pain Sympt Manag*, **12**(1), 47–51.

126. Li-Shan K, Tai-Yuan C, Su-Shun L, Wen-Yu H (2008) Knowledge, attitudes, and behavioral intentions of nurses toward providing artificial nutrition and hydration for terminal cancer patients in Taiwan. *Cancer Nurs*, **31**(1), 67–76.

127. Sprung C, Maia P, Bullow H, Ricou B, Armaganidis A (2007) The importance of religious affiliation and cultural on end of life decisions in European intensive care units. *Intens Care Med*, **33**, 1732–9.

128. Holden CM (1991) Anorexia in the terminally ill cancer patient: the emotional impact on the patient and the family. *Hospice J*, **7**, 73–84.

129. Oi-Ling K, Man-Wah D, Kam-Hung D (2005) Symptom distress as rated by advanced cancer patients, caregivers and physicians in the last week of life. *Palliat Med*, **19**, 228–33.

130. McClement S, Degner F, Harlos M (2003) Family beliefs regarding the nutritional care of a terminally ill relative: a qualitative study. *J Palliat Med*, **6**(5), 737–48.

131. McClement S, Woodgate RL (1997) Care of the terminally ill cachectic cancer patient: interface between nursing and psychological anthropology. *Eur J Cancer Care*, **6**, 295–303.

132. Poole K, Frogatt K (2002) Loss of weight and loss of appetite in advanced cancer: a problem for the patient, the carer, or the health professional? *Palliat Med*, **16**, 499–506.

133. McClement S (2005) Cancer anorexia–cachexia syndrome: psychological effect on the patient and family. *J Wound Ostomy Continence Nurs*, **32**(4), 264–8.

134. McClement S, Degner L (2004) Family responses to declining intake and weight loss in a terminally ill relative. Part 1: Fighting back. *J Palliat Care*, **20**(2), 93–100.

135. Pieper J (1997) Tod und Unsterblichkeit. In: Pieper J. *Schriften zür philosophischen Anthropologie und Ethik: Grundstrukturen menschlicher Existenz*, pp. 280–397. Hamburg: Meiner Verlag.

136. Miyashita M, Morita T, Shima Y, Kimura R, Takahashi M, Adachi I (2008) Nurse views of the adequacy of decision making and nurse distress regarding artificial hydration for terminally ill cancer patients: a nationwide survey. *Am J Hosp Palliat Care*, **24**(6), 463–9.

137. Van der Riet P, Good P, Higgins I, Sneesby L (2008) Palliative care professionals' perceptions of nutrition and hydration at the end of life. *Int J Palliat Nurs*, **14**(3), 145–51.

138. Sprung C, Maia P, Bullow H, Ricou B, Armaganidis A (2007) The importance of religious affiliation and cultural on end of life decisions in European intensive care units. *Intens Care Med*, **33**, 1732–9.

139. Council on Ethical and Judicial Affairs (1992) Decisions near the end of life. *J Am Med Assoc*, **267**, 2230–31.

140. Callahan D (1983) On feeding the dying. *Hastings Center Rep*, **13**, 22–7.

Chapter 24

Cultural and religious factors

Sarah Toule

Introduction

Dietary habits are largely defined by religious, social and economic factors and societies around the world have developed traditional eating patterns over centuries.

The extent to which traditional eating habits are retained varies greatly and it is generally during illness that such trends and traditional beliefs about diet and health gain importance.[1,2] Many patients feel a need to take responsibility for their health and manage their dietary intake because they want to improve their chances of recovery.

Patients facing the challenge of cancer often become nutritionally compromised and require nutritional intervention,[3] yet differences in cultural beliefs around health and treatments can impact on adherence to conventional treatment and medicines. With cancer, this is further exacerbated by the fact that the disease itself is a taboo subject in many cultures, with some patients further questioning the 'reasons' for developing the disease and how it should be treated. Often, patients will choose to complement conventional treatments with more traditional remedies or practices and it is therefore important that health professionals are aware of the self-prescribing behaviours of patients as well as their attitudes towards conventional methods.[4] Not only is this essential for improving adherence to treatment and avoiding undesirable pharmacological interactions that might reduce treatment efficacy, but it is also fundamental in responding to the needs of patients and ensuring that they receive culturally appropriate care and information.

There is currently little evidence-based literature that can inform clinical practice despite the recognition that there is a gap in the provision of culturally appropriate care.[5–8] This chapter will draw upon information gathered through the Diet and Cancer Information Project,[9] which aims to address the gap in provision of culturally appropriate dietary information for black and minority ethnic communities. The user-driven project requires consultation with the target communities as well as with health professionals with experience of working with these groups to ensure that the information resources produced are culturally appropriate and sensitive. The chapter will look at the issues that health professionals need to be aware of when providing dietetic advice for cancer patients from different cultural and religious backgrounds. It will also outline the most common religions that impose restrictions upon diet.

Traditional beliefs and cultural patterns

Knowledge and beliefs about health and disease vary across different ethnic groups and may be rooted in cultural traditions or shaped by religion. It is important to realize that what defines beliefs and food patterns is complex and multifactorial, resulting, for example, in various ethnic groups of the same religion practising different dietary patterns. For example, despite the proscription of fasting within Sikhism, many Sikhs in India will still practise this as a cultural tradition.

A health professional should be flexible in responding to patients' differing needs and traditions; demonstrating understanding of how these influence behaviour. Traditions will influence everyday habits such as cooking methods, meal times and choice of ingredients, as well as more overarching beliefs that will shape attitudes towards health, illness and treatments.

For example, traditional understandings of health underpin Chinese herbal medicine and Ayurveda. Both traditional practices are holistic healing systems which aim to maintain balanced energies within the body and mind. Diet is considered an important factor in maintaining this balance and foods are categorized according to the effects they have upon the body such as being warming (e.g. red meat) or cooling (e.g. vegetables). This belief may lower adherence to conventional dietary advice if it conflicts with what patients believe to be their elemental requirements. For example, increasing protein and fat may be advised for the involuntary weight loss that can accompany cancer cachexia but this may contrast with the plain foods that may traditionally be prescribed during illness.

Medicines are made from herbs, minerals, metals and animal-derived ingredients and there is little evidence to ensure that it is safe to take such medicines alongside conventional treatments. Additionally, the effectiveness of conventional treatment may be compromised when received simultaneously and it is particularly important to advise patients to avoid taking such medicines while receiving chemotherapy treatment.

Such deep-rooted beliefs all have an impact on a patient's willingness to adhere to conventional treatments.[10] Furthermore, lack of awareness of available services, frustration caused by language barriers and difficulties in understanding the principles of western medicine may also increase the tendency to turn to more traditional and familiar remedies.[7,11]

It is therefore important that health professionals take time to understand the cultural backgrounds of their patients, rather than make broad assumptions based on culture or religion. Patients must be approached in a sensitive manner which encourages honesty rather than the tendency to conceal traditional practices which they feel may be looked down upon by western medical professionals.

Culturally appropriate communication

Communication between health professionals and patients from different backgrounds poses a whole host of difficulties and challenges. Inappropriate communication is often highlighted as the main source of dissatisfaction in a patient's experience.[5,7,8] The problem is exacerbated by the general tradition within many ethnic minority groups not to question the professional and not to seek further information. Health professionals must encourage patients to voice any concerns and uncertainties and must not assume that all patients understand their entitlement to being involved with making certain decisions about their treatment and care.

Where language is an issue, interpreters and advocacy workers can serve as a valuable means of communication but must be chosen with care and sensitivity. Issues such as the interpreter's gender, knowledge of the medical subject as well as the choice of location for meetings are examples of issues that need consideration.

However, effective communication extends beyond the provision of information in appropriate languages. With written information, for example, many elderly people may speak, but not read, their native language. Alternatively, younger members of the family who may help to read information may speak the native language but only read English. For this reason, information provided in a bilingual or audio format is often more useful. Information providers must also pay attention to the cultural appropriateness of information materials in terms of the use of images, the level of language used and the amount of detail.

Religion and diet

Whereas cultural trends may influence behaviour and food preferences, stricter restrictions may be prescribed through religion. Adhering to such restrictions can be problematic when patients are offered food or nutritional supplements containing forbidden ingredients or when they are required to eat during a religious fasting period. For example, this can become particularly challenging when supporting patients with cachexia, when frequent snacking is recommended. Below, the main food restrictions instructed by some of the most common religions are outlined as well as important fasting periods, where relevant. Again, due to individual variations, it is useful to establish the level of a patient's adherence to religious laws.

Buddhism

Despite the common belief that Buddhism prescribes vegetarianism, there are in fact no laws regarding diet in Buddhism. Variations in diet tend to originate largely from cultural beliefs. However, the Buddhist precept 'do not harm' may have influenced the tendency amongst Buddhists to choose vegetarianism leading to the aforementioned misconception.

Buddhists will avoid alcohol and other stimulants to allow the mind to remain clear and alert.

Christianity

There are few restrictive dietary laws within the many branches of Christianity and these are adhered to in varying degrees.

Days of fasting

- Christians may fast during Lent, Holy Week, Good Friday, Fridays.

Orthodox Christianity specifies the avoidance of meat, dairy products, eggs and alcohol during some fasting seasons.

Hinduism

Hinduism teaches the importance of all creatures; humans and animals alike. In avoiding the harming of animals, vegetarianism is therefore encouraged, and common, but not obligatory.

Forbidden foods

- Pork and beef (due to the sacred status assigned to the cow).

Days of fasting

- Diwali, New Year, new moons, birthdays of Holy figures.

Fasting may be complete or involve a change of diet to more basic foods, adoption of a strict vegetarian diet or abstaining from favourite foods.

Judaism

Orthodox Jews follow the dietary laws and customs of Kasrut whereby permitted foods are termed *kosher* and forbidden foods *terefeh*.

Permitted foods

- Meat from animals with cloven hooves and that chew the cud. All meat must be slaughtered according to the Kasrut method of *shechitah* and bought from a kosher butcher (fats and sinews are forbidden and meat is salted to remove all traces of blood).

- Fish with fins and removable scales.
- Certain poultry: duck, chicken, goose and turkey.
- Kosher meals are available from certified providers.

Forbidden foods

- Pork and pork-derived products.
- All carnivorous animals and birds (other than poultry).
- Shellfish.
- Meat and dairy produce cannot be consumed within the same meal and must be kept separate in food preparation. This includes all utensils and working tops. After a meal containing meat, a period of 3 h must pass before dairy foods can be consumed.
- Grapes are viewed as a fruit of idolatry and therefore wine or other grape-derived products must be produced under supervision.

Days of fasting

- Yom Kippur and Tisha b'Av: eating and drinking are forbidden for a 25 h period, from sunset to sunset.
- Passover: during these 8 days in April, foods containing wheat, oats, barley or rye are forbidden. Unleavened bread is eaten instead or normal bread.
- Other religious days require partial fasting when no food or water is allowed from sunrise to sunset.

Islam

Food that can be consumed by Muslims and adheres to the Islamic dietary laws is referred to as *halal*. Proscribed foods are termed *haram*.

Permitted foods

- Halal meat must be slaughtered according to the traditional Islamic method.
- Fish with scales (the definitions for permitted seafood vary, with some forbidding shellfish).

Forbidden foods

- All meat from animals not slaughtered according to the Islamic method.
- Blood.
- Pork and pork-derived products.
- Carnivorous and omnivorous animals and birds of prey.
- Alcohol and other intoxicants.
- Insects apart from the locust.

Days of fasting

- Ramadan: Mandatory fasting period requiring abstinence from food and drink between the break of dawn and sunset.
- Shawwal: Muslims are encouraged to fast for 6 days.
- Other religious events require day-long fastings and many Muslims also choose to fast on Mondays and Thursdays.

Sikhism

Despite originating from a combination of Hinduism and Islam, Sikhism imposes fewer dietary restrictions.

Forbidden foods

- Halal and kosher meats (due to slaughtering methods being viewed as inhumane). Pork and beef (due to the sacred status assigned to the cow).
- Sikhs are expected to refrain from alcohol and drugs as these substances are believed to reduce physical and mental fitness.

Days of fasting

Fasting and other rituals are forbidden in Sikhism although in India fasting may still be practised as a cultural tradition.

Implications of religion and diet during illness

Additional to the challenge of patients needing to fast when treatment requires otherwise, many medications, nutritional supplements or nasogastric feeds may contain ingredients forbidden under certain religions. Feelings of obligation to adhere to such religious regulations may become even stronger during illness and can significantly impair a patient's adherence to treatment and thus chances of recovery. However, most religions and faiths consider the preservation of life as of utmost importance and it is generally acceptable during illness to break fasting periods and consume medication containing forbidden ingredients if not doing so may delay recovery or lead to further deterioration in health.

For example, in Judaism, whether a non-kosher product/ingredient may be taken depends largely on the degree of illness. When conditions are life-threatening or may become so if untreated, non-kosher medication is acceptable if no kosher alternative is available. With other levels of less-threatening illness, medication may be taken in an uncommon way of eating (e.g. swallowed without chewing) and without desirable flavours. Non-kosher products taken in a normal manner are normally forbidden in non-threatening conditions.

In Islam, breaking the fast is allowed if fasting may delay recovery or make illness worse and it is to be resumed when the patient has recovered. However, many may prefer to fast during the specified time due to the difficulties in fasting alone during a non-fasting period.

It is important that health professionals understand desires to adhere, but also to know and be able to communicate the conditions under which patients are exempt. Remember that some patients themselves may be unaware of these conditions and informing them may be the key to improved adherence to recommended treatments.

Local community and religious organizations can help with providing further information on religious laws and available certified alternatives. The useful contacts provided at the end of the chapter are sources of more detailed information.

Medication

Ingredients such as gelatine, stearates and certain vitamins may all be used in the manufacturing and preservation of tablets, capsules or syrups. If animal-derived, these will often conflict with numerous religious laws. Plant-derived ingredients will be acceptable but as the source is often unclear it is safer to choose kosher/halal-certified medicines where possible. Such alternatives are also recommended as alternatives to pleasant-tasting syrups which are forbidden in Judaism.

Nutritional supplements and nasogastric feeds

Beware of ingredients such as lactose and whey for those avoiding dairy produce and ensure that these are not taken within 3 h of consuming meat when treating Jewish patients.

Other ingredients such as rennet and vitamins A and D may be problematic if animal-derived. Plant-derived alternatives or kosher/halal certified options are available.

Conclusion

The provision of culturally appropriate care, in any setting, requires flexibility and being open to the multidimensional characteristics of patients with different backgrounds. The issues outlined above serve as a general indication of some of the issues that health professionals need to be aware of in the nutritional care of cancer patients, but it is important to avoid making assumptions based solely race or religion. It is only through individual assessment and tailored services that patients will receive the treatment, care and information appropriate to their needs.

United Kingdom useful contacts

Faith and Food

Information about dietary practices and beliefs of various religions.
Website: www.faithandfood.com

Multi-Cultural Nutrition Group, and The Oncology Group

The British Dietetic Association, 5th Floor Charles House, 148–149 Great Charles House, Queensway, Birmingham B3 3HT, UK
Website: www.bda.uk.com

London Beth Din (for kosher food enquiries)

735 High Road, London N12 0US, UK
Tel.: (0044) 208 343 6259
Website: www.kosher.org.uk

Muslim Food Board (UK)

PO Box 1786, Leicester LE5 5ZE, UK
Tel.: (0044) 116 273 8228
Website: www.halaal.org

Unites States of America useful contacts

American Dietetic Association

Headquarters American Dietetic Association
120 South Riverside Plaza, Suite 2000
Chicago, Illinois 60606-6995, USA
Tel.: (001) 800 8771600
Website: www.eatright.org

Oncology Nutrition Dietetic Practice Group

120 S. Riverside Plaza, Suite 2000
Chicago, IL 60606-6995, USA
Website: www.oncologynutrition.org/

Islamic Food and Nutrition Council of America

IFANCA Head Office
777 Busse Highway
Park Ridge, IL 60068, USA
Tel.: (001) 847 993 0034
Website: www.ifanca.org

Beth Din of America
305 Seventh Avenue
Twelfth Floor
New York, NY 10001-6008, USA
Tel.: (001) 212 8079042
Website: http://www.bethdin.org

References

1. Sheikh N, Thomas J (1994) Factors influencing food choice among ethnic minority adolescents. Part 2. *Curr Nutr Food Sci*, **5**, 29–35.
2. Henley A (1979) *Asian Patients in Hospital and at Home.* King Edward's Hospital Fund for London. Tunbridge Wells: Pitman Medical Publishing.
3. Ottery FD (1994) Cancer cachexia: prevention, early diagnosis, and management. *Cancer Pract*, **2**(2), 123–31.
4. Smaje C (1995) *Health, 'Race' and Ethnicity. Making Sense of the Evidence.* London: King's Fund Institute.
5. Deepak N (2004) *Beyond the Barriers: Providing Cancer Information and Support for Black & Minority Ethnic Communities.* London: CancerBACKUP.
6. Hartley BA, Hamid F (2002) Investigation into the suitability and accessibility of catering practices to inpatients from minority ethnic groups in Brent. *J Hum Nutr Diet*, **15**(3), 203–9.
7. Madhok R, Bhopal RS, Ramaiah RS (1992) Quality of hospital service: a study comparing 'Asian' and 'non-Asian' patients in Middlesbrough. *J Public Health Med*, **14**(3), 271–9.
8. Murphy K, Macleod Clark J (1993) Nurses' experiences of caring for ethnic-minority clients. *J Adv Nurs*, **18**(3), 442–50.
9. Cancer Equality. *Diet and Cancer BME Information Project 2005–2008.* Available at: http://www.cancerequality.org.uk/ (accessed 18 October 2008).
10. Thomas J (2002) Nutrition intervention in ethnic minority groups. *Proc Nutr Soc*, **61**, 559–67.
11. Kraus (1989) Sinking heart: a Punjabi communication of distress. *Soc Sci Med*, **29**(4), 536–75.

Part 8

Complementary and alternative medicine

Chapter 25

Nutrition and complementary and alternative medicine

Eran Ben-Arye, Dena Norton, Moshe Frenkel

Introduction

Alongside the outstanding development of scientifically and technologically oriented medicine, the second half of the twentieth century witnessed an increase in the public's interest in and use of complementary and alternative medicine (CAM). This trend of viewing alternative systems of medicine as complementary to conventional, scientifically based medicine was acknowledged in the 1950s–1970s by the establishment of homeopathic hospitals in the UK,[1] the regulation of herbal remedies in Germany,[2] and the use of traditional medicine in China[3] and India.[4] However, this concept was not officially accepted in the USA until October 1991 when the US Congress established the Office of Alternative Medicine within the National Institutes of Health to investigate and evaluate promising unconventional medical practices.[5,6] In October 1998, the US Congress upgraded this office to the National Center of Complementary and Alternative Medicine and charged it with exploring CAM healing practices in the context of rigorous science, training CAM researchers, and disseminating authoritative information to the public and medical professionals.[6] That same year, the Office of Cancer Complementary and Alternative Medicine was created to coordinate and enhance the CAM research activities of the National Cancer Institute.[7] The formation of these two centers made the USA a world leader in the promotion and financing of CAM education and research, particularly in the area of oncology.

By the early twenty-first century, the increasingly common use of complementary medicine in conjuction with conventional medicine led to the concept of 'integrative medicine': the integration of CAM and patient-centred care in conventional medical care.[8] For cancer patients, integrative medicine, or integrative oncology, indicates that conventional care is moving from a strict biomedical orientation to a bio-psycho-social-spiritual one, as manifested by concepts of palliative care, quality of life, spirituality, and narrative-based medicine.[9] Efficient doctor–CAM practitioner communication is one of the core issues in integrative oncology and is the basis for multidisciplinary collaboration between oncologists, CAM providers, nurses, social workers, family practitioners, and other health care providers.[10] The concept of integrative oncology is clinically practised and studied in the USA at academic oncology institutions such as The University of Texas M. D. Anderson Cancer Center and Memorial Sloan-Kettering Cancer Center.[11] Researchers at those sites and around the world are examining whether, why, and how patients with cancer use CAM, its implications on doctor–patient communication, and its impact on the efficacy and safety of conventional therapies. The main findings of these studies are as follows.

Prevalence of CAM use during cancer care

Forty to 80% of cancer patients use CAM, depending on gender, history of previous therapy, socio-economic status, cancer type, and the definition of CAM used in specific studies.[12–14] A high prevalence of CAM use is also evident during chemotherapy (e.g. 49% in Israel)[15] and radiation treatment.[16] In Canada, CAM use increased among patients with breast cancer from 66% in 1998 to 82% in 2005.[17] According to responses to the 2002 National Health Interview Survey, 40% of cancer survivors continue to use CAM.[18]

Cancer patients' motives for using CAM

In general, patients with cancer view CAM as complementary rather than alternative treatment and do not refrain from receiving conventional care. Typical reasons for CAM use by patients diagnosed with cancer are: conventional medicine does not meet all their needs; they feel helpless and desire to gain control and find hope; they do not completely trust their doctor; their diagnosis of cancer changed their outlook on life or their beliefs; and they have a strong belief in CAM.[19,20]

Doctor–patient communication concerning CAM use

Earlier studies found low rates of CAM disclosure in consultations with oncologists and other health care professionals,[21] but recent studies suggest that more than 50% of patients discuss their CAM use with physicians.[22] Richardson *et al.*[23] found discrepancies in the perspectives of physicians and patients identified as CAM users at M. D. Anderson Cancer Center. Physicians believed that patients thought that CAM discussions were unimportant and that as physicians they would not understand a patient's interest in CAM, would discontinue conventional treatment, or would discourage or disapprove of a patient's CAM use. Patients didn't discuss their use of CAM with their physicians because they were uncertain about its benefit and because their physician never asked.

Perspectives of patient and health care provider towards integrative cancer care

In the UK, Lewith *et al.*[24] evaluated attitudes toward CAM among patients and all health care staff at the Southampton Cancer Care Directorate and found that 99% of staff and patients wanted to see CAM treatments introduced into the service. Brazier *et al.*[25] qualitatively evaluated the impact of participating in an integrative cancer care programme in Vancouver, Canada, and found that participating patients gained a sense of empowerment, the means to create personal change, emotional support, and a sense of hope. Risberg *et al.*[26] conducted a large study in the five Norwegian university hospitals responsible for cancer treatment, and found that health care providers, including oncologists, expressed a positive attitude towards integrating CAM into oncological care.

CAM and nutrition in cancer care

Various CAM modalities view nutrition as an important element in the aetiology, diagnosis, treatment, and prognosis of cancer. CAM modalities relating to nutrition can be categorized into two main disciplines: traditional and systematic modalities that view food as an integral part of a broader philosophic, diagnostic, and therapeutic practice (Table 25.1) and other CAM modalities that specifically focus on nutrition, often in relation to cancer care (Table 25.2).

Table 25.1 Tips for nutritional counselling with cancer patients based on three CAM medical system perspectives

Symptom or question	Traditional Chinese medicine	Ayurvedic medicine	Anthroposophical medicine
Did I have cancer because of certain foods or eating behaviour?	Food is considered one of the 'other' causes of cancer development in addition to predisposing constitution, 'internal' emotional factors and numerous other pathogenic causes—do not blame yourself!	There are many reasons for cancer development and one should not blame oneself. Nevertheless, foods may promote health by matching the person's *dosha* status with specific food qualities that can increase or decrease specific dosha.	Foods may promote cancer growth by overburdening the body (eating too much, especially proteins, fats, refined carbohydrates); agriculture and food-preparing methods lower food vitality (fertilizers, food irradiation, food additives, deep-freezing)
What should I eat during chemotherapy?	Light frequent meals that include a variety of tastes and food ingredients, mixing cooked and fresh food. Consume cooked orange-coloured vegetables, whole and white rice, whole-wheat bread, legumes, fish and chicken, green leafy vegetables and spices with light pungent and bitter tastes, fresh ginger.	Beneficial nutrition depends on the cancer type, and the patient's specific dosha status. In the case of *kapha*-dominant cancer, recommendations are cooked vegetables and fruits with bitter, pungent and astringent tastes, decrease food quantity and sparse use of protein and fat in the diet.	Eat raw sprouted grains, high quality bread (wholewheat flour mixed with rye, barley and oats), culinary herbs (e.g. marjoram, basil, fennel) and spices, soured milk products, honey, vegetable roots and tubers (e.g. carrots, beetroots), leaves and stems (e.g. cabbage, fennel, lettuce), and vegetable flowers (e.g. broccoli, artichoke) and fruits (e.g. pumpkin). Advised to eat small meals at short intervals.
What food do I need to avoid during chemotherapy?	Avoid or decrease consumption of heavy full-size meals, red meat, carbohydrates with high glycaemic index, sweetening of hot and cold drinks.	In the case of *kapha*-dominant cancer, patients should avoid or decrease foods with sweet, sour and salty tastes.	Advised to avoid tomatoes and mushrooms, and reduce the amount of potatoes and meat.
Can food strengthen my body, soul or immunity to cope better with oncology treatment?	Indeed! Food and the way you relate to it can strengthen depleted vitality and *Qi*, thereby facilitating a balanced mind–body, and synergistic inter-relation of the vital organs	Food can strengthen the body vitality by decreasing waste products (*ama*) through reducing the volume and number of meals, using low fat and protein in the diet, drinking of boiled water and use of hot spices.	Food can nourish and vitalize the body, mind and soul and help the patient to cope better with chemotherapy and radiation treatment. Supplemented with herbal treatment (e.g. mistletoe) and artistic therapies, food can augment the higher bodies to take control of cancer.
How can I gain weight?	The above dietary recommendations will support your Spleen and Stomach Qi, decrease vomiting and diarrhoea and decrease weight loss	Reducing ama and supporting the dosha equilibrium will help achieve stable weight	Gaining weight may be assisted by eating bio-dynamic vegetarian food in a mindful and conscious context.

(Continued)

Table 25.1 (continued) Tips for nutritional counselling with cancer patients based on three CAM medical system perspectives

Symptom or question	Traditional Chinese medicine	Ayurvedic medicine	Anthroposophical medicine
Can I use dietary treatment to prevent cancer recurrence?	A balanced diet can help prevent cancer recurrence. Limit uncooked, raw and Cold food, excess of animal proteins, milk products and carbohydrates. Increase consumption of green fresh leafy vegetables with gentle pungent and bitter tastes. Avoid eating quickly and try to regard meals in a more 'nutritive' context supporting your mind and spirit.	Cancer secondary prevention can be supported by tuning the diet to the patient-specific dosha harmony and adapting a spiritual dimension to food and eating by practising meditation and yoga.	Consume organically grown food (preferably by bio-dynamic method). Avoid refined sugars. Adopt lifestyle attitude change and spiritual perspective to the meaning of food in your life. Avoid being overwhelmed by other impressions during meals (e.g. doing something else while eating, like watching TV). Eat mindfully, chew food thoroughly, to mix it well with saliva and taste it consciously.

The context of nutrition in various CAM modalities often differs from conventional ideas about nutrition. Traditional systems of medicine, such as Chinese and ayurvedic, view foods in correspondence with body organs and functions. In these systems, foods representing the macrocosm of nature may directly suppress or support the microcosm of the body. Mind–body and spiritual-oriented modalities, such as yoga, Tibetan medicine, and other schools of Buddhism, emphasize mindful eating. Monotheistic religions regard the spiritual meaning of food and eating, as reflected in prayer and blessing before and after eating. In all these modalities, fasting and avoiding or mixing certain foods can be regarded as part of a spiritual journey. Such a journey may be of particular interest to someone recently diagnosed with cancer, who faces the threat of death or disability and questions the meaning of life. The Judeo-Christian tradition recognizes whole foods as having been created by God who is responsible for physical and spiritual healing.

Discussing the spiritual and contextual dimensions regarding food and eating may be meaningful in the support and treatment of the near dying and patients with life-threatening symptoms or advanced disease. Likewise, communicating with patients and their caregivers about their concerns of weight loss and cachexia may lead discussion from caloric parameters to contextual aspects such as the meaningfulness of nutrition in life and disease.

Various foods and spices are important remedies used in herbal, homeopathic, and anthroposophical medicines to prevent and treat cancer symptoms and side-effects from chemotherapy and irradiation. For example, ginger is used in Asian cooking and to treat nausea;[34] turmeric (*Curcuma longa*) is used in curries and embolized curcuma aromatic oil is used to treat primary liver cancer;[35] and green tea, often drunk for refreshment, contains catechins that act as a chemopreventive agent against prostate cancer.[36]

CAM modalities such as naturopathy, the Ann Wigmore school (which extols the virtues of eating raw food and drinking wheat grass juice), and macrobiotics view nutrition as an integral part of a health-promoting philosophy and a way of living. Followers of these modalities typically view food as a whole that is more than the sum of its individual ingredients. Like herbs, foods are regarded as unique amalgams of elements that may benefit man not only by their nutritional content or active medicinal ingredients, but also by their synergistic interactions.

Table 25.2 Additional dietary practices that patients tend to explore

CAM modality	Conceptual agenda	Efficacy and safety issues
Raw food and Ann Wigmore approach	Wheatgrass refers to the sprouts/grass of the wheat plant, *Triticum aestivum*, that is freshly juiced. Proponents of wheatgrass juice (WGJ) claim that it may prevent cancer and improve quality of life during chemotherapy treatment. Drinking WGJ was promoted by Ann Wigmore, a holistic health practitioner, who founded the Hippocrates Health Institute in the USA. Wigmore's approach focuses on WGJ (daily drinking complemented occasionally with enemas), living organic whole and raw foods aimed at healing the body, mind, and spirit.[27]	In a prospective matched control study, 60 patients with breast carcinoma on FAC chemotherapy were assigned to WGJ 60 cc/day or control arm. The authors concluded that WGJ may reduce myelotoxicity, dose reductions, and need for GCSF support.[28] It should be noted that this was a pilot study with intention-to-treat analysis and a 20% attrition rate.
Macrobiotic diet	The macrobiotic diet is part of a way of life and is rooted in the Far East philosophy and Yin–Yang principles. Foods are recommended to be organically grown and minimally processed. The diet consists of 40–60% cereal grains, 20–30% vegetables (moistly cooked), 5–10% beans, consumption of sea vegetables, and occasional foods to be consumed on a weekly or monthly basis (e.g. fruit, fish, meat, seeds, nuts, dairy, sweets and eggs).[29]	Data concerning macrobiotic diet efficacy in cancer care are limited to retrospective studies and case studies.[30] Safety: it is advisable to monitor potential deficiencies in protein, vitamins D and B_{12}, iron, zinc and calcium.[31]
Gerson approach to cancer care	The therapy consists of high potassium, low sodium diet, with no fats or oils, and minimal animal protein. Juices of raw fruits and vegetables and raw liver are used in addition to iodine and niacin supplementation and caffeine enemas.[32]	In this diet, complete omission of dietary fat may result in fatty acid deficiencies and other deleterious impacts on health. Long term and frequent use of coffee enemas may cause serious fluid and electrolyte problems in addition to colitis. Serious infections and deaths from electrolyte imbalances have been reported. Also, thyroid supplementation has been associated with bleeding in patients with liver metastases.[33] In addition one needs to be aware that extreme caution is urged regarding supplementation with raw organ products.

Food as medicine

Epidemiological data demonstrate that a diet rich in a variety of plant foods and low in saturated fat, red meat, processed foods, and alcohol reduces the risk of cancer.[37,38] For example, increased consumption of Brassica vegetables (e.g. broccoli, cauliflower, cabbage, and kale) is linked to a decreased risk for cancers of the lung, oesophagus, stomach, colon, prostate, and breast, among other sites.[30,31] The methods by which the Brassica family of vegetables aid chemoprevention is complex, but it has been shown that sulphoraphane, indole-3-carbinol, and several other select compounds from this species beneficially interact with various human enzyme systems involved in cancer development.[39] This is particularly valuable information for individuals with a positive family history for these cancers who aim to reduce their personal cancer risk as much as possible. In fact, the field of nutrigenomics is rapidly expanding with the hope of providing 'nutrition prescriptions' based on one's genotype and resultant health risks.

Studying the individual and synergistic effects of phytochemicals in foods used as medicine is not only vital for chemoprevention but is also a powerful tool for those already diagnosed with cancer. One of many examples of phytochemicals known to affect existing cancer cell lines is resveratrol, the polyphenol found in red grapes, red wine, peanuts, blueberries, and various other plant foods. In the last two decades, research has shown that resveratrol reduces progression and increases apoptosis in numerous cancer cell lines (e.g. multiple myeloma, leukaemia, breast, prostate, stomach, colon, pancreas, and thyroid).[40] Studies in leukaemia and pancreatic cancer cell lines reveal that the beneficial effects of resveratrol are enhanced in the presence of the phytochemicals ellagic acid and quercetin.[41] Studies such as these indicate that consumption of whole foods rather than dietary supplements are the preferred source for optimal nutrient absorption and utilization. For example, consuming red grapes would provide the three beneficial phytochemicals already mentioned (resveratrol, ellagic acid, and quercetin) among a number of others, as well as fibre, potassium, and vitamin C.[42]

Several studies examined the possible medicinal benefits of foods in patients with breast cancer. In Canada, Seely *et al.*[43] summarized the epidemiological data concerning the consumption of five or more cups of green tea (*Camellia sinensis*) a day by Canadian patients with various stages of breast cancer and found a trend towards the prevention of breast cancer and a possible role in the prevention of recurrence in patients in remission from early-stage breast cancer. Cui *et al.*[44] studied a cohort of 1455 breast cancer patients in Shanghai, China, and found that regular ginseng users had a significantly reduced risk of death and better quality-of-life scores than did patients who never used ginseng. Trock *et al.*[45] performed a meta-analysis of 18 epidemiological studies examining the effect of soy intake on breast cancer risk. They concluded that the effect was small and advised readers to interpret their results with caution.

Additional studies have evaluated the efficacy of spices. Curcumin, a yellow colouring agent contained in turmeric, exhibits strong anti-inflammatory and antioxidant activities and modulates the expression of transcription factors, cell cycle proteins, and signal-transducing kinases.[46] In a clinical trial at M. D. Anderson Cancer Center, Dhillon *et al.*[47] examined the tolerance, absorption, and biological activity of curcumin in patients with pancreatic cancer. Interestingly, curcumin has poor bioavailability owing to its rapid metabolism in the liver and intestinal wall, but the addition of piperine, a major constituent of black pepper, which is commonly added to Indian curry spices, enhances the bioavailability of curcumin.[48] This traditional kitchen wisdom was also evident in a preliminary study suggesting that piperine also had a beneficial effect on 5-fluorouracil-induced leukopenia.[49] In a phase III placebo-controlled clinical trial of capsaicin cream, derived from hot chili peppers, Ellison *et al.*[50] found that the cream decreased postsurgical neuropathic pain in patients with cancer. In a recent study, Levine *et al.*[51] found that ginger reduced the delayed nausea of chemotherapy and the need for anti-emetic medications.

Individuals diagnosed with cancer are, more than ever, searching for practical and scientifically valid methods of assisting in the fight against their disease. Using current literature about a particular diagnosis to provide patients with a list of foods and nutrients for daily consumption is both prudent and safe. Furthermore, beyond the potential benefits with regard to cancer itself, tangible, active steps like these are welcomed by patients who often feel uninvolved in their cancer therapy. Therefore, the physical and psychological benefits of disease-specific diets outweigh any perceived risks.

Nutritional supplements

Another important approach to CAM and nutrition in cancer care is the use of nutritional supplements such as vitamins, minerals, and other dietary ingredients. Based on nationwide responses received for the National Cancer Institute's National Health Interview Survey, Millen *et al.*[52] found that the percentage of US adults taking a vitamin-and-mineral supplement daily increased from 23% in 1987 to 34% in 2000. The use of such supplements is usually not regarded in the context of a systematic or philosophic CAM background but is directed to specific clinical indications or to the overall well-being of patients with cancer. In the early 1970s, Cameron and Pauling[53] proposed the concept of 'orthomolecular medicine' to describe the use of megadoses of vitamins and other supplements to treat cancer, cardiovascular diseases, and other chronic conditions. In-depth reviews about the use of nutritional and dietary supplements in cancer care were recently published.[54,55]A systematic review of concurrent antioxidant supplementation with chemotherapy concluded that many studies showed either increased survival times, increased tumour responses, or both, as well as fewer toxicities than controls. The lack of adequate statistical power was a consistent limitation. Large, well-designed studies of antioxidant supplementation concurrent with chemotherapy were suggested. Antioxidants also hold the potential for reducing dose-limiting toxicities.

The prevalence of using CAM-oriented nutritional modalities in cancer care is not easy to estimate. In most studies, data regarding CAM nutritional use are limited to supplement use only. No study has yet observed the full spectrum of CAM nutritional use as part of the various CAM modalities. Appropriate research into the prevalence of CAM nutritional use should consider what patients purchase (e.g. nutritional supplements) or pay for (e.g. CAM providers' fees) but also whether a CAM philosophy or approach changed their attitudes regarding food preferences, preparation, and consumption. The magnitude of CAM influence on patients' care, especially during chemotherapy and radiation treatment, needs to be evaluated in terms of content, context, and spiritual perspective (the meaning of food and eating).

In their report on the American Cancer Society's studies of cancer survivors, Gansler *et al.*[56] found that nutritional supplements and vitamins were used by 40% of the respondents. In a previous chemoprevention trial on the use of vitamins, minerals, and nutritional supplements, Sandler *et al.*[57] found that 55% of the participants (mean number: 2.6) used such supplements (66% took more than one supplement and 13% took five or more daily). The researchers also found that vitamins, particularly vitamins C and E, were the most commonly used supplements (49% of participants), followed by minerals (22%), botanicals (13%), and others (5%). Kumar *et al.*[58] retrospectively studied nutritional therapies used during cancer treatment and found that 29% of patients reported using CAM nutritional therapies not prescribed by their physician. In a prospective pilot study from the Mayo Clinic, about 50% of patients with gastrointestinal or breast cancer who were undergoing active chemotherapy reported taking dietary supplements.[59]

The influence of cancer diagnosis extends not just to the use of nutritional supplements but also to food ingredients considered to be healthy. In a study from the University of Arizona, Thomson *et al.*[60] found that women who have had breast cancer reported higher intakes of fruits, vegetables, and fibre-rich foods and lower intakes of high fat foods, including fast foods, after diagnosis.[61] Similar findings were reported in a study from Finland in which 32% of the respondents changed their dietary habits after being diagnosed with breast cancer; this was particularly true for younger patients with higher educational backgrounds. The main changes they reported were decreased consumption of animal fat, sugar, and red meat and increased consumption of fruits, berries, and vegetables.

Several studies have examined patients' perspectives regarding dietary changes and nutritional supplement use as part of their cancer care. In a Norwegian study, 36% of patients with different cancers used herbs and dietary supplements to treat the cancer along with their conventional treatments. When asked about their motives for using these alternative treatments, 62% answered, 'I don't know,' whereas others believed that the products would strengthen their immune system or help fight the cancer.[62] In Seattle the predictors of changes in diet, physical activity, and dietary supplement use among cancer patients was investigated.[63] Forty per cent of patients made one or more dietary changes and 48% started taking new dietary supplements after their diagnosis. The researchers also found that having a strong desire for personal control or an internal locus of control predicted the use of new dietary supplements. In Hawaii, interviewed cancer survivors reported that the major themes for changing diet were the hopes that nutrition would increase well-being, maintain health, and prevent cancer recurrence, and the beliefs that foods that cause or prevent cancer should be avoided or increased, respectively.[64]

A Canadian qualitative study of women diagnosed with breast cancer[65] found that even though some women believed diet contributed to breast cancer, they made no dietary changes, whereas women who did not believe in such a relationship changed their diets after being diagnosed. The authors concluded that use of nutritional supplements appeared to be a common, although possibly temporary, response to a diagnosis of cancer. Another Canadian study in which researchers conducted semi-structured interviews with breast cancer survivors[66] concluded that, for women with breast cancer, food can be an important coping mechanism in gaining control, comfort, and hope. In the Finnish study, Salminen *et al.*[61] reported that 32% of patients (out of 123 participants) had changed their dietary habits after the diagnosis of breast cancer. The main reason for change in diet was the desire to be cured of cancer.

Limited research data are available on doctor–patient communication concerning nutritional supplements and cancer. Reedy[67] interviewed adults with and without a history of colorectal cancer regarding dietary choices and supplement use and found a lack of physician guidance in dietary supplement selection. Finnish patients with breast cancer noted a lack of precise dietary recommendations from their treatment centre for their individual disease situation and stated that they depended instead on information from other sources.[61] In Ohio,[68] the patterns of dietary supplement use in veterans with cancer indicated that 38% did not disclose dietary supplement use to their physicians and that a similar number of patients learned about dietary supplements from their physicians.

The perspectives of Canadian oncologists and naturopaths concerning the role of nutrition in cancer care were qualitatively compared by Novak and Chapman.[69] They found that oncologists believed little evidence existed about the role of diet in breast cancer prevention and treatment, so they provided only general advice about healthy eating to patients. By contrast, the naturopaths believed that diet was strongly implicated in breast cancer development, prevention, and treatment and provided patients with specific suggestions for foods to avoid or emphasize in their diets.

In summary, many cancer patients use nutritional supplements or modify their diet, but research supporting the efficacy of this behaviour is very limited. Patients often ask their clinical oncology physicians questions about what they should eat; which dietary supplements are the best to take in regard to benefit, quality, and cost; where reliable reading material on dietary approaches (with and without proven efficacy and safety) for their disease can be obtained; and whether they can be referred to a professional in CAM and nutrition. In addition, patients may regard the issue of nutrition and supplements on a much deeper and sometimes unconscious level. Patients may relate to nutrition in the context of self-blame, wondering whether their diet caused the cancer. At the same time, they may desire to be active and change their attitude about food and its meaning in life. Patients may also regard food and dietary supplements as external remedies for their feelings of deficiency and loss. They often yearn for something that will support them, and food is an intimate and immediate resource people identify with for nourishment, support, and health. Therefore, communicating with cancer patients about nutrition and dietary supplements should not be limited to research findings and cold facts alone but should extend to deeper emotional and psychological realms that are meaningful to both patients and health care providers.

Systematic and traditional medicine approaches to nutrition in cancer

Traditional systems of medicine often integrate dietary approaches into cancer treatment. The dietary consultation is usually incorporated into a larger therapeutic plan that typically also includes herbal, manual/touch, movement, and spiritual modalities. Here, we discuss dietary approaches to cancer originating from three main systematic CAM modalities: traditional Chinese medicine (TCM), Ayurveda, and Anthroposophy. TCM and Ayurveda are two of the most ancient and prominent traditional medical cultures, both arising during the first millennium BCE. The more recent anthroposophical medicine arose in central Europe in the early twentieth century. These modalities share a systematic analytic approach based on a thorough medical examination that leads to a diagnosis of a syndrome or patterns of disharmony rather than an isolated disease condition. Following this diagnostic procedure, a therapeutic plan is formulated that typically includes dietary recommendations. The dietary consultation focuses on specific foods to avoid or include as well as how to prepare and eat those foods. Although the three diagnostic systems approach nutrition counselling differently, they share the following perspectives regarding cancer care.

- Food is medicinal remedy that is meaningful in both primary and secondary prevention and in supporting patients during active conventional oncological treatment.
- Food is an image of other processes in nature and the human body: it corresponds to the fundamental cosmic elements (water, earth, fire, wood, and metal), and can be targeted to heal an imbalance (e.g. cancer) of these elements in the human body, soul, and spirit.
- The unique healing quality of food is determined by the synergism of its ingredients' qualitative aspects (cold–hot, taste qualities, etc.).
- The context of eating (e.g. daily, weekly, and seasonal rhythm of eating meals) is important for the healing effect.
- The practitioner identifies the disharmony pattern (disease) and strives to harmonize it by using foods with similar (strengthening) or contradictory (weakening) gestures (e.g. treating 'uprising' vomiting with food that has a 'downward' action in the stomach). Often, matching a specific food with a specific body action is based on a process of intuition, contemplation, and meditation that scholars of traditional medicine call 'the doctrine of signatures'.

Scientific research regarding the ayurvedic and traditional Chinese dietary approach to cancer is in its early stages. Preliminary evidence for the beneficial activity of multiple herbs and spices commonly used in the Indian and Chinese kitchen such as turmeric, ginger, black pepper (*Piper nigrum*), hot chilies, ginger and green tea are mentined in the 'Food as medicine' section.

In the following paragraphs, the basic philosophy, general practical dietary strategies, and other approaches to cancer treatment of the Chinese, ayurvedic, and anthroposophical methods are applied to the same case study. We suggest that the following sections be read with an open mind in regard to the taxonomies of the three systems. For example, Chinese concepts of organs and functions have broader interpretations than provided by conventional, modern, western vocabulary. Because we cannot discuss all aspects of such concepts here, we have used punctuation (initial capital letters or quotes) and font styles (italics) to indicate terms that generally reflect them, leaving it to the reader to explore the concepts more completely. For the purposes of this chapter, we suggest that readers view such terms as metaphors and acknowledge that they have a deeper and valid meaning within the philosophy of their respective medical system.

Case study: patient with ovarian carcinoma seeks dietary advice

Debbie is 40-year-old woman who was diagnosed 1 year ago with recurrent ovarian carcinoma involving the peritoneum. She is currently being treated with doxorubicin. Side-effects attributed to the chemotherapy include recurrent sore throat, severe nausea and vomiting that starts 1 day before chemotherapy treatment, weakness, and drowsiness. Debbie's oncologist referred her to an integrative CAM specialist working within the oncology service to help her find a way to decrease the anticipatory nausea and vomiting and to address the other gastrointestinal symptoms.

The integrative diagnostic work-up included a bio-psycho-social-spiritual history, questions regarding previous and current experience with CAM, expectations from the integrative treatment, and two brief structured questionnaires (the Edmonton Symptom Assessment System[70] and the Measure Yourself Concerns and Wellbeing.[71] On the first of these questionnaires, Debbie used a scale of 0–10 to rate the severity of ten symptoms common in cancer patients (pain, tiredness, nausea, depression, anxiety, drowsiness, appetite, well-being, and shortness of breath). On the second, she identified two personal concerns and then rated each on a scale of 0–6. During the integrative assessment, Debbie requested the goal of treatment be to alleviate her severe nausea and vomiting, which she linked to psychological considerations (she graded both anxiety and depression as 6 on a 10-point visual analogue scale). She spoke openly about the loss of her mother from cancer just before her own diagnosis of cancer. She expected holistic dietary advice regarding: what to eat ('How to eat appropriately'), what to avoid ('What foods can fuel my cancer?'), what to be careful with ('Can nutritional supplements decrease chemotherapy efficacy?'), and foods and supplements that may strengthen her body and soul, and help her to cope better with the cancer and the side-effects of chemotherapy. Debbie was also interested in changing her overall approach to the context of eating, her eating habits, and the meaning of food in her life, regardless of caloric intake and other quantifiable nutritional parameters.

Traditional Chinese medicine approach

Practitioners of TCM will approach Debbie's case along two parallel diagnostic lines: a cancer-centred approach based on the discipline's general perceptions of cancer, and a patient-centred approach that considers the individual characteristics of Debbie's symptoms and the way she copes with the side-effects of chemotherapy. The diagnostic work-up typically comprises a personal history that may include questions about the content and context of Debbie's diet and her lifestyle, and a thorough physical examination that focuses on the traditional Chinese tongue-and-pulse diagnosis. Next, the practitioner will use the discipline's rich nomenclature to diagnose patterns of illness and disharmony and to formulate a treatment plan. Treatment commonly includes acupuncture, herbal and dietary interventions, mind–body, manual, and movement therapies.

In this systematic diagnosis-based process, dietary considerations have meaning as both aetiological factors and potential therapeutics. In Debbie's case, because she is undergoing chemotherapy, the practitioner's contemplation about her perception of food and eating and formulation of a therapeutic nutritional strategy is aimed at alleviating the side-effects she experiences from chemotherapy and strengthening her physical and emotional abilities to cope with the conventional cancer treatment. Upon the successful termination of an active oncology treatment, the practitioner will consult with Debbie again about nutrition aimed at preventing the cancer from recurring or progressing.

The dietary approach to cancer in TCM is based on both practical and empirical knowledge gathered and distilled over thousands of years and the philosophical framework of two fundamental schools of thought: Yin and Yang and the five elements.[72]

Yin and Yang theory

Yin and Yang suggest the relativity and interrelation of two gestures, phases, or stages that define a whole by the dynamic balance of their opposing qualities, interdependence, mutual consumption, and transformation. The TCM practitioner may use Yin and Yang to describe two dietary qualities such as Cold and Hot. For example, cold and uncooked foods are perceived as more Yin, while hot and cooked foods are more Yang. The practitioner perceives healthy food and and a healthy diet as having balanced and harmonious Yin and Yang qualities. Interruption of this harmony may cause a relative excess of, or deficiency in, Yin or Yang and lead to disease formation. In terms of Chinese dietary therapy, Hot and Cold food qualities may increase or decrease the functions of internal organs. For example, Hot foods such as chilies may increase Heat, which causes body fluids in the Stomach to decrease, and cooling foods like cucumber may tonify these organs' fluids.[73] Cooking methods may also alter food properties. Frying foods increases their heating qualities, whereas freezing foods increases their cooling qualities. Considering cancer aetiology, eating too much cold or raw food produces warm-like Yang qualities and may eventually lead to Dampness, one of the important aetiological factors in cancer development. Eating is also regarded in terms of daily and seasonal rhythms, which also correspond to the Yin–Yang theory of Cold–Hot qualities. For example, noon is conceptualized as being relatively Yang and Hot, so lunch should be designed in accordance with these qualities.

Five elements/phases theory

This theory relates to the five fundamental macro- and microcosmic qualities (water, wood, fire, earth, and metal) in Chinese culture that correspond to body organs and tissues, emotions, stages of development, colours, sounds, tastes, etc. The five elements are often viewed in a sequential circle in which one element is generating another in a mother–child-like relationship (e.g. water generates wood which generates fire) while controlling or being controlled by the remaining elements in a grandparent–grandchild-like relationship (e.g. water controls fire and fire may 'insult' water). Figure 25.1 illustrates the correspondence among the five elements and the five internal organs (kidneys, liver, heart, spleen, and lungs), Chinese tastes (salty, sour, bitter, sweet, and pungent or hot), and common grains (millet, wheat, beans, rice, and hemp). Overconsumption or avoidance of food with a specific dominant taste may be interpreted as a causative factor for disease and may be used as a therapeutic modality to fine-tune, augment, or calm the activity of an organ. For example, a practitioner may suggest that Debbie consume green leaves that have a bitter taste during chemotherapy to enhance her splenic function. As Figure 25.1 shows, TCM attributes bitter taste with the Heart, which nourishes the Spleen, which has lessened activity in cancer.

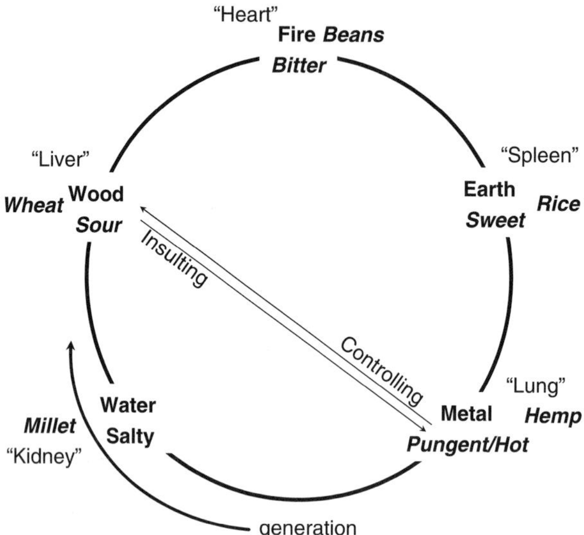

Fig. 25.1 Five elements in traditional Chinese medicine and correspondences to tastes and grains.

How these theories work together

According to this philosophy, cancer can develop from 'internal' causes (e.g. emotions such as anger, excessive excitement, worry, sadness, fear, and shock), 'external' causes (e.g. climatic factors such as wind and dampness), and other causes (e.g. diet, toxins, and weak constitution). Dietary factors in cancer development and recurrence are multifactorial.

- Consuming relatively too much uncooked, raw, and Cold food leads to deficient Yang.
- Consuming too much animal protein, milk products, and carbohydrates leads to food Stagnation and Dampness in the spleen. (In TCM, the Spleen governs the body's transformation and transportation of food and fluids; it controls the body's vital substances of *Qi*: energy or life force is the more Yang aspect of *Qi* and Blood, the dense and fluid form of *Qi*, is the more Yin aspect.)
- Consuming too few fresh green leafy vegetables with gentle pungent and bitter tastes causes stagnation because such vegetables purify the blood and facilitate *Qi* movement in the body.
- Eating too fast may cause incomplete food digestion, leading to Food Stagnation, Dampness, or Toxicity.
- Being too emotional during meals may also affect body organs, which according to the five elements theory correspond with specific emotions (anger corresponds with the Liver, sorrow with the Lungs, etc.). For example, repeated anger during family arguments over dinner may cause liver *Qi* to be stagnant, consequently affecting Spleen *Qi*, with resultant Dampness.

A cancer-related diagnosis in TCM is often viewed in relation to *Qi* and Blood deficiency, specifically with patterns of Spleen deficiency (e.g. fatigue and weight loss) and Stomach deficiency (e.g. fatigue and vomiting), which are related to Stagnation and Dampness.[74] Other disease patterns relate to the influence of Fire toxins such as chemotherapy, which can produce side-effects such as stomatitis and mucositis, and the emergence of emotions like anxiety and depression during the course of oncology treatment. Herbs and foods are used to move the Blood and *Qi* within the malignant tumour to 'soften and disperse' it.[75] In Debbie's case, the chemotherapy-associated vomiting, which includes an anticipatory psychological component, is viewed as a Fire toxin disrupting the Stomach's *Qi*. Nausea and vomiting are considered to be a failure of the Stomach to harmonize and pathologically ascends *Qi* upwards.

To control such Fire toxins, a dietary strategy during chemotherapy may include the following recommendations.

- Eat green leafy vegetables with light pungent and bitter tastes, orange-coloured vegetables, whole-grain or white rice, whole-wheat bread, legumes, fish, and chicken.
- Use spices such as ginger (preferably fresh, to control nausea and vomiting) and those with a light pungent or bitter taste (e.g. oregano and tumeric).
- Eat light, frequent small-portioned meals of minimally cooked (e.g. stir-fried in a small amount of oil) or fresh foods that reflect a variety of tastes, with a pleasant mood, in a pleasant environment, and with pleasant company (such as family and friends, particularly at lunch and dinner).
- Avoid or decrease consumption of heavy full-portioned meals, red meat, carbohydrates with a high glycaemic index, and sweetened hot and cold drinks.
- Perform mild physical activity, if desired, before breakfast

Table 25.1 summarizes useful tips for health care providers who are not familiar with TCM, but who are open-minded toward TCM-inspiring nutritional counselling for patients with cancer.

Ayurvedic medicine approach

Ayurveda, meaning the knowledge of life, stems from the Hindu philosophy and is the most prominent traditional medical system in India. Similar to Chinese medicine, Ayurveda regards macro- and microcosmic interrelations. The five ayurvedic elements of earth, water, fire, air, and ether are considered as both the building blocks of nature and of man and correspond to the five senses. The five elements create and conceptualize the three life forces (*doshas*) responsible for the activities of the body. Each dosha is characterized by typical gestures acting as physiological archetypes: *vata* is identified with movement, breathing, and secretion; *pitta* with digestion and heat; and *kapha* with holding, lubrication, and stability. Each of the three doshas corresponds with typical body tissues and functions as well as emotions and cognitive processes. Figure 25.2 illustrates the three doshas and their relation to the five elements and the six ayurvedic tastes (sweet, sour, salty, bitter, astringent, and pungent), which are intimately related to an increase or decrease of a specific dosha. Every person has a unique combination of the three doshas (referred to as constitution or *prakriti*), and disease is viewed as disharmony or out-of-equilibrium of the person's unique dosha balance.

Health

Health requires that the three doshas be in harmonious equilibrium. Disease is regarded as a disruption of this harmony, and therapy strives to return the patient to the prediseased state. The ayurvedic physician uses a sophisticated diagnostic system that includes history-taking and body examination to make an accurate doshic diagnosis. Nutrition is a highly valued therapeutic modality and is often combined with herbal medicine, manual practices, yoga, meditation, and other treatment modalities. Food has a major influence on health and disease because it nourishes, forms, and transforms the doshas and may influence the body's secretions and waste products.

One of the keys to understanding the connection between nutrition, health, and disease is to view the relationships among the six ayurvedic tastes (sweet, sour, salty, pungent, bitter and

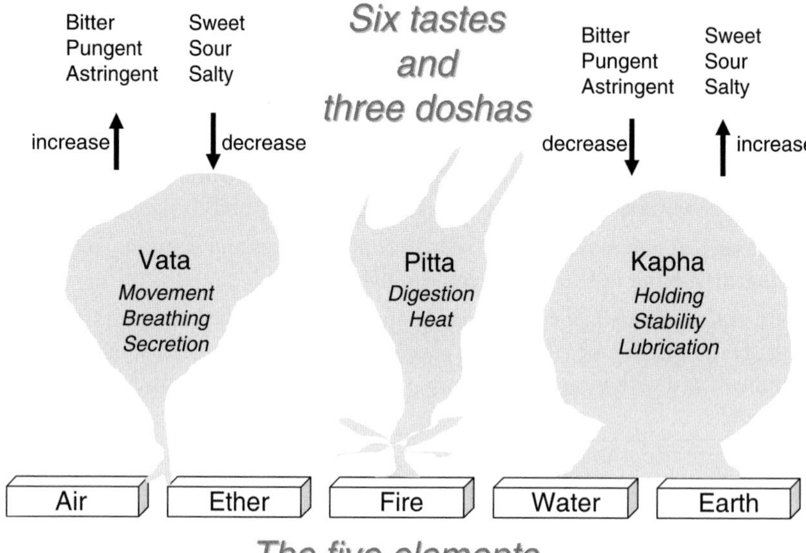

Fig. 25.2 Five elements, three doshas, and six tastes in Ayurvedic medicine.

astringent), the five elements, and the three doshas. In brief, every dosha is influenced by three tastes that increase it and three different tastes that decrease it. Foods such as medicinal herbs are viewed as powerful remedies that can be used to tune the doshas' harmony to promote health and longevity or to heal imbalance and disease. How foods restore harmony to the different doshas may also correspond to which part of a food is used for cooking (e.g. flowers and leaves relate to vata, oils and sap to pitta, and roots to kapha) and whether the food has a heating or cooling effect, is light or heavy, etc. A complex diagnosis defines the effects of various food parts for different dairy products, legumes, grains, vegetables, fruits, and spices and assigns them to the different doshas accordingly. The ayurvedic practitioner is expected to formulate an individual diet strategy for the patient according to that patient's present and prediseased dosha dispositions.

Cancer is a well-recognized disease in ayurvedic medicine. In the middle of the second millennium BCE, Sushruta, one of the leading ayurvedic founders, described cancer as a rounded immobile swelling giving rise to little pain with no associated inflammation. Contemporary ayurvedic physicians view cancer as a disruption of all the doshas, with accompanying low digestive 'fire' (*agni*), improper formation of tissues, and an accumulation of toxic waste products (*ama*).

Ayurvedic medicine postulates that there are specific dosha-type tumours such as the inflamed pitta type, and the slow-growing kapha type, all of which which are currently treated with both conventional oncological and complementary ayurvedic strategies.[76] Nutrition is an important supplemental therapy that is applied as medicinal herbs and accompanied by purification (*panchakarma*) and rejuvenation procedures aimed at increasing 'digestive fire', removing waste products (ama) and increasing immunity.

The ayurvedic nutritional strategy is concerned with restoring the patient's dosha constitution and generally reducing the waste products that accumulate in the body from the disease and the chemotherapy. An ayurvedic physician often advises patients with any dosha-type tumour to reduce the amount of food consumed and the number of meals eaten per day, to follow a diet low in fat and protein, to drink boiled water, and to use hot spices. Waste products from disease and chemotherapy are reduced in the body by consuming foods with bitter, astringent, and hot or pungent tastes. The physician will modify this nutritional strategy if the cancer is more of a vata type, in which case, the physician will suggest that the patient also eat spices and foods that have sweet, salty, and sour tastes.

An ayurvedic physician examining Debbie, who experiences severe anticipatory vomiting, would address her case according to the disease, her treatment-related symptoms, and her nutritional needs and goals, as described below.

Disease-oriented context

Recurrent ovarian carcinoma involving the peritoneum is related to kapha dominance. To decrease kapha dosha and ama, a typical nutritional approach would prescribe cooked vegetables and fruits with bitter, pungent, and astringent tastes, decreasing food quantities during meals, and including sparse amounts of protein and fat in the diet.

Symptoms-oriented context

Debbie's symptoms of nausea and vomiting, sore throat, weakness, and drowsiness are typical symptoms of ama accumulation in the body as a result of the disease and the chemotherapy. In addition to the classic ama-decreasing diet mentioned above, the ayurvedic physician may also suggest Debbie incorporate a yoga-related treatment, which stresses a few small-portioned meals that include cooked vegetables and wheatgrass juice.

Patient-centred context

The ayurvedic physician will attempt to diagnose her prediseased constitution and to direct individually designed dietary and herbal therapy to address the disharmony among Debbie's doshas, mental, emotional, and spiritual diagnostic keys. Debbie's psychological predisposition will be regarded as a pivotal expression of her *prana* (breathing-like vital energy). The ayurvedic physician may suggest yoga-related breathing exercises and meditation with the goal of achieving a sense of joy and presence in the 'here and now' in her daily activities, including eating.

Anthroposophical medicine approach

Anthroposophical medicine developed in the 1920s in Central Europe from the collaborative work of Dr Rudolf Steiner, who founded the School of Spiritual Science, and Dr Ita Wegman, a medical doctor who interpreted Steiner's stream of thought into medical terminology. Anthroposophical medicine was one of the first CAM systems to be integrated into European conventional hospitals, primary care settings, and oncology care. Anthroposophical physicians are required to be medical doctors and to view their work as an extension of conventional medicine. They perceive that understanding the essence and spiritual forces behind substance and illness is the key to healing. Therapy follows a salutogenic health orientation of self-healing aimed at strengthening the inner organism and instilling a sense of individuality and empowerment through self-responsibility.[77] Anthroposophical oncology, as well as other forms of anthroposophical medical care, relies on the collaborative teamwork of physicians, nurses, artistic therapists (mainly in Curative Eurythmy, an anthroposophical movement therapy, but also in music, painting, sculpturing, etc.), physical and massage therapists, and psychotherapy. Physicians and therapists share a similar understanding of anthroposophical diagnostic patterns, which consider the patient's individual patterns within the general anthroposophical understanding of the cancer process. Following a diagnosis, an anthroposophical physician may recommend nutritional, herbal, homeopathic, and other unique anthroposophical remedies. This may include preparations of the semiparasitic herb mistletoe (*Viscum album*), shown to possess some beneficial effects in cancer care, mostly related to improved quality of life during chemotherapy.[78]

Two fundamental models of this philosophy, the fourfold nature of the human organism and the threefold human being, are used in anthroposophical medicine. In the first, the anthroposophist perceives that the human organism has four members (bodies) that correspond to the four Greek medicinal elements of earth (mineral), water (fluid), air (gas), and fire (warmth) and are regarded as Lower or Upper bodies.[79] The Lower bodies include the Physical body, which correspondes to the material and measurable mineral realm, and the water-related Etheric body, which carries life and growth forces and is seen as the organizing principle in the plant kingdom, directing growth, regeneration, and reproduction. The Upper bodies include the air-related Astral body, which is the carrier of feelings (understood to exist in the animals as well as in humans) and is responsible for affect and consciousness, movement, desires, and emotions. The highest member of the Upper bodies, the I or Ego, is seen as a unique spark of divinity in humans and is associated with the warmth element and the human spirit that gives humans the abilities of self-reflection, thinking, creativity, and free will, which are related to idealistic actions.[73] In the second fundamental model, the threefold human being is characterized by two polar systems: an upper Nerve-sense system and a lower Metabolic-limb system.[80] The upper Nerve-sense system includes the brain, nerves, and sense organs and is identified with catabolism and cold sclerosing-like tendencies. The lower Metabolic-limb system, relating to the muscles, abdomen, and reproductive organs, corresponds to anabolism, warmth, and inflammation. These two polar systems are mediated by the Rhythmic system, which includes the heart and the lungs and maintains health through harmony and compensation.[74]

Anthroposophical medicine perceives cancer as a systemic illness that results from disharmony between the life-reproductive growth process originating in the Etheric body and the opposing formatting, limiting, and differentiated activities of the Ego. Tumour is regarded as rebellion of the cell element against the organism and as a 'disease of the organism and not a disease of the cells'.[81] Steiner suggested that cancer be viewed as a misplaced sense organ or a tendency to develop consciousness (emulating the Nerve-sense system) in the unconscious metabolic organs (Metabolic-limb system).[82] Anthroposophical physicians perceive cancer aetiology in relation to weakness of the formatting principle of the Ego in the body, which may be influenced by what is perceived as 'cooling' influences in childhood (growing up in an overstimulating environment, over-use of antipyretic drugs, etc.). In adulthood, the person may face the difficulty of having to 'dispel' the invading overstimulated modern environment and environmental pollutants such as agricultural fertilizers, pesticides, food preservatives, and colourants. Anthroposophical-oriented nutrition (biodynamic agriculture) and education (Waldorf schools) are regarded as modalities that can counteract modern life's 'carcinogenic' tendencies by nurturing humans and balancing the Nerve-sense, Metabolic-limb, and Rhythmic systems.

The aim of anthroposophical therapy in cancer care is to 'find ways of stimulating the form-giving activity of the Ego so that it regains mastery over the growth processes"'.[83] Nutrition is considered as a potential remedy or a risk factor for cancer development. Cancer may be prompted by eating too much (especially eating too many proteins, fats, and refined carbohydrates), by loss of rhythms in eating (e.g. lack of regular meals), and by agricultural (food fertilizers) and food-processing (food irradiation, additives, deep-freezing) methods that reduce food's natural vitality. The anthroposophical physician may recommend that patients eat foods with fewer odours and tastes, foods with fewer additives and artificial colouring, eat more conscientiously (e.g. chew food very thoroughly to mix it well with saliva and taste it consciously), and concentrate on eating (e.g. isolate the senses by not doing other things, like watching television, while eating).[84]

Certain foods, such as tomatoes, potatoes, and mushrooms, are considered potentially harmful in respect to cancer development. Anthroposophy advocates a vegetarian diet, but does not totally exclude meat. The nourishment of the body during cancer treatment is pivotal to the aim of supporting the human spirit. During cancer treatment, grains coupled with culinary herbs (e.g. herbs of the carrot family, Umbelliferae) are recommended as are soured and fermented milk products, which are preferred over fresh milk. During chemotherapy, patients are encouraged to eat bio-dynamic foods and are given specific recipes.[85]

In the case of nutritional counselling for our study patient, Debbie, the anthroposophical physician will not only focus on her anticipatory vomiting but also perceive her illness in the totality of body, mind, and soul. Symptoms of weakness, drowsiness, and depression will be associated with decreased life forces, and anxiety as expression of the Astral body. The physician will aim to empower Debbie's Ego forces by encouraging her interest in changing her overall approach to eating. The physician's suggestions of specific foods she add to her diet or avoid will be complemented by lifestyle changes regarding the context of eating and diminishing her burden of environmental stimuli. The anthroposophical physician may also suggest that Debbie recite a meditation or table prayer while preparing or eating the meal to connect her body and soul.[86]

Alongside nutritional counselling, the anthroposophical physician will often recommend remedies such as subcutaneous injections of mistletoe (*Viscum album*) to empower vitality (and strengthen the Ego) and to attenuate the side-effets of chemotherapy. Art therapies may be recommended to relieve the emotionally disturbed Astral body. In addition, psychotherapeutic 'biographical counselling' may be suggested to help Debbie cope with her mother's death from cancer just before her own cancer diagnosis and contemplate and define the meaning of her life and illness within her individual life journey.

Communicating with cancer patients about food, eating, and using nutritional supplments

A discussion with patients about their food and dietary lifestyle is one of the most relevant yet challenging topics in cancer care. Figure 25.3 suggests an algorithm that enables health care profesionals to approach this issue by using an integrative concept. The design of an integrated nutritional plan may begin by defining the therapeutic context, i.e. defining where the patient is on the path of cancer diagnosis and treatment. Patients near diagnosis or in the midst of chemotherapy and radiation treatment may face different dilemmas concerning nutrition. Patients encountering malignant life-threatening disease may be more willing to contemplate their lifestyle and the meaning of food in their life than are patients with limited disease. Patients who completed adjuvant chemotherapy or radiation treatment may feel a threshold experience of 'coming back to life' and seek dietary advice that will prevent cancer recurrence and enable them to feel more healthy and in control.

A second required step in the integrated nutritional plan design is to define the 'actors' who may be involved in the process: the patient, caregivers, and conventional and CAM health care providers. At first glance, some of these figures may be perceived as somehow irrelevant compared with the patient, the oncologist, and the surgeon. Caregivers are often as important because they are likely to be the ones addressing the patient's dietary concerns. Health care providers such as nurses, social workers, and family practitioners may add valuable perspectives in the process of weaving together a patient-centred dietary treatment plan. Caregivers may have noteworthy concerns regarding the patient's diet, weight loss, appetite, and nausea and other gastrointestinal symptoms. These concerns may affect the entire family perspective towards nutrition. Moreover, nutrition and dietary concerns may express deeper psychological, social, and spiritual aspects

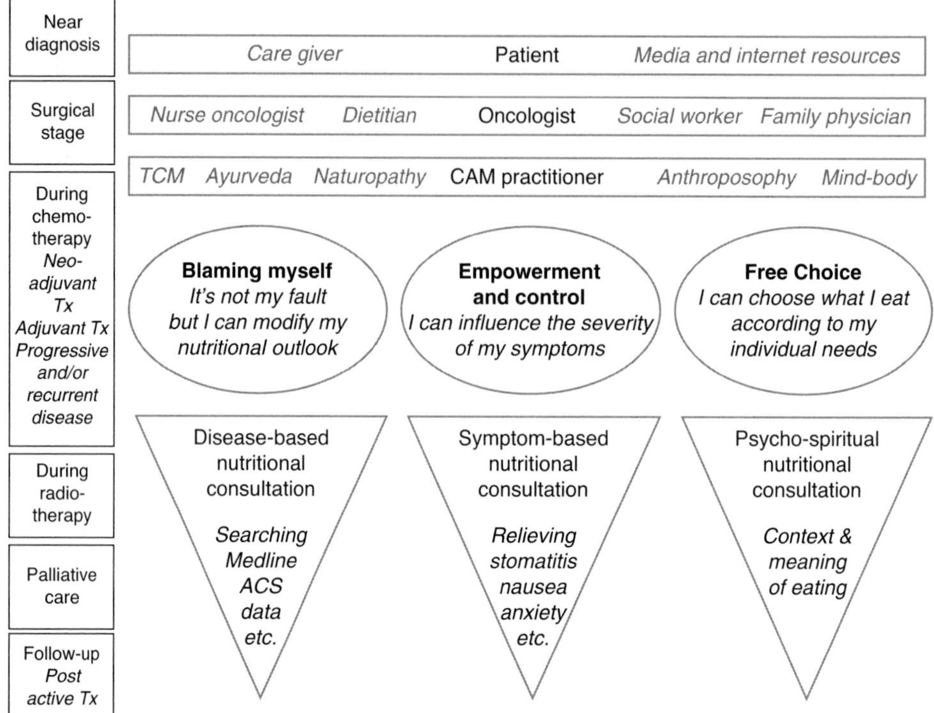

Fig. 25.3 Practical, patient-centred approach to nutritional consultation for cancer care in complementary and alternative medicine (CAM). TCM, traditional Chinese medicine; ACS, American Cancer Society.

concerning the patient's health deterioration. Weight loss and cachexia may be percieved as death-equivalent and promote caregivers to initiate an active fight ('doing') regarding calories rather than discussing their beloved's food desires or aversion ('being'). Defining the role of the caregivers concerning CAM and nutrition may be an important step in directing the integrative dietary treatment plan.

Nurses play a pivotal role during chemotherapy and often engage in an informal discussion with patients regarding food choices, preparation, and eating. Nurses and social workers may elicit the patient's outlook regarding food in the broad psychosocial context. Family practitioners and other primary care physicians may also add a valuable general perspective on the patient and the family. Family physicians may share their perception on the meaning of food and diet in the family context based on previous encounters with the patient and other family members concerning dietary management of chronic diseases, psychosomatic-based ailments, and previous cancer management of family relatives. Finally, yet importantly, CAM practitioners may have a unique role regarding nutrition counselling because of their CAM expertise, which may be augmented by a patient's expectations and association of CAM with concepts of healthy nutrition and lifestyle. Like family physicians, CAM practitioners may also have previous (before the cancer diagnosis) acquaintance with patients, for instance, acupuncture treatment for lower back pain. In the course of cancer treatment, patients may seek dietary advice from CAM practitioners who practice general systematic CAM modalities (e.g. ayurvedic, TCM, and anthroposophical medicine, among others) or from practitioners who practice a nutritional-focused approach (e.g. macrobiotics).

CAM practitioners, nurses, oncologists, social workers, family physicians, and other health care providers may contribute to the formation of a multidisciplinary team that can formulate an integrative nutritional approach tailored to the patient's and caregiver's needs and narratives. The three principal objectives that guide the integrative multidisciplinary team's approach concern providing patients with reassurance, a sense of empowerment and control, and a feeling of choice (Figure 25.3). Cancer patients require reassurance to counteract feelings of guilt. Patients may feel guilty or blame themselves, at least subconsciously, about having cancer because they indulged in 'wrong' dietary habits. These feelings may be augmented by the numerous publications in both conventional and CAM literature that associate lifestyle and various food consumptions or avoidance as reasons for cancer growth. A central objective of the integrative dietary plan is to teach patients to avoid self-accusation. That is, to reassure patients that it is not their fault that they have cancer, and to encourage them to take positive steps in the healing process by modifying their nutritional outlook.

A second objective is to suggest dietary and lifestyle modifications in the context of a patient's sense of empowerment and as a means by which they can gain more control and play an active role in the healing process. A patient's active involvement in the construction of their own dietary plan may increase their sense of responsibility and assertiveness. They may feel less passive and more like 'landlords' or navigators of the therapeutic process. Patients may perceive that the integrative dietary agenda either generally supports them during cancer treatment or alleviates specific symptoms caused by the disease (e.g. fatigue) or adverse effects of the oncology treatment (e.g. gastrointestinal symptoms).

The third important objective in constructing a dietary plan is to avoid using rigid nutritional guidelines that supposedly meet the needs of any patient or a specific cancer type. Although many CAM modalities recommend a nearly identical dietary strategy (whole cereals, low sugar intake, organic vegetarian food, plenty of vegetables, mindful eating, etc.), the integrative team should carefully study the individual patient's eating habits and dietary lifestyle as well as the patient's psychosocial, cultural, and spiritual context regarding food. The challenge of the integrative team in formulating a diet is to study the patient's narrative, to introduce CAM and evidence-based perspectives, and to create an individual treatment plan that respects the patient's free will and autonomy. Consideration of disease-based, symptom-based, and psycho-spiritual-based perspectives may enrich the practical core of the nutritional consultation.

A disease-based dietary outlook can be based on conventional research data, CAM research data, and nutritional guidelines (e.g. the American Cancer Society Guidelines on Nutrition and Physical Activity for Cancer Prevention).[87]

Various resources present scientific evidence about the foods and their constituents in relation to specific cancers (e.g. breast, colorectal, lung, and prostate)[88] and provide guidance for informed decision-making in primary to tertiary cancer prevention. Health care providers may also complement these structured guidelines with database (e.g. Medline) searches based on specific questions asked by patients and caregivers about food items and their role in cancer prevention. The use of specific and simple key words (e.g. the food item name + prevention + cancer + controlled) may offer preliminary information about the role of specific foods in cancer prevention and treatment. For example, a Medline search concerning tomatoes using these key words may reveal 13 references (as one search did in September 2008) and provide preliminary information on the role of tomatoes in cancer treatment or prevention. This search strategy is far from meeting the high methodological standards of systematic review but provides a practical starting point for an evidence-based dialogue with patients.

Table 25.3 provides selected research data categorized according to symptoms. Health care providers are encouraged to conduct frequent searches of references using databases such as

Table 25.3 Symptom-oriented complementary and alternative medicine (CAM) nutritional approaches in cancer care (limited review of selected articles)

Cancer-related symptom	CAM nutritional modality or supplement	Evidence for efficacy and safety
Fatigue	L-Carnitine	Prospective non-RCT: Patients with carnitine deficiency on either cisplatin or ifosfamide: treated with 3–4 g/day L-carnitine.[89]
		Phase I/II study: Patients with advanced cancer and carnitine deficiency experienced decreased fatigue with replacement doses up to 3 g/day. A subsequent double-blind placebo-controlled preliminary trial showed no benefit.[90,91]
	Vitamin C	Prospective non-RCT of terminal cancer patients: 10 g vitamin C twice with a 3-day interval and p.o. 4 g/day vitamin C for a week. Improved quality of life and decreased fatigue.[92]
	Omega-3 fish oil fatty acids	RCT: Cohort of 22 patients with advanced lung cancer and systemic immune–metabolic syndrome were randomly assigned to receive fish oil, 2 g tid + placebo vs fish oil + celecoxib 200 mg bid.[93]
		RCT: Supplement enriched with n-3 fatty acids is associated with an increase in physical activity in pancreatic cancer compared to an unenriched supplement.[94]
Weight loss	Omega-3 fish oil fatty acids	Systematic review: The authors suggest that administration of n-3 fatty acids (EPA and DHA) to patients with advanced cancer for prolonged periods (>8 weeks) in doses of at least 1.5 g/day are associated with increased weight and appetite, and improved QoL.[95]
	Glutamine and other amino acids	Retrospective study: Glutamine supplementation (10 g/8 h) may be beneficial in the prevention of acute radiation-induced oesophagitis and weight loss in lung cancer patients undergoing thoracic irradiation.[96]
		RCT: Combination of arginine, glutamine, HMB increased muscle mass within 4 weeks in patients with solid tumours.[97]
	ATP	RCT: 58 NSCLC patients randomized to ATP infusion or none. ATP improved weight, muscle strength, and QoL in patients with advanced NSCLC.[98]
Nausea and vomiting	Ginger	Two small studies of patients receiving chemotherapy: addition of ginger to standard anti-emetic medication reduced the severity of post-chemotherapy nausea.[27]

(Continued)

Table 25.3 (continued) Symptom-oriented complementary and alternative medicine (CAM) nutritional approaches in cancer care (limited review of selected articles)

Cancer-related symptom	CAM nutritional modality or supplement	Evidence for efficacy and safety
Stomatitis and mucositis	Glutamine	RCT (24 patients, 16 children, 8 adults): oral glutamine supplementation (2 g × 2/day swish and swallow) during and after chemotherapy significantly reduced both the duration and severity of chemotherapy-associated stomatitis.[99]
		RCT: 40 bone marrow transplantation patients received either intravenous alanyl-glutamine dipeptide or placebo: no benefit.[100]
Diarrhoea	Probiotics	RCT: Lactobacillus GG supplementation [1–2 × 10(10)/day] is well tolerated and may reduce the frequency of severe diarrhoea and abdominal discomfort related to 5FU-based chemotherapy.[101]
		RCT: Probiotic lactic acid-producing bacteria (VSL#3 one sachet tid) are an easy, safe, and feasible approach to protect patients undergoing adjuvant postoperative radiation therapy after surgery (sigmoid, rectal, or cervical cancer) against the risk of radiation-induced diarrhoea.[102]
Pain and neuropathy	vitamin E	RCT: vitamin E (300 mg/day) + cisplatin vs cisplatin alone. Supplementation of vitamin E decreased the incidence and severity of peripheral neurotoxicity.[103]

RCT, randomized controlled trial; EPA, eicosapentaenoic acid; DHA, docosahexaenoic acid; QoL, quality of life; HMB, β-hydroxy β-methylbutyric acid; NSCLC, non-small cell lung cancer; 5FU, 5-fluoruracil.

Medline and to organize their research data according to cancer sites and symptoms. Symptom-oriented data need to be further specified according to aetiology or association of the symptom to specific oncological treatments (e.g. glutamine treatment may be beneficial in radiation-induced mucositis as well as some chemotherapies[104] but did not alleviate 5-fluorouracil-induced mucositis in a phase III controlled study.[105] A symptom-based strategy for searching databases such as Medline might include keywords that identify the type of cancer and a specific symptom (e.g. fatigue) as well as a variety of CAM-related keywords associated with dietary themes such as complementary, alternative, CAM, TCM, ayurvedic, anthroposophical, macrobiotic, herbal, naturopathic, guided imagery, meditation, and many more.

Psycho-spiritual nutritional consultation focuses on the context and meaning of eating food and is primarily based on the unique contribution that every CAM modality offers to the concept of eating in one's life. Health care providers may refer patients to CAM practitioners who utilize one of the systematic and traditional medicine modalities such as TCM, ayurvedic medicine, or anthroposophical medicine, which illuminate various psycho-spiritual facets of nutrition. Other mind–body modalities may also contribute to the contextualization of nutrition. For example, Jon Kabat-Zinn proposed a 'raisin' meditation, based on Buddhist philosophy, that patients experience observing and eating a single raisin as completely and mindfully as though they had never eaten a raisin before.[106] Psycho-spiritual dietary consultation may complement patients' need for a very detailed and practical consultation regarding specific 'do' and 'don't do' dietary recommendations. Many of us, patients and health care providers, similarly hope for a 'magic pill', including one that might be found within a nutritional system to overcome cancer and its associated symptoms. The psycho-spiritual dimension may interpret such 'magic' as occurring in the kitchen or the dining realm, adding meaning to suffering and hope.

Acknowledgements

We thank Dr Elad Schiff, Ms Margalit Shilo, Mr Tal Avraham, and Dr Shahar Lev-Ari for their advice and appraisals concerning the TCM approach to nutrition; Dr Shai Pasternak for his advice and appraisals concerning the ayurvedic medicine approach to nutrition; and Drs Moti Levi, Tamar Shvat, Meiron Barak, Mariana Steiner, Ofer Lavie Avishai Gershoni, and Gil Bar-Sela for their advice and appraisals concerning the anthroposopical medicine approach to nutrition. And special thanks to Ms Kimberly Herrick for the extensive editorial review, suggestions and comments.

References

1. Fisher P (2005) Homeopathy and mainstream medicine: a dialogue of the deaf? *Wien Med Wochenschr*, **155**(21–22), 474–8.
2. Keller K (1991) Legal requirements for the use of phytopharmaceutical drugs in the Federal Republic of Germany. *J Ethnopharmacol*, **32**(1–3), 225–9.
3. Robinson N (2006) Integrated traditional Chinese medicine. *Complement Ther Clin Pract*, **12**(2), 132–40.
4. Srinivasan P (1995) National health policy for traditional medicine in India. *World Health Forum*, **16**(2), 190–3.
5. Jacobs JJ (1995) Building bridges between two worlds: the NIH's office of alternative medicine. *Acad Med*, **70**(1), 40–1.
6. National Center for Complementary and Alternative Medicine (http://www.nccam.nih.gov), National Institutes of Health, US Department of Health and Human Services, Bethesda, MD. *NCCAM History/ Chronology* (NIH Almanac) Available at: http://www.nih.gov/about/almanac/organization/NCCAM.htm (accessed 14 October 2008).
7. Office of Cancer Complementary and Alternative Medicine, National Cancer Institute, US National Institutes of Health, US Department of Health and Human Services, Bethesda, MD. *CAM at the NCI.* Available at: http://www.cancer.gov/cam/cam_at_nci.html (accessed 29 August 2008).
8. Boon H, Verhoef M, O'Hara D, Findlay B, Majid N (2004) Integrative healthcare: arriving at a working definition. *Altern Ther Health Med*, **10**(5), 48–56.
9. Deng GE, Cassileth BR, Cohen L, *et al.* (2007) Integrative oncology practice guidelines. *J Soc Integr Oncol*, **5**(2), 65–84.
10. Frenkel M, Ben-Arye E (2008) Communicating with patients about the use of complementary and integrative medicine in cancer care. In: Cohen L, Markman M (eds), *Integrative Oncology: Incorporating Complementary Medicine into Conventional Care.* Totowa, NJ: Humana Press.
11. Frenkel M, Cohen L (2008) Incorporating complementary and integrative medicine in a comprehensive cancer center. *Hematol Oncol Clin North Am*, **22**(4), 727–36.
12. Ernst E, Cassileth BR (1998) The prevalence of complementary/alternative medicine in cancer. *Cancer*, **83**(4) 777–82.
13. Richardson MA, Sanders T, Palmer JL, Greisinger A, Singletary SE (2005) Complementary/alternative medicine in a comprehensive cancer center and the implications for oncology. *J Clin Oncol*, **18**(13), 2505–14.
14. Vapiwala N, Mick R, Hampshire MK, Metz JM, DeNittis AS (2006) Patient initiation of complementary and alternative medical therapies (CAM) following cancer diagnosis. *Cancer J*, **12**(6), 467–74.

15. Ben-Arye E, Bar-Sela G, Frenkel M, Kuten A, Hermoni D (2006) Is a biopsychosocial–spiritual approach relevant to cancer treatment? A study of patients and oncology staff members on issues of complementary medicine and spirituality. *Support Care Cancer*, **14**(2), 147–52.
16. Yates JS, Mustian KM, Morrow GR, *et al.* (2005) Prevalence of complementary and alternative medicine use in cancer patients during treatment. *Support Care Cancer*, **13**(10), 806–11.
17. Boon HS, Olatunde F, Zick SM (2007) Trends in complementary/alternative medicine use by breast cancer survivors: comparing survey data from 1998 and 2005. *BMC Women's Health*, **7**, 4.
18. Mao JJ, Farrar JT, Xie SX, Bowman MA, Armstrong K (2007) Use of complementary and alternative medicine and prayer among a national sample of cancer survivors compared to other populations without cancer. *Complement Ther Med*, **15**(1), 21–9.
19. Verhoef MJ, Balneaves LG, Boon HS, Vroegindewey A (2005) Reasons for and characteristics associated with complementary and alternative medicine use among adult cancer patients: a systematic review. *Integr Cancer Ther*, **4**(4), 274–86.
20. Paltiel O, Avitzour M, Peretz T, *et al.* (2001) Determinants of the use of complementary therapies by patients with cancer. *J Clin Oncol*, **19**(9), 2439–48.
21. Von Gruenigen VE, White LJ, Kirven MS, Showalter AL, Hopkins MP, Jenison EL (2001) A comparison of complementary and alternative medicine use by gynecology and gynecologic oncology patients. *Int J Gynecol Cancer*, **11**(3), 205–9.
22. Eng J, Ramsum D, Verhoef M, Guns E, Davison J, Gallagher R (2003) A population-based survey of complementary and alternative medicine use in men recently diagnosed with prostate cancer. *Integr Cancer Ther*, **2**(3), 212–6.
23. Richardson MA, Mâsse LC, Nanny K, Sanders C (2004) Discrepant views of oncologists and cancer patients on complementary/alternative medicine. *Support Care Cancer*, **12**(11), 797–804.
24. Lewith GT, Broomfield J, Prescott P (2002) Complementary cancer care in Southampton: a survey of staff and patients. *Complement Ther Med*, **10**(2), 100–6.
25. Brazier A, Cooke K, Moravan V (2008) Using mixed methods for evaluating an integrative approach to cancer care: a case study. *Integr Cancer Ther*, **7**(1), 5–17.
26. Risberg T, Bremnes Y, Kolstad A, *et al.* (2004) [Should complementary therapies be offered in hospitals?] *Tidsskr Nor Laegeforen*, **124**(23), 3078–80.
27. Wigmore A (1984) *The Hippocrates Diet and Health Program: A Natural Diet and Health Program for Weight Control, Disease Prevention and Life Extension.* New York: Avery.
28. Bar-Sela G, Tsalic M, Fried G, Goldberg H (2007) Wheat grass juice may improve hematological toxicity related to chemotherapy in breast cancer patients: a pilot study. *Nutr Cancer*, **58**(1), 43–8.
29. Kushi LH, Cunningham JE, Hebert JR, Lerman RH, Bandera EV, Teas J (2001) The macrobiotic diet in cancer. *J Nutr*, **131**(11 Suppl), 3056S–64S.
30. Carter JP, Saxe GP, Newbold V, Peres CE, Campeau RJ, Bernal-Green L (1993) Hypothesis: dietary management may improve survival from nutritionally linked cancers based on analysis of representative cases. *J Am Coll Nutr*, **12**(3), 209–26.
31. Complementary/Integrative Medicine, The University of Texas M. D. Anderson Cancer Center. *Nutrition & Special Diets: Macrobiotics.* Available at: http://www.mdanderson.org/departments/cimer/display.cfm?id=24B21F93-82E8-4A5D-82032F14FCFA97DE&method=displayFull&pn=6EB86A59-EBD9-11D4-810100508B603A14 (accessed 29 August 2008).
32. Gerson M (1978) The cure of advanced cancer by diet therapy: a summary of 30 years of clinical experimentation. *Physiol Chem Phys*, **10**(5), 449–64.
33. Complementary/Integrative Medicine, The University of Texas M. D. Anderson Cancer Center. *Nutrition & Special Diets: Gerson Program.* Available at: http://www.mdanderson.org/departments/cimer/display.cfm?id=6293C02A-4E0E-11D5-811800508B603A14&method=displayFull&pn=6EB86A59-EBD9-11D4-810100508B603A14 (accessed 29 August 2008).

34. Hickok JT, Roscoe JA, Morrow GR, Ryan JL (2007) A phase II/III randomized, placebo-controlled, double-blind clinical trial of ginger (*Zingiber officinale*) for nausea caused by chemotherapy for cancer: a currently accruing URCC CCOP cancer control study. *Support Cancer Ther*, **4**(4), 247–50.
35. Cheng JH, Chang G, Wu WY (2001) A controlled clinical study between hepatic arterial infusion with embolized curcuma aromatic oil and chemical drugs in treating primary liver cancer. *Zhongguo Zhong Xi Yi Jie He Za Zhi*, **21**(3), 165–7.
36. Bettuzzi S, Brausi M, Rizzi F, Castagnetti G, Peracchia G, Corti A (2006) Chemoprevention of human prostate cancer by oral administration of green tea catechins in volunteers with high-grade prostate intraepithelial neoplasia: a preliminary report from a one-year proof-of-principle study. *Cancer Res*, **66**(2), 1234–40.
37. World Cancer Research Fund/American Institute for Cancer Research (2007) *Food, Nutrition, Physical Activity and the Prevention of Cancer: A Global Perspective*. Washington, DC: American Institute for Cancer Research.
38. Beliveau R, Gingras D (2007) Role of nutrition in preventing cancer. *Can Fam Physician*, **53**(11), 1905–11.
39. Park EJ, Pezzuto JM (2002) Botanicals in cancer chemoprevention, *Cancer Metastasis Rev*, **21**, 231–55.
40. Aggarwal BB, Bhardwaj A, Aggarwal RS, Seeram NP, Shishodia S, Takada Y (2004) Role of resveratrol in prevention and therapy of cancer: preclinical and clinical studies. *Anticancer Res*, **24**, 3–21.
41. Mertens-Talcott SU, Percival SS (2005) Ellagic acid and quercetin interact synergistically with resveratrol in the induction of apoptosis and cause transient cell cycle arrest in human leukemia cells. *Cancer Lett*, **218**, 141–51.
42. Agricultural Research Service, U.S. Department of Agriculture. *USDA National Nutrient Database for Standard Reference*, release 20 nutrient lists. Available at: http://www.ars.usda.gov/Main/docs.htm?docid=15869 (accessed 24 September 2008).
43. Seely D, Mills EJ, Wu P, Verma S, Guyatt GH (2005) The effects of green tea consumption on incidence of breast cancer and recurrence of breast cancer: a systematic review and meta-analysis. *Integr Cancer Ther*, **4**(2), 144–55.
44. Cui Y, Shu XO, Gao YT, Cai H, Tao MH, Zheng W (2006) Association of ginseng use with survival and quality of life among breast cancer patients. *Am J Epidemiol*, **163**(7), 645–53.
45. Trock BJ, Hilakivi-Clarke L, Clarke R (2006) Meta-analysis of soy intake and breast cancer risk. *J Natl Cancer Inst*, **98**(7), 459–71.
46. Gautam SC, Gao X, Dulchavsky S (2007) Immunomodulation by curcumin. *Adv Exp Med Biol*, **595**, 321–41.
47. Dhillon N, Aggarwal BB, Newman RA, *et al.* (2008) Phase II trial of curcumin in patients with advanced pancreatic cancer. *Clin Cancer Res*, **14**(14), 4491–9.
48. Shoba G, Joy D, Joseph T, Majeed M, Rajendran R, Srinivas PS (1998) Influence of piperine on the pharmacokinetics of curcumin in animals and human volunteers. *Planta Med*, **64**(4), 353–6.
49. Bezerra DP, de Castro FO, Alves AP, *et al.* (2008) In vitro and in vivo antitumor effect of 5-FU combined with piplartine and piperine. *J Appl Toxicol*, **28**(2), 156–63.
50. Ellison N, Loprinzi CL, Kugler J, *et al.* (1997) Phase III placebo-controlled trial of capsaicin cream in the management of surgical neuropathic pain in cancer patients. *J Clin Oncol*, **15**(8), 2974–80.
51. Levine ME, Gillis MG, Koch SY, Voss AC, Stern RM, Koch KL (2008) Protein and ginger for the treatment of chemotherapy-induced delayed nausea. *J Altern Complement Med*, **14**(5), 545–51.
52. Millen AE, Dodd KW, Subar AF (2004) Use of vitamin, mineral, nonvitamin, and nonmineral supplements in the United States: The 1987, 1992, and 2000 National Health Interview Survey results. *J Am Diet Assoc*, **104**(6), 942–50.
53. Cameron E, Pauling L (1973) Ascorbic acid and the glycosaminoglycans. An orthomolecular approach to cancer and other diseases. *Oncology*, **27**(2), 181–92.

54. Hardy ML (2008) Dietary supplement use in cancer care: help or harm. *Hematol Oncol Clin North Am*, **22**(4), 581–617.
55. Block KI, Koch AC, Mead MN, Tothy PK, Newman RA, Gyllenhaal C (2008) Impact of antioxidant supplementation on chemotherapeutic toxicity: a systematic review of the evidence from randomized controlled trials. *Int J Cancer*, **123**(6), 1227–39.
56. Gansler T, Kaw C, Crammer C, Smith T (2008) A population-based study of prevalence of complementary methods use by cancer survivors: a report from the American Cancer Society's studies of cancer survivors. Cancer, **113**(5), 1048–57.
57. Sandler RS, Halabi S, Kaplan EB, Baron JA, Paskett E, Petrelli NJ (2001) Use of vitamins, minerals, and nutritional supplements by participants in a chemoprevention trial. *Cancer*, **91**(5), 1040–5.
58. Kumar NB, Hopkins K, Allen K, Riccardi D, Besterman-Dahan K, Moyers S (2002) Use of complementary/integrative nutritional therapies during cancer treatment: implications in clinical practice. *Cancer Control*, **9**(3), 236–43.
59. Bardia A, Greeno E, Bauer BA (2007) Dietary supplement usage by patients with cancer undergoing chemotherapy: does prognosis or cancer symptoms predict usage? *J Support Oncol*, **5**(4), 195–8.
60. Thomson CA, Flatt SW, Rock CL, Ritenbaugh C, Newman V, Pierce JP (2002) Increased fruit, vegetable and fiber intake and lower fat intake reported among women previously treated for invasive breast cancer. *J Am Diet Assoc*, **102**(6), 801–8.
61. Salminen EK, Lagström HK, Heikkilä S, Salminen S (2000) Does breast cancer change patients' dietary habits? *Eur J Clin Nutr*, **54**(11), 844–8.
62. Johansen R, Toverud EL (2006) [Norwegian cancer patients and the health food market—what is used and why?] *Tidsskr Nor Laegeforen*, **126**(6), 773–5.
63. Patterson RE, Neuhouser ML, Hedderson MM, Schwartz SM, Standish LJ, Bowen DJ (2003) Changes in diet, physical activity, and supplement use among adults diagnosed with cancer. *J Am Diet Assoc*, **103**(3), 323–8.
64. Maskarinec G, Murphy S, Shumay DM, Kakai H (2002) A randomized isoflavone intervention among premenopausal women. *Cancer Epidemiol Biomarkers Prev*, **11**(2), 195–201.
65. Beagan BL, Chapman GE (2004) Eating after breast cancer: influences on women's actions. *J Nutr Educ Behav*, **36**(4), 181–8.
66. Adams C, Glanville NT (2005) The meaning of food to breast cancer survivors. *Can J Diet Pract Res*, **66**(2), 62–6.
67. Reedy J, Haines PS, Steckler A, Campbell MK (2005) Qualitative comparison of dietary choices and dietary supplement use among older adults with and without a history of colorectal cancer. *J Nutr Educ Behav*, **37**(5), 252–8.
68. Jazieh AR, Kopp M, Foraida M, *et al.* (2004)The use of dietary supplements by veterans with cancer. *J Altern Complement Med*, **10**(3), 560–4.
69. Novak KL, Chapman GE (2001) Oncologists' and naturopaths' nutrition beliefs and practices. *Cancer Pract*, **9**(3),141–6.
70. Bruera E, Kuehn N, Miller MJ, Selmser P, Macmillan K (1991) The Edmonton symptom assessment system (ESAS): a simple method for the assessment of palliative care patients. *J Palliat Care*, **7**(2), 6–9.
71. Paterson C, Thomas K, Manasse A, Cooke H, Peace G (2007) Measure yourself concerns and wellbeing (MYCaW): an individualized questionnaire for evaluating outcome in cancer support that includes complementary therapies. *Complement Ther Med*, **15**(1), 38–45.
72. Maciocia G (1989) *The Foundations of Chinese Medicine: A Comprehensive Text for Acupuncturists and Herbalists.* New York: Elsevier.
73. Ji-Lin Liu, Chi-lin Liu (eds) (1995) *Chinese dietary therapy*. New York: Churchill Livingstone.
74. Boik JC (1996) *Cancer and Natural Medicine: A Textbook of Basic Science and Clinical Research.* Portland: Oregon Medical Press.

75. Wong R, Sagar CM, Sagar SM (2001) Integration of Chinese medicine into supportive cancer care: a modern role for an ancient tradition. *Cancer Treat Rev*, **27**(4), 235–46.
76. Ranade S, Paranjape MH (1999) *Ayurvedic Treatment of Common Diseases*. Delhi: Sri Satguru Publications.
77. Kienle, G S, Kiene H, Albonico HU (2006) *Anthroposophic Medicine: Effectiveness, Utility, Costs, Safety*. Stuttgart: Schattauer Verlag.
78. Horneber MA, Bueschel G, Huber R, Linde K, Rostock M (2008) Mistletoe therapy in oncology. *Cochrane Database Syst Rev*, (2)CD003297.
79. Wolff O, Husemann F (1989) *The Anthroposophic Approach to Medicine*. New York: Anthroposophic Press.
80. Steiner R (1969) *Problems of Nutrition*. New York: Anthroposophic Press.
81. Smithers DW (1964) *On the Nature of Neoplasia in Man*. Edinburgh: Livingstone.
82. Twentyman R (1989) *The Science and Art of Healing*. Edinburgh: Floris Books.
83. Evans M, Rodger I (1998) *Anthroposophical Medicine*. Edinburgh: Floris Books.
84. Renzenbrink U (1990) *Diet and Cancer. An Anthroposophical Contribution to Cancer Prevention*. London: Rudolph Steiner Press.
85. Society for Cancer Research, Arlesheim, Switzerland (1988) *Cookery Book from the Lukas Clinic for Patients with Cancer or Precancerous Conditions*. London: Rudolph Steiner Press.
86. Schmidt G (1980) *The Dynamics of Nutrition*. Wyoming: Bio-dynamic Literature.
87. Kushi LH, Byers T, Doyle C, *et al.* (2006) American Cancer Society guidelines on nutrition and physical activity for cancer prevention: reducing the risk of cancer with healthy food choices and physical activity. *CA Cancer J Clin*, **56**(5), 254–81; quiz 313–4. Erratum (2007): *CA Cancer J Clin*, **57**(1), 66.
88. Brown JK, Byers T, Doyle C, *et al.* (2003) Nutrition and physical activity during and after cancer treatment: an American Cancer Society guide for informed choices. *CA Cancer J Clin*, **53**(5), 268–91.
89. Graziano F, Bisonni R, Catalano V, *et al.* (2002) Potential role of levocarnitine supplementation for the treatment of hemotherapy-induced fatigue in non-anaemic cancer patients. *Br J Cancer*, **86**(12),1854–7.
90. Cruciani RA, Dvorkin E, Homel P, *et al.* (2006) Safety, tolerability and symptom outcomes associated with L-carnitine supplementation in patients with cancer, fatigue, and carnitine deficiency: a phase I/II study. *J Pain Symptom Manag*, **32**(6), 551–9.
91. Cruciani RA, Dvorkin E, Homel P, *et al.*. L-Carnitine supplementation in patients with advanced cancer and carnitine deficiency: a double-blind, placebo-controlled study. *J Pain Sympt Manag*, 2008 Sep 20.
92. Yeom CH, Jung GC, Song KJ (2007) Changes of terminal cancer patients' health-related quality of life after high dose vitamin C administration. *J Korean Med Sci*, **22**(1), 7–11.
93. Cerchietti LC, Navigante AH, Castro MA (2007) Effects of eicosapentaenoic and docosahexaenoic n-3 fatty acids from fish oil and preferential Cox-2 inhibition on systemic syndromes in patients with advanced lung cancer. *Nutr Cancer*, **59**(1), 14–20.
94. Moses AW, Slater C, Preston T, Barber MD, Fearon KC (2004) Reduced total energy expenditure and physical activity in cachectic patients with pancreatic cancer can be modulated by an energy and protein dense oral supplement enriched with n-3 fatty acids. *Br J Cancer*, **90**(5), 996–1002.
95. Colomer R, Moreno-Nogueira JM, Garcia-Luna PP, *et al.* (2007) N-3 fatty acids, cancer and cachexia: a systematic review of the literature. *Br J Nutr*, **97**(5), 823–31.
96. Topkan E, Yavuz MN, Onal C, Yavuz AA (2008) Prevention of acute radiation-induced esophagitis with glutamine in non-small cell lung cancer patients treated with radiotherapy: evaluation of clinical and dosimetric parameters. *Lung Cancer* [Epub ahead of print].
97. May PE, Barber A, D'Olimpio JT, Hourihane A, Abumrad NN (2002) Reversal of cancer-related wasting using oral supplementation with a combination of beta-hydroxy-beta-methylbutyrate, arginine, and glutamine. *Am J Surg*, **183**(4), 471–9.

98. Agteresch HJ, Dagnelie PC, van der Gaast A, Stijnen T, Wilson JH (2000) Randomized clinical trial of adenosine 5'-triphosphate in patients with advanced non-small-cell lung cancer. *J Natl Cancer Inst*, **92**(4), 321–8.

99. Anderson PM, Schroeder G, Skubitz KM (1998) Oral glutamine reduces the duration and severity of stomatitis after cytotoxic cancer chemotherapy. *Cancer*, **83**(7), 1433–9.

100. Pytlik R, Benes P, Patorkova M, *et al.* (2002) Standardized parenteral alanyl-glutamine dipeptide supplementation is not beneficial in autologous transplant patients: a randomized, double-blind, placebo controlled study. *Bone Marrow Transplant*, **30**, 953–61.

101. Osterlund P, Ruotsalainen T, Korpela R, *et al.* (2007) Lactobacillus supplementation for diarrhoea related to chemotherapy of colorectal cancer: a randomised study. *Br J Cancer*, **97**(8), 1028–34.

102. Delia P, Sansotta G, Donato V, *et al.* (2007) Use of probiotics for prevention of radiation-induced diarrhea. *World J Gastroenterol*, **13**(6), 912–5.

103. Pace A, Savarese A, Picardo M, *et al.* (2003) Neuroprotective effect of vitamin E supplementation in patients treated with cisplatin chemotherapy. *J Clin Oncol*, **21**(5), 927–31.

104. Cerchietti LC, Navigante AH, Lutteral MA, *et al.* (2006) Double-blinded, placebo-controlled trial on intravenous L-alanyl-L-glutamine in the incidence of oral mucositis following chemoradiotherapy in patients with head-and-neck cancer. *Int J Radiat Oncol Biol Phys*, **65**(5), 1330–7.

105. Okuno SH, Woodhouse CO, Loprinzi CL, *et al.* (1999) Phase III controlled evaluation of glutamine for decreasing stomatitis in patients receiving fluorouracil (5-FU)-based chemotherapy. *Am J Clin Oncol*, **22**(3), 258–61.

106. Kabat-Zinn J (1990) *Full Catastrophe Living: Using the Wisdom of Your Body and Mind to Face Stress, Pain, and Illness.* New York: Delacorte Press.

Part 9

Exercise

Chapter 26

Exercise therapy

Lee W. Jones

Introduction

Regular exercise has been recognized to confer health benefits since antiquity.[1–4] Over the past century, a wealth of literature has accumulated describing the benefits of exercise in healthy as well as diseased adult populations.[5] The investigation of exercise in adults diagnosed with malignant diseases has received much less attention.[6] Over the past decade, however, there has been growing recognition and acceptance of the role of exercise following a cancer diagnosis. This chapter will provide a comprehensive overview of the research evidence supporting the role of exercise following a cancer diagnosis, with a view towards future directions in this rapidly growing area of research. Finally, exercise testing and prescription recommendations will be provided based on the current evidence base.

Physical activity, exercise, and cardiorespiratory fitness

The terms physical activity, exercise, and physical fitness are often used interchangeably in the literature, although these terms are distinct and describe different entities. Physical activity is defined as any bodily movement produced by the skeletal muscles which results in a substantial increase in energy expenditure over resting levels.[7] Leisure-time physical activity is defined as activity undertaken during discretionary time, with the key element being personal choice.[7] This form of physical activity is often contrasted with occupational and household physical activity. Exercise is defined as a form of leisure-time physical activity that is performed on a repeated basis over an extended period of time (i.e. exercise training) with the intention of improving fitness, performance, or health. An exercise training prescription typically includes activity mode (e.g. walking, running, swimming, etc.), volume (i.e. frequency, intensity, and duration), progression, and context (i.e. physical and social environment). Cardiorespiratory fitness is defined as the ability to perform muscular work satisfactorily and commonly includes components of body composition, cardiorespiratory fitness, muscular fitness, flexibility, and agility/balance.[7]

Health benefits of exercise

The first pioneering study indicating that a lifestyle encompassed by high levels of physical activity might protect against coronary heart disease was conducted in early 1950s. In this seminal 'natural experiment', Morris *et al.* studied the drivers and conductors of the famous London buses and found that the conductors, with physically active occupations, had significantly lower total incidence of coronary heart disease relative to the drivers, with physically inactive occupations.[8,9] Later, Paffenbarger *et al.* reported a strong inverse relationship between energy cost requirements of the San Francisco longshoremen (dock workers) and incidence of major risk factors for heart disease.[10] Since these early studies, numerous large-scale, prospective studies with long-term follow-up have investigated the relationship between self-reported physical activity as well as objective measures of cardiorespiratory fitness and the risk of cardiovascular and all-cause mortality across a broad range of apparently healthy populations as well as clinic diseased populations.[5] Overall, increased levels of physical activity and cardiorespiratory fitness are strongly inversely associated with the risk of cardiovascular and all-cause mortality, with average risk reductions between 20% and 50% relative to sedentary individuals for both men and women.[5] For example, Blair *et al.* found that age-adjusted all-cause mortality rates declined significantly across increasing physical fitness quintiles in both men and women.[11] These findings remained significant even after statistical adjustment for additional known risk factors for survival (e.g. age, smoking status, cholesterol level, systolic blood pressure, fasting blood glucose level, etc.).[11] Further investigations by Blair *et al.*[12] and Lee *et al.*[13] confirmed these observations. Myers *et al.*[14] confirmed and extended these earlier findings by examining the mortality rates in more than 6000 men referred for treadmill exercise testing. After adjustment for age, exercise capacity was the strongest predictor of risk of death among both normal subjects and those with cardiovascular disease. Moreover, each 1 MET (metabolic equivalent; 1 MET is defined as the energy expended in sitting quietly, which is the equivalent to a body oxygen consumption of about 3.5 ml/kg body weight/min for an average adult) increase in exercise capacity conferred a 12% improvement in survival. These findings were replicated among women by Gulati *et al.*[15,16] who reported that a 1-MET increase in cardiorespiratory fitness conferred a 17% improvement in survival.

The impressive prognostic ability of physical activity and cardiorespiratory fitness on mortality is mediated by favourable effects on cardiovascular risk factors. A wealth of epidemiological and experimental data exists demonstrating that regular physical activity and exercise training interventions cause significant improvements in body composition (e.g. reduced abdominal adiposity and improved weight control), lipid profile (e.g. reductions in triglyceride and low-density lipoprotein levels, increases in high-density lipoprotein, and decreased LDL:HDL ratio), blood pressure, markers of glucose–insulin homeostasis (e.g. insulin sensitivity, glycosylated haemoglobin, and fasting glucose), systemic inflammation, endothelial function, cardiac function, and blood coagulation.[5] Accordingly, regular exercise is of fundamental biological significance to maintain normal physiological genome regulation and optimize health and longevity in human beings.[4]

Exercise across the cancer continuum

Exercise and cancer prevention

More than 100 epidemiological studies have now been published investigating the association between occupational and non-occupational physical activity and the primary risk of several forms of cancer.[17–21] Overall, the putative evidence indicates that regular physical activity, achieved through occupational or non-occupational activity, is associated with reductions in the incidence of certain forms of cancer. The evidence is most compelling for breast and colon cancer.[22] Specifically, systematic reviews conclude that moderate intensity physical activity (>4.5 MET; e.g. brisk walking) confers greater risk reduction than physical activity performed at lower intensities. Physically active men and women exhibited a 30–40% reduction in the relative risk of colon cancer, and physically active women a 20–30% reduction in the relative risk of breast cancer compared with their sedentary counterparts.[22]

Commonly cited postulated mechanisms underlying the favourable effects of exercise on the prevention of cancer include modulation of metabolic (e.g. markers of insulin homeostasis) and sex steroid (e.g. estrogen) hormone levels, improvements in immune surveillance, and reduced systemic inflammation and oxidative damage.[23] However, direct evidence to support these mechanisms is currently lacking. As an initial step, McTiernan *et al.* investigated the effects of a one-year moderate intensity physical activity intervention on sex steroid hormone levels and multiple related markers (e.g. body weight, immune function, quality of life, etc.) in 168 women at high risk for breast cancer (i.e. sedentary, body mass index ≥25 kg/m^2).[24] The primary trial results demonstrated that physical activity was associated with non-significant reductions in serum estrogen levels at one year, although significant reductions were found for women who decreased body fat with estrogen reductions ranging from 11.9% to 16.7%.[25] Other key findings from this trial have also been published.[26–35] Several additional large-scale randomized controlled trials investigating the effects and underlying mechanisms of exercise on the prevention of breast and colon cancer in adults at high risk for these diseases are currently underway and results are eagerly anticipated.

Exercise following a cancer diagnosis

Exercise and symptom control

The use of conventional and novel therapies is associated with a diverse range of debilitating physiological (e.g. physical deconditioning, weight gain, cardiac and pulmonary dysfunction, etc.) and psychosocial (e.g. fatigue, nausea, depression, anxiety, etc.) symptoms that can have profound implications on quality of life.[6] To address these concerns, in the mid to late 1980s researchers initiated the first studies to explore whether exercise training may be an appropriate intervention to mitigate chemotherapy- and radiation-induced fatigue and loss of cardiorespiratory fitness among women with early-stage breast cancer. Since these early seminal studies, numerous research groups all over the world have started to examine the efficacy of physical activity and exercise training as an adjunct supportive care intervention before, during, or following cancer therapy. Several excellent systematic reviews and one meta-analysis have evaluated the pertinent literature.[6,36–40] To summarize, most studies were conducted in breast cancer survivors with fewer studies in colorectal, non-Hodgkin lymphoma, or mixed cancer populations. All studies either tested the effects of endurance or mixed (endurance combined with progressive resistance training) exercise training programmes prescribed at a moderate–vigorous intensity (50–75% of baseline exercise capacity), 3 or more days per week, for 10–60 min per exercise session. The length of the exercise programmes lasted from 2 to 24 weeks. Major outcomes of these reports were varied and included cardiorespiratory fitness, strength, quality of life, pain, immune parameters, and depression.[36–40] Overall, these reports conclude that exercise interventions following completion of primary treatment were associated with consistent and positive effects on the following outcomes: (i) vigor and vitality; (ii) cardiorespiratory fitness; (iii) quality of life; (iv) depression; (v) anxiety; and (vi) fatigue.[36–40] Specific details on several key trials are provided herein.

One of the earliest studies was conducted by MacVicar *et al.*[41] who investigated the effects of a 10-week aerobic interval training programme on cardiorespiratory fitness, as measured by a maximal cardiopulmonary exercise test to peak oxygen consumption (VO_{2peak}), in 62 women undergoing chemotherapy for early-stage breast cancer. Following baseline cardiopulmonary exercise testing, women were stratified by VO_{2peak} and randomly allocated to aerobic interval training, placebo control (i.e. flexibility and stretching exercises), or sedentary control. Women assigned to aerobic interval training performed intermittent bouts of aerobic exercise on a cycle ergometer in a ratio of high (exercise intensity performed at highest intensity achieved during baseline exercise test) to low (65–85% of heart-rate reserve) exercise, three times a week for 10 weeks. Women assigned to placebo control performed stretching and flexibility exercises three times a week for 10 weeks. The rationale for a placebo control group was to minimize the effects of social interaction on study endpoints. Finally, women assigned to sedentary control were instructed to maintain their normal levels of exercise and not to initiate a structured exercise programme. Forty-five women completed the study (a 27% drop-out rate); results were only presented for the 45 women who completed the study. Adherence rates in the exercise and placebo-control groups were not reported. The primary endpoint was change in VO_{2peak} over the course of the study. Results indicated a 40% relative pre-post improvement in VO_{2peak} for the interval training group compared with a non-significant improvement in placebo or sedentary control groups.[41]

Another early seminal contribution to the field was conducted by Dimeo *et al.* investigating the effects of exercise in patients undergoing high dose chemotherapy followed by autologous peripheral blood stem cell transplantation for solid malignancies.[42] In the week prior to hospital admission for high dose chemotherapy, all patients underwent baseline testing involving a 12-lead electrocardiogram (ECG)-monitored treadmill exercise test to assess maximal cardiorespiratory fitness. Seventy patients were deemed eligible for study participation and were randomly assigned to aerobic training or usual care group for the duration of hospitalization. Patients assigned to aerobic training performed daily supervised interval training on a supine cycle ergometer at an intensity of ≥50% of heart rate reserve. Patients in the control group were not provided with a supervised exercise programme. On the day of hospital discharge, all patients underwent a second exercise treadmill test. The primary endpoint was cardiorespiratory fitness assessed by maximal speed achieved on the treadmill exercise test. Secondary endpoints were the incidence and severity of complications assessed according to the World Health Organization criteria. Adherence rate in the exercise group was 82%. Authors reported a statistically significant improvement in cardiorespiratory fitness with walking speed increasing 13% in the exercise group relative to the control group. Specifically, cardiorespiratory fitness declined in both groups over the course of hospitalization but by a significantly lesser degree in the exercise group. Concerning secondary endpoints, reductions in the duration of neutropenia and thrombopenia, as well as platelet transfusion rate, duration of hospitalization, and severity of pain and diarrhoea were observed in the exercise group relative to the control group.[42]

Two trials of significance in breast cancer and prostate cancer patients were published by Courneya *et al.*[43] and Segal *et al.*[44] respectively in the same issue of the *Journal of the Clinical Oncology*, which is the official journal of the American Society of Clinical Oncology. Thus the publication of two exercise articles in the same issue (with an accompanying editorial) elevated the status and growing recognition of exercise as an important adjunct therapy for cancer patients. In the first study, Courneya *et al.*[43] sought to investigate the effects of 15 weeks of supervised aerobic training on quality of life and VO_{2peak} in 53 postmenopausal breast cancer patients at least one year post definitive adjuvant therapy (i.e. radiotherapy and chemotherapy). The exercise group trained on cycle ergometers three times per week at 60–80% of baseline VO_{2peak} progressing from 15 to 35 min over a 15-week period. The control group did not train. The primary outcomes were quality of life assessed by the Functional Assessment of Cancer Therapy—Breast (FACT-B) and VO_{2peak}.

Fifty-two participants completed the trial and the adherence rate in the exercise group was 98%. Intention-to-treat analyses (i.e. inclusion of data from all initially randomized patients) revealed statistically significant differences for VO_{2peak}, peak power output, overall quality of life, happiness, fatigue, and self-esteem that favoured the exercise group. Importantly, VO_{2peak} and quality of life increased 3.4 ml/kg/min and 8.8 points respectively, in the exercise group, both of which are considered a clinically important change.[43] As part of this trial, investigators also evaluated the effects of exercise on blood biomarkers proposed to influence risk of breast cancer recurrence and overall survival in early-stage breast cancer including sex steroid hormones (total estradiol, estrone, sex hormone binding globulin), metabolic peptide hormones (insulin, glucose, insulin-like growth factor-1, insulin-like growth factor binding protein-3, IGF-1:IGFBP-3 molar ratio), and immune function. Results indicated favourable improvements in several biomarkers and these results have been published.[45–47]

In the accompanying trial, Segal *et al.*[44] examined the effects of resistance training on muscular fitness and quality of life in men with prostate cancer undergoing androgen deprivation therapy. Following baseline assessments of strength and quality of life, eligible participants ($n = 155$) were randomly assigned to resistance training ($n = 82$) or usual care ($n = 73$). The resistance training group performed nine resistance exercises three times per week at 60–70% of 1-repetition maximum for 12 weeks. The primary endpoints were fatigue and quality of life as assessed by the FACT questionnaires. Secondary endpoints were upper and lower body muscular strength (as assessed by standard load tests). A total of 135 men completed the trial and the adherence rate was 79% in the resistance training group. Intention-to-treat analyses indicated statistically significant improvements in fatigue, overall quality of life, and upper and lower body muscular strength that favoured the resistance training group.[44]

An innovative study that adopted a different use of exercise in cancer patients was conducted by Jones *et al.*[48] This phase II pilot study investigated the feasibility of aerobic training on VO_{2peak} and 6-min walk distance (6MWD) test, health-related quality of life, and biochemical markers of inflammation in 20 patients with suspected non-small cell lung cancer prior to surgical resection. Presurgical VO_{2peak} is the strongest predictor of perioperative and postoperative surgical complications, thus interventions that can improve presurgical VO_{2peak} may lead to lower risk of complications. Exercise training consisted of stationary cycling, five times a week at 60–100% of VO_{2peak} until surgical resection. Participants underwent cardiopulmonary exercise testing, 6MWD, and pulmonary function testing at baseline, immediately before and 30 days after surgical resection. Follow-up assessments were obtained for 18 (90%) before resection and 13 (65%) patients post resection. The overall adherence rate was 72%. Intention-to-treat analysis indicated that mean VO_{2peak} increased by 2.4 ml/kg/min ($P = 0.002$) and 6MW distance increased 40 m ($P = 0.003$) baseline to presurgery. Per protocol analyses indicated that patients who attended ≥80% of prescribed sessions increased VO_{2peak} and 6MWD by 3.3 ml/kg/min ($P = 0.006$) and 49 m ($P = 0.013$), respectively. Exploratory analyses indicated that presurgical VO_{2peak} decreased post surgery, but did not decrease beyond baseline values.[48]

As part of this study, the investigators also examined the effects of exercise on systemic markers of proinflammation. Systemic proinflammatory markers included intracellular adhesion molecule (ICAM)-1, macrophage inflammatory protein-1α, interleukin (IL)-6, IL-8, monocyte chemotactic protein-1, C-reactive protein), and tumour necrosis factor-α. All systemic inflammatory markers were lower following exercise training although only the change in ICAM-1 reached statistical significance. Change in cardiorespiratory fitness was not associated with change in systemic inflammatory markers.[49]

Finally, in the largest study to date, by Courneya *et al.*,[50] investigated the effects of aerobic or resistance training relative to usual care control on VO_{2peak}, body composition, and quality of life among 242 breast cancer patients undergoing adjuvant chemotherapy. Following completion of the first cycle of chemotherapy, eligible patients were randomized to usual care ($n = 82$), supervised resistance exercise ($n = 82$), or supervised aerobic exercise ($n = 78$) for the duration of chemotherapy (median, 17 weeks). The primary endpoint was cancer-specific quality of life, as measured by the FACT-Anemia scale. Secondary endpoints included fatigue, VO_{2peak}, body composition, and lymphoedema. The adherence rate was 70%. Unadjusted and adjusted mixed-model analyses indicated that aerobic exercise was superior to usual care for improving self-esteem ($P = 0.015$), and VO_{2peak} ($P = 0.006$). Resistance exercise was superior to usual care for improving self-esteem ($P = 0.018$), muscular strength ($P < 0.001$), and lean body mass ($P = 0.015$). Neither form of exercise training was associated with lymphoedema.[50]

Collectively, the current putative literature provides promising preliminary evidence of the potential role of exercise in this setting and shows that additional large-scale, well-controlled intervention studies are required. Exercise also was generally associated with a small positive effect on other outcomes of interest, such as fatigue, anxiety, and depression. Importantly, no study reported any exercise-related adverse events. However, additional large-scale, well-controlled intervention studies in other cancer populations, as well as breast cancer survivors, are required that provide a comprehensive examination of safety issues.

Exercise and survival following a cancer diagnosis

Five recent epidemiological studies have provided the first important evidence that, similar to the primary prevention setting, regular exercise may be inversely associated with the risk of recurrence and cancer-specific and overall mortality following diagnosis, although these data are limited to early-stage breast and colorectal patients.[51–55] In the first published study, Holmes *et al.* examined the association between self-reported physical activity levels and breast cancer recurrence and mortality in a cohort of 2987 female nurses participating in the Nurses Health Study who had been diagnosed with early-stage breast cancer.[51] Results indicated that women who engaged in ≥9 MET-hours per week (equivalent to brisk walking for 1 h, 5 days/week) had an unadjusted absolute mortality risk reduction of 6% at 10 years compared with women who engaged in <3 MET-hours per week (equivalent to walking at an average pace for 1 h).[51] Three MET-hours is equivalent to walking at average pace of 2–2.9 mph for 1 h. Of interest, favourable effects of regular exercise were particularly strong for women with estrogen receptor (ER)-positive breast cancer. Women with ER-positive breast cancer who engaged in ≥9 MET-hours per week had a 50% reduced relative risk of breast cancer-specific mortality relative to women who engaged <9 MET-hours per week.

Next, Meyerhardt *et al.*'s two large-scale studies investigating the relationship between self-reported in the same issue of the *JCO*. In the first study, Meyerhardt *et al.*[53] examined the influence of self-reported physical activity on recurrence or overall survival in 832 patients with stage III colon cancer. After adjustment for medical and demographic variables, preliminary results indicated that men and women who engaged in >25 MET-hours of physical activity per week had a hazard ratio (HR) for disease-free survival of 0.65 (95% CI: 0.38–1.11; *P* for trend = 0.02) compared with patients who engaged in <3 MET-hours per week of physical activity. The second study examined the association between self-reported physical activity and colorectal-specific survival and overall survival in 573 women with stage I–III colorectal cancer.[54] Compared with women who engaged in <3 MET-hours per week of physical activity, those engaging in ≥18 MET-hours per week had an adjusted HR for colorectal cancer-specific mortality of 0.39 (95% CI: 0.18–0.82) and an adjusted HR for overall mortality of 0.43 (95% CI: 0.25–0.74). Interestingly, women who increased their activity (when comparing prediagnosis to postdiagnosis values) had a HR of 0.48 (95% CI: 0.24–0.97) for colorectal cancer deaths and a HR of 0.51 (95% CI: 0.30 to –0.85) for any-cause death, compared with those with no change in activity. Two additional epidemiological studies in breast cancer patients corroborate these findings.[52,55] It is noteworthy that all studies investigating the relationship between physical activity and cancer-specific survival have relied on subjective self-report retrospective recall of physical activity behaviour, which may be unreliable.

In other areas of medicine, formalized objective measures of exercise capacity or functional capacity through cardiopulmonary exercise testing or 6MWD tests, are widely used in everyday clinical practice and have been shown to be strong predictors of survival.[11,16,56] To date, the prognostic relevance of objective measures of exercise tolerance in cancer patients has not been investigated. Nevertheless, the initial epidemiological evidence indicates that regular exercise may be associated with improved clinical outcome in patients diagnosed with breast or colorectal cancer. On the basis of these data, two large-scale trials have been launched to confirm these findings using randomized, gold standard methodology. The first study, the Lifestyle Intervention Study in Adjuvant Treatment of Early Breast Cancer (LISA) trial, is a phase III trial investigating the effects of a lifestyle intervention (i.e. dietary and physical activity intervention) on weight management in women receiving hormone therapy for ER-positive early-stage breast cancer. The second study, Colon Health and Life-Long Exercise Change (CHALLENGE) trial, is a phase III trial investigating the effects of regular exercise on recurrence and cancer-specific mortality in colorectal cancer patients. The results of these studies will address many currently unanswered questions in the field of exercise oncology research.

Biological mechanisms underlying the effects of exercise on survival following a cancer diagnosis

Commonly cited postulated mechanisms underlying the effects of exercise on survival following a cancer diagnosis include modulation of metabolic (e.g. markers of glucose–insulin homeostasis) and sex steroid (e.g. estrogen) hormone levels, improvements in immune surveillance, and reduced systemic inflammation and oxidative damage.[23] However, direct evidence supporting the mechanistic association between exercise, proposed biological pathway(s), and cancer survival does not currently exist. As an initial step, two recent randomized trials investigated the effects of exercise on metabolic and immune function in early-stage breast cancer patients.

In the first trial, Fairey *et al.*[46] randomized 53 postmenopausal early breast cancer patients to a supervised 15-week aerobic training intervention or sedentary control. Results indicated significant improvements in IGF-1 and IGFBP-3 that favoured the exercise group. There were also reductions in fasting glucose, insulin, and insulin resistance although these differences did not reach statistical significance. Using the same data set, Fairey *et al.* also investigated the effects of exercise on blood immune function including natural killer cell cytotoxic activity, whole blood neutrophil function, the phenotypes of isolated mononuclear cells, estimations of unstimulated and phytohaemagglutinin-stimulated mononuclear cell function (rate of [^{3}H]thymidine uptake), and the production of proinflammatory [interleukin (IL)-1α, tumour necrosis factor-α, IL-6] and anti-inflammatory (IL-4, IL-10, transforming growth factor-β1) cytokines. Results indicated significant improvements in a range of study endpoints that favoured the exercise group. In the second study, Ligibel *et al.*[57] randomized 101 sedentary, overweight early breast cancer patients to a home-based aerobic and resistance training programme or sedentary control for 16 weeks. Exercise training was associated with a 28% reduction in fasting insulin and a non-significant improvement in insulin sensitivity.

Together, these early results provide initial insight into how exercise associated biological adaptations may influence the development and progression of cancer. Such studies are critical to optimize the efficacy and safety of exercise for cancer patients. Moreover, elucidation of the mechanisms underlying the effects of exercise on cancer biology may lead to discovery of new cancer targets and the development of novel pharmacological therapies that may lead to further improvements in cancer survival rates.

Exercise testing guidelines

The objective assessment of cardiorespiratory fitness is a recognized outcome of major importance in numerous clinical and research applications.[58] The measurement of cardiorespiratory fitness is most commonly determined during an incremental CPET to exhaustion or symptom limitation to assess VO_{2peak}. The measurement of VO_{2peak} supplies an objective measure of cardiorespiratory fitness which varies considerably between individuals.[59–61] Formalized exercise testing is widely used in numerous clinical settings and provides a wealth of diagnostic, prognostic, and decision-making information.[58] Guidelines for optimally conducting and/or interpreting exercise tests have been issued by several national and international organizations.[58,62–65]

By contrast, the assessment of cardiorespiratory fitness, and thus use of exercise testing, is not routinely used in the clinical management of cancer patients other than to determine the preoperative physiological status (i.e. operability) of patients with pulmonary malignancies.[66–69] Jones *et al.* recently conducted a systematic literature review of studies performing formal exercise testing among adults diagnosed with cancer. Studies were evaluated relative to the American Thoracic Society/American College of Chest Physicians (ATS/ACCP) recommendations for exercise testing.[56] Overall, the reporting of exercise testing methodology and data among adults with cancer suggests that the performance of these tests does not comply with national and international quality guidelines. A more recent clinical application of exercise testing in oncology settings has been to provide an objective measure of exercise capacity in studies investigating the role of exercise interventions in cancer control.[38,70,71] Unfortunately, few studies in this arena have employed 'symptom-limited' CPET with continuous gas exchange methodology and even fewer conducted physician-supervised, ECG-monitored protocols.[56] While current evidence suggests that the risk of an exercise-associated complication in early and advanced cancer patients may be low, a significant proportion of these patients will present with impaired exercise tolerance and significant underlying disease, thereby mandating appropriate testing procedures. To this end, Jones *et al.*[56] provided practice guidelines and recommendations for the use of exercise testing in cancer patients (see Table 26.1). These recommendations are briefly summarized here.

There are several methods available to investigators that enable the objective determination of cardiorespiratory fitness (see Table 26.1). Cardiorespiratory fitness can be measured using a maximal (with direct or estimated measurement of VO_{2peak}) or submaximal exercise test. Maximal tests can be divided into two distinct categories: (1) direct measurement of VO_{2peak} via incremental CPET with gas exchange measurement, or (2) estimated measurement of VO_{2peak} using standard formulas from the highest treadmill or cycle workload achieved. Both types of maximal tests are designed for the patient to achieve volitional exhaustion or symptom limitation; both provide accurate determination of cardioresiratory fitness. The decision to conduct maximal or submaximal exercise test should be determined by careful consideration of several factors including the purpose of the research investigation, the setting, and the patient population.[56]

Purpose

In cancer patients, exercise testing has been used predominately to provide: (1) an objective determination of VO_{2peak} or submaximal prediction of cardiorespiratory fitness, or (2) exercise training prescription and cardiorespiratory fitness evaluation following therapeutic intervention. For both indications, use of CPET is recommended since it provides the most accurate assessment of cardiorespiratory fitness.[56] Despite the stark advantages of CPET, submaximal testing (without gas exchange measurement) that typically measures cardiorespiratory fitness as time to achievement of a predetermined submaximal heart rate may also be of value in clinical oncology research. Such testing may be appropriate in frail or elderly patients, or when conducting a large number of tests in a non-clinic-based setting when appropriate medical supervision is not available. In addition to providing an evaluation of cardiorespiratory fitness, submaximal tests can also be used to assess functional capacity, in terms of distance walked or time to fatigue. For example, walk tests provide a simple, safe, and cheap objective assessment that can be performed in numerous clinical and research settings.[72] Distance covered has been demonstrated to be a significant predictor of morbidity and mortality in a wide range of clinical populations.[73–76]

Table 26.1 Guidelines for exercise test methodology and results reporting in clinical oncology research

	Maximal		**Submaximal**		
	CPET	**Stress test**	**Age-predicted HR**	**6 or 12 min walk test**	**Constant load test[a]**
Modality					
Purpose	Intervention Non-intervention Exercise limitation Diagnosis (CVD) Prognosis Cardiorespiratory fitness	Intervention Non-intervention Diagnosis (CVD)	Non-intervention	Intervention Non-intervention Prognosis	Intervention Non-intervention
Setting	Clinical	Clinical	Clinical Non-clinical	Clinical Non-clinical	Clinical Non-clinical
Patient population	Operable (early stage) Inoperable (advanced stage) Undergoing therapy Off therapy Pre surgery Pre BMT	Operable (early stage) Inoperable (advanced stage) Undergoing therapy Off therapy	Operable (early stage)	Inoperable (advanced stage) Undergoing therapy Frail, elderly	Inoperable (advanced stage) Undergoing therapy Frail, elderly Skeletal myopathy Respiratory limitation
Safety eligibility criteria	ATS/ACCP guidelines	ATS/ACCP guidelines	ATS/ACCP guidelines	ATS/ACCP guidelines	ATS/ACCP guidelines
Methodology					
Equipment	Cycle ergometer Treadmill Arm ergometer	Cycle ergometer Treadmill Arm ergometer	Cycle ergometer Treadmill Arm ergometer	Walking only	Cycle ergometer
Test protocol	Ramp, individualized workloads Ramp, set workloads	Ramp, individualized workloads Ramp, set workloads	Ramp, individualized workloads Ramp, set workloads	Not applicable	Constant workload
Monitoring of response	Physician monitored 12-lead ECG Blood pressure SpO_2 RER/RQ VO_2 Ventilatory parameters	Physician monitored 12-lead ECG Blood pressure SpO_2	Heart rate Blood pressure SpO_2	Heart rate SpO_2	Heart rate Blood pressure SpO_2

(Continued)

Table 26.1 (continued) Guidelines for exercise test methodology and results reporting in clinical oncology research

	Maximal		Submaximal		
	CPET	**Stress test**	**Age-predicted HR**	**6 or 12 min walk test**	**Constant load test[a]**
Results reporting	Heart rate Blood pressure SpO_2 RER/RQ VO_2 Ventricular tachycardia O_2 pulse Ventilatory parameters Symptoms/RPE Normative data Adverse events	Heart rate Blood pressure SpO_2 Time to exhaustion METs Predicted VO_2 Symptoms/RPE Normative data Adverse events	Heart rate Blood pressure SpO_2 Time to predicted HR Symptoms/RPE Adverse events	Heart rate Blood pressure SpO_2 Distance Normative data Adverse events	Heart rate Blood pressure SpO_2 Duration Symptoms/RPE Adverse events

CPET, cardiopulmonary exercise test; HR, heart rate; CVD, cardiovascular disease; BMT, bone marrow transplantation; ATS, American Thoracic Society; ACCP, American College of Chest Physicians; ECG, electrocardiogram; SpO_2, arterial oxygen saturation; RER, respiratory exchange ratio; RQ, respiratory quotient; VO_2, peak oxygen consumption; MET, metabolic equivalent; RPE, rate of perceived exertion.
[a]Can only be performed following a CPET.
Adapted from Jones *et al.* (Jones, Eves *et al.* 2008), with permission from Elsevier.

Setting

In non-clinical settings, submaximal tests may be desirable since CPETs are relatively expensive, require specialized personnel and equipment, and medical supervision. However, even submaximal tests should only be conducted among cancer patients at 'low risk' of exercise-related adverse event. Submaximal tests may also be particularly useful for exercise promotion studies to provide complementary, objective data on change in cardiorespiratory fitness/functional capacity associated with change in exercise behaviour (assessed by self-report or other tools).[56]

Patient population

CPET is the logical choice for the majority of cancer patients who typically are older and commonly present with concomitant comorbid disease that may limit exercise tolerance.[56,77] Further, oncology patients receive a broad range of locoregional and systemic therapies that may simultaneously adversely affect several steps in O_2 transport (i.e. pulmonary diffusion capacity, cardiovascular O_2 delivery, and oxidative phosphorylation).[78]

Exercise testing safety

Jones *et al.*[56] reported that maximal and submaximal exercise testing is a relatively safe procedure, with adverse events being reported <15% of all studies with no reported exercise test-related deaths. However, less than half have employed maximal CPET procedures and even fewer have conducted physician-monitored, ECG protocols. The ATS/ACCP report that the risk of death and life-threatening complications during exercise testing is 2–5 per 100 000 tests.[58] Maximal, particularly submaximal, exercise testing is a relatively safe procedure, especially in patients

Table 26.2 Relative intensities for aerobic exercise prescription (for activities lasting up to 60 min)

Intensity	%HRR	$\%HR_{max}$	RPE	RPE	Breathing rate	Body temperature	Example activity
Very light effort	<20	<50	<10	<2	Normal	Normal	Dusting
Light effort[a]	20–39	50–63	10–11	2–3	Slight increase	Start to feel warm	Light gardening
Moderate effort[a]	40–59	64–76	12–13	4–6	Greater increase	Warmer	Brisk walking
Vigorous effort[a]	60–84	77–93	14–16	7–8	More out of breath	Quite warm	Jogging
Very hard effort	>84	>93	17–19	9	Greater increase	Hot	Running fast
Maximal effort	100	100	20	10	Completely out of breath	Very hot/ perspiring heavily	Sprinting all-out

HRR, heart rate reserve; HR, heart rate; RPE, rate of perceived exertion.
[a]Range required for health.
Adapted from Warburton *et al.*;[79] Health Canada;[80] Medicine ACoS;[81] and Howley.[82]

without significant underlying disease. However, the risk of an exercise test-related event may be elevated in cancer patients due to the effects of the disease and related therapy on pathophysiological mechanisms of the exercise response and the high proportion of patients presenting with significant concomitant comorbid disease.[78] Thus, appropriate screening and testing procedures are mandated.[56]

Exercise prescription guidelines

No study to date has investigated the differential effects of exercise training performed at different intensities, duration, frequency, or length on cardiorespiratory fitness and related endpoints in cancer patients. There is currently no evidence to indicate that a higher frequency of exercise training, or interventions conducted for a greater length of time, result in more favourable outcomes. Based on current evidence, therefore, the application of standard exercise prescription guidelines for healthy adults issued by the American College of Sports Medicine (ASCM) and Centers for Disease Control and Prevention (CDC) (exercise on ≥5 days per week, for 30–45 min per session, at a moderate to vigorous intensity) appear prudent for cancer patients both during and following cancer therapy (see Tables 26.2–26.3). Clearly, much more research is required before the development of cancer-specific, treatment-specific, or cancer-site-specific exercise guidelines become a reality. In the interim, the development of any exercise prescription should be personalized to each individual based on the specific medical and demographic characteristics including the type of cancer, extent of disease, current cytotoxic or supportive care therapy, and concomitant comorbid disease.

Conclusions

Research as well as clinical interest in the role of exercise following a cancer diagnosis has increased remarkably and is likely to increase even further over the next decade with the emergence and increasing importance of cancer survivorship. Although much work remains to be done, the current literature provides sufficient evidence to suggest that exercise is a safe and well-tolerated supportive intervention that oncologists can recommend to their patients during and/or following

Table 26.3 General intensity classification for resistance activities and example activities of daily living for older adults

Intensity classification	Resistance activities (%1RM)	Example activities
Very light effort	<30	Watering the lawn or garden
Light effort	30–49	General house cleaning Ironing
Moderate effort	50–69	Raking leaves Vacuuming
Hard effort	70–84	Wood splitting Shovelling snow
Very hard effort	>84	Carrying groceries upstairs
Maximal effort	100	Lifting a heavy load that you can only lift once

%1RM, percentage of one repetition maximum.
Adapted from Warburton;[83] adapted from information provided by Warburton *et al.*[79] and ACSM.[83]

the completion of primary therapy. Building on the recent epidemiological findings indicating that exercise may be associated with substantial improvements in survival following a cancer diagnosis, the next generation of research using randomized designs to confirm these findings integrated with correlative science studies to elucidate underlying mechanisms should prove most exciting. These critical studies may provide the necessary evidence to convince policy-markers to include exercise rehabilitation as an integral component of comprehensive care for individuals diagnosed with cancer.

References

1. Booth FW, Laye MJ, Lees SJ, Spangenburg EE (2008) Reduced physical activity and risk of chronic disease: the biology behind the consequences. *Eur J Appl Physiol*, **102**(4), 381–90.
2. Lees SJ, Booth FW (2005) Physical inactivity is a disease. *World Rev Nutr Diet*, **95**, 73–9.
3. Lees SJ, Booth FW (2004) Sedentary death syndrome. *Can J Appl Physiol*, **29**(4), 447–60; discussion 444–6.
4. Booth FW, Chakravarthy MV, Spangenburg EE (2002) Exercise and gene expression: physiological regulation of the human genome through physical activity. *J Physiol* **543**, 399–411.
5. Warburton DE, Nicol CW, Bredin SS (2006) Health benefits of physical activity: the evidence. *Can Med Assoc J*, **174**(6), 801–9.
6. Jones LW, Demark-Wahnefried W (2006) Diet, exercise, and complementary therapies after primary treatment for cancer. *Lancet Oncol*, **7**(12), 1017–26.
7. Bouchard C, Shephard RJ, Stephens T (1994) *Physical activity, Fitness and Health. International Proceedings and Consenus Statement*. Champaign, IL: Human Kinetics.
8. Morris JN, Heady JA, Raffle PA, *et al.* (1953) Coronary heart-disease and physical activity of work. *Lancet*, **265**(6795), 1053–7; contd.
9. Morris JN, Heady JA, Raffle PA, *et al.* (1953) Coronary heart-disease and physical activity of work. *Lancet*, **265**(6796), 1111–20; concl.
10. Paffenbarger RS, Hale WE (1975) Work activity and coronary heart mortality. *N Engl J Med*, **292**(11), 545–50.
11. Blair SN, Kohl HW, 3rd, Barlow CE, *et al.* (1989) Physical fitness and all-cause mortality. A prospective study of healthy men and women. *J Am Med Assoc*, **262**(17), 2395–401.

12. Blair SN, Kohl HW, 3rd, Paffenbarger RS Jr, *et al.* (1995) Changes in physical fitness and all-cause mortality. A prospective study of healthy and unhealthy men. *J Am Med Assoc*, **273**(14), 1093–8.
13. Lee CD, Blair SN, Jackson AS (1999) Cardiorespiratory fitness, body composition, and all-cause and cardiovascular disease mortality in men. *Am J Clin Nutr*, **69**(3), 373–80.
14. Myers J, Prakash M, Froelicher V, *et al.* (2002) Exercise capacity and mortality among men referred for exercise testing. *N Engl J Med*, **346**(11), 793–801.
15. Gulati M, Pandey DK, Arnsdorf MF, *et al.* (2003) Exercise capacity and the risk of death in women: the St James Women Take Heart Project. *Circulation*, **108**(13), 1554–9.
16. Gulati M, Black HR, Shaw LJ, *et al.* (2005) The prognostic value of a nomogram for exercise capacity in women. *N Engl J Med*, **353**(5), 468–75.
17. Rogers CJ, Colbert LH, Greiner JW, *et al.* (2008) Physical activity and cancer prevention: pathways and targets for intervention. *Sports Med*, **38**(4), 271–96.
18. Friedenreich CM, Cust AE (2008) Physical activity and breast cancer risk: impact of timing, type and dose of activity and population subgroup effects. *Br J Sports Med*, **42**(8), 636–47.
19. Courneya KS, Friedenreich CM (2007) Physical activity and cancer control. *Semin Oncol Nurs*, **23**(4), 242–52.
20. Irwin ML (2006) Randomized controlled trials of physical activity and breast cancer prevention. *Exerc Sport Sci Rev*, **34**(4), 182–93.
21. Kruk J, Aboul-Enein HY (2006) Physical activity in the prevention of cancer. *Asian Pac J Cancer Prev*, **7**(1), 11–21.
22. Friedenreich CM, Orenstein MR (2002) Physical activity and cancer prevention: etiologic evidence and biological mechanisms. *J Nutr*, **132**(11 Suppl), 3456S–64S.
23. McTiernan A (2008) Mechanisms linking physical activity with cancer. *Nat Rev Cancer*, **8**(3), 205–11.
24. McTiernan A, Ulrich, Yancey D, *et al.* (1999) The Physical Activity for Total Health (PATH) Study: rationale and design. *Med Sci Sports Exerc*, **31**(9), 1307–12.
25. McTiernan A, Tworoger SS, Ulrich CM, *et al.* (2004) Effect of exercise on serum estrogens in postmenopausal women: a 12-month randomized clinical trial. *Cancer Res*, **64**(8), 2923–8.
26. McTiernan A, Wu L, Chen C, *et al.* (2006) Relation of BMI and physical activity to sex hormones in postmenopausal women. *Obesity (Silver Spring)*, **14**(9), 1662–77.
27. Atkinson C, Lampe JW, Tworoger SS, *et al.* (2004) Effects of a moderate intensity exercise intervention on estrogen metabolism in postmenopausal women. *Cancer Epidemiol Biomarkers Prev*, **13**(5), 868–74.
28. Campbell PT, Wener MH, Sorensen B, *et al.* (2008) Effect of exercise on in vitro immune function: a 12-month randomized, controlled trial among postmenopausal women. *J Appl Physiol*, **104**(6), 1648–55.
29. Tworoger SS, Sorensen B, Chubak J, *et al.* (2007) Effect of a 12-month randomized clinical trial of exercise on serum prolactin concentrations in postmenopausal women. *Cancer Epidemiol Biomarkers Prev*, **16**(5), 895–9.
30. Chubak J, McTiernan A, Sorensen B, *et al.* (2006) Moderate-intensity exercise reduces the incidence of colds among postmenopausal women. *Am J Med*, **119**(11), 937–42.
31. Chubak J, Ulrich CM, Tworoger SS, *et al.* (2006) Effect of exercise on bone mineral density and lean mass in postmenopausal women. *Med Sci Sports Exerc*, **38**(7), 1236–44.
32. Mohanka M, Irwin M, Heckbert SR, *et al.* (2006) Serum lipoproteins in overweight/obese postmenopausal women: a one-year exercise trial. *Med Sci Sports Exerc*, **38**(2), 231–9.
33. Frank LL, Sorensen BE, Yasui Y, *et al.* (2005) Effects of exercise on metabolic risk variables in overweight postmenopausal women: a randomized clinical trial. *Obes Res*, **13**(3), 615–25.
34. Aiello EJ, Yasui Y, Tworoger SS, *et al.* (2004) Effect of a yearlong, moderate-intensity exercise intervention on the occurrence and severity of menopause symptoms in postmenopausal women. *Menopause*, **11**(4), 382–8.
35. Irwin ML, Yasui Y, Ulrich CM, *et al.* (2003) Effect of exercise on total and intra-abdominal body fat in postmenopausal women: a randomized controlled trial. *J Am Med Assoc*, **289**(3), 323–30.

36. McNeely ML, Campbell KL, Rowe BH, *et al.* (2006) Effects of exercise on breast cancer patients and survivors: a systematic review and meta-analysis. *Can Med Assoc J*, **175**(1), 34–41.
37. Markes M, Brockow T, Resch KL, *et al.* (2006) Exercise for women receiving adjuvant therapy for breast cancer. *Cochrane Database Syst Rev* (4), CD005001.
38. Schmitz KH, Holtzman J, Courneya KS, *et al.* (2005) Controlled physical activity trials in cancer survivors: a systematic review and meta-analysis. *Cancer Epidemiol Biomarkers Prev*, **14**(7), 1588–95.
39. Friendenreich CM, Courneya KS (1996) Exercise as rehabilitation for cancer patients. *Clin J Sport Med*, **6**(4), 237–44.
40. Stevinson C, Lawlor DA, Fox KR, *et al.* (2004) Exercise interventions for cancer patients: systematic review of controlled trials. *Cancer Causes Control*, **15**(10), 1035–56.
41. MacVicar MG, Winningham ML, Nickel JL, *et al.* (1989) Effects of aerobic interval training on cancer patients' functional capacity. *Nurs Res*, **38**(6), 348–51.
42. Dimeo F, Fetscher S, Lange W, *et al.* (1997) Effects of aerobic exercise on the physical performance and incidence of treatment-related complications after high-dose chemotherapy. *Blood*, **90**(9), 3390–4.
43. Courneya KS, Mackey JR, Bell GJ, *et al.* (2003) Randomized controlled trial of exercise training in postmenopausal breast cancer survivors: cardiopulmonary and quality of life outcomes. *J Clin Oncol*, **21**(9), 1660–8.
44. Segal RJ, Reid RD, Courneya KS, *et al.* (2003) Resistance exercise in men receiving androgen deprivation therapy for prostate cancer. *J Clin Oncol*, **21**(9), 1653–9.
45. Fairey AS, Courneya KS, Field CJ, *et al.* (2005) Effect of exercise training on C-reactive protein in postmenopausal breast cancer survivors: a randomized controlled trial. *Brain Behav Immun*, **19**(5), 381–8.
46. Fairey AS, Courneya KS, Field CJ, *et al.* (2003) Effects of exercise training on fasting insulin, insulin resistance, insulin-like growth factors, and insulin-like growth factor binding proteins in postmenopausal breast cancer survivors: a randomized controlled trial. *Cancer Epidemiol Biomarkers Prev*, **12**(8), 721–7.
47. Fairey AS, Courneya KS, Field CJ, *et al.* (2005) Randomized controlled trial of exercise and blood immune function in postmenopausal breast cancer survivors. *J Appl Physiol*, **98**(4), 1534–40.
48. Jones LW, Peddle CJ, Eves ND, *et al.* (2007) Effects of presurgical exercise training on cardiorespiratory fitness among patients undergoing thoracic surgery for malignant lung lesions. *Cancer*, **110**(3), 590–8.
49. Jones LW, Eves ND, Peddle CJ, *et al.* (in press) Effects of presurgical exercise training on systemic inflammatory markers among patients with malignant lung lesions. *Appl Physiol Nutr Metab.*
50. Courneya KS, Segal RJ, Mackey JR, *et al.* (2007) Effects of aerobic and resistance exercise in breast cancer patients receiving adjuvant chemotherapy: a multicenter randomized controlled trial. *J Clin Oncol*, **25**(28), 4396–404.
51. Holmes MD, Chen WY, Feskanich D, *et al.* (2005) Physical activity and survival after breast cancer diagnosis. *J Am Med Assoc*, **293**(20), 2479–86.
52. Holick CN, Newcomb PA, Trentham-Dietz A, *et al.* (2008) Physical activity and survival after diagnosis of invasive breast cancer. *Cancer Epidemiol Biomarkers Prev*, **17**(2), 379–86.
53. Meyerhardt JA, Heseltine D, Niedzwiecki D, *et al.* (2006) Impact of physical activity on cancer recurrence and survival in patients with stage III colon cancer: findings from CALGB 89803. *J Clin Oncol*, **24**(22), 3535–41.
54. Meyerhardt JA, Giovannucci EL, Holmes MD, *et al.* (2006) Physical activity and survival after colorectal cancer diagnosis. *J Clin Oncol*, **24**(22), 3527–34.
55. Irwin ML, Smith AW, McTiernan A, *al.* (2008) Influence of pre- and postdiagnosis physical activity on mortality in breast cancer survivors: the health, eating, activity, and lifestyle study. *J Clin Oncol*, **26**(24), 3958–64.
56. Jones LW, Eves ND, Haykowsky M, *et al.* (2008) Cardiorespiratory exercise testing in clinical oncology research: systematic review and practice recommendations. *Lancet Oncol*, **9**(8), 757–65.
57. Ligibel JA, Campbell N, Partridge A, *et al.* (2008) Impact of a mixed strength and endurance exercise intervention on insulin levels in breast cancer survivors. *J Clin Oncol*, **26**(6), 907–12.

58. ATS/ACCP (2003) Statement on cardiopulmonary exercise testing. *Am J Respir Crit Care Med*, **167**(2), 211–77.
59. Wilson TM, Tanaka H (2000) Meta-analysis of the age-associated decline in maximal aerobic capacity in men: relation to training status. *Am J Physiol Heart Circ Physiol*, **278**(3), H829–34.
60. Tanaka H, Desouza CA, Jones PP, *et al.* (1997) Greater rate of decline in maximal aerobic capacity with age in physically active vs. sedentary healthy women. *J Appl Physiol*, **83**(6), 1947–53.
61. Fitzgerald MD, Tanaka H, Tran ZV, *et al.* (1997) Age-related declines in maximal aerobic capacity in regularly exercising vs. sedentary women: a meta-analysis. *J Appl Physiol*, **83**(1), 160–5.
62. Arena R, Myers J, Williams MA, *et al.* (2007) Assessment of functional capacity in clinical and research settings: a scientific statement from the American Heart Association Committee on Exercise, Rehabilitation, and Prevention of the Council on Clinical Cardiology and the Council on Cardiovascular Nursing. *Circulation*, **116**(3), 329–43.
63. Fleg JL, Pina IL, Balady GJ, *et al.* (2000) Assessment of functional capacity in clinical and research applications: An advisory from the Committee on Exercise, Rehabilitation, and Prevention, Council on Clinical Cardiology, American Heart Association. *Circulation*, **102**(13), 1591–7.
64. Palange P, Ward SA, Carlsen KH, *et al.* (2007) Recommendations on the use of exercise testing in clinical practice. *Eur Respir J*, **29**(1), 185–209.
65. Stein RA, Chaitman BR, Balady GJ, *et al.* (2000) Safety and utility of exercise testing in emergency room chest pain centers: An advisory from the Committee on Exercise, Rehabilitation, and Prevention, Council on Clinical Cardiology, American Heart Association. *Circulation*, **102**(12), 1463–7.
66. Beckles MA, Spiro SG, Colice GL, *et al.* (2003) The physiologic evaluation of patients with lung cancer being considered for resectional surgery. *Chest*, **123**(1 Suppl), 105S–114S.
67. Colice GL, Shafazand S, Griffin JP, *et al.* (2007) Physiologic evaluation of the patient with lung cancer being considered for resectional surgery: ACCP evidenced-based clinical practice guidelines (2nd edition). *Chest*, **132**(3 Suppl), 161S–77S.
68. Loewen GM, Watson D, Kohman L, *et al.* (2007) Preoperative exercise Vo2 measurement for lung resection candidates: results of Cancer and Leukemia Group B Protocol 9238. *J Thorac Oncol*, **2**(7), 619–25.
69. Wang JS, Abboud RT, Wang LM, *et al.* (2006) Effect of lung resection on exercise capacity and on carbon monoxide diffusing capacity during exercise. *Chest*, **129**(4), 863–72.
70. Knols R, Aaronson NK, Uebelhart D, *et al.* (2005) Physical exercise in cancer patients during and after medical treatment: a systematic review of randomized and controlled clinical trials. *J Clin Oncol*, **23**(16), 3830–42.
71. Galvao DA, Newton RU (2005) Review of exercise intervention studies in cancer patients. *J Clin Oncol*, **23**(4), 899–909.
72. Brooks D, Solway S, Gibbons WJ, *et al.* (2003) ATS statement on six-minute walk test. *Am J Respir Crit Care Med*, **167**(9), 1287.
73. Cahalin LP, Mathier MA, Semigran MJ, *et al.* (1996) The six-minute walk test predicts peak oxygen uptake and survival in patients with advanced heart failure. *Chest*, **110**(2), 325–32.
74. Celli BR, Cote CG, Marin JM, *et al.* (2004) The body-mass index, airflow obstruction, dyspnea, and exercise capacity index in chronic obstructive pulmonary disease. *N Engl J Med*, **350**(10), 1005–12.
75. Lederer DJ, Arcasoy SM, Wilt JS, *et al.* (2006) Six-minute-walk distance predicts waiting list survival in idiopathic pulmonary fibrosis. *Am J Respir Crit Care Med*, **174**(6), 659–64.
76. Paciocco G, Martinez FJ, Bossone E, *et al.* (2001) Oxygen desaturation on the six-minute walk test and mortality in untreated primary pulmonary hypertension. *Eur Respir J*, **17**(4), 647–52.
77. Jones LW, Eves ND, Mackey JR, *et al.* (2007) Safety and feasibility of cardiopulmonary exercise testing in patients with advanced cancer. *Lung Cancer*, **55**(2), 225–32.
78. Jones LW, Haykowsky MJ, Swartz JJ, *et al.* (2007) Early breast cancer therapy and cardiovascular injury. *J Am Coll Cardiol*, **50**(15), 1435–41.
79. Warburton DE, Nicol CW, Bredin SS, *et al.* (2006) Prescribing exercise as preventive therapy. *Can Med Assoc J*, **174**(7), 961–74.

80. Canada Health (1998) *Canada's Physical Actvity Guide to Healthy Active Living*. Ottawa.
81. Medicine ACoS (2000) *ACSM's Guidelines for Exercise Testing and Prescription*. Philadelphia: Lippincott, Williams, & Wilkins.
82. Howley ET (2001) Type of activity: resistance, aerobic and leisure versus occupational physical activity. *Med Sci Sports Exerc*, **33**(6 Suppl), S364–9; discussion S419–20.
83. Warburton DER (2008) *Laboratory Resource Manual for the Certified Personal Trainer*. Richmond, BC, Canada: Ascent Lifestyle Management Inc.
84. American College of Sports Medicine (1998) Position Stand. The recommended quantity and quality of exercise for developing and maintaining cardiorespiratory and muscular fitness, and flexibility in healthy adults. *Med Sci Sports Exerc*, **30**(6), 975–91.

Part 10

Clinical groups

Chapter 27

The cancer survivor

Wendy Demark-Wahnefried

Introduction

In 1986, the National Coalition for Cancer Survivorship defined a cancer survivor as any individual from 'the time of diagnosis, through the balance of his or her life.'[1] Given that family members, friends, and caregivers also are affected by the survivorship experience, the definition was further extended to include this broader population. In 2004, the National Cancer Institute's Office of Cancer Survivorship also formally adopted this definition, with the caveat that reports on prevalence, incidence, etc., would be confined to the proband.[1] Given this expanded definition, the entirety of this book relates to nutrition throughout the survivorship experience. Thus, to avoid overlap with other chapters, this chapter will focus exclusively on the more distal time points associated with the trajectory of early-stage disease within the cancer experience conceptual framework as outlined by Rose and O'Toole (see Figure 27.1), i.e. the stages of long term survivorship and health maintenance.[2] Indeed, the nutritional issues of these cancer survivors differ substantially from the more acute issues encountered during active treatment or those associated with end-stage cancer. Given trends toward ageing, as well as advances in early detection and treatment, the sheer number of long term cancer survivors is rapidly increasing, and the nutritional issues encountered in this patient population are fast becoming an increasingly important public health concern.

This year, approximately 1.44 million Americans will be diagnosed with cancer, and roughly two-thirds of these patients will survive at least five years. Although the latest results of the CONCORD study, a worldwide population-based study of survival from breast, prostate and colorectal cancer in 31 countries on five continents, suggest that survival rates are generally higher in the USA, as well as in greater North America, Australia, Japan and for most of Europe (Eastern Europe excluded) as compared to countries in Central and South America, Africa and Eastern Europe, these trends toward increasing survival are mirrored worldwide.[3] Indeed, it is good news that the clear majority of cancer patients, at least those diagnosed in developed countries, go on to 'cure'. However, the not-so-good news is that a substantial proportion of these survivors will return to the point of diagnosis, either via recurrence or the discovery of second malignancies.[4,5] In addition, many more will develop other comorbid conditions, such as cardiovascular disease (CVD), diabetes, or osteoporosis which also can significantly impact mortality.[4,6–12] As the number of cancer survivors increases, and as more data are gathered on the late effects associated with cancer and its treatment, the significance of health promotion within this high risk population becomes ever more important, not only to improve quality of life and reduce the burden of suffering, but also in terms of health care costs and economics.[4,13–15] In 2007, the economic burden of cancer in the USA alone totalled over US$219 billion, and while 40% of these costs were attributed to direct cancer care, the majority of expenses were related instead to increased morbidity, lost productivity, and premature mortality.[16] Therefore as the number of cancer survivors increases with each passing year, it is imperative that we address the long term health issues of

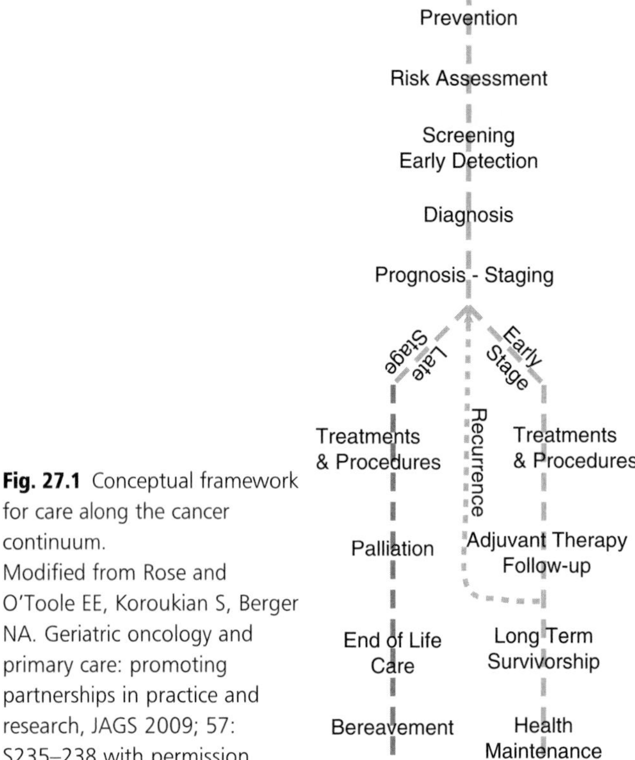

Fig. 27.1 Conceptual framework for care along the cancer continuum.
Modified from Rose and O'Toole EE, Koroukian S, Berger NA. Geriatric oncology and primary care: promoting partnerships in practice and research, JAGS 2009; 57: S235–238 with permission

cancer survivors and begin to deliver care that can prevent adverse sequelae and preserve or improve functional status and overall health.[7,17–19] Lifestyle factors, such as exercise (see Chapter 29), diet, and weight control are central to this effort.

Cancer survivors: a vulnerable and burgeoning population at increased risk

Currently, the most solid data regarding cancer survivorship derive from the US experience. In 2008, estimates indicate that cancer survivors comprise about 4% of the US population and number over 11 million.[20] This population segment is expanding rapidly owing to trends toward ageing, and advances in early detection and rates of cure.[4,9,16,20–23] Figure 27.2 illustrates the trend toward increasing numbers of cancer survivors over the past three decades; projections suggest that the number of cancer survivors will increase by roughly one million, annually.

Currently, more than half (54%) of cancer survivors are those who have had diagnoses of breast, prostate or colorectal cancer; reasons for this disease distribution are because these cancers are among the most common, and also have relatively high rates of cure (see Figure 27.3). In addition, because cancer is a disease associated with ageing, the majority (60%) of cancer survivors are aged ≥65 years (see Figure 27.4). The converging trends in cancer incidence, improved early detection and treatment, ageing, and differential mortality among genders work together to create the data shown in Figure 27.5: although most cancer survivors are within 5 years of diagnosis, cumulatively, the number of long term cancer survivors is greater and largely comprised of females (likely to be the survivors of breast cancer).

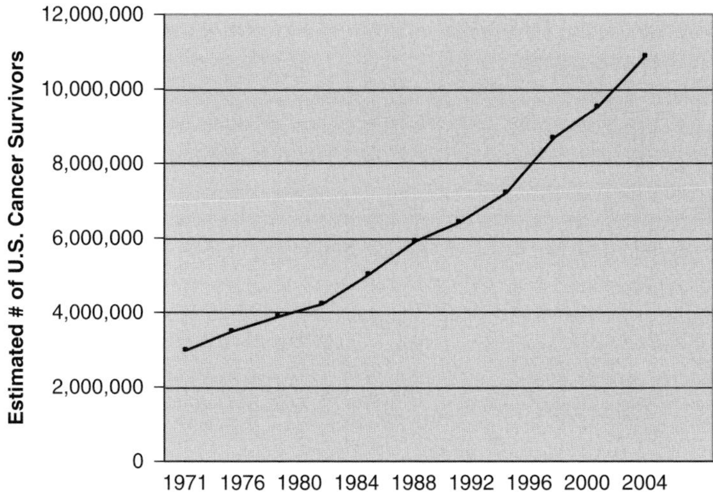

Fig. 27.2 Estimated number of cancer survivors in the USA from 1971 to 2005. Data source: Ries LAG, Melbert D, Krapcho M, *et al.* (eds), *SEER Cancer Statistics Review, 1975–2005*, National Cancer Institute, Bethesda, MD. http://seer.cancer.gov/csr/1975_2005, based on November 2007 SEER data submission, posted to the SEER website, 2008.

Survivorship should be celebrated, but it is important to acknowledge that the impact of cancer is significant and associated with several long term health and psychosocial sequelae.[4–6,9,11,16,21,24–36] Cancer survivors are high health care utilizers who have distinct health care needs.[12–15,37–42] Data clearly show that compared to others, cancer survivors are at greater risk for developing second cancers and other diseases, such as CVD, diabetes, and osteoporosis.[4–6,9,11,21,24–36] In a historic report, Brown *et al.*[38] compared more than 1.2 million patient records obtained from the Surveillance, Epidemiology, and End Results (SEER) database with those from the National Center for Health Statistics, and showed that 'the evidence that cancer patients die of non-cancer causes at a higher rate than persons in the general population was overwhelming.' In their data, the non-cancer relative hazard ratio (HR) for cancer patients was 1.37, with almost half of the

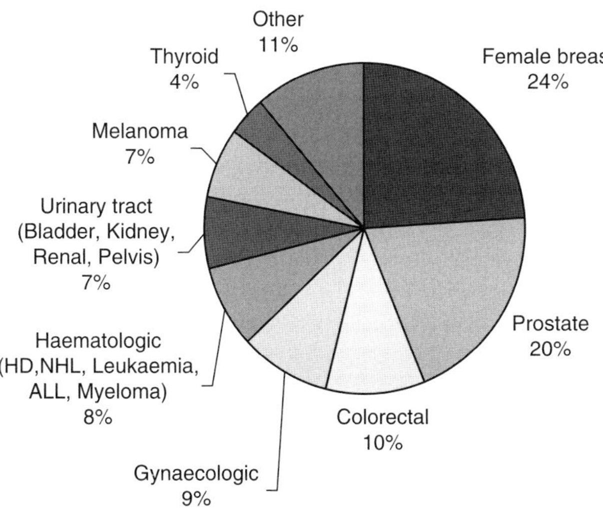

Fig. 27.3 Estimated number of cancer survivors in the USA by cancer site. Data source: see legend to Figure 27.2. HD, Hodgkin disease; NHL, non-Hodgkin lymphoma; ALL, acute lymphoblastic leukaemia.

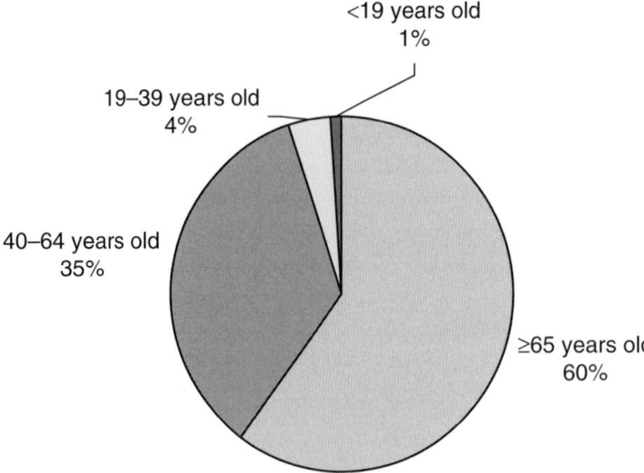

Fig. 27.4 Estimated number of cancer survivors in the USA by age. Data source: see legend to Figure 27.2.

deaths due to CVD. Data collected over the past decade confirm these findings.[12–15,37–42] Hewitt *et al.* and others[10,43–55] also report that cancer survivors have almost a two-fold increase in functional limitations which may threaten their ability to live, work and function independently, especially if they are elderly. Indeed, the costs of functional impairment alone have been estimated to 'exact an enormous toll each year on cancer survivors, their families and the American economy at large.'[39] High rates of functional decline, morbidity, and mortality among cancer survivors and their unmet needs for adequate health care ultimately culminated in a 2005 Institute of Medicine Report,[9] which called for increased efforts to this improve population's nutritional status and lifestyle factors, such as diet and physical activity.

Diet and weight control

The first nutrition guidelines that specifically addressed cancer survivors were established by the American Cancer Society (ACS) in 2003.[56] Three years later, these guidelines were updated.[57] In 2007, the American Institute for Cancer Research (AICR) in collaboration with the World Cancer Fund (WCF) updated their guidelines for cancer prevention and formally extended them for use in cancer survivors.[58] Because the risk of comorbid disease, including second cancers, is a significant concern for cancer survivors, both sets of guidelines are based heavily upon those used for

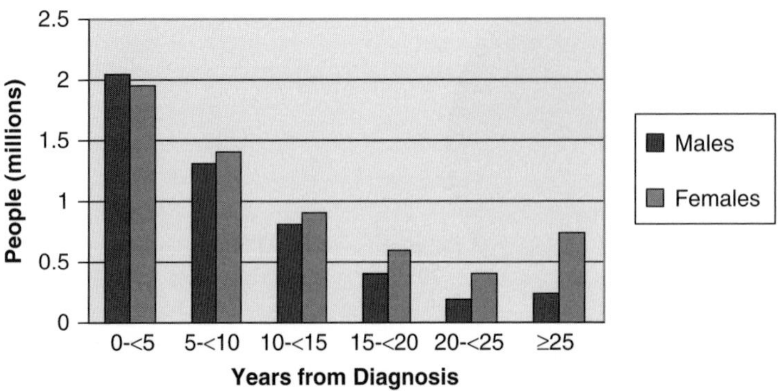

Fig. 27.5 Estimated number of cancer survivors in the USA by gender and time from diagnosis. Data source: see legend to Figure 27.2.

Table 27.1 Synthesis of nutrition guidelines for cancer survivors by the American Cancer Society (ACS) and the World Cancer Fund/American Institute of Cancer Research (WCF/AICR)[57,58]

		Recommendation
Weight	ACS	Maintain a healthy weight throughout life (balance caloric intake with physical activity, avoid excessive weight gain throughout the life cycle, and achieve and maintain a healthy weight if currently overweight or obese).
	WCF/AICR	Be as lean as possible without becoming underweight.
Dietary pattern	ACS	1. Choose foods and beverages in amounts that achieve and maintain a healthy weight. 2. Eat five or more servings of a variety of fruits and vegetables each day. 3. Choose whole grains in preference to processed (refined) grains. 4. Limit consumption of processed and red meats.
	WCF/AICR	1. Limit energy-dense foods; avoid sugary drinks. 2. Eat mostly foods of plant origin. 3. Limit intake of red meat and avoid processed meat. 4. Limit consumption of salt.
Alcohol	ACS	No more than one drink per day for women or two per day for men.
	WCF/AICR	Limit alcoholic drinks.
Supplements	ACS	Do not use supplements to protect against cancer.
	WCF/AICR	Aim to meet nutritional needs through diet alone.

primary cancer prevention, as well as those used for the prevention of other prevalent chronic diseases, such as cardiovascular disease and diabetes.[56–58] Of note, these guidelines also include recommendations for physical activity. Table 27.1 synthesizes the ACS guidelines and WCF/AICR recommendations according to common themes.

Weight management

It should be noted that weight management is the lead item in both sets of recommendations. This takes into account that although anorexia and cachexia may be of concern in selected subsets of cancer patients (i.e. those diagnosed with specific gastrointestinal, respiratory or head and neck cancers, or those diagnosed with late-stage disease) for the majority of cancer survivors, obesity and overweight are problems that are far more prevalent.[7,17–19,30,56,57,59] Indeed, data suggest that in the two largest segments of cancer survivors, i.e. survivors of breast and prostate cancer, the prevalence of overweight and obesity as indicated by a body mass index (BMI; kg/m^2) of >24.9 exceeds 70%, whereas the prevalence of underweight (BMI <18.5) is nil.[60] These data are not surprising given that obesity is a well-established risk factor for cancers of the breast (postmenopausal), colon, kidney (renal cell), oesophagus (adenocarcinoma), and endometrium.[61–63] Increased premorbid body weight and/or body weight at the time of diagnosis also has been associated with increased mortality (overall and cancer-specific) for all cancers combined, and specifically for non-Hodgkin lymphoma and multiple myeloma, as well as cancers of the breast, oesophagus, colon and rectum, cervix, uterus, liver, gallbladder, stomach, pancreas, prostate, and kidney.[64–66] Finally, additional weight gain is common during or after treatment for a variety of cancers.[30,56,57,59,67–73] Such weight gain has been found to reduce quality of life and exacerbate risk for functional decline, comorbidity, and perhaps even cancer recurrence and cancer-related death.[30,59,67,73,74] While data regarding associations between post-diagnosis weight gain and disease-free survival have been somewhat inconsistent,[56,57,59,62,68] a prospective observational study of more than 5000 women diagnosed with breast cancer within the Nurse's Health Study cohort found that breast cancer survivors who experienced increases in BMI post-diagnosis of at least 0.5 units had a significantly higher relative risk (RR) of recurrence and all-cause mortality.[74] This accumulating evidence of adverse effects of obesity in cancer survivors, plus evidence indicating that obesity has negative consequences for overall health and physical function, make weight management a priority for cancer survivors.[7,17,56–58,75–77] While the pursuit of a desirable weight can be postponed until primary treatment is complete, among patients who are overweight or obese there are no contraindications to a modest rate of weight loss (no more than two pounds per week) during treatment as long as the oncologist approves and it does not interfere with treatment.[56,57]

To date, a small number of studies have tested weight loss interventions among cancer survivors, one study being aimed at endometrial cancer survivors,[78] and the remainder targeting breast cancer survivors.[79–83] Generally these studies have been feasibility trials, with the largest enrolling 107 participants. While the earliest of these trials, conducted by de Waard *et al.*,[79] experienced difficulty with recruitment due to reported disbelief that obesity is a problem for cancer patients, more recent trials have found high levels of interest for weight loss interventions among cancer survivors, and specifically among women diagnosed with breast cancer.[73,80,81,84] In general, larger weight losses have been observed with interventions that utilize theory-driven behavioural models and group support.

Whereas energy restriction can be achieved by portion control and reducing the energy density of the diet via the substitution of low-energy density foods (e.g. water-rich vegetables, fruits, whole grains, and soups) for foods that are higher in calories,[85–87] more intensive programmes that promote energy deficits of up to 1000 calories/day may yield greater impact and improved weight status.[88] Therefore, overweight survivors may benefit from set reductions in energy intake, in combination with increased energy expenditure (via exercise).[80,81,83] Indeed, Goodwin *et al.*[81] found that exercise was the strongest predictor of weight loss among early-stage breast cancer patients who participated in a diet and exercise intervention in the year following diagnosis. A more recent observational study by Herman *et al.* found similar results.[30] Given evidence that sarcopenic obesity (gain of adipose tissue at the expense of lean body mass) is a documented side-effect of both chemotherapy and hormonal therapy,[71,73,89–92] exercise, especially resistance exercise, may be important for cancer survivors since it is considered the cornerstone of treatment for this condition. Until more is known, guidelines established for weight management in the general population should be applied to cancer survivors, and include not only dietary and exercise components, but also behaviour therapy.[56,57,62,93]

Dietary pattern

Previous research suggests that the choice of foods and their proportionate representation within an overall diet (dietary pattern) may be more important than absolute amounts.[58,59,94] Given that cancer survivors are at increased risk for other chronic diseases, guidelines suggest prudent diets that rely heavily on unrefined plant foods such as fruits, vegetables and whole grains, and in addition, the consumption of limited amounts of fat, simple sugars and red or processed meats.[9,56,57] Observational studies of breast cancer survivors (n = 2619) and colorectal cancer survivors (n = 1009) within the Nurse's Health Study cohort suggest that, as compared to survivors who reported a western-type diet (e.g. high proportional intakes of meat, refined grains, high fat dairy products, and desserts), those who reported a prudent diet (e.g. high proportional intakes of fruits, vegetables, whole grains and low-fat dairy products) had significantly better outcomes. Both studies found significant protective associations between the prudent diet and overall survival (likely owing to the impact of the low-fat, plant-based diet on CVD); however, the study by Meyerhardt *et al.* also found evidence of protection against colorectal cancer (CRC) recurrence and CRC specific mortality.[95,96]

Additional studies also suggest that diet quality during survivorship is significantly and positively associated with mental and/or physical functioning.[97,98] Such findings stem from a cross-sectional investigation on 714 breast cancer survivors participating in the Health, Eating, Activity and Lifestyle (HEAL) study, as well as another cross-sectional study of 688 elderly breast and prostate cancer survivors. Perhaps more compelling from the standpoint of being able to infer cause and effect, the results of a recent intervention trial that promoted improvements in diet quality and physical activity among 182 elderly breast and cancer survivors indeed found evidence of improved physical functioning with the multicomponent intervention.[99] While changes in functional status may be more attributed to the physical activity component of this intervention, it is important to note that these elders did not make significant improvements in their level of physical activity, whereas the intervention did result in significant improvements in diet quality.

In contrast, no differences were observed in either disease-free or overall survival in the recently completed Women's Healthy Eating and Living (WHEL) trial, which tested a low fat, high fiber and high fruit and vegetable (i.e. three fruit servings, five vegetable servings plus 16oz. of vegetable juice per day) diet against usual care among 3088 pre- and postmenopausal breast cancer patients followed over 7 years.[100] Null findings have been attributed to high baseline fruit and vegetable intakes in both study arms (mean of 7.4 servings/day), as well as an absence of weight loss, despite the low energy density diet.[101] Findings of WHEL differ markedly from the Women's Intervention Nutrition Study (WINS), in which the dietary intervention was solely focused on dietary fat restriction (<15% of total energy) and tested against a healthy diet. In WINS, 2437 postmenopausal breast cancer patients were followed for 5 years, and a significantly reduced risk of recurrence was observed [HR: 0.76; 95% confidence interval (CI): 0.60–0.98] among women assigned to the low fat diet, an effect which was even stronger among participants with estrogen-receptor-negative disease.[102] These findings, however, may have been confounded by the 6 lb weight loss observed within the low fat diet arm over the course of the study period (data which obviously reinforce the importance of weight control as a key lifestyle factor in cancer survivors).

In summary, a prudent dietary pattern may be important for quality of life and the prevention of various comorbid conditions among cancer survivors. Furthermore, the composition of the diet may also play a role in energy regulation and weight maintenance, which appears to be a key issue, not only for survivors, but also for the population as a whole.[62] Other recommendations that pertain to the avoidance of red and processed meats, as well as limiting the consumption of salty foods, are based more on the prevention of select cancers (i.e. colorectal and other aerodigestive cancers),[56–58] and for which survivors may be at greater risk given their increased susceptibility to second malignancies.[5]

Alcohol use

National data from the USA and Australia suggest that while moderate-to-heavy drinking is noted more frequently among select groups of cancer survivors (e.g. survivors of head, neck, lung and prostate cancers), alcohol consumption among cancer survivors overall is similar to that of the general population.[103–105] Furthermore, alcohol use diminishes significantly with age, and 'risky use', defined as more than two drinks per day for men and more than one drink per day for women, is noted among only 4.1% of cancer survivors aged ≥65 years.[103,104] The low prevalence of risky drinking among the majority of cancer survivors, plus the proven cardioprotective benefit of light alcohol consumption, form the basis of the recommendations established by both the ACS and the WCF/AICR.[57,58] However, continued alcohol use is strongly discouraged among survivors of renal and head and neck cancers due to significantly higher rates of treatment complications, comorbidity and second cancers.[106,107] Currently, the use of alcohol among breast cancer survivors is controversial.[57] On one hand, alcohol is associated with increased primary risk of breast cancer, in a population where risk is already high. However, data on breast cancer survivors show no increase in risk of recurrence or all-cause mortality.[57,59] Furthermore, recent findings suggest a 55% reduction in rates of ovarian cancer (95% CI: 0.2–1.0) among breast survivors who report continued alcohol use after diagnosis.[108]

Supplement use

Dietary recommendations from both the ACS and the WCF/AICR currently advocate food sources to supply needed nutrients, rather than the use of dietary supplements. Both organizations also recommend against the use of supplements for cancer control. These guidelines stem from the relatively poor performance of dietary supplements to date in clinical trials aimed at cancer prevention and control.[109] The Alpha Tocopherol and Beta Carotene (ATBC) Trial was one of the first trials to test whether dietary supplements afforded protection for individuals at high risk for cancer. After being launched on strong epidemiological evidence, as well as supportive preclinical studies, this trial was a major disappointment when findings showed that the beta-carotene arm, a food-related constituent in the same family as lycopene, was not only ineffective in reducing lung cancer incidence, it actually increased it. A second trial, the Carotene and Retinol Efficacy Trial (CARET), which had similar aims, also found similar results and was one of the few dietary intervention studies ever to employ stopping rules.[110] In another clinical trial conducted on 540 head and neck cancer patients receiving radiotherapy and randomized to 400 IU/day of vitamin E versus placebo, significantly higher all-cause mortality (HR: 1.38, 95% CI: 1.03–1.85), as well as increased cause-specific mortality was found in those who received vitamin E.[111] These findings ride on the heels of a meta-analysis by Miller *et al.*[112] which showed significantly higher ($P = 0.035$) all-cause mortality with ≥400 IU of vitamin E/day. Furthermore, recent clinical trials of folate supplementation to prevent breast cancer, as well as selenium and vitamin E to prevent prostate cancer, also have recently culminated in disappointing findings, either showing increased morbidity (in the worst case) or no harm (in the best case).[113] It is clear; however, that supplements have yet to show a protective effect in cancer populations. Some workers within the field of nutrition have speculated that single nutrient interventions may be similar to monotherapy in the treatment of cancer, and that while transformed or malignant cells might be held at bay for a brief period of time with such interventions, they are unlikely to work long term. Instead, more complex cocktails of nutrients might be needed and subsequently multivitamin preparations have become viewed as 'safer' options. However, such hypotheses were laid to rest with the reported findings from the National Institutes of Health (NIH)/American Association of Retired Persons (AARP) study ($n = 295\,344$), which found that multivitamin supplements were linked to increased risk of advanced [relative risk (RR): 1.32, 95% CI: 1.04–1.67] and fatal prostate cancer (RR: 1.98, 95% CI: 1.07–3.66) in men taking more than seven multivitamins per week.[114–117] This risk appeared strongest among men with a positive family history and those who took individual micronutrient supplements in addition to multivitamins.

In view of these research findings, clinicians should be circumspect regarding the endorsement of any nutritional supplements unless it is under the rubric of a clinical trial. Like pharmaceutical agents, it also must be borne in mind that nutritional supplements may carry a host of side-effects and cautions that may impact patient health in more immediate ways than affecting prostate cancer progression. Overdose can be dangerous, possibly fatal, particularly with trace elements and various fat-soluble vitamins. The National Institutes of Health Office of Dietary Supplements and the National Center for Alternative and Complementary Medicine (http://ods.od.nih.gov and http://nccam.nih.gov) provides a reliable source of information to both patients and providers regarding data on nutrient supplements, as well as functional foods and dietary regimens.

Survivors' health behaviour change and preferences for delivery

Levels of interest in dietary interventions

Research suggests that while most survivors attribute their cancer diagnosis to factors beyond their control (with the exception of tobacco use), they often become interested in modifying their diet and exercise behaviours post diagnosis in hopes of 'preventing recurrence'. [118–122] Surveys among adult survivor populations suggest 'extremely high to very high' levels of interest in dietary (54%) interventions.[60] These findings are remarkably similar in paediatric cancer survivor populations, with even higher levels of interest noted among their parents.[123] Thus, the cancer diagnosis may signal an opportune time or a 'teachable moment' for undertaking health behaviour change.[7,124,125] While some reviews and recent studies suggest that cancer survivors may begin to adopt healthier lifestyle practices on their own,[7,126,127] large population-based studies in the USA and Australia suggest that, for the most part, cancer survivors' health behaviours parallel those of the general population—a population marked by inactivity, overweight or obesity, suboptimal fruit, vegetable and fibre consumption, and high intakes of fat.[103–105] Similar results were found in another study that tracked lifestyle behaviours longitudinally over time in a cohort of women (n = 2321) with early-stage breast cancer.[68] These studies suggest that although many cancer patients report healthful lifestyle changes after diagnosis, these changes with may not generalize to all populations of cancer survivors, may be temporary, or may indicate that even after undertaking behaviour change, cancer survivors' behaviours are similar to those of the general population.[128] Given higher rates of comorbidity among survivors and evidence that diet affects the risk for other cancers and other chronic diseases, these recent data support a tremendous need for interventions that target the vulnerable population of cancer survivors.

Preferences, barriers and other considerations in delivering dietary interventions

While cancer survivors may have high levels of interest in dietary interventions, they may have special needs (i.e. food intolerances or digestive disorders, long term addictions to tobacco or alcohol, etc.) that must be considered if attempts to promote healthful lifestyle practices are to succeed.[129] Timing of interventions also may be of critical importance, since readiness to pursue various lifestyle changes may wax and wane along the survivorship continuum. Findings from a survey study of 978 breast and prostate cancer survivors suggest that while most survivors prefer lifestyle interventions that are initiated at the 'time of diagnosis or soon thereafter', interventions offered 'anytime' also garner high levels of interest.[60] Given evidence that levels of psychological distress after diagnosis differ in males (low initial levels which decrease significantly over time) versus females (high initial levels that decrease less precipitously), it is postulated that optimal intervention timing may differ between the sexes.[130] Thus, interventions that capitalize on moderate levels of distress (not too overwhelming, but enough to motivate behaviour change) may be gender dependent and yield the best results; however, this statement is speculative at best, and there are no firm data yet to support it. Other factors, such as concurrent demands of treatment and rehabilitation, are likely to play key roles influencing distress and readiness to pursue lifestyle change.[17,131,132] The targeted behaviour, the patients' self-efficacy in pursuing behaviour change, and various patient characteristics also are likely to influence uptake.[128,129,133] For example, in a recent study that tested the feasibility of a home-based diet and exercise intervention to prevent adverse body composition change among 90 breast cancer patients during active treatment, Demark-Wahnefried *et al.* found that whereas participants demonstrated excellent adherence to a low fat, high fruit and vegetable and calcium-rich diet, their adherence to strength training and aerobic exercise was much poorer.[134] These results differed remarkably from a smaller pilot study ($n = 10$) that tested the feasibility of a clinic-based diet and exercise programme, conducted by the same investigators, which found excellent adherence to both the diet and exercise components.[135] However, there was a much higher refusal rate for the clinic-based study (55% vs 19%), and the subjects who agreed to participate in the clinic-based programme also appeared much more fit, as indicated by a BMI mean of 24.1 vs 25.8. This comparison provides an overarching example of the biases that are inherent in conducting intervention research among cancer survivors or for that matter any population, i.e. the individuals who enroll are likely to be much different than the population for which you hope to generalize findings—bias that is accentuated with increasing demands placed on the study population (e.g. travel, time) and in accruing self-referrals vs population-based samples (i.e. those ascertained from cancer registries).[136,137]

As reviewed by Stull *et al.*,[129] most reported health behaviour interventions among cancer survivors have been conducted in self-referred or clinic-recruited samples and have utilized clinic-based interventions. Although the potential acceptability and reach for home-based interventions is notably greater than for clinic-based programmes, relatively few studies have employed this approach. Indeed, more research is necessary in this arena, especially since time and travel are well-recognized and significant barriers to participation and are likely to become even larger barriers as energy costs increase.[137] Telephone counselling has offered traditional means of addressing the barrier of distance and has been used with varying levels of success among cancer survivors, as well as in other high risk populations.[138–143] Web-based formats offer future promise; however, access issues may serve as barriers among cancer survivors who tend to be elderly.[144] Indeed, interventions that are delivered via mailed print materials receive the highest levels of interest, not only in a sample of 978 breast and prostate cancer survivors (mean age of 63 years), but also among 209 childhood cancer survivors (mean age of 19 years). Similarly, Rutten *et al.*[145] reported that cancer survivors were twice as likely to report reliance on print materials as sources of health information rather than the internet or other media sources. It is currently unknown whether these results are apt to change over time or whether there is a definite hard-set preference for print materials over computer-based venues. The salience of distance-medicine-based approaches, whether they are delivered via telephone, the mail, the web or via other home-based approaches is especially important for interventions that target highly mobile or geographically dispersed survivor populations (e.g. childhood cancer survivors) or those needing long term follow-up.

While the mode of intervention delivery is important, the use of behavioural theory to guide intervention development and evaluation is perhaps even more critical. Recent reviews however, of dietary, exercise and smoking cessation intervention trials suggest that less than one-third are theoretically based.[129] This is unfortunate since a solidly designed intervention that 'fits' behavioural theory to the targeted behaviour and the needs of the study sample not only has an increased probability of success, but also has the advantage of being perceived by participants as 'a well-conceived' study, and more likely to reduce attrition.[146–148] Among cancer survivors, the most frequently used theories for dietary interventions have been Social Cognitive Theory, the Theory of Planned Behaviour, and the Transtheoretical Model.[129,149–151] Multibehaviour interventions can particularly benefit from a solid and unified theoretical framework, which can enhance the organization and presentation of key components, and allow a systematic approach for testing issues such as behavioural sequencing.

Linking cancer survivors to diet-related interventions

The preceding sections of this chapter were devoted to reviewing some of the important health behaviours for cancer survivors, and then reviewed some of the 'what', 'where', 'when', and 'how' questions concerning intervention to improve health behaviours; the last topic remaining is 'who' should receive the intervention and 'who' should deliver it? In the realm of cancer survivorship, such interventions could benefit not only survivors (as a means of tertiary or quaternary prevention), but also family members who might be at increased risk and who may derive primary preventive benefit. In addition, family members, especially if they receive appropriate training, could serve as a source of support for interventions that target the cancer survivor.[152] Indeed, much more research is needed in both of these areas. Likewise, 'who' delivers the intervention also can make an impact, and also is an area where more research is needed. That being said, what is known is that the recommendation of the health care provider is a critical first step in motivating patients to consider lifestyle change.[153,154] Jones *et al.*[154] found that the oncologist's recommendation directly influenced perceived behavioural control and was associated with increased physical activity in a randomized controlled trial of 450 breast cancer survivors. Unfortunately, data suggest that only a minority of oncology care physicians appear to offer guidance regarding healthful lifestyle change, and report barriers, such as competing treatment or health concerns, time constraints, or uncertainty regarding the delivery of appropriate health behaviour messages.[60,155,156] Therefore, strategies are needed to efficiently and effectively bring to bear the motivational power of the physician.

Conclusions

The confluence of trends toward ageing and improved early detection and treatment have resulted in increasing numbers of cancer survivors, many of whom will become long term survivors in successive years. These trends have resulted in a paradigm shift of how the disease is viewed, as well as its nutritional management. Cancer increasingly is becoming viewed as a chronic disease. Nutrition management of the cancer survivor is still vitally important; however, the issues encountered in this population are distinctly different from those associated with acute care during active treatment or end-stage disease. The population of cancer survivors is marked, if anything, by overnutrition rather than undernutrition. The oncology care team should posture itself to capitalize on the teachable moment afforded by a cancer diagnosis to enforce the importance of weight management, and the need to obtain nutrients through a prudent, plant-based diet (not dietary supplements), in order to promote long term health and prevent comorbidity in this high risk population.

References

1. Twombley R (2004) What's in a name: who is a cancer survivor? *J Natl Cancer Inst*, **96**, 1414–15.
2. Rose JH, O'Toole EE, Koroukian S, Berger NA. Geriatric oncology and primary care: Promoting partnerships in practice and research, JAGS 2009; 57: S 235–238.
3. Coleman MP, Quaresma M, Berrino F, *et al.* (2008) Cancer survival in five continents: a worldwide population-based study (CONCORD), *Lancet Oncol*, **9**(8), 730–56.

4. Aziz NM (2007) Cancer survivorship research: state of knowledge, challenges and opportunities. *Acta Oncol*, **46**(4), 417–32.
5. Ng AK, Travis LB (2008) Second primary cancers: an overview. *Hematol Oncol Clin North Am*, **22**(2), 271–89.
6. Chapman JA, Meng D, Shepherd L, *et al.* (2008) Competing causes of death from a randomized trial of extended adjuvant endocrine therapy for breast cancer. *J Natl Cancer Inst*, **100**(4), 252–60.
7. Demark-Wahnefried W, Aziz NM, Rowland JH, Pinto BM (2005) Riding the crest of the teachable moment: promoting long-term health after the diagnosis of cancer. *J Clin Oncol*, **23**(24), 5814–30.
8. Ganz PA, Hahn EE (2008) Implementing a survivorship care plan for patients with breast cancer. *J Clin Oncol*, **26**(5), 759–67.
9. Hewitt M, Greenfield S, Stovall EL (2005) *Institute of Medicine and National Research Council: From Cancer Patient to Cancer Survivors: Lost in Transition*. Washington, DC: National Academies Press.
10. Hewitt M, Rowland JH, Yancik R (2003) Cancer survivors in the United States: age, health, and disability. *J Gerontol A Biol Sci Med Sci*, **58**(1), 82–91.
11. Oeffinger KC, Nathan PC, Kremer LC (2008) Challenges after curative treatment for childhood cancer and long-term follow up of survivors. *Pediatr Clin North Am*, **55**(1), 251–73.
12. Schultz PN, Beck ML, Stava C, Vassilopoulou-Sellin R (2003) Health profiles in 5836 long-term cancer survivors. *Int J Cancer*, **104**(4), 488–95.
13. Chang S, Long SR, Kutikova L, *et al.* (2004) Estimating the cost of cancer: results on the basis of claims data analyses for cancer patients diagnosed with seven types of cancer during 1999 to 2000. *J Clin Oncol*, **22**(17), 3524–30.
14. Ramsey SD, Berry K, Etzioni R (2002) Lifetime cancer-attributable cost of care for long term survivors of colorectal cancer. *Am J Gastroenterol*, **97**(2), 440–5.
15. Yabroff KR, Lawrence WF, Clauser S, Davis WW, Brown ML (2004) Burden of illness in cancer survivors: findings from a population-based national sample. *J Natl Cancer Inst*, **96**(17), 1322–30.
16. American Cancer Society. *Cancer Facts & Figures—2008*. Available at: http://www.cancer.org/docroot/MIT/content/MIT_3_2X_Costs_of_Cancer.asp.
17. Demark-Wahnefried W, Jones LW (2008) Promoting a healthy lifestyle among cancer survivors. *Hematol Oncol Clin North Am*, **22**(2), 319–42.
18. Jones LW, Demark-Wahnefried W (2006) Diet, exercise, and complementary therapies after primary treatment for cancer. *Lancet Oncol*, **7**(12), 1017–26.
19. Jones L, Demark-Wahnefried W (2007) Recommendations for health behavior and wellness following primary treatment for cancer. In: *Implementing Cancer Survivorship Care Planning: Workshop Summary*, pp. 166–205. Washington, DC: Institute of Medicine of the National Academies.
20. Centers for Disease Control (2008) Notice to readers: cancer survivorship. *Morb Mortal Wkly Rep*, **57**, 605–6.
21. Aziz NM, Rowland JH (2003) Trends and advances in cancer survivorship research: challenge and opportunity. *Semin Radiat Oncol*, **13**(3), 248–66.
22. Djulbegovic B, Kumar A, Soares HP, *et al.* (2008) Treatment success in cancer: new cancer treatment successes identified in phase 3 randomized controlled trials conducted by the National Cancer Institute-sponsored cooperative oncology groups, 1955 to 2006. *Arch Intern Med*, **168**(6), 632–42.
23. Ries LAG MD, Krapcho M, *et al.* (eds) (2004) *SEER Cancer Statistics Review, 1975–2004*. Available at: http://www.seer.cancer.gov/csr/1975_2004 (accessed 14 July 2008).
24. Brown BW, Brauner C, Minnotte MC (1993) Noncancer deaths in white adult cancer patients. *J Natl Cancer Inst*, **85**(12), 979–87.
25. Chen Z, Maricic M, Bassford T, *et al.* (2005) Fracture risk among breast cancer survivors: results from the Women's Health Initiative Observational Study. *Arch Intern Med*, **165**(5), 552–8.
26. Chen Z, Maricic M, Pettinger M, Ritenbaugh C, *et al.* (2005) Osteoporosis and rate of bone loss among postmenopausal survivors of breast cancer. *Cancer*, **104**(7), 1520–30.

27. Earle CC, Neville BA (2004) Under use of necessary care among cancer survivors. *Cancer*, **101**(8), 1712–9.
28. Fouad MN, Mayo CP, Funkhouser EM, Hall I, Urban DA, Kiefe CI (2004) Comorbidity independently predicted death in older prostate cancer patients, more of whom died with than from their disease. *J Clin Epidemiol*, **57**(7), 721–9.
29. Ganz PA (2001) Late effects of cancer and its treatment. *Semin Oncol Nurs*, **17**(4), 241–8.
30. Herman DR, Ganz PA, Petersen L, Greendale GA (2005) Obesity and cardiovascular risk factors in younger breast cancer survivors: The Cancer and Menopause Study (CAMS) *Breast Cancer Res Treat*, **93**(1), 13–23.
31. Jemal A, Clegg LX, Ward E, *et al.* (2004) Annual report to the nation on the status of cancer, 1975–2001, with a special feature regarding survival. *Cancer*, **101**(1), 3–27.
32. Ko C, Chaudhry S (2002) The need for a multidisciplinary approach to cancer care. *J Surg Res*, **105**(1), 53–7.
33. Meadows AT, Varricchio C, Crosson K, *et al.* (1998) Research issues in cancer survivorship. *Cancer Epidemiol Biomarkers Prev*, **7**(12), 1145–51.
34. Michaelson MD, Cotter SE, Gargollo PC, Zietman AL, Dahl DM, Smith MR (2008) Management of complications of prostate cancer treatment. *CA Cancer J Clin*, **58**(4), 196–213.
35. Rowland J, Mariotto A, Aziz N, Tesauro G, Feuer E (2004) Cancer Survivorship United Staes, 1971–2001. *Morb Mortal Wkly Rep* **53**, 526–9.
36. Schultz PN, Beck ML, Stava C, Sellin RV (2002) Cancer survivors. Work related issues. *Aohn J*, **50**(5), 220–6.
37. Arozullah AM, Calhoun EA, Wolf M, *et al.* (2004) The financial burden of cancer: estimates from a study of insured women with breast cancer. *J Support Oncol*, **2**(3), 271–8.
38. Brown ML, Riley GF, Potosky AL, Etzioni RD (1999) Obtaining long-term disease specific costs of care: application to Medicare enrollees diagnosed with colorectal cancer. *Med Care*, **37**(12), 1249–59.
39. Chirikos TN, Russell-Jacobs A, Jacobsen PB (2002) Functional impairment and the economic consequences of female breast cancer. *Women Health*, **36**(1), 1–20.
40. Lipscomb J, Gotay C, Snyder C (2005) Introduction to outcomes assessment in cancer. In: Lipscomb J, Gotay C, Snyder C, (eds), *Outcomes Assessment in Cancer: Measures, Methods, and Applications*, pp. 1–13. Cambridge: Cambridge University Press.
41. Stokes ME, Thompson D, Montoya EL, Weinstein MC, Winer EP, Earle CC (2008) Ten-year survival and cost following breast cancer recurrence: estimates from SEER-medicare data. *Value Health*, **11**(2), 213–20.
42. Wingo PA, Ries LA, Parker SL, Heath CW Jr (1998) Long-term cancer patient survival in the United States. *Cancer Epidemiol Biomarkers Prev*, **7**(4), 271–82.
43. Alfano CM, Smith AW, Irwin ML, *et al.* (2007) Physical activity, long-term symptoms, and physical health-related quality of life among breast cancer survivors: a prospective analysis. *J Cancer Surviv*, **1**(2), 116–28.
44. Ashing-Giwa K, Ganz PA, Petersen L (1999) Quality of life of African-American and white long term breast carcinoma survivors. *Cancer*, **85**(2), 418–26.
45. Baker F, Haffer SC, Denniston M (2003) Health-related quality of life of cancer and noncancer patients in Medicare managed care. *Cancer*, **97**(3), 674–81.
46. Bender CM, Engberg SJ, Donovan HS, *et al.* (2008) Symptom clusters in adults with chronic health problems and cancer as a comorbidity. *Oncol Nurs Forum*, **35**(1), E1–E11.
47. Bradley CJ, Neumark D, Luo Z, Bednarek H, Schenk M (2005) Employment outcomes of men treated for prostate cancer. *J Natl Cancer Inst*, **97**(13), 958–65.
48. Bylow K, Dale W, Mustian K, *et al.* (2008) Falls and physical performance deficits in older patients with prostate cancer undergoing androgen deprivation therapy. *Urology*, **72**(2), 422–7.
49. Deimling GT, Sterns S, Bowman KF, Kahana B (2007) Functioning and activity participation restrictions among older adult, long-term cancer survivors. *Cancer Invest*, **25**(2), 106–16.

50. Haab F, Meulemans A, Boccon-Gibod L, Dauge MC, Delmas V, Boccon-Gibod L (1995) Clearance of serum PSA after open surgery for benign prostatic hypertrophy, radical cystectomy, and radical prostatectomy. *Prostate*, **26**(6), 334–8.
51. Mandelblatt JS, Edge SB, Meropol NJ, *et al.* (2003) Predictors of long-term outcomes in older breast cancer survivors: perceptions versus patterns of care. *J Clin Oncol*, **21**(5), 855–63.
52. Nord C, Mykletun A, Thorsen L, Bjoro T, Fossa SD (2005) Self-reported health and use of health care services in long-term cancer survivors. *Int J Cancer*, **114**(2), 307–16.
53. Schmitz KH, Cappola AR, Stricker CT, Sweeney C, Norman SA (2007) The intersection of cancer and aging: establishing the need for breast cancer rehabilitation. *Cancer Epidemiol Biomarkers Prev*, **16**(5), 866–72.
54. Silliman RA, Prout MN, Field T, Kalish SC, Colton T (1999) Risk factors for a decline in upper body function following treatment for early stage breast cancer. *Breast Cancer Res Treat*, **54**(1), 25–30.
55. Williams ME (1987) Identifying the older person likely to require long-term care services. *J Am Geriatr Soc*, **35**(8), 761–6.
56. Brown JK, Byers T, Doyle C, *et al.* (2003) Nutrition and physical activity during and after cancer treatment: an American Cancer Society guide for informed choices. *CA Cancer J Clin*, **53**(5), 268–91.
57. Doyle C, Kushi LH, Byers T, *et al.* (2006) Nutrition and physical activity during and after cancer treatment: an American Cancer Society guide for informed choices. *CA Cancer J Clin*, **56**(6), 323–53.
58. World Cancer Fund; American Institute for Cancer Research (2007) *Food, Nutrition, Physical Activity and the Prevention of Cancer: A Global Perspective*, 2nd edn. Washington, DC: American Institute for Cancer Research.
59. Rock CL, Demark-Wahnefried W (2002) Nutrition and survival after the diagnosis of breast cancer: a review of the evidence. *J Clin Oncol*, **20**(15), 3302–16.
60. Demark-Wahnefried W, Peterson B, McBride C, Lipkus I, Clipp E (2000) Current health behaviors and readiness to pursue life-style changes among men and women diagnosed with early stage prostate and breast carcinomas. *Cancer*, **88**(3), 674–84.
61. Bergstrom A, Pisani P, Tenet V, Wolk A, Adami HO (2001) Overweight as an avoidable cause of cancer in Europe. *Int J Cancer*, **91**(3), 421–30.
62. Demark-Wahnefried W (2007) Diet: energy balance and obesity. In: *Cancer Prevention*, pp. 5.1–5.33. Alexandria, VA: American Society of Clinical Oncology.
63. International Agency for Research in Cancer (2002) *Handbook of Cancer Prevention*. Lyon: IARC.
64. Calle EE, Rodriguez C, Walker-Thurmond K, Thun MJ (2003) Overweight, obesity, and mortality from cancer in a prospectively studied cohort of U.S. adults. *N Engl J Med*, **348**(17), 1625–38.
65. Dawood S, Broglio K, Gonzalez-Angulo AM, *et al.* (2008) Prognostic value of body mass index in locally advanced breast cancer. *Clin Cancer Res*, **14**(6), 1718–25.
66. Efstathiou JA, Bae K, Shipley WU, *et al.* (2007) Obesity and mortality in men with locally advanced prostate cancer: analysis of RTOG 85-31. *Cancer*, **110**(12), 2691–9.
67. Demark-Wahnefried W, Winer EP, Rimer BK (1993) Why women gain weight with adjuvant chemotherapy for breast cancer. *J Clin Oncol*, **11**(7), 1418–29.
68. Caan B, Sternfeld B, Gunderson E, Coates A, Quesenberry C, Slattery ML (2005) Life After Cancer Epidemiology (LACE) Study: a cohort of early stage breast cancer survivors (United States). *Cancer Causes Contr*, **16**(5), 545–56.
69. Harvie MN, Howell A, Thatcher N, Baildam A, Campbell I (2005) Energy balance in patients with advanced NSCLC, metastatic melanoma and metastatic breast cancer receiving chemotherapy—a longitudinal study. *Br J Cancer*, **92**(4), 673–80.
70. Higano CS (2003) Side effects of androgen deprivation therapy: monitoring and minimizing toxicity. *Urol*, **61**(2 Suppl 1), 32–8.
71. Irwin ML, McTiernan A, Baumgartner RN, *et al.* (2005) Changes in body fat and weight after a breast cancer diagnosis: influence of demographic, prognostic, and lifestyle factors. *J Clin Oncol*, **23**(4), 774–82.

72. Strom SS, Wang X, Pettaway CA, *et al.* (2005) Obesity, weight gain, and risk of biochemical failure among prostate cancer patients following prostatectomy. *Clin Cancer Res*, **11**(19 Pt 1), 6889–94.
73. Demark-Wahnefried W, Rimer BK, Winer EP (1997) Weight gain in women diagnosed with breast cancer. *J Am Diet Assoc*, **97**(5), 519–26.
74. Kroenke CH, Chen WY, Rosner B, Holmes MD (2005) Weight, weight gain, and survival after breast cancer diagnosis. *J Clin Oncol*, **23**(7), 1370–8.
75. Chlebowski RT (2003) The American Cancer Society guide for nutrition and physical activity for cancer survivors: a call to action for clinical investigators. *CA Cancer J Clin*, **53**(5), 266–7.
76. Chlebowski RT, Aiello E, McTiernan A (2002) Weight loss in breast cancer patient management. *J Clin Oncol*, **20**(4), 1128–43.
77. Kristal AR, Gong Z (2007) Obesity and prostate cancer mortality. *Future Oncol*, **3**(5), 557–67.
78. von Gruenigen VE, Courneya KS, Gibbons HE, Kavanagh MB, Waggoner SE, Lerner E (2008) Feasibility and effectiveness of a lifestyle intervention program in obese endometrial cancer patients: a randomized trial. *Gynecol Oncol*, **109**(1), 19–26.
79. de Waard F, Ramlau R, Mulders Y, de Vries T, van Waveren S (1993) A feasibility study on weight reduction in obese postmenopausal breast cancer patients. *Eur J Cancer Prev*, **2**(3), 233–8.
80. Djuric Z, DiLaura NM, Jenkins I, *et al.* (2002) Combining weight-loss counseling with the weight watchers plan for obese breast cancer survivors. *Obes Res*, **10**(7), 657–65.
81. Goodwin P, Esplen MJ, Butler K, *et al.* (1998) Multidisciplinary weight management in locoregional breast cancer: results of a phase II study. *Breast Cancer Res Treat*, **48**(1), 53–64.
82. Loprinzi CL, Athmann LM, Kardinal CG, *et al.* (1996) Randomized trial of dietician counseling to try to prevent weight gain associated with breast cancer adjuvant chemotherapy. *Oncol*, **53**(3), 228–32.
83. Mefferd K, Nichols JF, Pakiz B, Rock CL (2007) A cognitive behavioral therapy intervention to promote weight loss improves body composition and blood lipid profiles among overweight breast cancer survivors. *Breast Cancer Res Treat*, **104**(2), 145–52.
84. Demark-Wahnefried W, Winer EP, Rimer BK (1993) Why women gain weight with adjuvant chemotherapy for breast cancer. *J Clin Oncol*, **11**(7), 1418–29.
85. Rolls BJ, Drewnowski A, Ledikwe JH (2005) Changing the energy density of the diet as a strategy for weight management. *J Am Diet Assoc*, **105**(5 Suppl 1), S98–103.
86. Rolls BJ, Roe LS, Meengs JS (2006) Reductions in portion size and energy density of foods are additive and lead to sustained decreases in energy intake. *Am J Clin Nutr*, **83**(1), 11–7.
87. Demark-Wahnefried W, Clipp EC, Lipkus IM, *et al.* (2007) Main outcomes of the FRESH START trial: a sequentially tailored, diet and exercise mailed print intervention among breast and prostate cancer survivors. *J Clin Oncol*, **25**(19), 2709–18.
88. Saquib N, Natarajan L, Rock CL, *et al.* (2008) The impact of a long-term reduction in dietary energy density on body weight within a randomized diet trial. *Nutr Cancer*, **60**(1), 31–8.
89. Demark-Wahnefried W, Peterson BL, Winer EP, *et al.* (2001) Changes in weight, body composition, and factors influencing energy balance among premenopausal breast cancer patients receiving adjuvant chemotherapy. *J Clin Oncol*, **19**(9), 2381–9.
90. Demark-Wahnefried W, Hars V, Conaway MR, *et al.* (1997) Reduced rates of metabolism and decreased physical activity in breast cancer patients receiving adjuvant chemotherapy. *Am J Clin Nutr*, **65**(5), 1495–501.
91. Rock CL, Demark-Wahnefried W (2002) Can lifestyle modification increase survival in women diagnosed with breast cancer? *J Nutr*, **132**(11 Suppl), 3504S–7S.
92. Smith MR (2003) Changes in body composition during hormonal therapy for prostate cancer. *Clin Prostate Cancer*, **2**(1), 18–21.
93. Expert Panel on the Identification, Evualation and Treatment of Overweight in Adults (2000) The practical guide: identification, evaluation, and treatment of overweight and obesity in adults. *Am J Clin Nutr*, **68**, 899–917.

94. Kennedy ET (2006) Evidence for nutritional benefits in prolonging wellness. *Am J Clin Nutr*, **83**(2), 410S–414S.
95. Kroenke CH, Fung TT, Hu FB, Holmes MD (2005) Dietary patterns and survival after breast cancer diagnosis. *J Clin Oncol*, **23**(36), 9295–303.
96. Meyerhardt JA, Niedzwiecki D, Hollis D, *et al.* (2007) Association of dietary patterns with cancer recurrence and survival in patients with stage III colon cancer. *J Am Med Assoc*, **298**(7), 754–64.
97. Demark-Wahnefried W, Clipp EC, *et al.* (2004) Physical function and associations with diet and exercise: results of a cross-sectional survey among elders with breast or prostate cancer. *Int J Behav Nutr Phys Act*, **1**(1), 16.
98. Wayne SJ, Baumgartner K, Baumgartner RN, Bernstein L, Bowen DJ, Ballard-Barbash R (2006) Diet quality is directly associated with quality of life in breast cancer survivors. *Breast Cancer Res Treat*, **96**(3), 227–32.
99. Demark-Wahnefried W, Morey MC, Clipp EC, *et al.* (2003) Leading the Way in Exercise and Diet (Project LEAD): intervening to improve function among older breast and prostate cancer survivors. *Contr Clin Trials*, **24**(2), 206–23.
100. Pierce JP, Natarajan L, Caan BJ, *et al.* (2007) Influence of a diet very high in vegetables, fruit, and fiber and low in fat on prognosis following treatment for breast cancer: the Women's Healthy Eating and Living (WHEL) randomized trial. *J Am Med Assoc*, **298**(3), 289–98.
101. Gapstur SM, Khan S (2007) Fat, fruits, vegetables, and breast cancer survivorship. *J Am Med Assoc*, **298**(3), 335–6.
102. Chlebowski RT, Blackburn GL, Thomson CA, *et al.* (2006) Dietary fat reduction and breast cancer outcome: interim efficacy results from the Women's Intervention Nutrition Study. *J Natl Cancer Inst*, **98**, 1767–76.
103. Bellizzi KM, Rowland JH, Jeffery DD, McNeel T (2005) Health behaviors of cancer survivors: examining opportunities for cancer control intervention. *J Clin Oncol*, **23**(34), 8884–93.
104. Coups EJ, Ostroff JS (2005) A population-based estimate of the prevalence of behavioral risk factors among adult cancer survivors and noncancer controls. *Prev Med*, **40**(6), 702–11.
105. Eakin EG, Youlden DR, Baade PD, *et al.* (2007) Health behaviors of cancer survivors: data from an Australian population-based survey. *Cancer Causes Contr*, **18**(8), 881–94.
106. Deleyiannis FW, Thomas DB, Vaughan TL, Davis S (1996) Alcoholism: independent predictor of survival in patients with head and neck cancer. *J Natl Cancer Inst*, **88**(8), 542–9.
107. Day GL, Blot WJ, Shore RE, *et al.* (1994) Second cancers following oral and pharyngeal cancers: role of tobacco and alcohol. *J Natl Cancer Inst*, **86**(2), 131–7.
108. Trentham-Dietz A, Newcomb PA, Nichols HB, Hampton JM (2007) Breast cancer risk factors and second primary malignancies among women with breast cancer. *Breast Cancer Res Treat*, **105**(2), 195–207.
109. Alpha-Tocopherol Beta Carotene Cancer Prevention Study Group (1994) The effect of vitamin E and beta carotene on the incidence of lung cancer and other cancers in male smokers. *N Engl J Med*, **330**(15), 1029–35.
110. Omenn GS, Goodman GE, Thornquist MD, *et al.* (1996) Risk factors for lung cancer and for intervention effects in CARET, the Beta-Carotene and Retinol Efficacy Trial. *J Natl Cancer Inst*, **88**(21), 1550–9.
111. Bairati I, Meyer F, Jobin E, *et al.* (2006) Antioxidant vitamins supplementation and mortality: a randomized trial in head and neck cancer patients. *Int J Cancer*, **119**(9), 2221–4.
112. Miller ER 3rd, Pastor-Barriuso R, Dalal D, Riemersma RA, Appel LJ, Guallar E (2005) Meta-analysis: high-dosage vitamin E supplementation may increase all-cause mortality. *Ann Intern Med*, **142**(1), 37–46.
113. *Selenium and Vitamin E Cancer Prevention Trial (SELECT)*. Available at: http://www.crab.org/select/ (accessed 11 June 2008).

114. Lawson KA, Wright ME, Subar A, *et al.* (2007) Multivitamin use and risk of prostate cancer in the National Institutes of Health–AARP Diet and Health Study. *J Natl Cancer Inst*, **99**(10), 754–64.

115. Food and Nutrition Board/National Academy of Sciences/Institutes of Medicine. *Dietary Reference Intakes*. Available at: http://www.iom.edu (accessed 10 January 2008).

116. Reid ME, Stratton MS, Lillico AJ, *et al.* (2004) A report of high-dose selenium supplementation: response and toxicities. *J Trace Elem Med Biol*, **18**(1), 69–74.

117. Williams R, Ansford A (2007) Acute selenium toxicity: Australia's second fatality. *Pathology*, **39**(2), 289–90.

118. Maskarinec G, Gotay CC, Tatsumura Y, Shumay DM, Kakai H (2001) Perceived cancer causes: use of complementary and alternative therapy. *Cancer Pract*, **9**(4), 183–90.

119. Wold KS, Byers T, Crane LA, Ahnen D (2005) What do cancer survivors believe causes cancer? (United States). *Cancer Causes Contr*, **16**(2), 115–23.

120. Linn MW, Linn BS, Stein SR (1982) Beliefs about causes of cancer in cancer patients. *Soc Sci Med*, **16**(7), 835–9.

121. Stewart DE, Cheung AM, Duff S, *et al.* (2001) Attributions of cause and recurrence in long-term breast cancer survivors. *Psycho-oncology*, **10**(2), 179–83.

122. Stewart DE, Wong F, Duff S, Melancon CH, Cheung AM (2001) What doesn't kill you makes you stronger: an ovarian cancer survivor survey. *Gynecol Oncol*, **83**(3), 537–42.

123. Demark-Wahnefried W, Werner C, Clipp EC, *et al.* (2005) Survivors of childhood cancer and their guardians. *Cancer*, **103**(10), 2171–80.

124. McBride CM, Emmons KM, Lipkus IM (2003) Understanding the potential of teachable moments: the case of smoking cessation. *Health Educ Res*, **18**(2), 156–70.

125. Gritz ER, Fingeret MC, Vidrine DJ, Lazev AB, Mehta NV, Reece GP (2006) Successes and failures of the teachable moment: smoking cessation in cancer patients. *Cancer*, **106**(1), 17–27.

126. Alfano CM, Day JM, Katz ML, *et al.* (2009) Exercise and dietary change after diagnosis and cancer-related symptoms in long-term survivors of breast cancer: CALGB 79804. *Psycho-oncology*, **18**(2), 128–33.

127. Humpel N, Magee C, Jones SC (2007) The impact of a cancer diagnosis on the health behaviors of cancer survivors and their family and friends. *Support Care Cancer*, **15**(6), 621–30.

128. Demark-Wahnefried W, Pinto BM, Gritz ER (2006) Promoting health and physical function among cancer survivors: potential for prevention and questions that remain. *J Clin Oncol*, **24**(32), 5125–31.

129. Stull VB, Snyder DC, Demark-Wahnefried W (2007) Lifestyle interventions in cancer survivors: designing programs that meet the needs of this vulnerable and growing population. *J Nutr* **137**, S243–248.

130. McBride CM, Clipp E, Peterson BL, Lipkus IM, Demark-Wahnefried W (2000) Psychological impact of diagnosis and risk reduction among cancer survivors. *Psycho-oncology*, **9**(5), 418–27.

131. Cleeland CS (2007) Symptom burden: multiple symptoms and their impact as patient-reported outcomes. *J Natl Cancer Inst Monogr*, (37), 16–21.

132. Ganz PA (2008) Psychological and social aspects of breast cancer. *Oncology (Williston Park)*, **22**(6), 642–50.

133. Pinto BM, Trunzo JJ (2005) Health behaviors during and after a cancer diagnosis. *Cancer*, **104**(11 Suppl), 2614–23.

134. Demark-Wahnefried W, Case LD, Blackwell K, *et al.* (2008) Results of a diet/exercise feasibility trial to prevent adverse body composition change in breast cancer patients on adjuvant chemotherapy. *Clin Breast Cancer*, **8**(1), 70–9.

135. Demark-Wahnefried W, Kenyon AJ, Eberle P, Skye A, Kraus WE (2002) Preventing sarcopenic obesity among breast cancer patients who receive adjuvant chemotherapy: results of a feasibility study. *Clin Exerc Physiol*, **4**(1), 44–9.

136. Snyder DC, Sloane R, Lobach D, *et al.* (2008) Differences in baseline characteristics and outcomes at 1- and 2-year follow-up of cancer survivors accrued via self-referral versus cancer registry in the FRESH START Diet and exercise trial. *Cancer Epidemiol Biomarkers Prev*, **17**(5), 1288–94.
137. Watson JM, Torgerson DJ (2006) Increasing recruitment to randomised trials: a review of randomised controlled trials. *BMC Med Res Methodol*, **6**, 34.
138. Pinto BM, Frierson GM, Rabin C, Trunzo JJ, Marcus BH (2005) Home-based physical activity intervention for breast cancer patients. *J Clin Oncol*, **23**(15), 3577–87.
139. Emmons KM, Puleo E, Park E, *et al.* (2005) Peer-delivered smoking counseling for childhood cancer survivors increases rate of cessation: the partnership for health study. *J Clin Oncol*, **23**(27), 6516–23.
140. Pierce JP, Newman VA, Flatt SW, *et al.* (2004) Telephone counseling intervention increases intakes of micronutrient- and phytochemical-rich vegetables, fruit and fiber in breast cancer survivors. *J Nutr*, **134**(2), 452–8.
141. Demark-Wahnefried W, Clipp EC, Morey M, *et al.* (2006) Lifestyle intervention development study to improve physical function in older adults with cancer: outcomes from Project LEAD. *J Clin Oncol*, **24**(21), 3465–73.
142. Hebert JR, Ebbeling CB, Olendzki BC, *et al.* (2001) Change in women's diet and body mass following intensive intervention for early-stage breast cancer. *J Am Diet Assoc*, **101**(4), 421–31.
143. Segal R, Evans W, Johnson D, *et al.* (2001) Structured exercise improves physical functioning in women with stages I and II breast cancer: results of a randomized controlled trial. *J Clin Oncol*, **19**(3), 657–65.
144. Pinto BM, Friedman R, Marcus BH, Kelley H, Tennstedt S, Gillman MW (2002) Effects of a computer-based, telephone-counseling system on physical activity. *Am J Prev Med*, **23**(2), 113–20.
145. Rutten LJ, Arora NK, Bakos AD, Aziz N, Rowland J (2005) Information needs and sources of information among cancer patients: a systematic review of research (1980–2003) *Patient Educ Couns*, **57**(3), 250–61.
146. Blue CL, Black DR (2005) Synthesis of intervention research to modify physical activity and dietary behaviors. *Res Theory Nurs Pract*, **19**(1), 25–61.
147. BootsMiller BJ, Ribisl KM, Mowbray CT, Davidson WS, Walton MA, Herman SE (1998) Methods of ensuring high follow-up rates: lessons from a longitudinal study of dual diagnosed participants. *Subst Use Misuse*, **33**(13), 2665–85.
148. Wilcox S, Parra-Medina D, Thompson-Robinson M, Will J (2001) Nutrition and physical activity interventions to reduce cardiovascular disease risk in health care settings: a quantitative review with a focus on women. *Nutr Rev*, **59**(7), 197–214.
149. Ajzen I (1985) From intentions to actions: a theory of planned behavior. In: Kuhl J, Beckman J, (eds), *Action-contro: From Cognition to Behavior*, pp. 11–39. Heidelberg: Springer.
150. Bandura A (1977) *Social Learning Theory*. Englewood Cliffs, NJ: Prentice-Hall.
151. Prochaska JO, DiClemente CC (1983) Stages and processes of self-change of smoking: toward an integrative model of change. *J Consult Clin Psychol*, **51**(3), 390–5.
152. Badr H, Taylor CL (2006) Social constraints and spousal communication in lung cancer. *Psycho-oncology*, **15**(8), 673–83.
153. Ahuja R, Weibel SB, Leone FT (2003) Lung cancer: the oncologist's role in smoking cessation. *Semin Oncol*, **30**(1), 94–103.
154. Jones LW, Courneya KS, Fairey AS, Mackey JR (2004) Effects of an oncologist's recommendation to exercise on self-reported exercise behavior in newly diagnosed breast cancer survivors: a single-blind, randomized controlled trial. *Ann Behav Med*, **28**(2), 105–13.
155. Jones LW, Courneya KS, Peddle C, Mackey JR (2005) Oncologists' opinions towards recommending exercise to patients with cancer: a Canadian national survey. *Support Care Cancer*, **13**(11), 929–37.
156. Sabatino SA, Coates RJ, Uhler RJ, Pollack LA, Alley LG, Zauderer LJ (2007) Provider counseling about health behaviors among cancer survivors in the United States. *J Clin Oncol*, **25**(15), 2100–6.

Chapter 28

Nutritional management of patients receiving primary cancer therapy

Richard D. Johnston, Rachel A. Barrett, and Tim E. Bowling

In 2004 there were 278 000 people diagnosed with cancer and 154 000 cancer-related deaths in the UK.[1] The three most common incident cancers were prostate, lung and colorectal among males, and breast, lung and colorectal among women. These cancers were also the most common causes of cancer-related deaths among each gender.

The interaction between cancer and nutrition is well established. Nutrition is implicated in the aetiology of developing certain tumours, for example, a high intake of red and processed meats and colon cancer.[2] Malnutrition at the outset of cancer diagnosis, or while undergoing its associated treatments, is a well-established poor prognostic indicator for survival.[3,4] Not only do malnourished cancer patients have a worse survival, but they also have a lower quality of life, reduced performance status and increased risk of treatment-related complications.[5,6] Optimizing and maintaining the nutritional status of cancer patients is consequently a critical area of their management, despite not being a primary focus of their cancer treatment.

Many cancer patients are malnourished at the time of diagnosis. Weight loss can be the first symptom of cancer development and a weight loss of more than 10% occurs in 15% of patients at the time of diagnosis.[7] There is also a strong association between the frequency and severity of weight loss and the tumour stage.[8] The incidence of malnutrition in patients undergoing cancer treatment depends on their premorbid nutritional state as well as other factors (Table 28.1). Preventing, where able, and/or managing these factors is critical in maintaining adequate nutrition in cancer patients.

General principles of nutritional support in cancer patients

The key aim of nutritional support in cancer patients is to revert or prevent the deleterious effects of malnutrition, i.e. to promote survival, quality of life, performance status, and reduce complication rates. The improvement in the physical health of the patient has been shown to translate into an improvement in quality of life.[9] Cancer patients place a high value on nutrition in determining their quality of life,[10] although the more invasive interventions have the potential to reduce quality of life through restricting mobility and independence from health care services.

Considering the need for and planning nutritional support requires an initial assessment of patients' current and predicted nutritional status. Supportive options include dietary counselling, oral nutritional supplements, enteral tube feeding, or parenteral nutrition. The response and compliance to such therapies needs regular reassessment. Patients with cancer are at a high risk of developing refeeding syndrome, and close monitoring of their biochemistry is required, especially if there has been marked recent weight loss or a prolonged period of minimal intake.

Table 28.1 Factors that influence the incidence of malnutrition in cancer patients undergoing treatment

Tumour-related factors	Systemic factors	Psychological factors	Treatment side-effects
Cachexia	Anorexia	Fear	Anorexia
Dysgeusia	Cachexia	Depression	Pain
Dysosmia	Hypermetabolism	Anxiety	Fatigue
Anorexia	Dysgeusia	Anger	Nausea
Odynophagia	Nausea		Vomiting
Dysphagia			Xerostomia
Gastrointestinal obstruction			Oral candidiasis
Early satiety			Dysgeusia
Biliary obstruction			Dysosmia
Malabsorption			Odynophagia
Pain			Dysphagia
			Mucositis
			Oesophagitis
			Gastric stasis
			Diarrhoea
			Constipation
			Malabsorption
			Enteritis

Dietary manipulations such as smaller and more frequent meals can help to increase dietary intake in patients with anorexia or early satiety. There is, however, no evidence that dietary modification improves cancer patients' survival or prognosis.[11]

The enteral route is preferred over parenteral for nutrition support due to its ease of administration, tolerability, cost and fewer metabolic disturbances such as hyperglycaemia, cholestasis, and fatty infiltration of the liver. Use of enteral tube feeding stimulates rather than suppresses appetite and improves voluntary food intake in malnourished patients.[12] Enteral nutrition also promotes gut mucosal growth and barrier function. Enteral support is limited where there is intestinal failure or functional (ileus) or mechanical obstruction of the gastrointestinal tract.

Parenteral nutrition is indicated in the presence of a failing intestinal tract either due to malabsorption or obstruction. Volume restrictions may well be required in fluid-overloaded patients and central venous access involves insertion complications and sepsis risk.[13] Long term parenteral nutrition results in low levels of hunger being reported.[14] This has been reported in short term use too. In a well-designed experiment, Gil *et al.*[15] blinded healthy volunteers as to the content of the infusion they were receiving. Oral intake was markedly reduced after 5 days in the parenterally fed individuals in proportion to the amount of energy and nitrogen infused. The anorectic effect persisted for 4 days after infusions were stopped. This effect is deleterious when attempting to reintroduce enteral nutrition to a patient following a period of parenteral nutrition.

Nutritional support should be commenced in all cancer patients if undernutrition is already present or if inadequate food intake is anticipated for more than 7 days, and should substitute the difference between actual intake and calculated requirements.[16]

This chapter addresses the practical issues surrounding the management of patients undergoing active therapy for cancer. Such therapy may be initiated with curative intent or merely to delay the disease progression. We also address the concept of malnutrition from a macronutrient perspective. Dietary exclusions and micronutrient replacements have also been developed for certain cancer therapies. Significant findings in this field are presented. The role of immunonutrition is covered in Chapter 11. The long term issues surrounding patients who either regain full health status, or have an impaired health as a consequence of the cancer or its therapy, or enter into a palliative stage following treatment, are discussed elsewhere.

Cancer therapies

The principal therapeutic strategies in cancer patients are surgery, radiotherapy, chemotherapy and stem-cell transplantation. Traditionally these therapies were used as sole agents, though they are increasingly being used in combination as our understanding of their adjunctive effects improves. Therapeutic strategies for cancer patients are therefore becoming increasingly varied. Given this complexity, one of the major recent developments in cancer management has been the widespread use of treatment planning by a multidisciplinary team. The close collaboration between pathologists and radiologists allows for an accurate diagnosis and staging. Medical, radiation and surgical oncologists are thus in a position to plan appropriate therapies. The principal factors determining such decisions are the tumour diagnosis and stage, the patient's prior medical and surgical history, the individual wishes of the patient, and their performance status.[17] The performance status of cancer patients is affected by their nutritional status.[7] Malnutrition is associated with an increased complication rate following surgery, chemotherapy and radiotherapy. Complications result in failure to complete such regimens and hence a poorer response.[3]

The increasing use of combination and adjunctive regimens results in cancer patients often undergoing a more aggressive, prolonged and potentially toxic course. Gone are the days when most tumours are solely treated by a brief surgical intervention or a single course of radiotherapy. The potential for malnutrition to occur during such prolonged therapies is therefore much greater, especially if complications or toxicity develop.

Chemotherapy

Medical oncologists have an ever-expanding arsenal of chemotherapeutic drugs. The traditional chemotherapy agents are the cytotoxic drugs. There is now an increasing array of hormonal and biological therapies. The lower incidence of gastrointestinal or anorectic side-effects in these newer agents has resulted in fewer nutritional complications, though they remain an issue.

Single agent chemotherapy remains the treatment of choice for some tumours, though frequently combination chemotherapy is prescribed. Options include combining the same class of drugs, for example cytotoxics, or combining a cytotoxic with a hormonal therapy, etc. Regimens involving combinations result in an enhanced tumour response, reduced development of drug resistance, and an increased patient survival in certain tumours. However, this is at the expense of an increased likelihood of toxicity developing. The side-effect profile of combination therapy is generally predictable and based upon the side-effects of the individual therapies.

Cytotoxic agents

Cytotoxics are antiproliferative, inducing direct damage to the DNA of dividing cells. They are therefore not tumour-specific and have the potential to damage both tumour and normal cells. Normal tissues that are particularly vulnerable are those with a high rate of cell turnover, such as bone marrow, gastrointestinal tract, hair follicles and the ovary and testes. The antiproliferative side-effect profile of most cytotoxic drugs therefore predominantly originates from these organs, including myelosuppression, oral and/or intestinal mucositis, alopecia and teratogenicity. The individual medications also have their own individual side-effect profile separate from their antiproliferative toxicities. Frequently cytotoxics stimulate the chemoreceptor region of the brainstem, inducing vomiting, as will be discussed further.

Tumours with a high cell turnover, such as some of the haematological malignancies, are generally more responsive to cytotoxic agents than the more indolent or slow-growing tumours. Other factors that determine response include the degree of differentiation and size of the tumour. Poorly differentiated tumours lose the tissues' normal growth-regulating mechanisms, and hence are less cytotoxic responsive. Large tumours commonly have poor central vascular supply, limiting cytotoxic access and efficacy. It is in such tumour types that combination with radiotherapy can overcome these issues and hence improve results.

Hormonal therapies

Hormonal therapies are predominantly prescribed for the hormonally driven prostate and breast cancers. Tamoxifen is an anti-estrogen and the aromatase inhibitors block the peripheral conversion of androgens to estrogen. Neither tamoxifen nor the aromatase inhibitors have any significant gastrointestinal side-effects.[18] Anti-androgen therapies are utilized in metastatic prostate cancer. They have no reported gastrointestinal side-effects, bar mild diarrhoea noted in patients taking flutamide.[19]

Biological therapy

Monoclonal antibodies, and the so-called 'small molecule' therapies (e.g. tyrosine kinase inhibitors) target specific molecular factors that are both overexpressed by tumour cells and central to their growth and progression. As compared to cytotoxic therapies these agents are highly tumour specific. Biological agents are highly effective when treating differentiated tumours that continue to express these targets. Systemic side-effects do, however, still occur. Epidermal growth factor receptor (EGFR) is the molecular target of gefitinib, erlotinib, cetuximab, panitumamab and lapatinib. Skin toxicity is the most frequent side-effect of such agents, though epidermal growth factor is also involved in maintaining intestinal and gastric mucosa.[20] As a result these therapies commonly result in abdominal pain, oral mucositis and diarrhoea. Such symptoms are normally mild and self-limiting.

Nutritionally related side-effects of chemotherapy

Chemotherapy-induced nausea and vomiting (CINV)

Nausea and vomiting are among the most feared symptoms by chemotherapy patients.[21] The pathogenesis of CINV is poorly understood, with several factors involved. The emetic centre and the chemoreceptor trigger zone within the brainstem regulate nausea and vomiting. These regions receive central signals from other regions of the brain and peripheral signals from the gastrointestinal system. Drugs and hormones within the systemic circulation cross the incomplete blood–brain barrier of the area postrema to affect these brainstem regions.[22]

The onset of the nausea and vomiting can be acute (within 24 h of administration), delayed (between 24 h and several days later) and anticipatory. Sensations such as taste, odour or sight, along with anxiety, are the common triggers for anticipatory symptoms.[23]

The main factor in determining the likelihood of a regimen inducing vomiting is the emetogenicity of the chemotherapeutic agents, determined by their effect on the area postrema and the gastrointestinal tract. The reported risk of nausea or vomiting following administration of each individual chemotherapeutic agent without anti-emetics has recently been published by the American Society of Clinical Oncology (ASCO)[24] (Table 28.2). This table is of great use as it facilitates prophylactic strategies and patient education. Some caution has to be used, however, as the risk attributable to each drug is affected by the dose, route and rate of drug administration,[25]

Table 28.2 Emetic risk of intravenously administered antineoplastic agents (incidence of emesis without anti-emetics)[24]

<10%	10–30%	30–90%	>90%
Bevacizumab	Docetaxel	Oxaliplatin	Cisplatin
Bleomycin	Paclitaxel	Carboplatin	Streptozocin
Rituximab	Mitoxantrone	Ifosfamide	Cyclophosphamide >1500 mgmg/m^2
Vinblastine	Topotecan	Cyclophosphamide <1500 mg/m^2	Carmustine
Vincristine	Etoposide	Doxorubicin	Dacarbazine
Vinorelbine	Methotrexate	Epirubicin	Dactinomycin
	Mitomycin C	Irinotecan	
	Gemcitabine		
	Fluorouracil		
	Cetuximab		
	Trastuzumab		

and non-drug-related factors are not included. The full details of the 2006 guidelines devised by the ASCO are beyond the scope of this chapter. In brief, however, no routine prophylaxis is advised for agents with a <10% risk. Agents with a risk of 10–30% are advised to have dexamethasone co-prescribed. Dexamethasone plus one or two anti-emetics is recommended pre chemotherapy in the 30–90% and >90% categories respectively. Sedatives, in particular lorazepam, are efficacious in reducing the incidence of anticipatory nausea. Medication may also be prescribed post therapy to prevent delayed reactions.

The development of serotonin ($5HT_3$) receptor antagonists in the early 1990s substantially reduced the incidence of CINV. Today, compliance with anti-emetic guidelines prevents vomiting in 70–80% of patients despite receiving highly emetogenic therapies.[26] It is crucial to control these symptoms, as otherwise malnutrition, dehydration and electrolyte imbalances occur, resulting in prolonged hospital admissions and failure to complete the chemotherapy regimen.

Other critical factors in the development of nausea and vomiting include the frequency of the chemotherapeutic cycle and patient-related factors such as female gender, younger age and a past history of motion sickness, hyperemesis gravidarum or alcohol abuse.[26] Psychological interventions and relaxation techniques have been shown to be efficacious in this setting.[27,28]

Chemotherapy-related diarrhoea

Chemotherapy-related diarrhoea results from drug-specific toxicities, the development of intestinal mucositis and opportunistic infections in the presence of immunosuppression. The latter needs to be screened for, prior to routine use of antidiarrhoeal agents. Chemotherapeutic agents that are prone to inducing significant diarrhoea include capecitabine, cisplatin, fluorouracil, irinotecan, liposomal doxorubicin, raltitrexed and streptozocin.[29] Profuse acute diarrhoea frequently occurs with use of fluorouracil and raltitrexed, whereas irinotecan commonly produces a delayed diarrhoea. As previously described, mild diarrhoea is a common side-effect of biological agents that act on EGFR. Fluid and electrolyte balance needs to be closely monitored in the presence of diarrhoea as otherwise toxic side-effects can develop from the chemotherapeutic agents.

Chemotherapy-related constipation

Significant constipation and hence a reduced nutritional intake can result from excessive opiate and antidiarrhoeal agent use during the chemotherapy regimen.[3] Specific to chemotherapy, the vinca alkaloids can cause an adynamic ileus that presents with pain, bloating and constipation. The elderly are most susceptible to this side-effect.

Mucositis

Chemotherapy and radiotherapy are frequently complicated by oral and/or intestinal mucositis. The development of mucositis is multifactorial. The initial trigger is disruption or loss of the rapidly dividing surface layer. This disruption results in a mucosa that is vulnerable to further injury, either by immune responses or by colonization by local pathogenic bacteria or fungi. This further injury results in mucosal ulceration, which can in turn lead to pain and bleeding. The risk of developing mucositis depends upon the integrity of the patient's immune system, the presence of opportunistic pathogens and the nature of the regimen. An increased risk of mucositis occurs with certain therapies, as shown in Table 28.3, following high or accelerated doses of chemotherapy, and following combined chemo-radiotherapy.

Around half a million people suffer from mucositis each year[30] and it is not infrequently the cause for cancer therapy cessation. Oral mucositis results in a reduction of food and fluid intake whereas intestinal mucositis results in malabsorption, nausea, vomiting, diarrhoea and abdominal pain or distension.[30]

There is limited evidence in the prevention and management of mucositis. The 2007 American Cancer Society guidelines advise maintaining oral hygiene, the use of targeted radiotherapy to limit intestinal exposure, and symptomatic control with the use of systemic and topical oral analgesia, proton pump inhibitors and loperamide.[31] Other mucositis strategies include antibiotics and antifungals if there is evidence of superadded infection, and reduced doses or longer recovery intervals between the anticancer treatments. Such modifications of the anticancer regimen, however, risk the survival or recovery of neoplastic cells and hence a reduced treatment efficacy. Glutamine supplementation has been shown to be beneficial in controlling the duration and incidence of chemotherapy-induced diarrhoea but has no effect on the incidence of nausea or vomiting.[30]

Table 28.3 Mucositis risk of antineoplastic agents

Low risk	Intermediate	High	Very high
Aldesleukin Carboplatin Carmustine Cetuximab Cisplatin Dacarbazine Gemcitabine Ifosfamide Irinotecan Melphalan Mitomycin C Oxaliplatin Raltitrexed Streptozocin Thiotepa Topotecan Treosulfan Vindesine	Bevacizumab Bleomycin Capecitabine Mitoxantrone Paclitaxel Vinblastine Vincristine	Cyclophosphamide Dactinomycin Docetaxel Etoposide Fluorouracil (5FU) Liposomal doxorubicin Methotrexate	Doxorubicin Epirubicin

[a]Data adapted from Stanley.(29)

Effect of pre-chemotherapy malnutrition

Dewys *et al.*[7] analysed the prognostic effect of weight loss pre chemotherapy in 3047 patients. The majority had lost weight and its presence was predictive of a shorter survival and a worse performance status. These effects were not independent of tumour stage and so this study does not support routine nutritional support pre chemotherapy. However, the presence of malnutrition and low nutrient intake has been shown to be a predictor for the development of side-effects from chemotherapy despite such patients receiving lower doses.[5,32]

Energy requirements and chemotherapy

Weight loss during chemotherapy is rarely reported despite significant reductions in dietary energy. This is due to a matched reduction in physical activity and resting energy expenditure (REE).[33] The main consequence of this is a loss of lean body mass due to the reduced activity.

Weight gain commonly occurs during breast cancer chemotherapy with the increased body fat and a loss of lean body mass resulting in sarcopenic obesity. This effect is often attributed to the use of steroids as anti-emetics, though it has been shown to develop in the absence of nutritional supplements or steroid use. Harvie *et al.*[34] studied body composition, energy intakes, energy requirements and activity levels for a year following adjuvant chemotherapy for early breast cancer. Physical activity decreased during chemotherapy and for the following three months, resulting in a significantly reduced REE. However, there was an increased energy intake during this time period. The combined outcome was a 15% increase in total body fat and a small reduction in fat-free mass. At 1 year post chemotherapy there was a 28% increase in body fat and a 4% reduction in fat-free mass. Similar changes in body composition and energy intakes have been documented in those undergoing chemotherapy for advanced cancers.[35] Management strategies for such patients should logically involve increased levels of physical activity and a degree of calorie restriction in those at risk of obesity. Such strategies have not, however, been shown to be effective in controlling weight gain.[36,37]

Protein requirements and chemotherapy

Chemotherapy does not affect overall nitrogen balance in the majority of patients, though a negative balance does occur in those who lose weight.[38] Studies frequently note reductions in lean body mass during chemotherapy, and so it is important to advise maintenance of regular physical activity and intake of the protein dietary reference values. Trials of arginine and glutamine supplementation in order to maintain protein status have only been performed in cancer cachexia patients, with no such data in chemotherapy patients.

Nutritional interventions and chemotherapy

Varying effects on metabolism, energy balances and body composition have been demonstrated with chemotherapy. Such studies are difficult to design and frequently suffer from a selection bias, with healthier patients tending to enroll for the baseline investigations and drop-outs tending to occur among those with deteriorating health. As a result the data are often conflicting and tend to describe those with the least metabolic or nutritional risk.

Little benefit in terms of outcome has been shown with nutritional support in chemotherapy. Retrospective and unadjusted analyses have shown an increased rate of toxicity from chemotherapy in patients with a reduced calorie and protein intake.[32] Intakes of <10.1 MJ (2400 kcal)/day in men and <8.8 MJ (2100 kcal)/day in women were associated with a doubled toxicity rate.

A three-fold increased risk of chemotherapy side-effects was noted with intake of <70 g of protein per day in men, and <65 g in women.

Oral nutritional supplements and chemotherapy

Given the low incidence of malnutrition that has been shown to develop as a consequence of chemotherapy, it is not surprising that there are few supportive data for supplementation. Importantly no beneficial effect on the response rate or side-effect profile of chemotherapy has ever been clearly documented. Many of the studies involve non-randomized interventions and again have been hampered as the most nutritionally vulnerable patients are rarely recruited. A review of 11 studies assessing the effects of oral supplement use in cancer patients failed to show any benefit in body weight, composition or illness outcome.[39] The 2006 European Society for Clinical Nutrition and Metabolism (ESPEN) guidelines consequently state that there is no indication for routine enteral nutritional support during chemotherapy.[16]

Enteral tube feeding and chemotherapy

Enteral tube feeding may benefit patients with severe malnutrition or in whom chemotherapy-related toxicities will prevent adequate oral intake for more than a week. Such intervention is not evidence-based and there is a need for studies to address this issue.

Parenteral nutrition and chemotherapy

The role of routine parenteral nutrition was assessed in early studies and shown to be detrimental.[40] Many of these problems were due to sepsis and hyperalimentation, issues that have been improved with modern management. A recent meta-analysis however still failed to demonstrate a benefit in 3-month survival, whereas a significant, four-fold increased risk for developing a significant infection was demonstrated with parenteral nutrition.[41] Such analyses were recognized by the author as being limited by the poor descriptive and analytical details presented in the original papers. Another major flaw in these studies was that few patients were malnourished at study inclusion and many had concurrent adequate oral intake. These patients would not ordinarily receive, and potentially benefit from, parenteral nutrition in modern clinical practice.

Parenteral nutrition may well have a non-evidence-based place in patients with severe malnutrition and temporary intestinal failure. Such patients are few and will benefit from a multidisciplinary decision. Again, further evidence in this area is required.

Dietary counselling and chemotherapy

Fortnightly dietetic counselling structured to encourage the recommended daily intake of calories and protein has been shown to result in significant increases in intake of energy by 1 MJ and protein by 10 g per day during chemotherapy.[42] This did not translate into clinical benefit, however, with no significant weight gain at 5 months, no changes in therapy response rates, quality of life or survival.

Weekly dietetic counselling and advice to consume an energy- and protein-dense supplement along with 1.1 g of eicosapentaenoic acid (EPA) was assessed in breast and non-small cell lung cancer chemotherapy patients.[43] It resulted in gains in weight and fat mass following chemotherapy, though critically failed to prevent loss of fat-free mass. These weight changes correlated strongly with changes in energy intake.

Neutropenic diet and chemotherapy

A 'neutropenic diet', otherwise referred to as a clean or low bacterial diet, is often used in the prevention of food- and/or water-borne infection. Although evidence for its use is not in existence, nor is it likely to be obtained, it seems prudent to not expose neutropenic patients to potential sources of infection. In practice, neutropenic diets are predominantly used in patients with haematological malignancies; however similar precautions are advised in patients with solid tumours who develop neutropenia. This is discussed further, below, in patients undergoing haematopoietic stem cell transplantation.

Nutrient supplements and chemotherapy

Antioxidants have been shown to be used by 60% of patients undergoing chemotherapy or radiotherapy.[44] Most are self-prescribed and frequently without the oncologist's knowledge.[45] The antineoplastic efficacy of chemotherapy and radiotherapy requires free radical generation. There are therefore theoretical concerns that the binding of free radicals by dietary antioxidants may prevent the desired oxidative damage within tumour cells. The conflicting clinical and laboratory data in this field have resulted in opposing expert advice being generated: some authors advocate antioxidant use, others warn against it.[46,47] Definitive studies would require massive patient cohorts, and have not been done. The use of chemical radio-sensitizers to enhance the effects of radiotherapy by promoting free-radical activity is showing promising results.[48] At this stage it therefore seems counterintuitive to advise supplementing antioxidants greater than the dietary reference values, though neither can dietary restriction of foodstuffs containing antioxidants be advised.

Oral glutamine, 15 g twice a day, has been shown to prevent oxaliplatin-induced neuropathy,[49] and non-randomized data support the use of glutamine supplementation in prophylaxis for paclitaxel-induced peripheral neuropathies,[50] myalgias and neuralgias.[51]

Oral L-carnitine, 6 g per day for 4 weeks, improved the functional status of patients undergoing chemotherapy for a variety of advanced tumours.[52] There was a significant reduction in fatigue scores and an increase in lean body mass and appetite. These are non-controlled data and further studies are required.

Radiotherapy

Ionizing radiation generates toxic free radicals and induces double-strand breaks in the DNA of irradiated cells. The repair process results in arrested cellular proliferation and as a result apoptosis, necrosis, or mitotic mutations occur.[53] This, along with the generation of free radicals, accounts for the cytotoxic effect of radiotherapy. Tumour cells are highly proliferative and hence susceptible to such radiation-induced DNA damage.

Radiotherapy can be prescribed as a curative, adjuvant, neo-adjuvant, or palliative therapy. Determining factors include the tumour type, stage, local effects (e.g. spinal cord compression) and the general health of the patient. Radiotherapy can be administered externally, termed external-beam radiotherapy, or internally. Radiotherapy may be prescribed in conjunction with surgery either preoperatively as a neo-adjuvant, intraoperatively with internal administration or postoperatively. It is also commonly co-prescribed with chemotherapy.

External beam radiotherapy

External beam radiotherapy is predominantly targeted at the tumour site, though it may be directed to the lymphatic drainage as well. It is usually delivered in single daily doses, termed

Table 28.4 Acute side-effects of external beam radiotherapy

Radiotherapy site	Acute symptoms	Acute pathological findings
General effects	Anorexia Lethargy Skin changes Hair loss	Local inflammatory response Systemic release of inflammatory cytokines
Central nervous system	Sleepiness Headache Seizures Nausea/vomiting Dysphagia	Raised intracranial pressure Inflammatory response and oedema Focal neurological scarring
Head and neck	Dry mouth Sore mouth Dysphagia Aspiration	Reduced saliva production Mucositis Oesophagitis
Breast	Breathlessness and cough Dysphagia	Pneumonitis Oesophagitis
Cardiac	Breathlessness Palpitations Oedema	Pericardial effusion Congestive heart failure Arrhythmias
Oesophagus	Sore mouth Dysphagia Aspiration Heartburn	Mucositis Oesophagitis
Genitourinary	Frequency Dysuria Urgency Haematuria	Cystitis
Lung	Breathlessness and cough Sore mouth Dysphagia Heartburn	Pneumonitis Mucositis Oesophagitis
Upper GI tract	Anorexia Nausea/vomiting Abdominal pain GI bleed	Radiation enteritis Ileus Subacute or acute obstruction
Pelvis	Diarrhoea Abdominal pain GI bleed Vomiting	Radiation enteritis Ileus Subacute or acute obstruction

GI, gastrointestinal.

fractions, over several weeks though differing regimens exist. Hyperfractionation regimens involve daily increments over the time period in order to allow tolerance to the toxic effects (Table 28.4). Accelerated fractionation delivers relatively high doses in an intensive and shortened schedule. The rationale behind this approach is to overcome the possibility of tumour proliferation during a therapeutic course. It also allows the delivery of the therapy prior to the development of any localized reactions, such that symptoms develop following the end of the course. This reduces the incidence of incomplete therapy due to symptom development.

Use of external beam radiotherapy has been greatly advanced recently. The technique of intensity-modulated radiation therapy (IMRT) involves treatment planning using three-dimensional computed tomography (CT) images and computer-generated algorithms.[54] IMRT allows for targeted precision to within a 1 mm radius, and for differing intensity exposures within the lesion. IMRT therefore minimzes the exposure to normal structures.[53] The organs most commonly treated with IMRT are: prostate, spine, lung, breast, kidney, pancreas, liver, larynx, tongue, and sinus.

Internal radiotherapy

Internal radiotherapy comprises both brachytherapy and radioisotope therapy (Table 28.5). Brachytherapy involves placing solid radioactive material in the form of needles, wires or tubes close to or inside the tumour under sedation or general anaesthesia. These radiation-delivering devices may be removed after a few days if the treatment is given as an adjuvant to external therapy, or up to 1 week if it is the sole therapy to be given. Permanent radioactive seed implants can be placed under general anaesthetic into the prostate. The radioactivity from these seeds persists for around a year and they are not removed. The implants only transmit to a depth of a few millimetres and so the local effects are minimal.

Radioisotopes can be administered orally or intravenously. Strontium-89 and samarium-153 are radioisotopes, which have been investigated for their use in palliation of metastatic bone cancer pain, though their precise indications and role are yet to be fully determined. Response rates have been shown to vary from 40% to 95%, with an onset after 1–4 weeks.[55] Mild and reversible thrombocytopenia or neutropenia commonly occur.

Chemo-radiotherapy

The concurrent use of systemic hormonal or chemotherapy has been a major advance in the field of radiotherapy. The evidence for this is strongest for locally advanced head and neck cancer patients.[56] It is, however, widely used in patients with gastrointestinal cancers including oesophageal, rectal, pancreatic and gastric. Chemo-radiotherapy results in increased tumour sensitization to radiotherapy. This results in either a greater clinical outcome or a reduced radiotherapy exposure requirement for the same effect. The toxicity that arises from combined chemo-radiotherapy is predictable and based on the individual therapies. Of note, the prevalence of mucositis is increased due to dual effects on the mucosal layer.

Nutritionally related side-effects of radiotherapy

The main acute nutritional side-effects occur in patients receiving head and neck and abdominal/pelvic radiotherapy (Table 28.4). This chapter will therefore primarily focus on these patients.

Table 28.5 Internal radiotherapy and radioisotopes

Caesium applicator	Caesium or iridium wires	Radioisotope
Cervical	Oral	Thyroid
Vaginal	Head and neck	(iodine-131)
	Breast	Metastatic prostate
	Anal	(strontium-89 or radium-233)
	Oesophageal	Polycythaemia
	Lung	(phosphorus-32)
	Penile	
	Bile duct	
	Urethra	

Head and neck radiotherapy

Head and neck cancers originate from the oral cavity, nasopharynx, oropharynx, hypopharynx and the larynx. The majority are squamous cell carcinomas. Radiotherapy for head and neck cancer may be a primary therapy, adjunctive or increasingly in combination with chemotherapy.

It is important to remember that many head and neck patients may well be malnourished even before the onset of their cancer. There is a 125-fold increased risk of head and neck cancer among alcoholics even after adjusting for tobacco use.[57] At the time of diagnosis, and prior to radiotherapy, many patients have been shown to be malnourished. Pre treatment there is a mean weight loss of 4%, with dysphagia, dysgeusia and anorexia as predictive symptoms.[58] Critical weight loss, defined as a loss >5% of the original body weight in 1 month or >10% in 6 months, is present in 19% of pre-radiotherapy head and neck patients.[59]

Further weight loss occurs during radiotherapy. A mean loss of around 6% occurs in the first 3 months following radiotherapy. This is predominantly a loss of lean body mass.[60] Beaver *et al.*[61] noted that 33% of patients developed critical weight loss during radiotherapy. Intake of fluids is impaired, with more than half of patients developing biochemical evidence of dehydration during chemo-radiotherapy with cisplatin.[62] This results in hospital inpatient admissions for dehydration in 11% of head and neck radiotherapy patients who have no route of enteral support.[61] Critical factors for this reduction in oral intake are the development of xerostomia, symptomatic mucositis and dysphagia. Salivary flow rates reduce by 62% following a course of radiotherapy and incompletely recover.[63] Xerostomic patients have a delayed swallow, especially with dry absorbent foodstuffs, as assessed by videofluoroscopy.[64]

Symptomatic oral mucositis starts to develop within 2 weeks of the onset of a radiotherapy course. It is present in roughly a half of those undergoing standard radiotherapy and in three-quarters of those undergoing the more intensive continuous, hyperfractionated, accelerated radiotherapy (CHART) regimen.[65] The onset of symptomatic dysphagia following head and neck radiotherapy starts at 2 weeks,[66] and occurs in up to 50% of patients receiving head and neck chemo-radiotherapy.[67] Oral, oesophageal or pharyngeal mucositis results in acute dysphagia and odynophagia. Chronic dysphagia results from fibrosis, strictures and a diminished pharyngeal sensation.

Pelvic radiotherapy complications

Radiation enteritis The intestinal tract is frequently exposed to radiotherapy targeted for gynaecological, abdominal, rectal or prostatic malignancies. Following exposure there are three possible gastrointestinal clinical outcomes, no clinical effect (which is rare), an acute enteropathy or a chronic enteropathy. The most frequently affected sections of the gastrointestinal tract are the terminal ileum, sigmoid colon and rectum. The mobile jejunum and proximal ileum are seldom involved.

Factors that increase the risk of developing radiation enteritis include:

- concurrent chemotherapy, in particular with adriamycin, methotrexate, fluorouracil or bleomycin;
- high dose or accelerated fractionation radiotherapy regimens;
- intestinal adhesions from prior abdominal surgery;
- diabetes, hypertension and other risk factors for vascular occlusive disease;
- thin patients with limited abdominal wall or intra-abdominal fat.

Acute radiation enteritis Acute radiation enteritis develops due to damage to cells undergoing mitosis, resulting in apoptosis or necrosis. The intestinal mucosa repopulates its cellular structure every 5 days and so is particularly vulnerable to radiation damage. The resultant mucosal denuding takes 10–15 days to fully resolve. Accelerated radiotherapy regimens allow insufficient time for mucosal healing and regeneration in between doses and so there is an increased prevalence of enteritis.

The loss of the mucosal lining causes diarrhoea, which may be bloody if ulceration occurs, and ileal involvement can result in bile salt malabsorption. Up to 70% of patients develop acute radiation enteritis symptoms. Symptoms are normally temporary and resolve within a fortnight of the end of the course. As a result, weight loss due to acute enteritis is rare.[68] The loss of intestinal barrier function increases gut permeability such that systemic bacteraemia and toxaemia can develop. A greater prevalence of toxic symptoms is noted following higher radiation doses.[69]

Chronic radiation enteritis Fifty per cent of exposed patients develop a chronic enteropathy following 6 months to 30 years after the initial radiation exposure. Serious gastrointestinal complications including obstruction, fistulation and colitis occur in 5–10%.[68] As opposed to the damage to the mitotically active cells in acute radiation enteritis, chronic enteritis results from damage to the vascular endothelial and connective tissue cells. A progressive and occlusive vasculitis develops, resulting in arterial or venous thromboses and consequently a chronic ischaemia.

Effect of pre-radiotherapy malnutrition

The presence of malnutrition pre-radiotherapy has been shown to be a poor prognostic indicator. A body mass index (BMI; kg/m^2) <18 and a plasma albumin <35 g/l are strongly predictive of a poor outcome with chemo-radiotherapy for oesophageal cancer.[4]

Energy requirements and radiotherapy

De la Maza *et al.*[70] rigorously assessed the nutritional effects of external pelvic radiotherapy in women undergoing a 5-week regimen entailing 45–50 Gy for gynaecological malignancy. The majority reported non-persistent diarrhoea and abdominal pain, which were associated with a significant reduction in documented intestinal transit times and increases in intestinal permeability. Their reduction in dietary energy intake and physical activity resulted in a predominant loss of lean body mass. Using the Subjective Global Assessment tool (SGA), a third of patients became moderately malnourished.

The energy requirements of head and neck patients undergoing radiotherapy alone have not been studied, though it has been in chemo-radiotherapy. Garcia-Peres *et al.*[71] showed a 12% reduction in REE, using indirect calorimetry, from baseline to 4 weeks following the start of the regimen. Following this, the REE started to normalize and formed a U-shaped curve. The Harris–Benedict formula was shown to underestimate the requirements of these patients by 10% as compared to indirect calorimetry. Silver *et al.*[72] assessed a similar cohort of patients but also assessed exercise levels. Weight fell after 1 week of treatment and 11% was lost at 1 month. Of this 11%, 70% was a reduction in lean body mass. No significant change in the calculated REE was noted on indirect calorimetry, though there were significant reductions in physical activity.

It is widely believed that a reduced calorific intake occurs in head and neck patients undergoing radiotherapy, and that this accounts for the majority of their weight loss.[16] Sadly, substantive evidence for this viewpoint is lacking. In the absence of dietary supplementation, both significant increases and decreases in calorific intake have been described.[73,74] The reasons for these diverging findings are unclear. Silver *et al.*[72] in their thorough study showed a non-significant reduction from a mean intake of 10.3 MJ (2454 kcal)/24 h to 8.8 MJ (2108 kcal)/24 h despite the instigation of supplementation in those with significant reductions in oral intake. As there was no change in these patients' REE and their activity levels decreased, then one assumes that the reductions in calorific intake contribute substantially to their observed weight loss.

Protein requirements and radiotherapy

As radiotherapy induces cellular destruction, it is widely assumed that protein requirements increase during therapy. The evidence to support this is limited. Formal nitrogen balance studies have not been done in patients undergoing radiotherapy, though significant losses of lean body mass have been shown.[72,73] Unfortunately it is unclear whether these losses were due to their reduced dietary nitrogen intake, reduced levels of physical activity or catabolic state.

Nutritional interventions and radiotherapy

All patients due to undergo a course of radiotherapy should be screened for nutritional risk at the time of diagnosis.[3] The goal of nutritional management in this setting is to improve and maintain dietary intake with the aim of maintaining quality of life, physical function and reducing treatment-related complications. Quality of life has been shown to correlate strongly with the amount of nutritional intake during radiotherapy.[73] There is little evidence, however, that nutritional therapy impacts on tumour response, complication rates or patient survival.[6] A multidisciplinary approach is required, as poorly controlled symptoms are the principal factor that accounts for the reduction of oral intake in most patients. Specific attention needs to be paid to dentition, salivary dysfunction, pain, dysphagia and the development of increased nutritional losses due to diarrhoea.

Oral nutritional support and radiotherapy

A recent meta-analysis of three randomized controlled trials showed that oral nutritional support, as compared to routine care, in radiotherapy patients results in a significantly increased dietary energy intake by nearly 1.7 MJ (400 kcal)/day.[6] Oral nutritional supplementation does not appear to reduce intake of calories and protein from foodstuffs in head and neck[76] and general radiotherapy patients,[77] and hence results in increased overall intakes. Despite this, no changes in body composition, plasma albumin levels or outcome have been shown.[6]

Enteral tube feeding and radiotherapy

Enteral tube feeding in non-dysphagic oesophageal cancer patients undergoing chemo-radiotherapy has been shown to result in less weight loss than standard diet.[78] However, no comparisons were made between the total macronutrient intakes in this non-randomized study and so it has limited practical implications.

Head and neck radiotherapy patients often struggle symptomatically to meet their dietary needs, and their oral intake is frequently unsafe due to the development of strictures and neuromuscular incoordination. Barium swallow assessments performed 3 months following chemoradiotherapy show a moderate-to-severely impaired swallow in three-quarters of patients and evidence of silent aspiration in more than a third.[79]

The elective placement of enteral tubes pre head and neck radiotherapy has been shown to be safe[80] and result in fewer treatment delays.[81] Unfortunately there are no prospective randomized data to support the use of electively placed pre-radiotherapy enteral feeding tubes. Enteral tube placement pre-radiotherapy is advised if a severe oral or pharyngeal mucositis is predicted either due to either the intensity of the radiotherapy regimen or if it is to be combined with chemotherapy.[16] Use of a percutaneous enteral gastrostomy (PEG) tube is normally preferred as it bypasses the oral, pharyngeal and oesophageal mucosa. There are no randomized controlled trials comparing use of PEGs and nasogastric feeding tubes. Retrospective data demonstrate patient preference for PEGs[82] with better cosmesis, independence and mobility.

Lee *et al.*[83] placed prophylactic PEG tubes pre head and neck chemo-radiotherapy. 98% of the tubes were subsequently used either due to resultant poor oral intake or weight loss. The PEG tubes allowed patients to receive all of their prescribed radiotherapy and 72% of their prescribed chemotherapy. Patients with locally advanced stage 3 or 4 oropharyngeal tumours frequently undergo aggressive chemo-radiotherapy regimens and so have a high prevalence of symptomatology. Enteral support is therefore frequently employed. Three months following the onset of such a therapeutic regimen only a third of patients maintain all their nutritional requirements orally and nearly a quarter take nil orally.[84]Oral intake normally regains at a year post therapy, but a half of patients have been shown to require continued enteral support to meet their nutritional requirements.

Parenteral nutrition and radiotherapy

Parenteral nutrition may be indicated in patients with chronic radiation enteritis. The role of parenteral nutrition around the time of the radiotherapy itself has neither been prospectively studied nor widely described. There are case reports of its use during severe mucositis.[85] Routine use cannot therefore be recommended. It appears to be indicated only in the rare situation where enteral access and absorption is impossible and continued radiotherapy is felt to be beneficial.

Dietary counselling and radiotherapy

Dietary intake in head and neck radiotherapy patients changes as a consequence of impaired salivary flow, dysgeusia, mucositis and impaired swallow. During radiotherapy, patients consume an increased amount of carbohydrates, which are relatively easy to consume orally, and a reduced amount of protein.[66,74] This is potentially deleterious due to the presumed increased nitrogen requirement following radiotherapy.

There are strong data supporting the role of dietetic counselling for those undergoing pelvic radiotherapy as opposed to the sole use of written advice or liquid supplementation. Raasco *et al.*[74] prospectively randomized head and neck radiotherapy patients into three groups. The first group received dietary counselling, the second were supplied high-protein liquid supplements and the third received no dietetic advice or support. Dietary counselling resulted in increased total energy and protein intakes for 3 months following radiotherapy. High-protein liquid supplements resulted in initial increases, though these levels fell to baseline by 3 months. Those offered no dietetic support or advice had reduced intakes post radiotherapy. Crucially these changes in nutritional intakes between the groups reflected functional and symptomatic quality of life, which increased most significantly with dietary counselling and worsened markedly in the non-interventional group. Isenring *et al.*[86] showed that the combination of intensive nutritional counselling and oral nutritional supplements results in less weight loss, malnutrition and quality-of-life impairment in patients undergoing pelvic and head and neck radiotherapy. The control arm received the usual local practice of general advice and a nutrition booklet.

The role of elemental diets has been studied in radiotherapy. In a small and early study, the use of an isocaloric semi-elemental diet resulted in greater weight maintenance in patients undergoing abdominal or pelvic radiotherapy than a standard diet.[86] Elemental diets reduce the frequency of leukopenia in patients undergoing pelvic radiotherapy as compared to matched controls on a standard diet,[88] though these effects were not noted in oesophageal radiotherapy patients.[78]

There is no conclusive benefit from the wide variety of other nutritional interventions that have been trialled during pelvic radiotherapy including restriction of lactose, fat, fibre and caffeine.[68]

The rationale behind lactose restriction is the theory that the radiation-induced mucosal damage will result in damage to the brush border enzymes and hence an acquired lactose intolerance. A prospectively randomized study of either a low fat, low lactose diet or standard diet showed a significant initial benefit with the restricted diet, though no such benefit was maintained at 12 weeks.[89]

Diet supplements and radiotherapy

The controversial role of antioxidant use in radiotherapy is discussed in the chemotherapy section of this chapter. The benefit of probiotics as a diarrhoeal prophylaxis in pelvic radiotherapy has long been known[90] and repeatedly shown. Use of VSL#3 (Ferring Pharmaceuticals, Slough, UK) three times daily resulted in a significant reduction in the diarrhoeal frequency and severity.[91] A recent Cochrane review analysed the findings of four placebo-controlled studies of the use of glutamine in mucositis prevention during radiotherapy.[92] No beneficial effect was demonstrated.

Bone marrow and haematopoietic stem cell transplantation

In recent times there has been an increase in the use of bone marrow transplant (BMT) or haematopoietic stem cell transplant (HSCT) as therapy for both haematological malignancies such as leukaemia, lymphoma, and myeloma, and some solid tumour types. In part, the reduced toxicities following the advent of reduced intensity conditioning regimens based on chemotherapy agents alone have resulted in these therapies being more acceptable. The theory behind using non-myeloablative conditioning regimens is that their curative potential is mediated by a graft-versus-host disease (GVHD; tumour versus leukaemia) effect, rather than from the myeloablative effects of high dose chemotherapy and/or total body irradiation (TBI).[93]

Table 28.6 summarizes the different transplant types, the composition of the conditioning regimens and cell type used. The development of using peripheral haematopoietic stem cells in preference to bone marrow has led to shorter engraftment times.[94] Both this, and the availability and routine use of growth factors such as granulocyte colony-stimulating factors, has substantially reduced the duration of neutropenia, and therefore decreased the risk of infectious complications.[95] The use of cord blood in transplantation has also been developed over the past 30 years, although currently this is a relatively rare source of stem cells.[96]

Table 28.7 highlights each stage of the inpatient BMT/HSCT treatment process; however, increasingly transplantation is being performed in the outpatient setting. The timings are not exact, but more an approximation of what happens at each stage, as patients with differing diagnoses undergo a variety of conditioning regimens and transplant types.

Nutritional complications of BMT/HSCT

During the conditioning phase, the majority of patients are well, although prophylactic anti-emetics such as ondansetron, granisetron and low dose steroids are often used to prevent nausea and vomiting brought on by high dose chemotherapy infusion and/or TBI. The side-effects of these treatment modalities are highlighted in Tables 28.2–28.4. In addition, antifungal, antiviral and antibacterial prophylaxis is commenced along with regular mouthcare using teeth cleaning and mouthwashes up to six times per day. Despite the availability of numerous antimicrobial mouthwash agents, studies to date have not demonstrated any greater benefit of these over the use of saline as a prophylactic measure.[98] Patients usually remain asymptomatic until they become neutropenic, especially when neutrophils reach $<0.5 \times 10^9$/L, at which point the patient usually

Table 28.6 Main transplant types, conditioning regimens and cell type

Transplant type	Conditioning and cell type
Reduced intensity conditioning autograft	High dose chemotherapy Patient's own cells
Full intensity autograft	High dose chemotherapy Total body irradiation Patient's own cells
Reduced intensity conditioning sibling allograft	High dose chemotherapy Sibling donor cells
Full intensity sibling allograft	High dose chemotherapy Total body irradiation Sibling donor cells
Reduced intensity conditioning voluntary unrelated donor allograft	High dose chemotherapy Unrelated donor cells
Full intensity voluntary unrelated donor allograft	High dose chemotherapy Total body irradiation Unrelated donor cells

requires protective isolation. Around day +5 onwards, signs of mucositis arise in the form of stomatitis, ulceration, glossitis, xerostomia, odynophagia, dysphagia, oesophagitis, abdominal cramping or pain and profuse watery, often secretory diarrhoea.[99]

The impact therefore of such treatment on nutritional status can be catastrophic. A BMT/HSCT can lead to complete intestinal failure post bone marrow or stem cell return. At the same time as neutropenia occurs, mucositis worsens, and infectious complications develop as a result of bacterial translocation, the placement of multiple lumen central venous catheters and viral reactivations. The potential development of GVHD, presenting in the gut, liver and skin, can also further compromise nutritional status.

Table 28.7 BMT/HSCT process[a]

Time period	Stage of the BMT/HSCT process
Days –2 to –7	Conditioning with chemotherapy ± total body irradiation.
Day 0	Transplantation: infusion of bone marrow or haematopoietic stem cells via a central venous catheter.
Day +5 to +15	Mucositis, diarrhoea, leukopenia, thrombocytopenia, pancytopenia, high risk of infection.
Day +15 onwards	Recovery, with resumption of a normal oral dietary intake providing there are no other complications; potential for infectious complications remains.
1–18 months	Immune function gradually restored.

BMT, bone marrow transplant; HSCT, haematopoietic stem cell transplant.
[a]Data adapted from Steward *et al.*[96]

Mucositis and intestinal symptoms

According to Stiff,[100] studies have demonstrated that significant oral mucositis occurs in about 75% of patients undergoing BMT/HSCT, particularly in those receiving TBI-based conditioning regimens and high dose etoposide and melphalan. Such patients often report significant changes in their saliva, including a decline in or absent production of saliva, increased viscosity of the saliva causing a 'sticky' or even 'stringy' mouth, and the enzyme composition appears to alter.[101] This results in a reduced ability to tolerate starchy carbohydrates and prevents regular toothpaste from foaming in the mouth.

The combination of high dose chemotherapy and/or TBI can contribute to gut stasis and even the formation of an ileus, resulting in early satiety, anorexia, nausea and vomiting.[102] Patients undergoing BMT/HSCT are required to take multiple medications throughout a 24 h period, which is also thought to impact on satiety.[103] Some of these medications, particularly if changed to liquid preparations if patients have a degree of dysphagia secondary to mucositis, are poorly tolerated orally and can often cause nausea and vomiting. The extreme fatigue that patients also report leads to reduced desire to eat and drink.

Graft-versus-host disease

An often complex and potentially fatal complication of allogeneic BMT/HSCT is the development of GVHD whereby the immunocompetent cells in the graft specifically target the antigens on the recipients' cells.[95] There are two types of GVHD, acute and chronic. Both forms differ in onset, and clinical features post allogeneic BMT/HSCT (Table 28.8). Treatment includes a combination of immunosuppressive drugs including corticosteroids such as methylprednisolone, and immunosuppressants such as cyclosporin, tacrolimus, and mycophenolate mofetil.[95,96] In cases of steroid refractory GVHD, additional treatment options include: monoclonal antibodies, i.e. daclizumab, infliximab and entanercept, antithymocyte globulin, extracorporeal photopheresis or an infusion of mesenchymal stem cells.[96]

The nutritional management of GVHD is poorly studied. Enteral and oral nutritional support should be optimized in these patients. Manipulation of dietary fibre, fat and sugar, particularly lactose, needs to be considered so as not to worsen diarrhoea and promote absorption.[104] Those patients with severe intestinal GVHD often defined by the colour, consistency and volume of diarrhoea should be considered for parenteral nutrition.[105] They may require intestinal failure-type pharmaceutical management, using antidiarrhoeal agents, proton pump inhibitors to reduce

Table 28.8 Comparison of the features of acute and chronic graft-versus-host diease (GVHD)

	Acute GVHD	**Chronic GVHD**
Onset	<100 days post transplant	>100 days
Natural history	Can occur immediately post BMT/HSCT	Occurs after the onset of, or previous resolution of, acute GVHD.
Clinical features	Erythematous dermatitis	Sclerodermatous skin changes.
	Diarrhoea	Malabsorption.
	Transaminitis	Obstructive hepatitis.
		Can be extensive and affect eyes, salivary glands, oral mucosa and other organs.

BMT, bone marrow transplant; HSCT, haematopoietic stem cell transplant.

gastric acid secretion, oral rehydration solution, pancreatic enzymes and bile sequestrants to reduce volume output and electrolyte disturbances.

Hepatic complications of BMT/HSCT

The use of certain antifungals as prophylaxis or treatment for infection along with prolonged periods of not eating and drinking can contribute to the derangement of liver enzymes and the onset of cholestasis. Further complications of the BMT/HSCT process include the development of GVHD, as previously mentioned, or veno-occlusive disease (VOD) of the liver. GVHD is discussed in greater detail later in this chapter. VOD arises secondarily to the effects of the conditioning regimen with both chemotherapy and irradiation causing a vascular endothelial injury. Hepatic VOD is characterized by a tender hepatomegaly, jaundice and ascites.[106] This potentially life-threatening complication has no optimal therapeutic strategy and poorly understood preventive measures.[107]

Neutropenia and immunocompromisation

As part of the work-up pre BMT/HSCT, discussions on the need for a neutropenic diet during the transplant process should be undertaken. The neutropenic diet, as previously highlighted in this chapter, should be used when the patient's neutrophil counts decrease to $\leq 0.5 \times 10^9$/l. This diet is also referred to as a low microbial, low bacterial, sterile or clean diet, and such diets often appear in the methodology of published BMT/HSCT studies; however, no agreed definition or precise composition of a neutropenic diet has yet been agreed.[108]

In the USA, Karras[109] reported that the commonest sources of food- and water-borne infections are undercooked poultry and eggs, and fresh water. This situation is likely to be in line with that of the UK and Europe. The most frequently isolated organisms in cases of food poisoning among the general population are *Campylobacter*, *Shigella* and *Salmonella*,[109,110] but these are not the pathogens routinely isolated in patients with neutropenic sepsis.[111] The common causes of Gram-negative sepsis in the immunocompromised patient population are *Pseudomonas*, *Enterobacter* and *Klebsiella* species. Interestingly, the microbiological testing of foods served in the hospital environment and other public settings demonstrates colonization by large numbers of such pathogens.[110] Two scientific groups have suggested that these pathogens are likely to arise from translocation from dormant colonization of the gastrointestinal tract aided by mucositis.[111,112]

The neutropenic diet should encompass both strict food safety practices and additional dietary restrictions of the specific foodstuffs that potentially contain bacteria, yeasts, moulds, parasites and viruses.[113] However, it is recognized that such restrictions can impact on an already nutritionally compromised population[108,114,115] and no association has yet been shown between adherence to a neutropenic diet and chemotherapy-related infection rates.[116] Although the use of neutropenic diets in the immunosuppressed patient population remains something of a controversy, it would appear prudent to limit the diet where necessary to reduce the risk of acquiring food- or water-borne infections. Current practice in the UK, while not as yet nationally accepted, is in line with the recommendations made by Dykewicz[117] for the prevention of opportunistic infections in patients undergoing BMT/SCT.

Box 28.1 provides recommendations on the high risk foods to avoid in the neutropenic patient;[109] these concern foodstuffs that are likely to be from unpasteurized sources, purposefully contain bacteria or moulds, or are known recognized sources of bacteria or food-borne infections.

Box 28.1 High risk foods to be avoided by all immunocompromised patients[a]

- All unpasteurized dairy products, i.e. farm fresh milk, Parmesan cheese
- Soft mould-ripened cheese, i.e. Brie, Camembert, goat's cheese
- Blue-veined cheese, i.e. Danish blue, Stilton
- Raw or undercooked eggs, i.e. homemade mayonnaise, mousse, egg nog, meringue or hollandaise sauce
- Raw or under cooked shellfish, i.e. prawns, mussels, etc.
- Raw or undercooked meat, poultry or fish, i.e. rare meat, sushi, smoked meats/fish, e.g. parma ham, smoked salmon
- Pate and fish paste
- Probiotics, live or bio products, i.e. live yoghurts, probiotic-containing supplements and drinks.

[a]Adapted from Rees.[108]

The US Centers for Disease Control and Prevention published a slightly more restrictive set of dietary guidelines for BMT/SCT, specifying the avoidance of both raspberries and vegetable sprouts due to published case reports.[118] Uncooked foods are a well-recognized source of Gram-negative bacteria, which include: *Pseudomonas aeruginosa*, *Klebsiella*, *Serratia*, and *Enterobacter* spp.[119] Not surprisingly, there are no controlled studies that have evaluated the effect of salads on infection rates in neutropenic patients. Many clinicians, however, do advise patients experiencing neutropenia to avoid fresh fruits, vegetables, and store-bought perishables.[120] Such advice is routinely reported in the literature,[121] and appears to be good practice,[119] although it remains to be studied in this population group.

Invasive mould infections are identified as important causes of morbidity and mortality in patients who are undergoing BMT.[122] Gangneux *et al.*[123] and Beyer *et al.*[124] have reported that certain foodstuffs should not be offered to patients at risk of developing invasive pulmonary aspergillosis and other mould infections as these have been isolated in the following: pepper, spices, nuts, black and herbal teas, corn, coconut, cashew nuts, coffee, beans, soya, cheese, smoked meat, downy-skinned fruits (apricots, kiwis, and peaches), smooth-skinned fruits (apples, bananas, lemons, and oranges), and freeze-dried soups.

With the greater use of probiotic agents in the medical setting, concerns surrounding the risk of sepsis should be considered with this particular patient group. Case reports in humans with haematological disease have been described.[125–128] Boyle *et al.*[125] concluded that probiotics are generally safe to use in healthy individuals, but that they should be used with caution in patients with immune compromise.

In addition to food sources, the most overlooked but potentially controllable source of nosocomial pathogens is the hospital water supply.[129] Water provides a medium in which organisms can replicate;[112] these primarily are *Enterobacter*, *Pseudomonas*, and *Klebsiella* spp., which have been isolated from both tap water and ice.[130] The UK 'Boucheir Report'[131] provided guidance around the provision of water for immunocompromised patients and states that 'all water, from whatever source, that might be consumed by immunocompromised persons should be brought to the boil and allowed to cool before use.' Tap water in the UK remains the commonest source of drinking water provision in the hospital setting.[108] This routine use of tap water has been previously questioned[132] and both water and ice sources have been implicated as the cause of nosocomial infection outbreaks in immunocompromised individuals.[129,133–138]

It is recognized that although no existing method of water treatment is guaranteed to provide an entirely microbe-free product,[139] the use of natural mineral water in immunocompromised patients is potentially dangerous since 'natural mineral water is not sterilized, pasteurized, or otherwise treated to remove or destroy micro-organisms'.[140] A variety of organisms, including *Campylobacter* spp. and coliforms, have been found in mineral water and these survive a considerable length of time, particularly in plastic bottles of uncarbonated water.[141,142] Sterile, filtered, cool boiled, freshly run tap and carbonated mineral waters have all been cited in the literature as options for water provision in the immunocompromised patient following a neutropenic diet.[135] Problems with patient palatability, especially with sterile and cool boiled tap waters have also been highlighted, which can have a significant impact on the maintenance of adequate hydration. It is recommended that immunocompromised patients should avoid both tap water and ice made from tap water.[112] Disposable point-of-use filters have been suggested as the optimal means to provide drinking water for immunocompromised patients in hospital.[135]

Effect of pre BMT/HSCT malnutrition

Both previous treatments and the underlying effects of the disease process can result in a suboptimal nutritional status prior to transplant.[143] On admission for transplant the patient has often had previous chemotherapy, radiotherapy and possibly immunotherapy with the use of monoclonal antibodies, to induce remission or de-bulk the malignant disease. As the patient needs to be medically fit for the transplant process, an optimal nutritional status is therefore an important contributory factor in the preparatory work-up phase.[115]

Patients undergoing BMT/HSCT rarely enter such treatment with malnutrition or apparent cachexia or anorexia.[97,144] Well-nourished patients have a significantly lower post-transplant length of stay as compared to malnourished patients[144] and a better survival rate.[145–147]

Energy and protein requirements of the BMT/HSCT patient

Muscaritoli *et al.*[95] provided an overview of the literature concerning energy and protein requirements in BMT/HSCT. This group reported that from studies in BMT patients, a consensus suggests that this patient group requires energy between 130 and 150% of their basal metabolic rate equating to energy being provided at 0.147–0.126 MJ (30–35 kcal)/kg. Protein requirements are reportedly elevated and should potentially be provided adequately by 1.4–1.5 g/kg. However, in a study of children undergoing allografts, a significant decline in REE was found, which may be attributable to changes in lean body mass and activity levels post transplant, and that care should be taken not to overfeed, which could lead to further complications.[148]

Nutritional management of the BMT/HSCT patient

There remain no standards for nutritional assessment, follow-up or management of the BMT/HSCT patient.[147] As part of the pre-transplant work-up, all patients being prepared for a BMT/HSCT should be nutritionally assessed to establish a baseline to allow for monitoring throughout the transplant process,[99,144,147,149] although at present time this is not routine practice in the transplant setting. Should a patient present at work-up with malnutrition, ideally a programme of nutritional support using a combination of dietary counselling, oral or enteral nutritional support methods should be commenced to maintain or improve nutritional status prior to the transplant process being undertaken, although time may be a limiting factor.

Irrespective of nutritional status, nutritional support should be delivered routinely following BMT/HSCT to prevent malnutrition. Malnutrition can develop due to gastrointestinal toxicity related to conditioning regimens or as a result of increased nutrient requirements.[95] Since most patients are well nourished at the start of treatment, the goal of nutritional support is to maintain nutritional status rather than to achieve nutritional repletion.[97]

Oral nutritional support, dietary counselling and BMT/HSCT

Nutritional support should be initiated prior to all patients commencing the conditioning regimen while their appetites remain unaffected. First-line nutritional support in the form of dietary counselling and/or the use of oral nutrition supplements (ONS) should be offered. Such simple methods can be effective and tend to be of greater benefit in patients undergoing autografts and reduced intensity conditioning regimens. These patients often have fewer side-effects and a shorter duration of neutropenia. However, consideration should be given to providing variety, and to the fact that many patients report taste fatigue secondary to previous or long term ONS use. Treatment-related dysosmia (altered smell) and dysgeusia (altered taste), salivary changes and the development of oral mucositis can result in the failure of these methods of nutritional support to be effective, and ultimately there should be a low threshold for managing these patients more aggressively.

Enteral tube feeding and BMT/HSCT

Like many aspects of nutritional support, the evidence for artificial nutritional support in the BMT/HSCT is lacking, particularly when looking at enteral nutrition feeding methods. As well as the previously described benefits of enteral feeding, a tube also provides a suitable route for additional hydration and administering medications in the sick BMT/HSCT patient. However, due to the lack of demonstrated effects on tumour response, therapy-associated side-effects, graft survival, GVHD or overall survival, Arends *et al.*[16] concluded that tube feeding is not routinely indicated during autologous or allogeneic BMT/HSCT. At present there is a lack of evaluable data available concerning the relative effectiveness of enteral tube feeding versus parenteral nutrition.[150]

Despite the lack of published evidence deemed adequately supportive for enteral nutrition in this patient group, the use of this feeding route in the BMT/HSCT population, anecdotally, is rising. In the UK particularly, there appears to be increasing use of enteral nutrition such as that demonstrated by Sefcick *et al.*[143] and Papadopoulou *et al.*[151] However, it is acknowledged that sample sizes are small. The risk of bleeding secondary to pancytopenia is often cited as a reason for not considering the enteral route; however, a retrospective case note audit at a UK transplant centre of nasogastric tube (NGT) insertions in BMT/HSCT found that only a single case in a sample of 23 adult patients reported a nose bleed post-insertion despite adequate platelets.[152] Tubes do get placed with platelets <50, although this is likely to be dependent on the centre, and advice on platelet cover for insertion should be discussed with the haematology team.[153]

By placing a prophylactic enteral feeding tube in the patient undergoing a BMT/HSCT, not only can an adequate nutritional intake be maintained via the oral and/or enteral route when mucositis develops, but this route can also ensure delivery of additional hydration and medications that are tolerated poorly orally. Since gastric stasis can often occur, it has been suggested that a nasojejunal tube (NJT) may be preferable to a NGT in these patients.[99,143] Preferred practice would be to insert a prophylactic NGT or NJT on admission for BMT/HSCT or by day +1 post stem cell return[143] and no later than day +4 due to the severity of mucositis because enteric tubes are difficult to insert when mucositis is established. An anti-emetic policy should be instituted to prevent displacement and facilitate optimal enteral nutrition.[143,153] Some centres use longer term feeding tubes, i.e. PEGs or percutaneous endoscopic gastrojejunostomy (PEGJ) tubes,[99] particularly in paediatrics or young adults. Such tubes require early insertion to allow adequate healing. Diarrhoea may be associated with enteral nutrition, and theoretically may be reduced with the use of peptide or semi-elemental feeds. The osmolarity of such feeds, however, is often significantly higher than that of standard polymeric enteral feeds, and as a result they can be poorly tolerated. Practical advice would suggest that if the patient is malabsorbing feed, this would be the point at which to consider the use of parenteral nutrition. Arends *et al.*[16] also felt that the increased risk of haemorrhage and infections associated with enteral tube placement in immunocompromised and thrombocytopenic patients has to be considered; and therefore in certain situations, parenteral nutrition may be preferred to enteral nutrition. However, clinical studies using the enteral route for feeding do not support this statement.[153] In the paediatric BMT/HSCT population, longer term enteral feeding is more commonly used,[151] to ensure that nutritional status is maintained, and to provide adequate nutrients for growth.

Parenteral nutrition and BMT/HSCT

Both the literature and historical clinical practice in many transplant centres demonstrate a preference for parenteral over enteral nutrition.[99] This in part is likely to be due to the fact that parenteral nutrition is easy to administer, since this patient group already have a central venous catheter *in situ*, which ensures the reliable delivery of nutrients. It is also easier to manipulate fluid and electrolytes via this feeding method. However, it does ultimately require forward planning with the transplant team since dedicated central line luminal access is required and therefore a triple lumen central venous catheter is likely to be required. Although parenteral nutrition is not without its problems, potentially every additional lumen is an additional infection risk. It also can result in hepatic steatosis and cholestasis and hepatic dysfunction is common in BMT/HSCT secondary to the process itself or the side-effects of medications, particularly antifungals.

Nutritional supplementation and BMT/HSCT

Murray and Pindoria[150] reported that parenteral nutrition supplemented with glutamine versus standard therapy showed a trend towards a reduced length of stay and a reduced incidence of positive blood cultures. There is some supportive data for the use of EPA in BMT/HSCT, with significant reductions in mortality, complications, and improvements in inflammatory markers observed with the use of EPA capsules. This resulted in the trials being suspended early due to the marked differences in survival observed between the groups.[154,155]

The ESPEN expert group reached a consensus not to recommend the enteral administration of glutamine or EPA in patients undergoing BMT/HSCT as they felt that the data were inconclusive.[16] Since then a reduction in short-term mortality in allogeneic HSCT recipients fed glutamine supplemented parenteral nutrition has been demonstrated.[156]

Post-BMT/HSCT transplant

Patients often leave hospital with ongoing symptoms of xerostomia, dysosmia, dysgeusia, early satiety, nausea and extreme fatigue, which in no doubt continue to impact on both nutritional intake and status. Various authors have suggested that the severity and duration of gastrointestinal toxicity may differ among individuals and that this condition significantly affects both food intake and absorption for up to 2–3 weeks post BMT/HSCT.[157–159] However, in practice the recovery to full health and improved appetite can take up to a year, particularly in those who have undergone an allograft.[132] Patients therefore should be kept under nutritional/dietetic review while they remain symptomatic.

Cancer surgery

Compared with other cancer therapies, there is a lot of interest in optimizing patients' nutritional status prior to surgical interventions. The main nutritional issues relate to abdominal surgery, which will be the focus of this section. Elective abdominal surgery was traditionally performed by an open procedure following mechanical bowel preparation. It was accompanied by periods of nil-by-mouth pre and post procedure, and postoperative nasogastric tube decompression.[169] All of these management practices have recently been challenged with a view to promoting the functional recovery of the patient. Perioperative nutritional optimization is central to these new practices.[161] The role of immunonutrition has been assessed extensively in upper gastrointestinal and colorectal surgery and is discussed in Chapter 11.

Energy requirements and surgery

Energy requirements vary during the postoperative period with differing rates of physical exertion and tissue healing. The first few days are characterized by the greatest energy expenditure.[162] As a general rule, uncomplicated surgery results in minimal elevations of the basal metabolic rate (BMR) between 1.0- and 1.15-fold, whereas more complicated surgery can elevate the BMR by up to 1.5.[163]

Protein requirements and surgery

Preoperative protein depletion has been shown to predict for operative complications.[164] Protein requirements are estimated to be between 1.5 and 2 g/kg/day.[165] In the absence of supplementation, a significantly negative protein balance, with consequent loss of muscle mass and function has been shown to occur following major abdominal surgery. Mathur *et al.*[166] assessed patients undergoing a radical cystectomy for their REE, total body nitrogen, fat-free mass and muscle strength using indirect calorimetry, neutron activation analysis, tritium dilution and hand grip dynamometry respectively. At day 14 post surgery, there was a non-significant increase in REE as compared to baseline, whereas there were around 10% reductions noted in all three other variables. At 6 months, grip strength had returned to preoperative values whereas there was an incomplete recovery in the fat-free mass and total body nitrogen.

Preoperative malnutrition

Accurate nutritional assessment in the surgical patient is challenging, as both anthropometric and biochemical measurements are affected by the disease state and its treatment.[164] Preoperative malnutrition has been repeatedly shown, in both benign and malignant disease, to predict for an increased risk of postsurgical morbidity.[167] Malnourished patients have a three-fold increased risk of postoperative nosocomial infections, multiorgan dysfunction, impaired wound healing and a prolonged functional recovery.[168,169] The aim of nutritional support in the perioperative period is to preoperatively correct malnutrition and to maintain nutritional health and aid recovery following surgery.

Preoperative nutritional interventions

There is limited evidence to support the routine use of ONS in well-nourished patients prior to elective cancer surgery. MacFie *et al.*[170] showed no benefit in 100 patients undergoing elective laparotomies. Smedley *et al.*[171] assessed the outcome of standard care versus oral supplements taken pre- and postoperatively in 179 unselected patients undergoing colorectal surgery. Supplementation reduced weight loss, incidence of minor complications and inpatient stay duration.

The management of malnourished patients prior to elective cancer surgery has been infrequently studied. At least 10 days of ONS taken as an outpatient prior to surgery halved operative complication rates in malnourished head and neck cancer patients.[172] There is limited evidence to support the use of enteral tube feeding. Shukla *et al.*[173] demonstrated a reduction in major complication rates from 30% to 10% in patients with gastrointestinal, breast and head and neck disease. Von Meyenfeldt *et al.*[174] showed only non-significant reductions in major complication rates in gastric and colorectal cancer patients with preoperative tube feeding. Wu *et al.*[175] randomized 468 elective patients with gastric or colorectal cancers with moderate or severe malnutrition to either 7 days of preoperative and 7 days of postoperative nutritional support or a standard hospital diet. Parenteral nutrition was initiated in those with intestinal failure. Significant reductions in complication rates, mortality and hospital stay were shown with nutritional support. Unfortunately the outcomes for parenteral and enteral support are jointly presented in the paper, limiting its interpretation.

The largest single study to date assessing preoperative parenteral nutrition involved 395 patients undergoing major abdominal or non-cardiac thoracic surgery.[176] Preoperative parenteral nutrition was given for 7–15 days at a rate of 0.168 MJ (40 kcal)/kg/day, and continued for 3 days postoperatively. A reduced overall complication rate was shown in the severely malnourished group of patients (BMI <17), but in the rest the parenterally fed were disadvantaged, with an overall increase in parenteral nutrition-related infectious complications.

Overall, preoperative nutrition support studies are quite historic, with most of the evidence base published well before 2000, using nutritional regimes which are no longer being used, and preceding other improvements in surgical practice, including recognition of the importance of glycaemic control, earlier mobilization and the cessation of routine preoperative bowel preparation and postoperative nasogastric decompression (see below). This all makes interpretation of the evidence more difficult, and decisions on best practice more challenging. Recent consensus guidelines state that in patients with BMI >18.5 preoperative nutritional support is not required, and surgery should not be delayed. For those with a BMI <18.5 and/or weight loss of >10–15% over 6 months and/or serum albumin <30 g/l (without liver or renal dysfunction), preoperative optimization of nutrition should be attempted for 10–14 days by oral/enteral means, and only parenterally if this is not possible.[167]

Postoperative nutritional support

There is a period of gastro- and colonoparesis following abdominal surgery that can last for several days.[160] However, small intestinal motility usually returns within 8–24 h. Traditional surgical practice involved NGT placement to decompress the upper gastrointestinal tract and to limit enteral feeding until there was objective evidence of a return of gastrointestinal function, either with the passage of flatus or defecation.[177] It was believed that this practice would reduce the risk of pulmonary aspiration and distension and hence dehiscence of the anastamosis. A recent Cochrane review on the routine use of NGTs following abdominal surgery showed that rather than benefiting the situation, it results in significant delays in the return of bowel function, increased patient discomfort and increased pulmonary complications.[176] The evidence is therefore quite clear that routine nasogastric decompression is not indicated.

Early feeding following gastrointestinal resection has been shown to prevent a negative nitrogen balance developing and maintains gut mucosal integrity, and is something that all surgeons should endeavour to achieve.[177] The options are oral feeding, enteral tube feeding and parenteral feeding.

Oral feeding

Reissman *et al.*[180] prospectively randomized 161 patients undergoing elective colorectal surgery to a clear liquid diet on day 1 with increased intakes as tolerated, or standard care (nil by mouth until bowel sounds). There was no difference in the complication rate between the groups, whereas those fed early tolerated a regular diet 2 days earlier than the standard group. Feo *et al.*[181] randomized 100 colorectal cancer patients to a similar regimen, and again demonstrated an earlier return to normal diet and no differences in terms of outcomes and complications. There have been many other studies of oral diet started within 24 h of surgery, and the results are consistent and clearly show that early feeding is safe with no jeopardy to anastamoses or any other complications. Given that earlier feeding assists other aspects of recovery (see Enhanced Recovery After Surgery: ERAS, see below), this is now an approach being widely encouraged to all surgeons.

Enteral tube feeding

Similar favourable outcomes have been shown with tube feeding in many studies, and this is clearly demonstrated in a meta-analysis[182] and a more recent Cochrane review.[183] Because of this widely held consensus and the recognition that small intestinal motility recovers quickly, surgeons are now more inclined to place jejunal tubes perioperatively to allow for the commencement of feeding within the first 24 h. A more detailed exposition of current practice guidelines can be found in Weimann *et al.*[167]

Parenteral nutrition

Parenteral nutrition following gastrointestinal surgery has been compared to standard care in nine studies involving over 700 patients, and overall the parenteral nutrition group had a 10% increase in complications.[161] Many studies comparing postoperative enteral and parenteral nutrition have been undertaken in different patient groups, using different caloric regimes and with different outcomes. Overall the conclusions are consistent that enteral feeding is better. Therefore the place for parenteral nutrition postoperatively remains consigned only to those in whom the gastrointestinal tract is either not working (e.g. prolonged ileus), inaccessible (widespread intra-abdominal sepsis) or absent (excised gut or proximal fistulae).

Post-discharge nutritional management

It takes around 3 months for patients to regain their weight following gastrointestinal cancer surgery.[184] Eighty-seven patients randomized to receive either dietetic advice and an oral protein-rich nutritional supplement or standard care following intestinal resection had significantly greater increases in their lean body mass at both 2 and 4 months,[185] although these changes did not translate into functional benefits.[186] Beattie *et al.*[187] prospectively randomized 101 malnourished post-operative patients to receive either 400 ml of an oral nutritional support or standard care for 10 weeks. The intervention group had a significant increase in weight at 2 weeks, and by week 10 the difference was >4 kg. This was accompanied by significantly improved anthropometry, grip strength and quality of life at week 10. Despite the recognition that weight loss and nutritional compromise persist long after surgery, there are no other studies on post-discharge nutritional support. In the absence of an evidence base, we would recommend that patients be given appropriate dietary counselling prior to hospital discharge and encouraged to keep up with adequate intakes.

Other relevant surgical factors

There are a number of other important factors in surgical practice that have direct implications on the effectiveness of any nutritional support that may be considered. These include the following.

Minimally invasive surgery

The advent of the laparoscopic technique has revolutionized abdominal surgery. It results in reduced rates and duration of ileus formation thus facilitating earlier postoperative feeding.[188] As opposed to an open procedure, laparoscopic resection results in fewer wound infections and pulmonary complications,[189] as well as reductions in postoperative pain and length of hospital stay.[190] There have been concerns relating to the abilities to adequately stage the disease and sample enough lymph nodes, and also fears over tumour dissemination especially at the port-sites. However, as practice has advanced these issues are becoming less of a concern, and there are now published complications rates showing little differences compared to open procedures.[191,192]

Bowel preparation

Recently the traditional dogma over the requirement for bowel preparation prior to elective colorectal surgery has been questioned. It was believed to reduce the incidence of infectious complications, anastomotic dehiscence and intraoperative bowel handling.[193] Preparation remains standard practice in many centers despite a lack of evidence to support these claims.[194] Furthermore, it results in low intakes of nutrition preoperatively and risks dehydration and electrolyte imbalances,[195] and is also associated with bacterial translocation through the gut wall, which may promote infectious complications.[196] A recent Cochrane review of 1592 patients found a doubling in anastomotic leak rates and a non-significant increase in wound infections following bowel preparation prior to colorectal surgery.[194] As with nasogastric decompression, the evidence for the routine use of bowel preparation is overwhelmingly in favour of its abandonment.

Preoperative fluids and carbohydrate loading

Overnight fasting results in dehydration by around 1 litre, which is commonly replaced intravenously during surgery.[197] The American Society of Anaesthesiologists' (ASA) guidelines state that patients may drink clear fluids up to 2 h prior to elective anaesthesia, unless there is a documented problem with gastric emptying.[198] These guidelines have been shown to be safe with no resultant increased aspiration reporting.[199]

Preoperative fasting increases the degree of insulin resistance, which develops as part of the stress response to surgery, and this has been shown to correlate with postoperative complications.[200] Oral loading with carbohydrates the night before and 2 h prior to surgery has been shown to decrease insulin resistance.[201] In addition to symptomatically reducing thirst, anxiety and hunger,[202] this also preserves muscle mass[203] and strength[204] following major abdominal surgery, with a resulting reduction in postoperative stay.[205]

Enhanced Recovery After Surgery (ERAS)

The ERAS approach has been developed initially for elective colorectal surgery, but is now being rolled out to other surgical disciplines. It aims to promote a speedier postoperative recovery and discharge using a multimodal approach focusing on the issues mentioned above, i.e. preoperative carbohydrate loading, omitting bowel preparation and a decompressing NGT, along with optimizing the judicious use of perioperative fluid, early feeding and mobilization, and prompt attention to nausea and postoperative pain with epidural anaesthesia and avoidance, where possible, of opiates.[206] This protocol has allowed lengths of stay to be halved with no increase in long-term complications or readmission rates.[207] ERAS is therefore being widely encouraged within the surgical community as an approach that not only benefits the patients, but also substantially decreases the costs of care.

Conclusions

Nutritional support is considered to be an integral part of the supportive care of patients undergoing cancer therapy. It is recognized that optimum nutrition improves therapeutic modalities, the clinical course of disease and the outcome of patients with cancer.[208] The key issue, however, has not been conclusively addressed. That is, are malnutrition and recent weight loss early markers for a poor outcome with cancer therapy, regardless of their subsequent care? Or does poor outcome arise from the failure to adequately correct these factors? Potentially weight loss and malnutrition may represent a more aggressive tumour, or they may result in patients receiving a less aggressive therapeutic regimen.[5] Prospectively randomized studies are needed to definitively answer these issues, and such studies are lacking.[6]

Such awareness of the role of nutrition in improving therapeutic outcomes has brought many traditional practices under scrutiny. Some of the main recent changes have been in abdominal surgical practice. A recent survey demonstrated wide differences in colorectal surgical practice in five northern European countries.[209] This variation in practice occurred despite abundant high quality evidence and international guidelines.[210] Thirty per cent reported routinely leaving NGTs *in situ* for at least 1 day postoperatively, more than 50% restricted the intake of solid foodstuffs until the onset of bowel sounds and 5% kept patients routinely nil by mouth for at least 3 days.

Rest was historically prescribed to treat a plethora of medical and surgical conditions including myocardial infarction, back pain, stroke and repaired hernias. Such therapy has no place in modern day management, with the advent of rehabilitation and day case procedures. The concept of therapeutic gut rest appears equally to have no place in modern day medical and surgical practice although, despite strong evidence, it may take time before this becomes the accepted norm.[211] The recent ESPEN guidelines recommend the initiation of enteral nutrition within 24 h of all gastrointestinal surgery, and tube feeding in all patients who were obviously undernourished at the time of any surgery.[167]

Nationally run integrated programmes involving translational education and practice feedback have been shown to markedly improve cancer outcomes.[212] This is an exciting period for nutrition in cancer therapy, though perhaps the greatest challenge is to translate good quality evidence into widespread practice.

Case study

Mr N was a 51-year-old, married man with two teenage children. He was self-employed, a non-smoker and enjoyed the occasional glass of wine. His previous medical history included testicular carcinoma treated with a radical orchidectomy. He was diagnosed with chronic lymphocytic leukaemia in 2005 and initially was treated with three different combination chemotherapy regimens.

This gentleman was first referred to the dietitian in a pretransplant assessment clinic in early April 2007 as part of his work-up for a reduced intensity conditioning, voluntary unrelated donor allograft. Baseline nutritional status was assessed with a weight of 74.4 kg, BMI 22.2 kg/m^2, and a hand grip strength of 40.1 kg (normal for an adult male). Mr N reported eating three good meals a day with regular snacks and drinking on average 2 l daily. A discussion was had around a prophylactic NGT, and Mr N consented to this post stem cell return. His main concern was nausea and vomiting since this had been a repeated difficulty with every chemotherapy agent he had previously received. Mr N was electively admitted for his reduced intensity conditioning, voluntary unrelated donor allograft with fludarabine/melphalan/campath as conditioning on 10 April (day –9), his baseline weight 74 kg. Nausea and vomiting started the next day, but symptom control did improve with a review of anti-emetics. However, nausea continued and both his appetite and weight began to decline.

Day 0: The donor stem cells were infused. His weight decreased to 69 kg. He was commenced Fortisip (Nutricia, Trowbridge, UK) twice daily, in addition to oral intake as tolerated.

Day +1: NGT placed and feeding started with Nutrison Standard (Nutricia) at 30 ml/h, with ongoing oral intake encouraged. This continued until day +4 when dietetic review suggested increasing the feed to 50 ml/h. Overnight Mr N vomited out his NGT. There were early signs of oral mucositis and diarrhoea started.

Day +5: NGT was replaced, his feed restarted at 50 ml/h and Mr N was managing half of his meals.

Day +8: Mr N was barely eating or drinking, but was tolerating NG feeding at 100 ml/h, although reporting ongoing nausea. Plans were made to set up an anti-emetic subcutaneous pump.

Day +10: NGT was vomited out again, secondary to an oral antifungal liquid suspension, and Mr N was anxious about eating solids due to nausea and vomiting. He was keen to try NG feeding again, since he now had no appetite and significant taste changes and it was agreed that the palliative care team should review his symptom control. His weight was now 76.4 kg, much of this due to fluid retention/overload.

Day +12: NG feeding was re-established and tolerated well at 100 ml/h overnight (weight 70.2 kg). A subcutaneous pump remained *in situ* with anti-emetics. Engraftment had occurred. The diarrhoea began to worsen, with liquid motions 5–6 times daily and Mr N reported retching with anything orally.

Day +20: Mr N's weight had decreased to 67 kg and the NGT was vomited out again. Xerostomia was now a problem, and a significant skin rash had occurred suggestive of skin GVHD. Artificial saliva, methylprednisolone and topical steroids were commenced and the diarrhoea improved. Dietetic review suggested a change of tube to NJT, although a likely delay in time to placement in endoscopy/radiology was highlighted. In the interim a further NGT was placed (day +23, weight 65.4 kg) and metoclopramide added to encourage gut motility. At this stage the diarrhoea was no longer a problem and feeding was restarted at 50 ml/h.

Day +34: Mr N was discharged home with full NG feeding tolerated, although oral intake of diet and fluids was minimal.

Day +38: Mr N was readmitted with intractable nausea, vomiting and diarrhoea and intestinal GVHD was suggested, his weight now at 60.2 kg. A palliative care review for symptom control was undertaken, his steroid dose increased and an NJT placed on day +40, post upper gastrointestinal endoscopy, where multiple biopsies where taken.

Day +52: His gastrointestinal symptoms had worsened, and intestinal GVHD was histologically confirmed. His weight decreased to 55.8 kg and it was decided to give parenteral nutrition (PN) via a peripherally inserted central catheter (PICC) line. Patient care for nutritional support was handed over to the nutrition team.

Day +74: Mr N's weight had declined to 52.5 kg despite PN and managing Fortisip three times daily orally without nausea or vomiting and semi-formed stools. It was noted that Mr N's fasting blood glucose levels were 24 mmol/l, and steroid-induced diabetes was diagnosed. It was also noted that the patient was receiving excess energy and protein for his requirements from his PN and Fortisip intake.

Day +77: PN continued but NGT feeding was recommenced to attempt to wean off PN.

Day +84: Weight 59.5 kg, PN discontinued as full requirements were being provided by the overnight NG feeding, Fortisip twice a day and oral diet.

Day +90: Discharged home with NGT *in situ* for ongoing feeding. Weight 57.5 kg (22% weight loss). Dietetic review proposed PEG tube insertion in view of longer term need for feeding to replete loss of body mass.

Day +154: Ongoing review by the dietitian continued in the transplant outpatient clinic. NG overnight feeding continued and oral intake remained poor, but was slowly improving. In light of the poor oral intake, a PEG tube was placed. Repeat anthropometry documented a weight of 55.4 kg, BMI of 16.5 (severely underweight), and a hand grip strength of 17.4 kg (about 40% of normal), suggestive of protein-energy malnutrition. Overnight feeding was commenced with 1 litre Nutrison Energy Multi Fibre, in addition to energy- and protein-dense oral intake at 3 meal times daily.

Day +434: PEG removed as patient was eating 3 meals a day, snacks and managing Fortisip twice daily. Weight increased to 67.2 kg (BMI 20.1) hand grip improved to 30.8 kg (about 80% of normal).

Mr N has since returned to work full-time and is now embarking on intensive physiotherapy and an exercise programme to increase his muscle mass. Whereas his intestinal GVHD has resolved, his skin remains a problem and there are plans for him to receive further treatment with extracorporeal photopheresis.

References

1. Westlake S, Cooper N, Rowan S (2007) *Cancer incidence and mortality in the United Kingdom 2002–04*. London: National Cancer Intelligence Centre, Office for National Statistics.
2. Johnson IT, Lund EK (2007) Review article: nutrition, obesity and colorectal cancer. *Aliment Pharmacol Ther*, **26**(2), 161–81.
3. Capra S, Ferguson M, Ried K (2001) Cancer: impact of nutrtion intervention outcome—nutrition issues for patients. *Nutrition*, **17**, 769–72.
4. Di Fiore F, Lecleire S, Pop D, *et al.* (2007) Baseline nutritional status is predictive of response to treatment and survival in patients treated by definitive chemoradiotherapy for a locally advanced esophageal cancer. *Am J Gastroenterol*, **102**, 2557–63.
5. Andreyev HJN, Norman AR, Oates J, Cunningham D (1998) Why do patients with weight loss have a worse outcome when undergoing chemotherapy for gastrointestinal malignancies? *Eur J Cancer*, **34**, 503–09.
6. Elia M, Van Bokhurst-De Van Der Schueren MAE, Garvey J, *et al.* (2006), Enteral (oral or tube administration) nutritional support and eicosapentaenoic acid in patients with cancer: a systematic review. *Int J Oncol*, **28**, 5–23.
7. Dewys WD, Begg C, Lavin PT, *et al.* (1980) Prognostic effect of weight loss prior to chemotherapy in cancer patients. *Am J Med*, **69**, 491–97.
8. Bozzetti F, Migliavacca S, Scotti A, *et al.* (1982) Impact of cancer, type, site, stage and treatment on the nutritional status of patients. *Ann Surg*, **196**, 170–9.
9. Caro MMM, Laviano A, Pichard C (2007) Nutritional intervention and quality of life in adult oncology patients. *Clin Nutr*, **26**, 289–301.
10. Ravasco P, Monteiro-Grillo I, Vidal PM, Camilo ME (2004) Cancer: disease and nutrition are key determinants of patients' quality of life. *Support Care Cancer*, **12**, 246–52.
11. Davies AA, Smith GD, Harbord R, *et al.* (2006) Nutritional Interventions and Outcome in Patients With Cancer or Pre-invasive Lesions: Systematic Review. *J Nat Cancer Institute*, **98**, 961–73.
12. Stratton RJ, Elia M (1999) The effects of enteral tube feeding and parenteral nutrition on appetite sensations and food intake in health and disease. *Clin Nutr*, **18**, 63–70.
13. Szeluga DJ, Stuart RK, Brookmeyer R, Utermohlen V, Santos GW (1987) Nutritional support of bone marrow recipients: a prospective, randomized clinical trial comparing total parenteral nutrition to an enteral feeding program. *Cancer Res*, **47**, 3309–16.
14. McCutcheon NB, Tennissen AM (1989) Hunger and appetitive factors during total parenteral nutrition. *Appetite*, **13**, 129–41.
15. Gil KM, Skeie B, Kvetan V, *et al.* (1991) Parenteral nutrition and oral intake: effect of glucose and fat infusions. *JPEN*, **15**, 426–32.
16. Arends J, Bodoky G, Bozzetti F, *et al.* (2006) ESPEN guidelines on enteral nutrition: non-surgical oncology. *Clin Nutr*, **25**, 245–59.
17. Blazeby JM, Wilson L, Metaclfe C, Nicklin J, English R, Donovan JL (2006) Analysis of clinical decision-making in multi-disciplinary cancer teams. *Annal Oncol*, **17**, 457–60.
18. Perez EA (2007) Safety profiles of tamoxifen and the aromatase inhibitors in adjuvant therapy of hormone-responsive early breast cancer. *Annals Oncol*, **18**, viii26–viii35.
19. Gillatt D (2006) Antiandrogen treatments in locally advanced prostate cancer: are they all the same? *J Cancer Res Clin Oncol*, **132**, S17–S26.
20. Widakowich C, De Castro G, De Azambuja E, Dinh P, Awada A (2007) Side effects of approved molecular targeted therapies in solid cancers. *The Oncologist*, **12**, 1443–5.
21. Laszlo J (1983) Nausea and vomiting as major complications of cancer chemotherapy. *Drugs*, **25**, 1–7.
22. Hesketh PJ (2004) Understanding pathobiology of chemotherapy-induced nausea and vomiting. Providing a basis for therapeutic progress. *Oncology (Williston Park)*, **18**, 9–14.

23. Aapro MS, Molassiotis A, Olver I (2005) Anticipatory nausea and vomiting. *Support Care Cancer*, **10**, 88–95.
24. Kris MG, Hesketh PJ, Somerfield MR, *et al.* (2006) American Society of Clinical Oncology guideline for antiemetics in clinical oncology: update 2006. *J Clin Oncol*, **24**, 2932–47.
25. Divall MV, Cerosimo RJ (2007) Prevention and treatment of chemotherapy-induced nausea and vomiting: a review. *Formulary*, **42**, 378–88.
26. Jordan K, Kasper C, Schmoll HJ (2005) Chemotherapy-induced nausea and vomiting: current and new standards in the antiemetic prophylaxis and treatment. *Eur J Cancer*, **41**,199–205.
27. Marchioro G, Azzarello G, Viviani F, *et al.* (2000) Hypnosis in the treatment of anticipatory nausea and vomiting in patients receiving cancer chemotherapy. *Oncology*, **59**, 100–4.
28. Mundy EA, DuHamel KN, Montgomery GH (2003) The efficacy of behavioural interventions for cancer treatment-related side effects. *Semin Clin Neuropsychiatry*, **8**, 253–75.
29. Stanley A (2002) Monitoring and treatment of adverse effects in cancer chemotherapy. In: Allwood M, Stanley A, Wright P (eds), *The Cytotoxics Handbook*, 4th edn, pp. 203–53. Abingdon: Radcliffe Medical Press.
30. Duncan M, Grant G (2003) Review article: oral and intestinal mucositis—causes and possible treatments. *Aliment Pharmacol Ther*, **18**, 853–74.
31. Keefe DM, Schubert MM, Elting LS, *et al.* (2007) Updated clinical guidelines for the prevention and treatment of mucositis. *Cancer*, **109**, 820–31.
32. Tian J, Chen ZC, Hang LF (2007) Effects of nutritional and psychological status in gastrointestinal cancer patients on tolerance of treatment. *World J Gastroenterol*, **13**, 4136–40.
33. Demark-Wahnefried W, Hars V, Conaway MR, *et al.* (1997) Reduced rates of metabolism and decreased physical activity in breast cancer patients receiving adjuvant chemotherapy. *Am J Clin Nutr*, **65**, 1495–501.
34. Harvie MN, Campbell IT, Baildam A, Howell A (2004) Energy balance in early breast cancer patients receiving adjuvant chemotherapy. *Breast Cancer Res Treat*, **83**, 201–10.
35. Harvie MN, Campbell IT, Thatcher N, Baildam A (2003) Changes in body composition in men and women with advanced non-small cell lung cancer (NSCLC) undergoing chemotherapy. *J Hum Nutr Diet*, **16**, 323–6.
36. Segal R, Evans W, Johnson D, *et al.* (2001) Structured exercise improves physical functioning in women with stages I and II breast cancer: results of a randomized controlled trial. *J Clin Oncol*, **19**, 657–65.
37. Loprinzi CL, Athmann LM, Kardinal CG, *et al.* (1996) Randomized trial of dietician counselling to try to prevent weight gain associated with breast cancer adjuvant chemotherapy. *Oncology*, **53**, 228–32.
38. Ollenschlaeger G, Konkol K, Wickramanayake PD, Schrappe-Baecher M, Mueller JM (1989) Nutrient intake and nitrogen metabolism in cancer patients during oncological chemotherapy. *Am J Clin Nutr*, **50**, 454–9.
39. Stratton RJ, Elia M (1999) A critical, systematic analysis of the use of oral nutritional supplements in the community. *Clin Nutr*, **18**, S29–84.
40. American College of Physicians (1989) Position paper: Parenteral nutrition in patients receiving cancer chemotherapy. *Ann Intern Med*, **110**,734–6.
41. Peltz G (2002) Nutrition support in cancer patients: a brief review and suggestion for standard indications criteria. *Nutr J*, **1**, 1–5.
42. Ovesen L, Allingstrup L, Hannibal J, Mortensen EL, Hansen OP (1993) Effect of dietary counselling on food intake, body weight, response rate, survival, and quality of life in cancer patients undergoing chemotherapy: a prospective, randomized study. *J Clin Oncol*, **11**, 2043–9.
43. Bauer JD, Capra S (2005) Nutrition intervention improves outcome in patients with cancer cachexia receiving chemotherapy—a pilot study. *Support Care Cancer*, **13**, 270–4.

44. Prasad KN (2004) Rationale for using high-dose multiple dietary antioxidants as an adjunct to radiation therapy and chemotherapy. *J Nutr*, **134**, 3182S–3.
45. Burstein HJ, Gelber S, Guadagnoli E, Weeks JC (1999) Use of alternative medicine by women with early-stage breast cancer. *New Eng J Med*, **340**, 1733–9.
46. D'Andrea GM (2005) Use of antioxidants during chemotherapy and radiotherapy should be avoided. *CA Cancer J Clin*, **55**, 319–21.
47. Moss RW (2006) Should patients undergoing chemotherapy and radiotherapy be prescribed antioxidants? *Integrative Cancer Therapies*, **5**, 63–82.
48. Wardman P (2007) Chemical radiosensitizers for use in radiotherapy. *Clin Oncol*, **19**, 397–417.
49. Wang WS, Lin JK, Lin TC, *et al.* (2007) Oral glutamine is effective for preventing oxaliplatin-induced neuropathy in colorectal cancer patients. *The Oncologist*, **12**, 312–9.
50. Vahdat L, Papadopoulos K, Lange D, *et al.* (2001) Reduction of paclitaxel-induced peripheral neuropathy with glutamine. *Clin Cancer Res*, **7**(5), 1192–7.
51. Savarese D, Boucher J, Corey B (1998) Glutamine treatment of paclitaxel-induced myalgias and arthralgias. *J Clin Oncol*, **16**, 3918–9.
52. Gramignano G, Lusso MR, Madeddu C, *et al.* (2006) Efficacy of L-carnitine administration on fatigue, nutritional status, oxidative stress, and related quality of life in 12 advanced cancer patients undergoing anticancer therapy. *Nutrition*, **22**, 136–45.
53. Elshaikh M, Ljungman M, Haken RT, Lichter AS (2006) Advances in radiation oncology. *Annu Rev Med*, **57**, 19–31.
54. Morris MM, Schmidt-Ullrich R, Johnson CR (2000) Advances in radiotherapy for carcinoma of the head and neck. *Surg Oncol Clin N Am*, **9**, 563–75.
55. Finlay IG, Mason MD, Shelley M (2005) Radioisotopes for the palliation of metastatic bone cancer: a systematic review. *Lancet Oncol*, **6**, 392–400.
56. Cooper JS, Pajak TF, Forastiere AA, *et al.* (2004) Post-operative concurrent radiation therapy and chemotherapy for high-risk squamous cell carcinoma of the head and neck. *N Engl J Med*, **350**, 1937–44.
57. Maier H, Seeewald E, Wolf-Dieter-Heller GF *et al.* (1994) Chronic alcohol consumption—the key risk factor for pharyngeal cancer. *Otolaryngol Head Neck Surg*, **110**, 168–73.
58. Lees J (1999) Incidence of weight loss in head and neck cancer patients on commencing radiotherapy treatment at a regional oncology centre. *Eur J Cancer*, **8**, 133–36.
59. Jager-Wittenaar H, Dijkstra PU, Vissink A, Van Der Laan BF, Van Oort RP, Roodenburg JLN (2007) Critical weight loss in head and neck cancer–prevalence and risk factors at diagnosis: an explorative study. *Support Care Cancer*, **15**, 1045–50.
60. Isenring EA, Capra S, Bauer J, Davies PSW (2003) The impact of nutrition support on body composition in cancer outpatients receiving radiotherapy. *Acta Diabetol*, **40**, S162–4.
61. Beaver ME, Matheny KE, Roberts DB, Myers JN (2001) Predictors of weight loss during radiation therapy. *Otolaryngol Head Neck Surg*, **125**, 645–8.
62. Lin A, Jabbari S, Worden FP, *et al.* (2005) Metabolic abnormalities associated with weight loss during chemoirradiation of head-and-neck cancer. *Int J Radiat Oncol Biol Phys*, **63**, 1413–8.
63. Bonan PRF, Pires FR, Lopes MA, Di Hipolito O (2003) Evaluation of salivary flow in patients during head and neck radiotherapy. *Pesqui Odontol Bras*, **17**, 156–60.
64. Hamlet S, Faull J, Klein B, *et al.* (1997) Mastication and swallowing in patients with post irradiation xerostomia. *Int J Radiat Oncol Biol Phys*, **37**, 789–96.
65. Bentzen SM, Saunders MI, Dische S, Bond SJ (2001) Radiotherapy-related early morbidity in head and neck cancer: quantitative clinical radiobiology as deduced from the CHART trial. *Radiother Oncol*, **60**(2), 123–35.
66. Chencharick JD, Mossman KL (1983) Nutritional consequences of the radiotherapy of head and neck cancer. *Cancer*, **51**, 811–5.

67. Nguyen NP, Sallah S, Karlsson U, *et al.* (2002) Combined chemotherapy and radiation therapy for head and neck malignancies: quality of life issues. *Cancer*, **94**, 1131–41.
68. McGough C, Baldwin C, Frost G, Andreyev HJN (2004) Role of nutritional intervention in patients treated with radiotherapy for pelvic malignancy. *Br J Cancer*, **90**, 2278–87.
69. Dorr W, Kost S, Keinert K, Glaser F, Endert G, Herrmann T (2006) Early intestinal changes following abdominal radiotherapy. Comparison of endpoints. *Strahlenther Onkol*, **182**, 1–8
70. De La Maza P, Gotteland M, Ramirez C (2001) Acute nutritional and intestinal changes after pelvic radiation. *J Am Coll Nutr*, **20**, 637–42.
71. García-Peris P, Lozano MA, Velasco C, *et al.* (2005) Prospective study of resting energy expenditure changes in head and neck cancer patients treated with chemoradiotherapy measured by indirect calorimetry. *Nutrition*, **21**(11–12), 1107–12.
72. Silver HJ, Dietrich MS, Murphy BA (2007) Changes in body mass, energy balance, physical function, and inflammatory state in patients with locally advanced head and neck cancer treated with concurrent chemoradiation after low-dose induction chemotherapy. *Head Neck*, **29**, 893–900.
73. Ravasco P, Monteiro-Grillo I, Camilo ME (2003) Does nutrition influence quality of life in cancer patients undergoing radiotherapy? *Radio Oncol*, **67**, 213–20.
74. Ravasco P, Monteiro-Grillo I, Vidal PM, Camilo ME (2005) Impact of nutrition on outcome: a prospective randomized controlled trial in patients with head and neck cancer undergoing radiotherapy. *Head Neck*, **27**, 659–68.
75. Ng K, Leung SF, Johnson PJ, Woo J (2004) Nutritional consequences of radiotherapy in nasopharynx cancer patients. *Nutr Cancer*, **49**, 156–61.
76. Arnold C, Richter MP (1989) The effect of oral nutritional supplements on head and neck cancer. *Int J Radiat Oncol Biol Phys*, **16**, 1595–9.
77. McCarthy D, Weihofen D (1999) The effect of nutritional supplements on food intake in patients undergoing radiotherapy. *Oncol Nurs Forum*, **26**, 897–900.
78. Bozzetti F, Cozzaglio L, Gavazzi C, *et al.* (1998) Nutritional support in patients with cancer of the esophagus: impact on nutritional status, patient compliance to therapy, and survival. *Tumori*, **84**, 681–6.
79. Goguen L, Posner MR, Norris CM, *et al.* (2006) Dysphagia after sequential chemoradiation therapy for advanced head and neck cancer. *Otolaryngol Head Neck Surg*, **134**, 916–22.
80. Nguyen NP, North D, Smith HJ (2006) Safety and effectiveness of prophylactic gastrostomy tubes for head and neck cancer patients undergoing chemoradiation. *Surg Oncol*, **15**, 199–203.
81. Daly JM, Weintraub FN, Shou J, Rosato EF, Lucia M (1995) Enteral nutrition during multimodality therapy in upper gastrointestinal cancer patients. *Ann Surg*, **221**, 327–38.
82. Ohrn KEO, Wahlin YB, Sjoden PO (2001) Oral status during radiotherapy and chemotherapy: a descriptive study of patient experiences and the occurrence of oral complications. *Support Care Cancer*, **9**, 247–57.
83. Lee JH, Machtay M, Unger LD, *et al.* (1998) Prophylactic gastrostomy tubes in patients undergoing intensive irradiation for cancer of the head and neck. *Arch Otolaryngol Head Neck Surg*, **124**, 871–5.
84. Shiley SG, Hargunani CA, Skoner JM, Holland JM, Wax MK (2006) Swallowing function after chemoradiation for advanced stage oropharyngeal cancer. *Otolaryngol Head Neck Surg*, **134**, 455–9.
85. Treister N, Sonis S (2007) Mucositis: biology and management. *Curr Opin Otolaryngol Head Neck Surg*, **15**, 123–9.
86. Isenring EA, Capra S, Bauer JD (2004) Nutrition intervention is beneficial in oncology outpatients receiving radiotherapy to the gastrointestinal or head and neck area. *Br J Cancer*, **91**, 447–52.
87. Bounous G, LeBel E, Shuster J, Gold P, Tahan WT, Bastin E (1975) Dietary protection during radiation therapy. *Strahlentherapie*, **149**, 476–83.
88. Foster KJ, Brown MS, Alberti KG, *et al.* (1980) The metabolic effects of abdominal irradiation in man with and without dietary therapy with an elemental diet. *Clin Radiol*, **31**, 13–7.

89. Bye A, Kaasa A, Ose T, Sundfor K, Trope C (1992) The influence of low fat, low lactose diet on diarrhoea during pelvic radiotherapy. *Clin Nutr*, **11**, 147–53.
90. Salminen E, Elomaa I, Minkkinen J, Vapaatalo H, Salminen S (1988) Preservation of intestinal integrity during radiotherapy using live *Lactobacillus acidophilus* cultures. *Clin Radiol*, **39**, 435–7.
91. Delia P, Sansotta G, Donato V, *et al.* (2007) Use of probiotics for prevention of radiation-induced diarrhoea. *World J Gastroenterol*, **13**, 912–5.
92. Worthington HW, Clarkson JE, Eden OB (2007) Interventions for preventing oral mucositis for patients with cancer receiving treatment. *Cochrane Database Syst Rev*, Issue 4.
93. Johansson JE, Brune M, Ekman T (2001) The gut mucosa barrier is preserved during allogeneic, haemopoietic stem cell transplantation with reduced intensity conditioning. *Bone Marrow Transplant*, **28**, 737–742.
94. Soutar RL, King DJ (1995) Fortnightly review: Bone marrow transplantation. *Br Med J*, **310**, 31–6.
95. Muscaritoli M, Grieco G, Capria S, Iori AP, Fanelli FR (2002) Nutritional and metabolic support in patients undergoing bone marrow transplantation. *Am J Clin Nutr*, **75**, 183–90.
96. Apperley J, Carreras E, Gluckman E, Gratwohl A, Masszi T (2008) *The EBMT Handbook*, 5th edn. Haematopoietic Stem Cell Transplantation. Genoa: Forum Service Editore.
97. Steward W, Hunter A, O'Byrne K, Snowden J (2001) Chemotherapy and haematological stem cell transplantation. In: Nightingale J (ed.), *Intestinal Failure*, pp. 65–86. London: Greenwich Medical Media.
98. Vokurka S, Bystřická E, Koza V, *et al.* (2005) The comparative effects of povidone-iodine and normal saline mouthwashes on oral mucositis in patients after high-dose chemotherapy and APBSCT—results of a randomized multicentre study. *Support Care Cancer*, **13**, 554–8.
99. Martin-Salces M, de Paz R, Canales MA, Mesejo A, Hernandez-Navarro F (2008) Nutritional recommendations in hematopoietic stem cell transplantation. *Nutrition*, **24**, 769–75.
100. Stiff P (2001) Mucositis associated with stem cell transplantation: current status and innovative approaches to management. *Bone Marrow Transplant*, **27**(Suppl 2), S3–S11.
101. Franca CM, Domingues-Martins M, Filho RSP, Soares de Araujo N (2001) Severe oral manifestations of chronic graft-vs.-host disease. *J Am Dental Assoc*, **132**, 1124–7.
102. Johansson JE, Abrahamsson H, Ekman T (2003) Gastric emptying after autologus haemopoietic stem-cell transplantation: a prospective trial. *Bone Marrow Transplant*, **32**, 815–9.
103. Eagle DA, Gian V, Lauwers GY, *et al.* (2001) Gastroparesis following bone marrow transplantation. *Bone Marrow Transplant*, **28**, 59–62.
104. Stern JM (2002) Nutritional assessment and management of malabsorption of the hematopoietic stem cell transplant patient. *J Am Diet Assoc*, **102**, 1812–5.
105. Imataki O, Nakatani S, Hasegawa T, *et al.* (2006) Nutritional support for patients suffering from intestinal graft-versus-host disease after allogeneic hematopoietic stem cell transplantation. *Am J Hematol*, **81**, 747–52.
106. Wadleigh M, Ho V, Momtaz P, Richardson P (2003) Hepatic veno-occlusive disease: pathogenesis, diagnosis and treatment. *Curr Opin Hematol*, **10**, 51–462.
107. Tay J, Tinmouth A, Fergusson D, Huebsch L, Allan DS (2007) Systematic review of controlled clinical trials on the use orsodeoxycholic acid for the prevention of hepatic veno-occlusive disease in hematopoietic stem cell transplantation. *Biol Blood Marrow Transplant*, **13**, 206–17.
108. Rees W (2005) Low microbial diets in immunocompromised patients. *Br J Cancer Manag*, **2**, 21–3.
109. Karras DJ (2000) Incidence of food borne illnesses: preliminary data from the foodbourne diseases active surveillance network. *Ann Emerg Med*, **35**, 92–3.
110. Moody K, Charlson M, Finlay J (2002) The neutropenic diet: what's the evidence? *J Ped Hematol Oncol*, **24**, 717–21.
111. Hughes WT, Armstrong D, Bodey GP, *et al.* (2002) Guidelines for the use of antimicrobial agents in neutropenic patients with cancer. *Clin Infect Dis*, **34**, 730–51.

112. Risi GF, Tomascak V (1998) Prevention of infection in the immunocompromised host. *Am J Infect Control*, **26**, 594–604.
113. Centres for Disease Control and Prevention, Infectious Disease Society of America, American Society of Blood and Marrow Transplantation. Guidelines for preventing opportunistic infections among hematopoietic stem transplant recipients (2000) *Morb Mortal Recomm Rep*, **49**(RR10), 46–9.
114. Mank A, Davies M, Langeveld N, van de Wetering M, van der Lelie H (2007) Low bacterial diet to prevent infection in neutropenic patients. *The Cochrane Library*, Issue 4, 1–7.
115. Sheean PM (2005) Nutrition support of blood or marrow transplant recipients: how much do we really know? *Pract Gastroenterol*, **26**, 84–97.
116. Wilson BJ (2002) Dietary recommendations for neutropenic patients. *Semin Oncol Nurs*, **18**, 44–9.
117. Dykewicz CA (2001) Summary of the guidelines for preventing opportunistic infections among hematopoietic stem cell transplant recipients. *Clin Infect Dis*, **33**,139–44.
118. Moody K, Finlay J, Mancuso C, Charlson M (2006) Feasibility and safety of a pilot randomised trial of infection rate: neutropenic diet versus standard food safety guidelines. *J Ped Hematol Oncol*, **28**, 126–33.
119. Fenlon LE (1995) Protective isolation: who needs it? *J Hosp Infect*, **30** (Suppl), 218–22.
120. Shelton BK (2003) Evidence-based care for the neutropenic patients with leukaemia. *Semin Onc Nurs* **19**, 133–41.
121. Ninin E, Milpied N, Moreau P *et al.* (2001) Longitudinal study of bacterial, viral, and fungal infections in adult recipients of bone marrow transplants. *Clin Infect Dis*, **33**, 41–7.
122. Baddley JW, Stroud TP, Salzman D, Pappas PG (2000) Invasive mould infections in allogeneic bone marrow transplant recipients. *Clin Infect Dis*, **32**, 1319–24.
123. Gangneux J-P, Noussair L, Bouakline A, Roux N, Lacroix C, Derouin F (2004) Experimental assessment of disinfection procedures for eradication of Aspergillus fumigatus in food. *Blood*, **104**, 2000–2.
124. Beyer J, Schwartz S, Heinemann V, Siegert W (1994) Strategies in prevention of invasive pulmonary aspergillosis in immunosuppressed or neutropenic patients. *Antimicro Agents Chemo*, **38**, 911–7.
125. Boyle RJ, Robins-Browne RM, Tang MLK (2006) Probiotic use in clinical practice: what are the risks? *Am J Clin Nutr*, **83**, 1256–64.
126. Olver WJ, James SA, Lennard A, *et al.* (2002) Nosocomial transmission of *Saccharomyces cerevisiae* in bone marrow transplant patients. *J Hosp Infect*, **52**, 268–72.
127. Cesaro S, Chinello P, Rossi L, Zanesco L (2000) Saccharomyces cerevisiae fungemia in a neutropenic patient treated with Saccharomyces boulardii. *Support Care Cancer*, **8**, 504–5.
128. Oggioni MR, Pozzi G, Valensin PE, Galieni P, Bigazzi C (1998) Recurrent septicaemia in an immunocompromised patient due to probiotic strains of Bacillus subtilis. *J Clin Microbiol*, **36**, 325–6.
129. Anaissie EJ, Penzak SR, Dignani MC (2002) The hospital water supply as a source of nosocomial infections. *Arch Intern Med*, **162**, 1483–92.
130. Aker SN, Cheney CL (1983) The use of sterile diets and low microbial diets in ultra-isolation environments. *J Parenter Enter Nutr*, **7**, 390–7.
131. Department of the Environment, Transport and the Regions and Department of Health (1998) Cryptosporidium and water supplies (The 'Bouchier Report'). London: HMSO. http:/www.dwi.gov.uk/pubs/bouchier/index.htm.
132. Henry L (1997) Immunocompromised patients and nutrition. *Prof Nurse*, **12**, 655–9.
133. Vianelli N, Giannini MB, Quarti C, *et al.* (2006) Resolution of a *Pseudomonas aeruginosa* outbreak in a haematology unit with the use of disposable sterile water filters. *Haematologica*, **91**, 983–5.
134. Hayes-Lattin B, Leis JF, Maziarz RT (2005) Isolation in the allogeneic transplant environment: how protective is it? *Bone Marrow Transplant*, **36**, 373–81.
135. Hall J, Hodgson G, Kerr KG (2004) Provision of safe potable water for immunocompromised patients in hospital. *J Hosp Infect*, **58**, 155–8.

136. McCann S, Byrne JL, Rovira M, *et al.* for the Infectious Diseases Working Party of the EBMT (2004) Outbreaks of infectious diseases in stem cell transplant units: a silent cause of death for patients and transplant programmes. *Bone Marrow Transplant*, **33**, 519–29.
137. Engelhart S, Krizek L, Glasmachery A, Fischnaller E, Markleinz G, Exner M (2002) *Pseudomonas aeruginosa* outbreak in a haematology-oncology unit associated with contaminated surface cleaning equipment. *J Hosp Infect*, **52**, 93–8.
138. King D (2001) Ice machines—an audit of their use in clinical practice. *Comm Dis Publ Health*, **4**, 49–52.
139. Leising LK, McCarthy PL, Hahn T, Dunfold L, McKernon M (2007) Bottled water myths: separating fact from fiction. *Pract Gastroenterol*, **5**, 87–93.
140. Bernito-Armas B, Sutherland JP (1999) A survey of the microbiological quality of bottled water sold in the UK and changes during storage. *Int J Food Microbiol*, **48**, 59–65.
141. Evans MR, Ribeiro D, Salmon RL (2003) Hazards of healthy living: bottled water and salad vegetables as risk factors for campylobacter infection. *Emerg Infect Dis*, **9**, 1219–25.
142. Hunter PR (1993) The microbiology of bottled natural mineral waters. *J Appl Bacteriol*, **74**, 345–52.
143. Sefcick A, Anderton D, Byrne JL, Teahon K, Russell NH (2001) Naso-jejunal feeding in allogeneic bone marrow transplant recipients: results of a pilot study. *Bone Marrow Transplant*, **28**, 1135–9.
144. Horsley P, Bauer J, Gallagher B (2005) Poor nutritional status prior to peripheral blood stem cell transplantation is associated with increased length of hospital stay. *Bone Marrow Transplant*, **35**, 1113–6.
145. Coghlin Dickson TM, Kusnierz-Glaz CR, Blume KG, *et al.* (1999) Impact of admission body weight and chemotherapy dose adjustment on the outcome of autologous bone marrow transplantation. *Bio Blood Marrow Transplant*, **5**, 299–305.
146. Deeg HJ, Seidel K, Bruemmer B, Pepe MS, Appelbaum FR (1995) Impact of patient weight on non-relapse mortality after marrow transplantation. *Bone Marrow Transplant*, **15**, 461–8.
147. Raynard B, Nitenberg G, Gory-Delabaere G, *et al.* (2003) Summary of the standards, options and recommendations for nutritional support in patients undergoing bone marrow transplantation. *Br J Cancer*, **89**(1), S101–6.
148. Duggan C, Bechard L, Donovan K, *et al.* (2003) Changes in resting energy expenditure among children undergoing allogeneic stem cell transplantation. *Am J Clin Nutr*, **78**, 104–9.
149. Aldamiz-Echerarria L, Bachiller MP, Ariz MC, Gimenez A, Barcia MJ, Marin M (1996) Continuous versus cyclic parenteral nutrition during bone marrow transplantation: assessment and follow up. *Clin Nutr*, **15**, 333–6.
150. Murray SM, Pindoria S (2004) Nutrition support for bone marrow transplant patients. *Cochrane Library*, Issue 3.
151. Papadopoulou A, MacDonald A, Williams MD, Darbyshire PJ, Booth IW (1997) Enteral nutrition after bone marrow transplantation. *Arch Dis Child*, **77**, 131–6.
152. Barrett RA (2008) A review of enteral feeding practice in allogeneic haematopoietic stem cell transplant patients. *Bone Marrow Transplant*, **41**, S378.
153. Langdana A, Tully N, Molloy E, Bourke B, O'Meara A (2001) Invasive enteral nutrition support in paediatric bone marrow transplantation. *Bone Marrow Transplant*, **27**, 741–6.
154. Takatsuka H, Takemoto Y, Yamada S, *et al.* (2002) Oral eicosapentaenoic acid for acute colonic graft-versus-host disease after bone marrow transplantation. *Drugs Exp Clin Res*, **28**, 121–5.
155. Takatsuka H, Takemoto Y, Iwata N, *et al.* (2001) Oral eicosapentaenoic acid for complications of bone marrow transplantation. *Bone Marrow Transplant*, **28**, 769–74.
156. Da Gama Torres HO, Vilela EG, da Cunha AS, *et al.* (2008) Efficacy of glutamine-supplemented parenteral nutrition on short-term survival following Allo-SCT: a randomized study. *Bone Marrow Transplant*, **27**, 1–7.

157. Luger SM, Stadmauer EA (1994) Noninfectious complications of bone marrow transplantation. In: Mandell BF (ed.), *Acute Rheumatic and Immunological Diseases. Management of the Critically Ill Patient*, pp. 239–56. New York: Marcel Dekker.

158. Keenan AM (1989) Nutritional support of the bone marrow transplant patient. *Nurs Clin North Am*, **24**, 383–93.

159. Wolford JL, McDonald GB (1988) A problem-orientated approach to intestinal and liver disease after marrow transplantation. *J Clin Gastroenterol*, **10**, 419–33.

160. Catchpole BN (1989) Smooth muscle and the surgeon. *Aust NZ J Surg*, **59**, 199–208.

161. Howard L, Ashley C (2003) Nutrition in the perioperative patient. *Annu Rev Nutr*, **23**, 263–82.

162. Ishikawa M, Nishioka M, Hanaki N, *et al.* (2006) Postoperative host responses in elderly patients after gastrointestinal surgery. *Hepatogastroenterology*, **53**(71), 730–5.

163. Reid CL (2004) Nutritional requirements of surgical and critically-ill patients: do we really know what they need? *Proc Nutr Soc*, **63**(3), 467–72.

164. Windsor JA, Hill GL (1988) Protein depletion and surgical risk. *Aust NZ J Surg*, **58**(9), 711–5.

165. Salvino RM, Dechicco RS, Seidner DL (2004) Perioperative nutrition support: who and how? *Cleveland Clin J Med*, **71**(4), 345–51.

166. Mathur S, Plank LD, Hill AG, Rice MA, Hill GL (2008) Changes in body composition, muscle function and energy expenditure after radical cystectomy. *BJU Int*, **101**(8), 973–7.

167. Weimann A, Braga M, Harsanyi L, *et al.* (2006) ESPEN Guidelines on Enteral Nutrition: Surgery including organ transplantation. *Clin Nutr*, **25**(2), 224–44.

168. McClave SA, Snider HL, Spain DA (1999) Preoperative issues in clinical nutrition. *Chest*, **115**, 64S–70S.

169. Kuzu MA, Terzioglu H, Genc V, *et al.* (2006) Preoperative nutritional risk assessment in predicting postoperative outcome in patients undergoing major surgery. *World J Surg*, **30**(3), 378–90.

170. MacFie J, Woodcock NP, Palmer MD, Walker A, Townsend S, Mitchell CJ (2000) Oral dietary supplements in pre- and postoperative surgical patients: a prospective and randomized clinical trial. *Nutrition*, **16**(9), 723–8.

171. Smedley F, Bowling T, James M, *et al.* (2004) Randomized clinical trial of the effects of preoperative and postoperative oral nutritional supplements on clinical course and cost of care. *Br J Surg*, **91**, 983–90.

172. Flynn MB, Leightty FF (1987) Preoperative outpatient nutritional support of patients with squamous cancer of the upper aerodigestive tract. *Am J Surg*, **154**(4), 359–62.

173. Shukla HS, Rao RR, Banu N, *et al.* (1984) Enteral hyperalimentation in malnourished surgical patients. *Indian J Med Res*, **80**, 339–46.

174. Von Meyenfeldt MF, Meijerink W, Roufflart M, Builmaassen M, Soeters P (1992) Perioperative nutritional support: a randomized clinical trial. *Clin Nutr*, **11**, 180–6.

175. Wu GH, Liu ZH, Wu ZH, Wu ZG (2006) Perioperative artificial nutrition in malnourished gastrointestinal cancer patients. *World J Gastroenterol*, **12**(15), 2441–4.

176. Veterans Study Group (1991) Perioperative total parenteral nutrition in surgical patients. *N Engl J Med*, **325**(8), 525–32.

177. Sands DR, Wexner SD (1999) Nasogastric tubes and dietary advancement after laparoscopic and open colorectal surgery. *Nutrition*, **15**(5), 347–50.

178. Nelson H, Edwards S, Tse B (2007) Prophylactic nasogastric decompression after abdominal surgery. *Cochrane Database Syst Rev*, (3)CD004929.

179. Carr CS, Ling KD, Boulos P, Singer M (1996) Randomised trial of safety and efficacy of immediate postoperative enteral feeding in patients undergoing gastrointestinal resection. *Br Med J*, **312**, 869–71.

180. Reissman P, Teoh TA, Cohen SM, Weiss EG, Nogueras JJ, Wexner SD (1995) Is early oral feeding safe after elective colorectal surgery? A prospective randomized trial. *Ann Surg*, **222**(1), 73–7.

181. Feo CV, Romanini B, Sortini D, *et al.* (2004) Early oral feeding after colorectal resection: a randomized controlled study. *Aust NZ J Surg*, **74**(5), 298-301.

182. Lewis SJ, Egger M, Sylvester PA, Thomas S (2001) Early enteral feeding versus "nil by mouth" after gastrointestinal surgery: systematic review and meta-analysis of controlled trials. *Br Med J*, **323**, 773–6.

183. Andersen HK, Lewis SJ, Thomas S (2006) Early enteral nutrition within 24h of colorectal surgery versus later commencement of feeding for postoperative complications. *Cochrane Database Syst Rev*, (4)CD004080.

184. Hill GL, Douglas RG, Schroeder D (1993) Metabolic basis for the management of patients undergoing major surgery. *World J Surg*, **17**, 146.

185. Jenson MB, Hessov I (1997) Dietary supplementation at home improves the regain of lean body mass after surgery. *Nutrition*, **13**(5), 422–30.

186. Jenson MB, Hessov I (1997) Randomization to nutritional intervention at home did not improve postoperative function, fatigue or well-being. *Br J Surg*, **84**(1), 113–8.

187. Beattie AH, Prach AT, Baxter JP, Pennington CR (2000) A randomised controlled trial evaluating the use of enteral nutritional supplements postoperatively in malnourished surgical patients. *Gut*, **46**(6), 813–8.

188. Chen HH, Wexner SD, Iroatulam AJ (2000) Laparoscopic colectomy compares favorably with colectomy by laparotomy for reduction of postoperative ileus. *Dis Colon Rectum*, **43**(1), 61–5.

189. Jenkins NL, Roth JS, Johnson JO, Pofahl WE (2005) Laparoscopic colorectal surgery: indications and techniques. *Curr Surg*, **62**(3), 319–23.

190. Rovera F, Dionigi G, Boni L, *et al.* (2007) Colorectal cancer: the role of laparoscopy. *Surg Oncol*, **16**, S65–7.

191. Ziprin P, Ridgway PF, Peck DH, Darzi AW (2002) The theories and realities of port-site metastases: a critical appraisal. *J Am Coll Surg*, **195**(3), 395–408.

192. Nelson H, Sargent DJ, Wieand HS, *et al.* (2004) A comparison of laparoscopically assisted and open colectomy for colon cancer. *N Eng J Med*, **350**(20), 2050–9.

193. McCoubrey AS (2007) The use of mechanical bowel preparation in elective colorectal surgery. *Ulster Med J*, **76**(3), 127–30.

194. Guenaga KF, Matos D, Castro AA, Atallah AN, Wille-Jorgensen P (2005) Mechanical bowel preparation for elective colorectal surgery. *Cochrane Database Syst Rev*, (1)CD001544.

195. Holte K, Nielsen KG, Madsen JL, Kehlet H (2004) Physiologic effects of bowel preparation. *Dis Colon Rectum*, **47**, 1397–1402.

196. Reddy BS, MacFie J, Gatt M, Larsen CN, Jensen SS, Leser TD (2006) Randomized clinical trial of effect of synbiotics, neomycin and mechanical bowel preparation on intestinal barrier function in patients undergoing colectomy. *Br J Surg*, **94**(5), 546–54.

197. Holte K, Kehlet H (2002) Compensatory fluid administration for preoperative dehydration: does it improve outcome? *Acta Anaesthesiol Scand*, **46**, 1089–93.

198. Warner MA, Caplan RA, Epstein BS, *et al.* (1999) Practice guidelines for preoperative fasting and the use of pharmacologic agents to reduce the risk of pulmonary aspiration: application to healthy patients undergoing elective procedures: a report by the American Society of Anesthesiologist Task Force on Preoperative Fasting. *Anesthesiology*, **90**(3), 896–905.

199. Brady M, Kinn S, Stuart P (2003) Preoperative fasting for adults to prevent perioperative complications. *Cochrane Database Syst Rev*, (4)CD004423.

200. Svanfeldt M, Thorell A, Hausel J, *et al.* (2005) Effect of 'preoperative' oral carbohydrate treatment on insulin action: a randomised cross-over unblinded study in healthy subjects. *Clin Nutr*, **24**, 815–21.

201. Nygren J, Soop M, Thorell A, Efendic S, Nair KS, Ljungqvist O (1998) Preoperative oral carbohydrate administration reduces postoperative insulin resistance. *Clin Nutr*, **17**(2), 65–71.

202. Hausel J, Nygren J, Lagerkranser M, *et al.* (2001) A carbohydrate-rich drink reduces preoperative discomfort in elective surgery patients. *Anesth Analg*, **93**, 1344–50.

203. Yuill KA, Richardson RA, Davidson HI, Garden OJ, Parks RW (2005) The administration of an oral carbohydrate-containing fluid prior to major elective upper-gastrointestinal surgery preserves skeletal muscle mass postoperatively—a randomised clinical trial. *Clin Nutr*, **24**(1), 32–7.

204. Henriksen MG, Hessov I, Dela F, *et al.* (2003) Effects of preoperative oral carbohydrates and peptides on postoperative endocrine response, mobilization, nutrition and muscle function in abdominal surgery. *Acta Anaesthesiol Scand*, **47**, 191–9.

205. Noblett SE, Watson DS, Huong H, Davison B, Hainsworth PJ, Horgan AF (2006) Pre-operative oral carbohydrate loading in colorectal surgery: a randomized controlled trial. *Colorectal Dis*, **8**(7), 563–9.

206. Basse L, Hjort Jakobsen D, Billesbolle P, Werner M, Kehlet H (2000) A clinical pathway to accelerate recovery after colonic resection. *Ann Surg*, **232**(1), 51–7.

207. King PM, Blazeby JM, Ewings P, *et al.* (2006) The influence of an enhanced recovery programme on clinical outcomes, costs and quality of life after surgery for colorectal cancer. *Colorectal Dis*, **8**(6), 506–13.

208. Rivadeneira DE, Evoy D, Fahey TJ, Lieberman MD, Daly JM (1998) Nutritional support of the cancer patient. *Clin J Cancer*, **48**, 69–80.

209. Lassen K, Hannemann P, Ljungqvist O, *et al.* (2005) Patterns in current perioperative practice: survey of colorectal surgeons in five northern European countries. *BMJ*, **330**, 1420–1.

210. Urbach DR, Baxter NN (2005) Reducing variation in surgical care. *Br Med J*, **330**, 1401–2.

211. Schulman AS, Sawyer RG (2005) Have you passed gas yet? Time for a new approach to feeding patients postoperatively. *Pract Gastroenterol*, **10**, 82–8.

212. Wibe A, Eriksen MT, Syse A, Myrvold HE, Søreide O (2003) Total mesorectal excision for rectal cancer—what can be achieved by a national audit? *Colorectal Dis*, **5**, 471–7.

Chapter 29

Nutritional management in recurrent, advanced or metastatic cancer

Shalini Dalal

Introduction

The majority (50–80%) of patients with advanced cancer become cachectic, with higher prevalence in patients with gastrointestinal and pancreatic tumours. Patients with involuntary weight loss have decreased benefit from cancer therapies (such as chemotherapy, radiation or surgery) and experience significantly more toxicities from such therapies. They have lower performance status, quality of life (QoL), and increased morbidity and mortality.[1,2]

We now consider four patient scenarios to illustrate the clinical issues pertinent to nutrition and cachexia in advanced cancer patients.

Case 1. D.A., a 65-year-old male with metastatic non-small lung cancer

D.A. is a 65-year-old male diagnosed 6 months ago with stage IV non-small cell lung cancer, involving lungs, thoracic spine and left hip. He received three cycles of chemotherapy and recently completed palliative radiation to the hip and thoracic spine (T4–T10). In the outpatient clinic he complains of mid-chest pain radiating to his epigastrium (rates it as 7 on a scale of 0–10), odynophagia, and fatigue. His hip pain is well controlled on morphine. The review of systems is significant for constipation, early satiety and decreased appetite. His past medical history is significant for gout and obesity. One year ago he weighed 135 kg and at the time of cancer diagnosis, 120 kg. On physical examination, D.A. appears well nourished. His vital signs reveal tachycardia (pulse 114), BP 125/66, weight 97 kg, BMI 29 kg/m^2. Home medications include morphine, sennoside tablets, and sucralfate suspension four times per day.

Case 2. G.R., a 55-year-old female with advanced ovarian cancer

G.R. was diagnosed with ovarian cancer 10 years ago. Her initial treatment included surgery (total abdominal hysterectomy, bilateral salpingo-ophorectimy, and tumour reduction) followed by chemotherapy. Unfortunately her disease recurred 1 year ago, with peritoneal implants and lung metastases. While receiving chemotherapy as an outpatient, she developed intractable nausea, abdominal pain and dehydration which required admission to hospital. Other symptoms include anorexia, early satiety, fatigue and constipation (last bowel movement was 6 days ago). Review of her records reveals weight loss of 5 kg over the past 3 months. On examination, she appears frail, and has temporal muscle wasting and poor skin turgor. Vital signs: pulse 120/min, BP 105/56, respiratory rate 20/min, weight 66 kg. Chest auscultation reveals decreased breath sounds at both lung bases. Her abdomen is distended, and has a well-healed midline incision with mild tenderness to palpation. There is evidence of moderate ascites despite a recent paracentesis, and pitting oedema of her lower extremities.

Case 3. P.S., a 70-year-old male with unresectable advanced pancreatic cancer

P.S. approached his general practitioner a month ago, complaining of weight loss (15 kg over 4 months), anorexia, dyspnoea and fatigue. Further investigation reveals a locally advanced pancreatic cancer complicated by pulmonary embolism. He is treated with single agent gemcitabine because of his relatively poor performance status. After two cycles and a decrease in CA19-9 levels, he reports continued weight loss, anorexia and fatigue, requiring postponement of his next chemotherapy cycle. He is referred to the palliative care department for symptom management. On examination, P.S. is a tall cachectic male who appears fatigued and withdrawn. He weighs 58 kg (BMI 17 kg/m^2), and has an ECOG performance status of 2. He reports fullness and bloating after eating small amounts of food as well as chronic nausea, diarrhoea, depressed mood and insomnia. His wife is very anxious because he shows no interest in food, is socially withdrawn, and appears 'all skin and bones'. She is hopeful his weight and fatigue improve as soon as possible, so that he can continue to receive further chemotherapy

Case 4. L.M., a 61-year-old male with invasive squamous cell carcinoma base of tongue

L.M. presented initially with oral pain and weight loss of 12 kg over 6 months. He was found to have locally advanced carcinoma of the base of the tongue and treated with concurrent chemotherapy and radiation.After completing 3 weeks of radiation therapy, he reports severe odynophagia, constipation and persistent pain despite use of morphine every 4 h. His physical examination is remarkable for muscle wasting and a Karnofsky performance status of 2.

All four case scenarios are examples of presentations by patients with advanced cancer. Cachexia, secondary nutrition impact symptoms (refer to Chapter 12) and secondary cachexia may all contribute to the weight loss experienced by an individual patient. Whereas all the patients share features of involuntary weight loss and/or wasting, they differ considerably in their clinical presentations and symptoms. These four cases are used to illustrate the discussions below.

What causes weight loss and nutritional decline in advanced cancer patients?

Research suggests the dominant mechanism for cachexia is an interaction between the tumor and host. A state of chronic systemic inflammation influences central and peripheral regulatory systems, such as appetite regulation, endocrine homeostasis, hepatic acute phase protein response, adipose and muscle metabolism. Cachexia caused by these mechanisms could be referred to as 'primary cachexia'. (Refer to Part 2 for further discussion.)

In addition to the primary mechanism of cachexia, weight loss in cancer patients can arise from one or multiple coexisting symptoms that contribute to decreased nutritional intake. These 'secondary nutrition impact symptoms', include early satiety, nausea, anorexia, taste alterations, dry mouth, dysphagia, depressed mood, odynophagia and constipation. The symptoms are caused by the direct effects of the tumour or side-effects of cancer treatment. Patients might have coexisting comorbidities or conditions that also contribute to wasting and poor appetite. The weight loss resulting from these factors could be referred to as 'secondary cachexia'.

Only a few studies have evaluated symptoms that may contribute to cachexia. A prospective longitudinal survey in medical oncology patients reported that the most common 'nutrition impact' symptoms were dry mouth, nausea, and constipation. The most distressing symptoms were dry mouth, diarrhoea, and stomach pain. These symptoms were commonly experienced, even 12 months after initiation of chemotherapy, and were associated with poorer QoL and performance status.[3] Another study reported anorexia, early satiety and pain as most common among patients with gastrointestinal and lung cancers.[4] Patients with reduced food intake had more symptoms than patients who had not lost weight. A recent retrospective review of 50 cachectic cancer patients from a clinic at a cancer hospital found that the vast majority of patients presented with two or more of factors[5] that could contribute to cachexia. Most common symptoms were early satiety, constipation, pain and depression.

In our case examples, all appear to have primary cachexia and secondary conditions or symptoms contributing to inadequate caloric intake. Case 1 (D.A.) experienced progressive weight loss over the year prior to his diagnosis of cancer. Later, he developed symptoms of odynophagia and dysphagia because of radiation-induced oesophagitis which severely limited his oral intake and contributed to further weight loss. In addition, his constipation (aggravated by opioid use), probably exacerbated his early satiety and abdominal pain. Because of his pre-existing obesity, his muscle atrophy is not readily apparent on physical examination. Case 2 (G.R.) has uncontrolled chronic nausea which appears to be aggravated by chemotherapy. She has significant abdominal disease and ascites which contribute to nausea and early satiety. Case 3 (P.S.) has metastatic pancreatic cancer and cachexia, but is also depressed and sleeping poorly. Depression is a likely contributor to his poor appetite and weight loss. Case 4 (J.L.) has significant weight loss related to severe uncontrolled pain when swallowing. The side-effects of chemo-radiation and inadequate pain control are the main reasons for his poor oral intake.

How is cachexia diagnosed?

The most easily recognizable sign of cancer cachexia is an unintentional loss of body weight. Weight loss of ≥5% over the preceding 6 months is commonly used to define cachexia in cancer patients, and has been associated with decreased survival.[6] Although cachexia usually conjures up an image of 'skin and bones', it is important to note that the dynamic 'loss' of weight is more important than the weight at clinical presentation, especially for many patients who have baseline obesity. Because of the high frequency of obesity in the USA and western world, many cancer patients, such as case 1 (D.A.) in our example, may appear to be 'well nourished' despite progressive weight loss and muscle wasting.

Obtaining a weight loss history is necessary, and key characteristics of the cachexia syndrome need to be considered, including muscle wasting, decreased oral intake and the presence of inflammation. For instance, in advanced pancreatic cancer patients, Fearon *et al.* showed that weight loss alone could not explain the full effect of cachexia on physical function and also was not a prognostic variable.[7] A three-factor profile (weight loss, reduced food intake and systemic inflammation) was more useful in identification of patients with both adverse function and prognosis. Serum C-reactive protein (CRP) is a surrogate marker of systemic inflammation and levels of ≥10 mg/l correlate with weight loss, poor appetite and hypermetabolism, as well as negative clinical outcomes such as tumour recurrence and poor survival.[8,9]

Assessment and management of cachexia in advanced cancer patients

As illustrated in our four case examples, cachexia is a complex and multifaceted syndrome that varies widely in its presentation, aetiology (contributing factors) and impact. Although no two patients are alike, a standardized approach to assessment can be adopted by the medical team, one that systematically assesses the various facets of the syndrome. Such an assessment should be followed by a decision-making process that formulates an individualized treatment plan for nutritional care and cachexia management (Figure 29.1). Ideally, an interdisciplinary, collaborative approach, and validated assessment tools should be adopted.

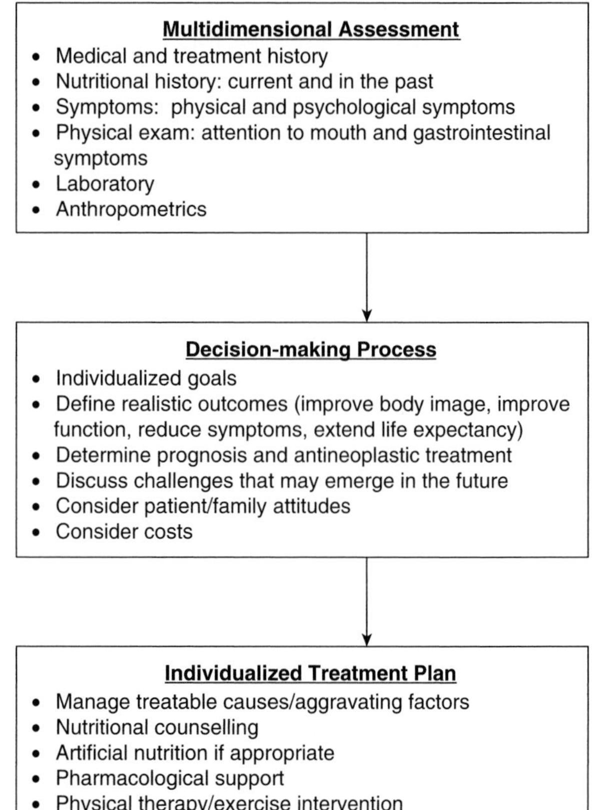

Fig. 29.1 Recommended approach to cachexia assessment and management.

Nutritional assessment

All cancer patients should undergo nutritional screening at the time of cancer diagnosis to identify patients at risk of malnutrition or cachexia. A number of validated nutritional screening assessment tools (such as the Malnutrition Screening Tool)[10] are available, and can easily be incorporated into the routine forms used in outpatient or inpatient settings. For those patients who have more than a low risk of malnutrition/cachexia, a comprehensive nutritional assessment and consultation with a nutritionist is necessary.

A comprehensive assessment of nutritional status comprises several domains and includes a medical and nutritional history, symptom assessment, physical examination, functional status, anthropometric measurements and laboratory data. These components are key to treating symptoms contributing to nutritional decline, formulating realistic treatment and nutritional interventions, and in identifying future care needs.

Symptom assessment

As discussed previously, advanced cancer patients may have one or more concurrent symptoms that compromise oral intake. Many symptoms such as depression are 'silent' symptoms, because patients may not volunteer this information unless specifically asked. A validated, simple tool such as the Edmonton Symptom Assessment Scale (ESAS) can be used to assess the severity of common symptoms such as anorexia, nausea, depression and fatigue. A careful history should be performed with attention to the mouth and gastrointestinal system including taste changes, dental problems, and the presence of early satiety and constipation.

Laboratory assessment

Several laboratory abnormalities are frequently noted in advanced cancer patients but none are specific for cachexia, and may be influenced by the status of cancer, related organ dysfunction or treatment toxicities. For instance, in addition to poor nutritional intake, low serum albumin might indicate impaired liver function. Serum albumin is a negative acute-phase protein, decreases with chronic inflammation and is an independent prognostic variable for survival in patients with cancer.[11] A high serum CRP is a well-established surrogate marker of inflammation and directly correlates with cachexia and poor outcomes. Patients with raised serum CRP levels have lower energy intake than those with normal levels[12] and there is some evidence that resting energy expenditure may be increased in these patients.[13] A more detailed laboratory work-up could include a complete blood count, liver function tests, albumin, CRP, vitamin levels (D and B_{12}), testosterone, thyroid-stimulating hormone and cortisol. Hypogonadism is common in patients with advanced cancer, particularly those on opioids, megestrol and corticosteroids.

Body composition assessment

Whereas there is loss of both fat and lean body mass (LBM) in cachexia, the early and predominant loss of LBM is in contrast to simple starvation where LBM is relatively conserved in early stages.[14] Several methods of measuring body composition such as whole-body potassium, densitometry, anthropometrics [e.g. triceps skinfold thickness (TSF), arm muscle area]; bioelectrical impedance, magnetic resonance imaging, and computed tomography (CT) have been evaluated in cancer patients.[15] Many of these modalities are not practical due to cost or availability. Some of the methods (bioelectrical impedance, whole-body potassium) do not distinguish skeletal muscle from other non-adipose tissues,[16–19] whereas others such as plain anthropometrics are cumbersome and operator dependent, making comparisons difficult between studies. CT is emerging as the gold standard in body composition analysis. CT imaging techniques allow for assessment of regional muscle and adipose tissue depots, including the separation of adipose tissue into subcutaneous (SAT), and visceral (VAT) compartments.[21–24] Since CT imaging in cancer patients is often considered standard care, the use of this modality for body composition analysis is attractive, both in practical terms and because of the precision of data that can be obtained. Despite their wide availability and the importance attributed to lean tissue loss there are few clinical studies. Several trials are currently evaluating the potential role of CT imaging in cachexia management.

The decision-making process

Following the multidimensional assessment, a frank discussion with the patient and caregivers is important to address their goals and to define realistic outcomes (Figure 29.1). The discussion will be influenced by the patient's cancer stage, comorbidities, and overall prognosis. A comprehensive treatment approach must be emphasized since no single therapy will be consistently effective. Furthermore, although weight gain is usually desired, it may not be the primary goal of the treatment intervention. Improvement of physical function, QoL or increased LBM may be the desired outcome for many patients.

An individualized treatment plan

Following the decision-making process, an individualized treatment plan should be formulated (Figure 29.1).

Nutritional intervention

In cancer patients, nutrition intervention in the form of counselling, with or without high protein-energy supplementation, can improve QoL, symptoms, increase oral intake and attenuate weight loss.[25–29] A recent systematic review did not find any benefits regarding survival[30] but several national practice guidelines support nutritional counselling in cancer patients.[31–32] There are four key steps (ABCD) in nutritional counselling that are shown in Box 29.1 and briefly discussed below.

Assessment of current intake

In patients with advanced cancer dietary records, detailing nutrient intakes and meal patterns for 3 consecutive days (including 1 weekend day) has been shown to reflect adequately dietary intake.[33] Depending on the setting, this may not be practical and a 24–48 h food diary can be recorded instead. The frequency and size of meals, snacks, beverages, dietary preferences, food allergies, as well as recent changes in dietary patterns, should be noted. Energy and protein intake estimates can be calculated from the food intake, and serve as a baseline. For a 3-day calorie count, the average for 24 h is obtained.

Barriers to nutritional intake

The nutritionist should identify barriers to adequate dietary intake, including issues of food availability and preparation, companionship during meal times, relationships in the home, and presence of physical and psychological symptoms. Alterations in taste, presence of mucositis, dysphagia, dry mouth, early satiety, bloating sensation, nausea, constipation, depressed mood, and anxiety are common causes of poor nutritional intake. Treatment of these symptoms are discussed in detail in Part 4.

Calculation of energy and protein requirements

The exact energy and protein needs of weight-losing cancer patients are not clear. In cancer patients, energy intake >120 kJ/kg/day and protein intake >1.2–1.4 g/kg/day may be required for weight maintenance.[34,35] Due to the high variation in basal energy requirements, a more accurate method for measuring individual energy expenditure is via indirect calorimetry. If indirect calorimetry is not available, an energy intake >120 kJ/kg/day can be estimated.

Dietary recommendations

An individualized nutritional plan should be formulated based on the prior steps, patient preferences and goals of care. A Canadian study of dietary patterns in cachectic advanced cancer patients

Box 29.1 Key domains in individual nutritional counselling

A **Assessment** of current nutritional intake
B Identification of **barriers** that impact adequate nutritional intake
C **Calculation** of energy and protein requirements for the patient
D Individualized **dietary** recommendations

found that 'normal foods' rather than commercially available nutritional supplements were preferred by the majority (70%) of patients.[36] The frequency of eating was an important variable in total energy intake, and greater total caloric intake was largely derived from the consumption of food outside of the three main meals of the day. A supportive environment for snacking behaviour, and use of snacks with high nutritional value were important. The relationship of the nutritionist with the patient should not be imposing, and small efforts by the patient and family should be validated. Frequent reinforcement and modifications of care plans based on overall medical goals and tolerance may be required.

Symptom management

Advanced cancer patients may have one or multiple concurrent symptoms that compromise oral intake. These are discussed in further detail in Part 4.

Early satiety and nausea

As noted in all our patients, early satiety and chronic nausea are common symptoms in cachectic cancer patients, and can be treated with oral metoclopramide, starting with doses of 10 mg every 4 h, and increasing up to a maximum of 120 mg per day. Constipation (often as a result of opioids) may also contribute to early satiety and/or nausea.

Depression

Depressed mood can lead to decreased oral intake, and should be managed with counselling, and antidepressants if indicated. There are anecdotes to suggest that mirtazapine improves appetite and weight gain, and it is currently undergoing study in cancer patients.

Mucositis, xerostomia, and odynophagia

These symptoms are commonly experienced in patients undergoing combined chemoradiation treatment and are frequently severe enough to require treatment interruptions or delays, such as our patient in case 4. Opioids are usually required in order to achieve adequate pain control and immediate release formulations can be administered an hour prior to meals. Side-effects of these medications such as constipation should be managed with adequate doses of daily laxatives.

Is there a role for enteral or parenteral nutrition? (see Part 6)

Although it would seem that caloric replacement via artificial means (either with enteral or parenteral routes), should help improve the nutritional status of advanced cancer patients, there is a large body of evidence suggesting that artificial nutrition does not improve patient survival, performance status, QoL, treatment toxicity or psychological well-being for the majority of patients.[37–39] Enteral nutrition via gastrostomy tubes may be appropriate for patients with predominant starvation component due to dysphagia or obstruction caused by the primary location of their tumours (such as cancer of the esophagus, head and neck). This therapy is most appropriate for L.M. (case 4) who requires short term nutritional support while he completes radiation therapy and heals from toxic side-effects. Aspiration pneumonia, nausea, and diarrhoea are some of the complications of enteral nutrition therapy.

Specific pharmacological therapies

A number of active trials are evaluating pharmacological agents such as thalidomide, melatonin, androgens, ghrelin/ghrelin agonists and non-steroidal anti-inflammatory drugs for use in advanced cancer patients with cachexia. More evidence is required regarding their efficacy and safety. As cachexia is a multidimensional syndrome, a multimodality intervention that includes a combination of pharmacological agents, exercise, nutrition, and symptom management is likely to be the most effective approach.

Monitoring response to therapy

Ongoing attention to optimal management of symptoms remains a key component. Whereas weight gain is often a desired outcome, it may not be the sole focus of intervention. Further, body weight may not accurately reflect changes in nutritional status due to the presence of ascites or oedema. In patients with advanced cancer and predominantly primary cachexia, weight stabilization is associated with improved QoL and survival, and is an appropriate goal in advanced cancer patients who have life expectancy estimated in months. For those patients whose life expectancy is limited to weeks or months, goals of therapy should focus on alleviating distressful symptoms. In this setting, additional measures of nutritional assessment are less important than indicators of QoL, such as activity level, stamina, mood, and sense of well-being.

Summary

Alterations in nutritional status are common in advanced cancer patients. Attention to nutritional status should begin early, at the time of cancer diagnosis, and continue throughout the cancer trajectory. Patients vary widely in their presentation. Efforts to maintain adequate nutrition require effective control of symptoms that contribute to poor intake. For patients with advanced cancer, a standardized assessment should be followed by an individualized management plan.

References

1. Andreyev HJ, Norman AR, Oates J, *et al.* (1998) Why do patients with weight loss have a worse outcome when undergoing chemotherapy for gastrointestinal malignancies? *Eur J Cancer*, **34**, 503–9.
2. Dewys WD, Begg C, Lavin PT, *et al.* (1980) Prognostic effect of weight loss prior to chemotherapy in cancer patients. Eastern Cooperative Oncology Group. *Am J Med*, **69**, 491–7.
3. Tong H, Isenring E, Yates P (2009) The prevalence of nutrition impact symptoms and their relationship to quality of life and clinical outcomes in medical oncology patients. *Support Care Cancer*, **17**, 83–90.
4. Khalid U, Spiro A, Baldwin C, *et al.* (2007) Symptoms and weight loss in patients with gastrointestinal and lung cancer at presentation. *Support Care Cancer*, **15**, 39–46.
5. Del Fabbro E, Dalal S, Delgado M, Freer G, Bruera E (2007) Secondary vs. primary cachexia in patients with advanced cancer. *J Clin Oncol*, **25**, 9128.
6. Dewys WD, Begg C, Lavin PT, *et al.* (1980) Prognostic effect of weight loss prior to chemotherapy in cancer patients. Eastern Cooperative Oncology Group. *Am J Med*, **69**, 491–7.
7. Fearon KC, Voss AC, Hustead DS, Cancer Cachexia Study Group (2006) Definition of cancer cachexia: effect of weight loss, reduced food intake, and systemic inflammation on functional status and prognosis. *Am J Clin Nutr*, **83**, 1345–50.
8. Falconer JS, Fearon KC, Ross JA, *et al.* (1995) Acute-phase protein response and survival duration of patients with pancreatic cancer. *Cancer*, **75**, 2077–82.
9. McMillan DC, Watson WS, O'Gorman P, Preston T, Scott HR, McArdle CS (2001) Albumin concentrations are primarily determined by the body cell mass and the systemic inflammatory response in cancer patients with weight loss. *Nutr Cancer*, **39**, 210–13.
10. Ferguson ML, Bauer J, Gallagher B, Capra S, Christie DR, Mason BR (1999) Validation of a malnutrition screening tool for patients receiving radiotherapy. *Australas Radiol*, **43**, 325–7.

11. Evans WK, Nixon DW, Daly JM, *et al.* (1987) A randomized study of oral nutritional support versus ad lib nutritional intake during chemotherapy for advanced colorectal and non small cell lung cancer. *J Clin Oncol*, **5**, 113–24.
12. Wigmore SJ, Plester CE, Ross JA, Fearon KC (1997) Contribution of anorexia and hypermetabolism to weight loss in anicteric patients with pancreatic cancer. *Br J Surg*, **84**, 196–7.
13. Falconer JS, Fearon KC, Plester CE, Ross JA, Carter DC (1994) Cytokines, the acute-phase response, and resting energy expenditure in cachectic patients with pancreatic cancer. *Ann Surg*, **219**, 325–31.
14. Keys A, Brozek J, Henschel A, *et al.* (1950) *The Biology of Human Starvation*. St Paul, MN: University of Minnesota Press.
15. Lukaski HC (1987) Methods for the assessment of human body composition: traditional and new. *Am J Clin Nutr*, **46**, 537–56.
16. Jatoi A, Daly BD, Hughes VA, *et al.* (2001) Do patients with nonmetastatic non-small cell lung cancer demonstrate altered resting energy expenditure? *Ann Thorac Surg*, **72**, 348–51.
17. Mcmillan DC, Watson WS, Preston T, *et al.* (2000) Lean body mass changes in cancer patients with weight loss. *Clin Nutr*, **19**, 403–6.
18. Moley JF, Aamodt R, Rumble W, *et al.* (1987) Body cell mass in cancer-bearing and anorexic patients. *J Parenter Enteral Nutr*, **11**, 219–22.
19. Pichard C, Kyle UG (1998) Body composition measurements during wasting diseases. *Curr Opin Clin Nutr Metab Care*, **1**, 357–61.
20. Pietrobelli A, Wang Z, Heymsfield SB (1998) Techniques used in measuring human body composition. *Curr Opin Clin Nutr Metab Care*, **1**, 439–48.
21. Heymsfield SB, Wang Z, Baumgartner RN, *et al.* (1997) Human body composition: advances in models and methods. *Annu Rev Nutr*, **17**, 527–58.
22. Mitsiopoulos N, Baumgartner RN, Heymsfield SB, *et al.* (1998) Cadaver validation of skeletal muscle measurement by magnetic resonance imaging and computerized tomography. *J Appl Physiol*, **85**, 115–22.
23. Janssen I, Heymsfield SB, Wang ZM, *et al.* (2000) Skeletal muscle mass and distribution in 468 men and women aged 18–88 yr. *J Appl Physiol*, **89**, 81–8.
24. Janssen I, Ross R (1999) Effects of sex on the change in visceral, subcutaneous adipose tissue and skeletal muscle in response to weight loss. *Int J Obes Relat Metab Disord*, **23**, 1035–46.
25. Ollenschlager G, Thomas W, Konkol K, Diehl V, Roth E (1991) Nutritional behavior and quality of life during oncological polychemotherapy: results of a prospective study on the efficacy of oral nutrition therapy in patients with acute leukemia. *Eur J Clin Invest*, **22**, 546–53.
26. Ovesen L, Allingstrup L, Hannibal J, Mortensen EL, Hansen OP (1993) Effect of dietary counseling on food intake, body weight, response rate, survival, and quality of life in cancer patients undergoing chemotherapy: a prospective, randomized study. *J Clin Oncol*, **11**, 2043–9.
27. Ravasco P, Monteiro-Grillo I, Vidal PM, Camilo ME (2005) Dietary counseling improves patient outcomes: a prospective, randomized, controlled trial in colorectal cancer patients undergoing radiotherapy. *J Clin Oncol*, **23**, 1431–8.
28. Isenring E, Capra S, Bauer J (2004) Nutrition intervention is beneficial in oncology outpatients receiving radiotherapy to the gastrointestinal, head or neck area. *Br J Cancer*, **91**, 447–52.
29. Ravasco P, Monteiro-Grillo I, Vidal PM, Camilo ME (2005) Dietary counseling improves patient outcomes: a prospective, randomized, controlled trial in colorectal cancer patients undergoing radiotherapy. *J Clin Oncol*, **23**, 1431–8.
30. Davies AA, Davey SG, Harbord R, *et al.* (2006) Nutritional interventions and outcome in patients with cancer or preinvasive lesions: systematic review. *J Natl Cancer Inst*, **19**, 961–73.
31. Ladas EJ, Sacks N, Meacham L, *et al.* (2005) A multidisciplinary review of nutrition considerations in the pediatric oncology population: a perspective from children's oncology group. *Nutr Clin Pract*, **20**, 377–93.

32. Bauer JD, Ash S, Davidson WL, *et al.* (2006) Evidence based practice guidelines for the nutritional management of cancer cachexia. *Nut Dietet*, **63**, S3–S32.
33. Posner BM, Martin-Munley SS, Smigelski C, *et al.* (1992) Comparison of techniques for estimating nutrient intake: the Framingham Study. *Epidemiology*, **3**, 171–7.
34. Bauer JD, Capra S (2005) Nutrition intervention improves outcomes in patients with cancer cachexia receiving chemotherapy—a pilot study. *Support Care Cancer*, **13**, 270–4.
35. Davidson W, Ash S, Capra S, Bauer J (2004) Weight stabilisation is associated with improved survival duration and quality of life in unresectable pancreatic cancer. *Clin Nutr*, **23**, 239–47.
36. Hutton JL, Martin L, Field CJ, Wismer WV, Bruera ED, Watanabe SM, Baracos VE (2006) Dietary patterns in patients with advanced cancer: implications for anorexia–cachexia therapy. *Am J Clin Nutr*, **84**, 1163–70.
37. Klein S, Koretz RL (1994) Nutrition support in patients with cancer: what do the data really show? *Nutr Clin Pract*, **9**, 91–100.
38. Koretz RL, Avenell A, Lipman TO, Braunschweig CL, Milne AC (2007) Does enteral nutrition affect clinical outcome? A systematic review of the randomized trials. *Am J Gastroenterol* **102**, 412–29.
39. McGeer AJ, Detsky AS, O'Rourke K (1990) Parenteral nutrition in cancer patients undergoing chemotherapy: a meta-analysis. *Nutrition*, **6**, 233–40.

Chapter 30

Patients at the end of life

Egidio Del Fabbro

Introduction

Effective communication and symptom management are essential components of end of life care. They are also important when addressing the nutritional concerns experienced by palliative care patients. In this chapter clinical case studies are used to illustrate some of the fundamentals necessary to provide comprehensive interdisciplinary care for patients and their families. The management of bowel obstruction and the indications for parenteral nutrition (PN) and hydration are discussed while the treatment of specific nutritional impact symptoms appears in Part 4 of this book.

What the patient and family need to know

An open, honest dialogue between patients, their families and the interdisciplinary health care team is crucial at the end of life if the expectations and perceptions of family members are to be fully appreciated. Specific concerns regarding nutrition and hydration need to be addressed, as well as other medical, social and spiritual issues common to palliative care.

Family members providing care are concerned about nutrition and may perceive the loss of appetite by a loved one as the most burdensome issue at the end of life,[1] often more so than pain. For the family, food and eating may be symbolic of nurturing and compassion as well as 'not letting go'.[2] Although high importance is placed by families on patients' ability to eat and maintain weight, this aspect of care is sometimes neglected by health care providers. Physicians and nurses may not wish to engage in a lengthy discussion about poor appetite and weight loss because of the belief that this is an inevitable outcome of the cancer and no effective therapeutic options are available. Unfortunately, the consequences of avoiding this dialogue could include resentment on the part of families, who might perceive that important aspects of patient care have been neglected. Families in turn may feel frustrated by their failure to increase a patient's oral intake despite the best of efforts. They could also inadvertently worsen symptoms such as early satiety, nausea, abdominal distention, and pain by pressuring patients to increase their oral intake. Families need to understand that providing more calories or improving oral intake will not reverse cachexia towards the end of life and may in fact cause unnecessary gastrointestinal distress due to bloating, cramping and nausea. Having to explain this difficult, counterintuitive concept may pose a challenge for many health care providers. Usually an empathic and straightforward explanation of the widespread, overwhelming nature of the cancer and its effect on muscle and appetite will allay concerns of starvation and reassure families that useful therapy is not being withheld. The body's inability to utilize protein and calories, coupled with the continued breakdown of muscle and fat by tumour products and inflammatory factors, needs to be explained without medical jargon. Sometimes the use of an analogy describing a metabolic 'factory' that is 'on strike' and unable to manufacture products despite a steady supply of raw material may facilitate understanding of the aberrant pathophysiology associated with cachexia. The difficulties facing the dysfunctional metabolic 'factory' may be compounded when the 'raw material' is also in short supply because of inadequate caloric intake. It helps to remind families that loved ones are not suffering because their calorie intake has declined, and that patients almost universally report no hunger at the end of life. To the contrary, aggressive oral feeding as well as tube feeds may exacerbate distressing symptoms such as nausea and increase the risk for aspiration pneumonia. It may be necessary to explain that PN also carries potential for severe side-effects and possibly limited benefit, particularly in rapidly progressive cancers where there is unlikely to be a significant 'starvation' component. Discussion should not be limited to nutrition, since a family meeting often presents an appropriate opportunity for the palliative care team to facilitate decisions surrounding cardiopulmonary resuscitation and ventilator support. An interdisciplinary team (see Chapter 19) can address issues concerning resuscitation that may not have been discussed earlier in the disease trajectory. Also, patients' decision-making preferences often change and the goals of care may evolve toward comfort and symptom management at the end of life. Surprisingly, cancer patients are less likely to have had documented advanced care planning discussions despite worse survival than other chronic incurable diseases such as amyotrophic lateral sclerosis.[3]

Case 1

History

A 51-year-old accountant (Mr J), diagnosed with a high grade intra-abdominal sarcoma and treated with surgical resection and chemotherapy, presents to the emergency center complaining of abdominal pain and nausea. Complications since his initial diagnosis include local recurrence of the sarcoma, surgery for a colo-cutaneous fistula, splenectomy, lysis of adhesions and the creation of an ileostomy. During this period, care is provided in both inpatient and outpatient settings by his primary medical oncologist, surgeon and a multi-disciplinary team. More recently, he is referred to the palliative care clinic for management of poor appetite and abdominal pain.

On his final admission to hospital, he reports a 3-day history of increased abdominal pain, nausea and profound fatigue. His oral intake has decreased progressively in the weeks preceding his admission, and for the past 48 h he has not been able to eat or drink because of persistent nausea and emesis. Prior to admission he experienced excellent pain control on methadone scheduled every 8 h and one or two doses of oral hydromorphone daily for breakthrough pain. In the emergency centre, intravenous opioids provide rapid pain relief, and a nasogastric tube (NGT) inserted to suction drains a litre of bile-stained fluid, alleviating his nausea immediately and further reducing his abdominal discomfort.

Home medications include opioids, scheduled laxatives, 5 mg methylphenidate twice daily as needed for fatigue and 100 mg thalidomide once daily for a symptom cluster of weight loss, early satiety and insomnia.

Physical examination reveals an underweight male with NGT in place to suction. He is afebrile, normotensive, attentive and displays no evidence of disorganized thoughts. On inspection his oral mucosa is dry, chest is clear to auscultation, and other than tachycardia, his cardiac examination is normal. Examination also reveals a distended, diffusely tender abdomen, with no guarding and scanty bowel sounds. Several hard masses are appreciated in the left flank, measuring 3–12 cm in diameter.

Laboratory tests reveal a normal amylase and lipase, hypoalbuminaemia, normal liver function tests, normal blood urea nitrogen (BUN) and creatinine, hypokalaemia (2.9 mmol/l), anaemia (haemoglobin: 9 g/dl) and leukocytosis 12.5 (white cell count: $12.5 \times 10^3/\mu l$).

Computed tomography (CT) of the abdomen and pelvis demonstrates marked progression of retroperitoneal and intraperitoneal tumour implants and interval dilatation of the small bowel representing mechanical obstruction due to suspected invasion of distal ileum by tumour. The right kidney is markedly displaced and obstructed by tumour, and multiple tumour implants directly invade the abdominal wall muscles. There is also loss of subcutaneous and intra-abdominal fat since a prior CT scan 3 months ago, and development of a small amount of ascites.

Management

A discussion is held in the emergency centre with Mr J and his family regarding cardiopulmonary resuscitation and ventilator support should his condition deteriorate. All are in agreement that interventions such as intubation, cardioversion and chest compressions are likely to cause discomfort without altering the course of the aggressive, rapidly progressing disease. Additionally, in the event of a cardiopulmonary arrest and successful attempt at resuscitation, transfer to the intensive care unit (ICU) would be mandatory. Interaction between Mr J and family members would be limited because of increased sedation while on mechanical ventilation and restricted access to the ICU.

Intravenous (i.v.) opioids and fluids are continued after admission to the palliative care unit, and i.v. haloperidol is administered for nausea as needed. The following day his symptoms are much improved and he is eager for the NGT to be removed as soon as possible. He now rates both nausea and pain intensity as 3/10 on a numerical rating scale of 0–10 (10 being worst), compared to 10/10 and 8/10 respectively on arrival in the emergency centre. Ice chips and cold water are allowed orally in order to soothe his dry mouth and throat irritation. Mr J's surgeon is of the opinion that surgery is not feasible because of the increased disease burden and multiple new peritoneal implants. A lengthy discussion held with patient, spouse and their two adult children explores the possible non-surgical options for treating bowel obstruction as well as their concerns regarding nutritional support and hydration. Mr J's medical oncologist is present at the family meeting and confirms that any benefits of surgical intervention are doubtful. He notes that in addition to the high risk of intraoperative mortality, a prolonged postoperative recovery period will probably extend beyond the anticipated duration of survival. Endoscopic stent placement is also not possible because of the obstruction site and presence of extensive peritoneal carcinomatosis. Medical management of bowel obstruction with anti-emetics (e.g. haloperidol) and antisecretory medications (e.g. octreotide) are discussed, as well as the option of percutaneous gastrostomy tube (G-tube) placement for venting purposes. Mr J elects to have a G-tube placed because of the tremendous symptomatic relief he experiences when swallowing liquids.

A day later, he undergoes a fluoroscopically guided G-tube placement by the interventional radiology service. Although he reports relief of dry mouth and satiation of hunger, he is aware that the G-tube is primarily for venting purposes and that absorption of nutrients is very unlikely.

During a meeting to discuss transition to hospice care, tearful family members are reassured by the interdisciplinary team that PN will not improve survival or quality of life in the face of a rapidly progressive cancer. Continued symptom control and comfort are, however, attainable goals that will continue to be the focus of care on discharge from hospital. The placement of a subcutaneous line is initiated in anticipation of the need for opioids, anti-emetics and fluids under the care of home hospice.

Malignant bowel obstruction

Inoperable malignant bowel obstruction (MBO) can produce bloating, pain and emesis. Treatment approaches towards the end of life for relief of these symptoms include mechanical drainage via nasogastric or gastrostomy tube and combinations of antisecretory/anti-emetic medications. NGT is uncomfortable, unsightly and should be considered a temporary measure until replaced by medical management or a venting gastrostomy. There are few randomized trials in MBO comparing the commonly used drugs, such as octreotide, anticholinergics (e.g. hyoscine butylbromide) and dexamethasone. A prospective trial[2] of patients with inoperable bowel obstruction managed by a decompressive NGT successfully used octreotide 300 μg daily or scopolamine butylbromide 60 mg daily via subcutaneous infusion to reduce secretions, enabling removal of the NGT in the majority of patients. The sustained release formulation[3] of octreotide also appears to be effective in decreasing secretions and relieving symptoms. Corticosteroids may have a theoretical benefit by decreasing peritumoral inflammation and temporarily relieving the obstruction and accompanying symptoms. A systematic review[4] concluded that the role of corticosteroids remains debatable, but that octreotide can be considered more effective than hyoscine butylbromide in relieving symptoms and reducing secretions. Although trial data are lacking, anticholinergic drugs are more likely to produce somnolence and confusion than octreotide. Haloperidol is usually an effective anti-emetic in these patients and can safely be administered by the subcutaneous route (see Chapter 14).

G-tube placement for decompression of the stomach and small bowel is an alternative approach to medications that may be especially useful for those patients wanting oral liquids for comfort (e.g. Mr J, case 1). A venting G-tube should also be considered if drugs fail to reduce secretions or vomiting to an acceptable level. Recent studies indicate that neither ascites nor tumour encasement of the stomach is a contraindication to G-tube placement.[5]

Case 2

History

A 67-year-old retired schoolteacher (Mrs B) with a history of carcinoid syndrome due to metastatic neuroendocrine carcinoma originating from the small bowel presents to the palliative care clinic with complaints of fatigue and increased intensity of chronic right upper quadrant pain. Her daughter notes that Mrs B has been intermittently confused over the past week and unable to transfer independently from her bed to chair. Her oral intake has also declined considerably during this period.

The primary carcinoid tumour was resected 10 years ago but recurred 4 years later, requiring cytoreductive surgery of her small bowel and liver metastases. Her last cancer treatment comprised an experimental oral chemotherapeutic agent in combination with long-acting octreotide. Unfortunately, the tumour progressed and all chemotherapy was discontinued except octreotide for her symptoms of flushing and diarrhoea. The chronic right upper quadrant pain due to large liver metastases has been well controlled on low dose methadone. Poor appetite and weight loss are persistent problems managed in the past by calorie-dense supplements, dietary counselling and trials of various pharmacological agents, including melatonin, thalidomide and mirtazapine.

Mrs B has also required prolonged hospital stays over the past 6 months because of complications including obstructive uropathy, deep vein thrombosis and recurrent infections (candidaemia, empyema and hepatic abscess) often accompanied by delirium.

Home medications include a multivitamin and 5 mg of methadone every 12 h for pain. She has been taking non-prescription diphenhydramine for insomnia over the past few weeks as well as multiple extra doses of methadone for breakthrough pain.

Physical examination reveals a frail, cachectic woman, sitting upright in bed. Severe wasting of her upper limbs is apparent, and her lower extremities are edematous. Her abdomen appears distended and hepatomegaly is palpable 10 cm below the costal margin. She is afebrile, systolic blood pressure is 90 mmHg, and her chest is clear to auscultation bilaterally, with decreased breath sounds at the right base. Chest X-ray reveals a right pleural effusion with associated atelectasis. She is inattentive during the interview and displays impaired short-term memory on a brief screening test for delirium. No other neurological abnormalities are identified, except for an impaired gag reflex.

Laboratory tests are remarkable for an elevated BUN and a normal creatinine suggestive of hypovolaemia. She has mild anaemia, leukopenia, normocalcaemia and mildly elevated liver enzymes (alanine aminotransferase 2× > normal). Blood and urine cultures are obtained but reveal no growth after 24 h, and a chest X-ray is unchanged in comparison to a prior examination 3 weeks ago.

CT scan of the abdomen and pelvis reveals a large retroperitoneal mass in the upper abdomen and liver metastases which are increased in size compared to previous imaging studies.

Management

In the palliative care unit intravenous rehydration is initiated and it is anticipated that Mrs B's mild delirium and severe fatigue will improve after administration of fluids, adjustment of opioid analgesics and discontinuation of diphenhydramine. Her daughter is counselled that attempts will be made to limit breakthrough doses of methadone, since Mrs B's expression of pain is thought to be amplified by disinhibition due to delirium. Family members always need to be forewarned when opioid analgesics are to be limited, since such a measure in response to increased pain expression is counterintuitive at first glance. While the cause of the delirium is probably multifactorial, an unnecessary dose escalation of methadone could produce opioid-induced neurotoxicity and an exacerbation of delirium. Mrs B becomes more attentive over the next 48 h, displaying organized thoughts and decreased pain despite only requiring one breakthrough dose of methadone. She is now able to provide a complete history and reports difficulty swallowing both solid foods and liquids over the preceding 2 weeks. She has a history of gastro-oesophageal reflux and an endoscopy 1 year previously showed no stricture or metastatic disease. After discussion with Mrs B and her daughter, an aggressive work-up (CT imaging and repeat endoscopic evaluation) is not pursued. Instead, speech therapy is requested to perform a bedside swallowing evaluation.

The speech therapist's examination reveals mild hypernasality of spontaneous speech, moderately reduced labial and lingual strength and an absent gag reflex. There is no evidence of oropharyngeal candidiasis. Swallowing is observed with cup sips of thin liquids, teaspoons of purées and soft mixed solid consistencies while seated in the upright position in bed. Subtle oral holding with liquids and prolonged oral preparation with solid consistencies is noted.

The pharyngeal phase of swallowing evaluated with bolus trials of liquids and purées is prolonged due to a reported foreign body sensation with masticated consistencies. No coughing, choking or additional voice quality changes are noted. Utilizing a liquid wash with chewed consistencies eliminates the perceived bolus sensation. Mild oropharyngeal dysphagia is identified with no overt clinical indicators of aspiration, although silent aspiration cannot be excluded at bedside. The patient expresses her preference for oral intake for pleasure and comfort, and requests that no further assessments such as modified barium swallow are pursued.

Strategies to overcome her difficulties include the use of soft solids, sitting upright at 90 degrees, taking small bites and sips at a slow rate, utilizing liquid wash (alternate liquids with solids) and sitting upright about 10–50 min after meals. Mrs B, her nurse and primary caregiver (daughter) receive instruction at bedside from the speech therapist.

Although clinically improved after 48 h, Mrs B still requires assistance for transfers from her bed to chair. She also reports intermittent nausea despite scheduled haloperidol and complains of continued poor appetite and severe fatigue. Dexamethasone, 8 mg daily, is started and appears to attenuate this cluster of symptoms. It is apparent that continued care at home by a medical assistant during daytime hours and her daughter during the evening hours (after returning from work) is no longer practical. Her daughter reluctantly agrees to transfer Mrs B to a nearby inpatient hospice facility that will provide 24 h nursing and medical care.

Providing nutrition and fluid at the end of life

Patients at the end of life (such as Mrs B) often experience early satiety, poor appetite, and progressive difficulty in swallowing. Using pharmacological agents to stimulate appetite and alleviate other symptoms such as early satiety, pain and depression may improve oral intake, but non-pharmacological management by a multidisciplinary team may be just as important. Specific nutritional goals and the psychosocial aspects of palliative care need to be addressed in order to ease the suffering experienced by many patients and their families. The roles of other members within this team are discussed in Chapter 19.

By mouth

Severe skeletal muscle loss impairs function and independence, and the wasting of respiratory muscles may directly shorten survival. Unfortunately, cachexia is less responsive to therapy towards the end of the disease trajectory. Since improvement of lean body mass is not realistic within the last few weeks of life, intervention could be targeted toward improving appetite and associated symptoms such as fatigue, depression and early satiety. Better functional outcomes and increased lean body mass may assume a lower priority at this stage. A randomized placebo-controlled trial of megestrol acetate[6] (480 mg daily) and an open label trial of thalidomide (100 mg daily) in patients with cancer cachexia improved appetite and well-being within 10 days of treatment. Side-effects appeared to be insignificant in these trials, perhaps because of the fairly low doses of these drugs and the short duration of treatment. In spite of these positive results, corticosteroids might be the preferred pharmacological option for appetite stimulation in the last few weeks of life. Corticosteroids are inexpensive, well tolerated during short term use[7] and also rapidly effective for a variety of symptoms, including nausea and fatigue.

Up to two-thirds of patients with advanced cancer exhibit autonomic dysfunction, which may contribute to gastroparesis and early satiety.[8] Metoclopramide's anti-emetic and prokinetic actions can improve appetite[9] in this patient group and should be prescribed at a dose of 10 mg every 4 h if possible. Head and neck cancers can cause swallowing difficulties because of disrupted normal anatomy; however, even when anatomic integrity is preserved, functional impairment is frequent and can provoke aspiration pneumonia.[10] Similarly, autonomic dysfunction may contribute to dysphagia in patients without any direct tumour involvement of the head and neck. A swallowing evaluation by a speech therapist is useful to identify specific impairments of the complex swallowing process so that non-invasive therapeutic strategies can be implemented to overcome the problem. If this is not possible, consideration can be given to alternate enteral and parenteral routes for caloric or fluid administration. When patients elect not to receive nutrition or hydration at the end of life, their decision to forgo therapy should be supported by the health care team (please refer to Chapter 23).

Parenteral nutrition (see Chapter 22)

Families and patients may inquire about the value of PN when the enteral route is impossible or ineffective at stabilizing a patient's weight. Health care professionals need to address the concerns in an empathic manner and relay the risks and benefits of such therapy with a clear understanding. In general, patients at the end of life are unlikely to benefit from PN; however, qualitative research[11] suggests that patients and their families experience physical, social and psychological benefits from home parenteral nutrition (HPN) treatment. In an earlier study[12] the same group of researchers reported that family members felt powerless and frustrated when facing a loved one's inability to eat. There was also a perception that health care providers neglected nutritional problems. Since patients and families were no longer able to solve the nutritional problems within the family, the offer of HPN was viewed as a 'positive' alternative.

The health care team needs to be aware that once PN is initiated in the hospital, families may have difficulty accepting the lack of an 'alternative', and that withdrawal of PN on discharge could have a considerable psychological impact.[13]

In clinical circumstances when the tumour is slow growing and there is mechanical obstruction, PN may be indicated to treat the starvation component of the cachectic patient. It should be emphasized that clinical guidelines[14] from the European Association for Palliative Care suggest that PN should be considered only for a subset of patients with a good performance status who may die of starvation rather than their cancer. A retrospective review from one centre[15] in the USA found that any benefits of home PN were confined to a small subset of patients with slow-growing tumours (e.g. carcinoid). Practical guidelines[16] proposed over the past 25 years are fairly consistent and include the following: PN should be considered if the expected survival of the patient is more than 3 months and enteral feeding is impossible. Patients must be aware of their diagnosis, desire PN, spend more than 50% of the time out of bed and be able to manage intravenous infusions. Patients and family members must be made aware of the potential complications[17] such as sepsis and thrombosis of catheters. As always, the evaluation and treatment of each patient should be individualized, weighing the benefits against potential harm. A recent study of patients with advanced cancer on home PN indicated that performance status [Karnofsky Performance Status (KPS) >50] was an important determinant of survival (median 6 months). Those patients with a KPS <50 had a median survival of 3 months. In addition to the difficult clinical decisions regarding PN, there are reimbursement issues to consider in the USA when a patient is transferred to hospice care. PN might not be covered by health insurance, thereby hindering appropriate transition to hospice care.

Parenteral hydration

In both clinical cases patients experienced a decline in their ability to take fluids enterally. Mr J experienced this abruptly after he developed MBO, and in Ms B's case progression occurred over several days or weeks. Hypovolaemia and dehydration are likely to recur after discharge from hospital, so decisions need to be made regarding the desirability and potential benefit of continuing parenteral fluids. These decisions may be influenced by various factors, including the presence of comorbidities such as cardiomyopathy or renal failure which increase the propensity for volume overload. The financial cost and burden of administering PH also affects patients, their families and health care systems.

A distinction should be made between the use of PN and hydration. There are clinical situations where patients with advanced cancer may benefit from parenteral hydration even though PN is not indicated. The consequences of dehydration in terminally ill cancer patients have provoked strong debate and elicited divergent opinions among physicians,[18] with arguments for and against fluid administration. Unfortunately, the debate is hampered by an absence of randomized controlled trials evaluating the benefits and risks of parenteral hydration. There are enormous variations in hydration practice among palliative care centres. A survey of Canadian palliative care physicians[19] found use of parenteral hydration to be quite low (median of 6–10%) with a wide range from 0 to 100%. Japanese oncologists perceived intravenous hydration to be more effective for symptom management and less harmful in terminally ill patients than did palliative care physicians and nurses.[20] There is some research exploring the attitudes of patients and families towards hydration. An Israeli study revealed that an overwhelming majority (95%) of patients and families was not involved in decision-making.[21] Most patients receiving parenteral hydration in an Italian palliative care unit perceived hydration to be beneficial, wanted to continue at home and preferred the intravenous route.[22]

The reasons for a decline in oral intake may be multiple, including profound anorexia, odynophagia, oral lesions, dysphagia, nausea, delayed gastric emptying, bowel obstruction and severe depression. Ascribing symptoms to dehydration is problematic in terminally ill cancer patients because these symptoms can be produced by the cancer itself or by medications.[23] In the last few days of life biochemically documented hypovolaemia (increased osmolality or BUN) is found in a minority of patients.[24] Although one study found thirst to be associated with dehydration (hyperosmolality) and water depletion (measured by atrial natriuretic peptide), thirst was also associated with opioids and anticholinergic medications, mouth breathing and stomatitis.[25] Thirst symptoms can be alleviated by simple measures (oral care, small sips of water, lubrication)[26] and a small randomized controlled trial during the last 4 days of life found no benefit of parenteral hydration for the relief of thirst.[27] Dry mouth is a symptom often encountered early in the disease trajectory, suggesting that conditions other than dehydration (e.g. the cancer itself or medications) may contribute to its origin.

Several preliminary trials in cancer and in elderly patients suggest that hydration may help in preventing neuropsychiatric conditions such as delirium.[28] Depletion of intravascular and intracellular volumes, complicated by impaired renal function, may hasten the onset of delirium and coma. Almost 80% of patients with cancer experience at least one episode of delirium before the end of life. The aetiology is usually multifactorial and includes medication side-effects, metabolic disturbances, hypoxia or infection. While there are no controlled trials of patients with opioid-induced neurotoxicity, observational studies suggest that fluid deficits are associated with delirium reversibility[29] and that hydration therapy (along with opioid adjustment/rotation) may be beneficial. Adoption of a vigorous hydration policy in a Canadian palliative care unit was associated with decreased frequency of delirium episodes.[30] Hydration appeared to reverse or improve symptoms of delirium in 30–70% of patients. A recent randomized, double-blind study of parenteral hydration (1000 vs 100 ml/day of normal saline), administered intravenously or subcutaneously, showed a rapid decrease in degree of sedation, myoclonus and a trend toward decreased hallucinations in patients with advanced cancer.[31] These benefits may have resulted from hydration or simply from an increased elimination of active opioid metabolites from patients (all were receiving opioids for their pain). Although the preliminary findings from this prospective trial suggest that clinical symptom improvement can be achieved with a volume of about 1000 ml/day, these results are far from conclusive and need to be confirmed by larger studies. By contrast, at least two studies show no benefit of parenteral hydration for the treatment of delirium at the end of life. A multicentre observational study of cancer patients in the last 3 weeks of life[32] did not identify any neuropsychiatric benefits arising from hydration therapy. A prospective randomized controlled trial of hypodermoclysis (1000 ml/day) plus subcutaneous haloperidol in advanced cancer patients[22] showed no improvement of delirium compared to those receiving only subcutaneous medications.

Parenteral hydration could increase the risk for oedema and respiratory distress in those patients with comorbidities such as congestive heart failure and renal failure. However, patients treated by palliative care teams usually receive significantly smaller volumes of hydration (<1000 ml) compared with those admitted to cancer centres[33] and a multicentre observational study[34] revealed no association between the development of bronchial secretions and hydration volume. Disadvantages of intravenous hydration include the relatively high cost, need for venepunctures and attachment to an infusion device. Intravenous administration is difficult to maintain at home and consequently may lead to an unnecessarily prolonged stay in hospital. Patients with advanced cancer and decreased oral intake are unlikely to receive any parenteral hydration after admission to home hospice in the USA.

Subcutaneous hydration or hypodermoclysis is an alternative method of fluid hydration for palliative care patients and has many potential advantages.[35] Hypodermoclysis may be started without risk of thrombosis or bleeding and is easier to manage in the home setting, since family members (or patients) are adept after minimal training. Subcutaneous hydration with a daily volume of 1000 ml can be administered independently, and preliminary findings suggest a measurable symptomatic improvement.[36] Infusions can be easily administered by gravity, avoiding the need for infusion pumps, and the same infusion site can be used for many days. Proctoclysis[37] is also feasible, since fluids can be absorbed via the rectum with minimal discomfort in most cases. The cost of relatively inexpensive equipment required for hypodermoclysis (sterile needles, tubing and sterile fluids) may be prohibitive for developing countries. By using nasogastric catheters and tap water, inexpensive, effective hydration can be safely delivered to terminally ill cancer patients.

Conclusion

Even at the end of life, patients and their families place a high value on nutrition, especially the ability to eat and maintain weight. Therapeutic options are limited, and patients and families may perceive that important aspects of care have been neglected. Discussion of the risks and benefits of specific treatments with patients and their families might allay these fears and also avoid the use of reactive, inappropriate interventions. PN is seldom indicated in patients at the end of life, although there may be some symptomatic benefit from parenteral hydration (including hypodermoclysis).The symptoms of MBO can be managed effectively with medications such as octreotide and haloperidol or venting G-tubes when surgery is not an option.

References

1. Suarez-Almazor ME, Newman C, Hanson J, Bruera E (2002) Attitudes of terminally ill cancer patients about euthanasia and assisted suicide: predominance of psychosocial determinants and beliefs over symptom distress and subsequent survival. *J Clin Oncol*, **20**(8), 2134–41.
2. Vander riet (2008) Palliative care professionals' perceptions of nutrition and hydration at the end of life *Int J Palliat Nurs*, **14**(3), 145–51.
3. Astrow AB, Sood JR, Nolan MT (2008) Decision-making in patients with advanced cancer compared with amyotrophic lateral sclerosis. *J Med Ethics*, **34**, 664–8.
4. Ripamonti C, Mercadante S, Groff L, Zecca E, De Conno F, Casuccio A (2000) Role of octreotide, scopolamine butylbromide, and hydration in symptom control of patients with inoperable bowel obstruction and nasogastric tubes: a prospective randomized trial. *J Pain Sympt Manag*, **19**(1), 23–34.
5. Massacesi C, Galeazzi G (2006) Sustained release octreotide may have a role in the treatment of malignant bowel obstruction. *Palliat Med*, **20**(7), 715–16.
6. Mercadante S, Casuccio A, Mangione S (2007) Medical treatment for inoperable malignant bowel obstruction: a qualitative systematic review. *J Pain Sympt Manag*, **33**(2), 217–23.
7. Pothuri B, Montemarano M, Gerardi M, *et al.* (2005) Percutaneous endoscopic gastrostomy tube placement in patients with malignant bowel obstruction due to ovarian carcinoma. *Gynecol Oncol*, **96**, 330–4.
8. Bruera E, Ernst S, Hagen N, *et al.* (1998) Effectiveness of megestrol acetate in patients with advanced cancer: a randomized, double-blind, crossover study. *Cancer Prev Control*, **2**, 74–8.
9. Bruera E, Roca E, Cedaro L, Carraro S, Chacon R (1985) Action of oral methylprednisolone in terminal cancer patients: a prospective randomized double-blind study. *Cancer Treat Rep*, **69**(8), 751–4.
10. Bruera E, Catz Z, Hooper R, *et al.* (1987) Chronic nausea and anorexia in advanced cancer patients: a possible role for autonomic dysfunction. *J Pain Sympt Manag*, **2**, 19–21.
11. Nelson KA, Walsh TD (1993) Metoclopramide in anorexia caused by cancer-associated dyspepsia syndrome (CADS). *J Palliat Care*, **9**(2), 14–18.
12. Nguyen NP, Moltz CC, Frank C, Vos P (2006) Evolution of chronic dysphagia following treatment for head and neck cancer. *Oral Oncol*, **42**(4), 374–80.
13. Orrevall Y, Tishelman C, Permert J (2005) Home parenteral nutrition: a qualitative interview study of the experiences of advanced cancer patients and their families. *Clin Nutr*, **24**(6), 961–70.
14. Orrevall Y, Tishelman C, Herrington MK, Permert J (2004) The path from oral nutrition to home parenteral nutrition: a qualitative interview study of the experiences of advanced cancer patients and their families. *Clin Nutr*, **23**(6), 1280-7.
15. Strasser F (2003) Eating-related disorders in patients with advanced cancer. *Support Care Cancer*, **11**(1), 11–20.

16. Ripamonti C, Twycross R, Baines M, *et al.* (2001)Working Group of the European Association for Palliative Care. Clinical-practice recommendations for the management of bowel obstruction in patients with end-stage cancer. *Support Care Cancer*, **9**(4), 223–33.
17. Hoda D, Jatoi A, Burnes J, Loprinzi C, Kelly D (2005) Should patients with advanced, incurable cancers ever be sent home with total parenteral nutrition? A single institution's 20-year experience. *Cancer*, **103**(4), 863–8.
18. McKinlay AW (2004) Nutritional support in patients with advanced cancer: permission to fall out? *Proc Nutr Soc*, **63**(3), 431–5.
19. Mullady D, O'Keefe S (2006) Treatment of intestinal failure: home parenteral nutrition. *Nat Clin Prac Gastroenterol Hepatol*, **3**, 492–504.
20. Morita T, Shima Y, Adachi I (2002) Japan Palliative Oncology Study Group. Attitudes of Japanese physicians toward terminal dehydration: a nationwide survey. *J Clin Oncol*, **20**(24), 4699–704.
21. Lanuke K, Fainsinger RL (2003) Hydration management in palliative care settings—a survey of experts. *J Palliat Care*, **19**(4), 278–9.
22. Morita T, Shima Y, Miyashita M, Kimura R, Adachi I (2004) Japan Palliative Oncology Study Group. Physician- and nurse-reported effects of intravenous hydration therapy on symptoms of terminally ill patients with cancer. *J Palliat Med*, **7**(5), 683–93.
23. Musgrave CF, Bartal N, Opstad J (1996) Intravenous hydration for terminal patients: what are the attitudes of Israeli terminal patients, their families, and their health professionals? *J Pain Sympt Manag*, **12**(1), 47–51.
24. Mercadante S, Ferrera P, Girelli D, *et al.* (2005) Patients' and relatives' perceptions about intravenous and subcutaneous hydration. *J Pain Sympt Manag*, **30**, 354–8.
25. Steiner N, Bruera E (1998) Methods of hydration in palliative care patients. *J Palliat Care*, **14**, 6–13.
26. Ellershaw JE, Sutcliffe JM, Saunders CM (1995) Dehydration and the dying patient *J Pain Sympt Manag*, **10**(3), 192–7.
27. Morita T, Tei Y, Tsunoda J, *et al.* (2001) Determinants of the sensation of thirst in terminally ill cancer patients. *Support Care Cancer*, **9**, 177–86.
28. McCann RM, Hall WJ, Groth-Juncker A (1994) Comfort care for terminally ill patients. The appropriate use of nutrition and hydration. *J Am Med Assoc*, **272**(16), 1263–6.
29. Cerchietti L, Navigante A, Sauri A, *et al.* (2000) Hypodermoclysis for control of dehydration in terminal-stage cancer *Int J Palliat Nurs*, **6**, 370–4.
30. Lawlor PG, Gagnon B, Mancini IL, *et al.* (2000) Occurrence, causes, and outcome of delirium in patients with advanced cancer: a prospective study. *Arch Intern Med*, **160**, 786–94.
31. Yan E, Bruera E (1991) Parenteral hydration of terminally ill cancer patients. *J Palliat Care*, **7**, 40–3.
32. Bruera E, Franco JJ, Maltoni M, *et al.* (1995) Changing pattern of agitated impaired mental status in patients with advanced cancer: association with cognitive monitoring, hydration, and opioid rotation. *J Pain Sympt Manag*, **10**, 287–91.
33. Bruera E, Sala R, Rico MA, *et al.* (2005) Effects of parenteral hydration in terminally ill cancer patients: a preliminary study. *J Clin Oncol*, **23**(10), 2366–71.
34. Morita T, Hyodo I, Yoshimi T, *et al.* (2005) Japan Palliative Oncology Study Group: Association between hydration volume and symptoms in terminally ill cancer patients with abdominal malignancies. *Ann Oncol*, **16**, 640–7.
35. Bruera E, Belzile M, Watanabe S, *et al.* (1996) Volume of hydration in terminal cancer patients. *Support Care Cancer*, **4**, 147–50.
36. Morita T, Hyodo I, Yoshimi T, *et al.* (2004) Japan Palliative Oncology Study Group. Incidence and underlying etiologies of bronchial secretion in terminally ill cancer patients: a multicenter, prospective, observational study. *J Pain Sympt Manag*, **27**(6), 533–9.

37. Fainsinger RL, MacEachern T, Miller MJ, *et al.* (1994) The use of hypodermoclysis for rehydration in terminally ill cancer patients. *J Pain Sympt Manag*, **9**(5), 298–302.
38. Bruera E, MacDonald N (2000) To hydrate or not to hydrate: how should it be? *J Clin Oncol*, **18**, 1156–8.
39. Bruera E, Pruvost M, Schoeller T, Montejo G, Watanabe S (1998) Proctoclysis for hydration of terminally ill cancer patients. *J Pain Sympt Manag*, **15**(4), 216–9.

Part 11

Special populations

Chapter 31

Paediatric patients

Sian Kirkham and Martin Hewitt

Nutrition support in the child with cancer encompasses all aspects of cancer control: prevention, treatment, supportive care, delayed effects and even palliative care.
(*Rogers et al.*[1])

Introduction

Nutrition support is a core component of the care of a child affected with cancer. However, there is a perception that this has, until recently, been under-recognized.[2] Improved survival rates in children affected with cancer have shifted our focus to a more holistic model of care. This improvement has been a result of national and international cooperation with randomized group clinical trials in paediatric oncology which continue to refine treatment protocols and standards of care.

Malnutrition at diagnosis in the child affected with cancer is variable (6–50%) and dependent on disease stage and location.[3,4] There is evidence in the literature that malnutrition is associated with increased infection rates and reduced chemotherapy tolerance and quality-of-life indices.[3,5,6] Malnutrition (under- or overnutrition) has also been linked with reduced survival although this evidence is more controversial.[7,8] It is widely recognized that childhood obesity is becoming an increasing problem in both America and Europe. Obesity at diagnosis is associated with a poor prognosis in children with acute myeloid leukaemia and teenage girls with acute lymphoblastic leukaemia (ALL).[7] This may be due to incorrect dosing of chemotherapy. Malnutrition ultimately, therefore, has the potential to influence long term effects of both the disease and the treatment.[9]

A recent survey of standards of practice within 233 participating institutions within the Children's Oncology Group consortium demonstrated no uniform approach to nutritional assessment or intervention.[10,11] There are a few published guidelines relating to nutritional intervention, including a recent American Society for Parenteral and Enteral Nutrition review,[12–14] but no clinical studies assessing their efficacy in children with cancer. The effects of varied nutrition practice on the quality of life and outcome of children with cancer are unknown and now the focus of the Children's Oncology Group.[1]

The Children's Oncology Group Nutrition Committee (National Cancer Institute, USA) has been established to further the knowledge of nutrition in children with cancer. The Committee aims to promote and conduct clinical studies in order that standardized methods of nutritional assessment and evidence-based nutritional interventions for children with cancer can be defined.[1]

In this chapter we present the current literature informing practice relating to nutritional assessment and intervention in children with cancer. An understanding of the epidemiology of cancer in childhood, in particular malignancies associated with a high nutrition risk, is key to identifying children who will benefit from nutritional intervention. An overview of the tools currently available for nutritional assessment in children and factors influencing their application in paediatric oncology is given. Finally the nutritional interventions available and a review of the limited data relating to their efficacy in children with cancer are considered.

Epidemiology

In Great Britain during 1991–2000, the incidence of cancer [including non-malignant central nervous system (CNS) tumours] among children aged <15 years was just under 140 per million.[15] Hence about 1500 new cases of childhood cancer are diagnosed each year in the UK. Of these, around 32% have leukaemia, of which ALL is the most predominant form. Some 26% of the total have CNS tumours, among which the most frequent are astrocytomas and other gliomas (13% of all cancers) and primitive neuroectodermal tumours (5%). Lymphomas account for 10% (Hodgkin lymphoma, 4%; non-Hodgkin lymphoma, 6%). Other solid tumours account for the remaining 33%, including neuroblastoma (6%), retinoblastoma (3%), renal tumours (6%), bone tumours (4%), and soft tissue sarcomas (7%).

Survival rates have improved markedly over the last 25 years due to many reasons[15] but there is no doubt that an improved understanding of supportive care has made a significant contribution. Blood product support, antimicrobial policies and proactive nutritional programmes must take their place alongside improved chemotherapy regimens, tailored radiotherapy and improved surgical techniques.

Children with ALL treated on national trials have seen their 5-year survival chances improve from 60% to 85% over the last 30 years. Those with acute myeloid leukaemia have seen an even greater change with 5-year survival moving from 25% to around 70%. Children with solid tumours have seen similar changes, with some diseases having 5-year survival of >90%.

Some tumour types present specific problems with regard to their nutritional demands. Most children will present with some degree of weight loss due simply to their inanition. Those with CNS tumours may present with raised intracranial pressure, with both emesis and headache making adequate oral intake difficult. Some may have specific problems of pharyngeal coordination which may make subsequent management difficult. Children with large intra-abdominal masses may clearly have difficulty in establishing adequate volumes of enteral feeding, as can be seen with neuroblastomas, nephroblastomas, hepatoblastomas and B-cell lymphomas. Although the latter tend to respond very quickly to chemotherapy the other tumours usually take longer to reduce, and therefore can create difficulties in nutritional management at presentation. Primary tumours of the oesophagus, stomach and intestines are extremely rare in children and young adults.

Nutritional assessment

There are no published guidelines relating to nutritional assessment of the child with cancer and current practice is diverse.[8,11,12] There is a general consensus, however, that children with cancer should be screened for nutrition risk at diagnosis and during therapy.[16,17]

Nutrition assessment should include a comprehensive medical and surgical history, dietary history, medical treatment plan, anthropometric measurements, screening biochemical markers and an estimate of resting energy expenditure and nutritional requirement.[18] Research methods of evaluating nutritional status (dual-energy X-ray absorptiometry, bioelectrical impedance) are covered elsewhere in this book. In this chapter we focus on clinical measures of nutritional status relating specifically to paediatric practice.

Anthropometric data

One of the most sensitive indices of nutritional status in a child is growth. Longitudinal data on weight, length or height for age, head circumference and body mass index (BMI; kg/m^2) should be recorded at diagnosis and at intervals during therapy to allow growth velocity to be calculated. The appropriate growth chart for age and sex should be completed: UK90 reference chart (UK),[19] National Center for Health Statistics growth chart (USA)[20] and Euro Growth References.[21]

Initial assessment should also include some measure that is independent of tumour mass in children with solid tumours. Arm anthropometry (biceps and triceps skinfold thickness and mid–upper arm circumference) can provide a reliable baseline measurement of nutritional status that can be followed longitudinally to measure response to a given nutrition intervention.[22,23]

Clinical/physical examination

Clinical and physical examination combined with nutritional assessment and monitoring techniques all form part of a paediatric assessment.

A. Clinical observations:
  - (i) Change in appetite/nutrient intake.
  - (ii) Gastrointestinal problems such as nausea, vomiting, diarrhoea, constipation, mucositis, dysphagia.
  - (iii) Energy levels and activity.

B. Physical observations:
  - (i) Condition of hair, teeth, tongue, nails, breath.
  - (ii) Impression of preservation or wasting of fat and protein mass.
  - (iii) Oedema.
  - (iv) Blood pressure.

Biochemical markers

Patient plasma values compared with normal age-specific reference ranges can also be used in determining the nutrition status of children with cancer. Serum pre-albumin and albumin levels give a measure of protein status. Caution is required, however, as hydration status and liver function affect these values.[18] Turnover for pre-albumin is 2–3 days versus 21 days for albumin, which make it potentially a more reliable measure of the efficacy of any nutrition intervention.[18] Insulin growth factor-1 relates to arm anthropometry as an index of nutritional status.[24]

Patients with chronic malnutrition are at risk of biochemical imbalance during nutrition intervention. The collective term used for this in current practice is refeeding syndrome. Fluid balance, calcium, magnesium, phosphate and potassium should be closely monitored and actively corrected as calories are cautiously increased.[25]

Resting energy expenditure and nutritional requirements

Standard dietary reference values are available in the UK[26] and USA[27] to define baseline nutritional requirements. There is some evidence that basal metabolic rate and resting energy expenditure is increased in children with cancer, affecting in turn nutritional requirement.[28,29] However, there are no guidelines currently relating to its application in clinical practice. Standard dietary reference values are therefore the clinical benchmark.

Nutritional screening tools

STAMP is a new Screening Tool for the Assessment of Malnutrition in Paediatrics. It is a simple way of determining whether a child is at risk of malnutrition and encompasses the more detailed assessment parameters outlined above.[30]

It is likely to be adopted nationally in the UK in the same way as the Malnutrition Universal Screening Tool (MUST), Mini Nutritional Assessment (MNA) and NRS used in adult practice.[31] It could provide a standardised method of nutritional screening at the point of initial and follow-up hospital admission in children with cancer to prompt appropriate further investigation and nutritional intervention.

In the USA, the Children's Oncology Group (COG) Nutrition Committee has recently defined specific categories of malnutrition (underweight or overweight) based on ideal body weight or BMI. An algorithm has been developed as a guideline for nutritional intervention specific to children with cancer.[1] This will be used within the COG to develop standardized nutritional guidelines for children on COG clinical trials.

Nutritional intervention

The main aim of nutritional intervention in children with cancer is to optimize nutrition and to maintain normal growth and development during cancer treatment. If protein-energy malnutrition is present the nutritional deficit must first be addressed and future malnutrition prevented. The intervention of choice is that which meets the child's nutrition requirement with the minimum associated risk.[4]

Nutrition advice and oral feeding

The state-registered dietitian plays a vital role in educating children and families, medical and nursing staff on the impact of cancer and its treatment on nutritional status. The oral route should always be the first to be considered in nutritional supplementation. Favourite nutrient-rich foods and nutritional supplements can be offered (Table 31.1). A dietitian should guide the choice of appropriate supplement.

Enteral tube feeding

Early initiation of enteral nutrition support with the use of nutritional supplements via an enteral tube (gastrostomy or nasogastric tube) should be considered when:

- the child's oral intake fails to meet recommended nutritional intake; and/or
- the child fails to maintain an adequate growth velocity;
- other non-nutritional causes are excluded.

Studies have demonstrated that tube feeding is successful in maintaining adequate nutrition and reversing malnutrition in the paediatric oncology population.[32,33]

The use of enteral tube feeding is inconsistent in children with cancer.[11] Effects of treatment such as neutropenia, thrombocytopenia, and mucositis have previously been thought to lead to a high risk of bleeding with enteral tube insertion, although clinical trials have shown that this is not evidence-based.[32–34] There is some experience that pre-emptive enteral tube feeding in nutritionally high risk populations, such as children undergoing bone marrow transplantation, improves outcome.[35] Percutaneous gastrostomy insertion has also been demonstrated to be safe and effective in children with cancer and is a route to be considered where longer term enteral tube feeding is required, e.g. children with head and neck tumours.[36]

Advantages of enteral tube feeding for nutrition support include lower cost compared to parenteral nutrition, decreased risk of infection, and maintenance of the integrity of the intestinal

Table 31.1 Examples of nutritional supplements available in the UK

Supplement	Suggested use
Glucose polymers	Add to infant formula milk, baby juice, cow's milk, water, squash, tea, lollies
Powder, e.g. Maxijul (SHS Ltd),	
Polycose (Abbott labs), Vitajoule (Vitaflo)	
Liquid, e.g. Polycal (Nutricia Ltd), Maxijul (SHS Ltd)	
Fat emulsion	Add to infant formula, cow's milk
E.g. Calogen, Liquigen (SHS Ltd)	
Combined fat and carbohydrate	
E.g. Duocal (SHS limited), QuickCal (Vitaflo)	
Protein	Add to infant formula, liquid Duocal
Powder	
Protifar (Nutricia)	
Pro-cal (Vitaflo)	Not for children <1 year
Liquid	
Pro-cal shot (Vitaflo)	Not for children <1 year
Nutritionally complete	For oral or enteral tube feeding in children
Nutrini (1 kcal/ml), Nutrini Energy (1.5 kcal/ml) (Nutricia Ltd)	>1 year/>8 kg
Frebini (1 kcal/ml), Frebini Energy (1.5 kcal/ml) (Fresenius)	1–10 years (8–30 kg)
Tentrini (1 kcal/ml), Tentrini Energy, (1.5 kcal/ml) (Nutricia)	6–12 years (20–45 kg)
All ± fibre	
Sip feeds:	
Fortini (1.5 kcal/ml) (Nutricia)	
Paediasure (1 kcal/ml) (Abbott)	1–6 years (8–20 kg)
Paediasure plus (1.5 kcal/ml) (Abbott)	1–10 years (8–30 kg)
Fortijuce (1.5 kcal/ml) (Nutricia Ltd)	
Fortisip (1.5 kcal/ml) (Nutricia Ltd)	≥12 years (>45 kg)
Ensure/Ensure plus (1 kcal/1.5 kcal/ml) (Abbot)	
Fortisip yoghurt style (1.5 kcal/ml) (Nutricia Ltd)	

mucosa.[37] Selection of a formula should be guided by a paediatric dietitian according to age, gastrointestinal function and local guidelines. Age-appropriate whole-protein nutritionally complete formulae can be used for patients with normal gastrointestinal and renal function. Pre-digested or elemental formulae are appropriate for children who demonstrate poor tolerance of nutritionally complete formulae.

Enteral feeds can be delivered as a continuous feed, intermittent bolus feed or as a combination. Continuous feeds may be better tolerated than bolus regimes where chemotherapy-induced nausea and vomiting is an issue. Bolus feeds are more physiological. Combining a nocturnal continuous feed with daytime oral or bolus feeds is a common approach. If feeds are not tolerated a trial of a 20 h continuous feed is indicated. Anti-emetics and prokinetics can improve tolerance. Where this fails, post-pyloric feeding via a jejunal tube may improve tolerance and avoid the need for parenteral nutrition.

Parenteral nutrition

Parenteral nutrition (PN) is the intravenous administration of macronutrients, vitamins and minerals. It is used to treat children who cannot be fully fed by the enteral route, for example due to intestinal failure. This is the where ingestion, digestion or absorption of macronutrients is insufficient to maintain health and growth. Appropriate efforts to avoid PN with the consideration and use of specialized feeds and artificial enteral feeding devices should be made before its use.[38]

High dose chemotherapy regimens and radiotherapy can damage the gastrointestinal tract causing mucositis and enteritis resulting in difficulty establishing enteral feeds, thereby necessitating the introduction of PN. The PN prescription should be determined by those with appropriate expertise after a comprehensive nutritional assessment, and subsequently reviewed with regular biochemical and nutritional parameters. The enteral route should be used as soon as practicable and the child transitioned on to enteral feeding.

Care of the child on PN requires a multidisciplinary approach. Hospital nutrition teams have been shown to optimize the treatment of hospitalized patients and where available can provide advice and support on transitioning the child to enteral feeding as quickly as possible.[39]

Refeeding syndrome is a serious complication of PN. Rapid feeding in the presence of malnutrition can result in electrolyte disturbance (potassium, magnesium and phosphate), fluid imbalance and associated cardiovascular, pulmonary and neurological symptoms. Many of the commonly used therapeutic agents used in oncology can also cause electrolyte depletion, e.g. cisplatin and magnesium loss, and this also needs to be taken into consideration. Children with cancer are at increased risk of refeeding syndrome and associated electrolyte disturbance.[25] Parenteral calories should be slowly advanced with close monitoring.

Other complications of parenteral nutrition include sepsis and cholestasis. Infusion of a nutrient-rich mixture provides a culture medium for bacteria and children receiving PN should be closely monitored, the central line cultured and prompt treatment initiated if they develop signs of sepsis. PN can also induce cholestasis, especially in the absence of any enteral stimulus, recurrent episodes of sepsis and longer duration of PN.[34] Long term PN use (>1 month) is associated with cholestasis in 30–60% of children. PN-induced liver dysfunction can progress to hepatic fibrosis and liver failure.[35] It is therefore important to cycle PN where possible and advance enteral feeding as soon as practicable.

There are limited studies looking at the use of PN in the paediatric oncology population. Benefits reported include improvement in treatment tolerance, decreased delays in therapy and provision of a reliable source of nutrients.[1] Fears that nutrition provision might stimulate tumour growth and promote metastasis, or significantly increase the risk of infection in immunosuppressed patients, have not been substantiated.[1]

Psychosocial intervention

Psychosocial support is essential in the care of the child with cancer, particularly in relation to facilitation of nutrition support and intervention.

Parents' instinct-led desire to feed their children is very strong and can lead to an excessive focus on food. This can have deleterious effects on the children who have lost the desire to eat due to side-effects of anticancer therapy.[40] The psychosocial team can work with the parent and child to reduce the tension around food and prepare the child for invasive procedures such as nasogastric tube insertion if required.

Case histories

The cases below illustrate in practice the systematic approach to nutrition assessment and intervention in children with cancer outlined in this chapter.

Case study 1

A 14-year-old girl presented with swelling of the left calf. Imaging confirmed a mass in the soleus muscle and biopsy showed that this was a Ewing's sarcoma. The tumour was of small volume and there was no evidence of metastatic disease. She commenced six cycles of chemotherapy which included vincristine, ifosphamide, doxorubicin and etoposide at 3-week intervals. The latter three drugs have significant emetogenic potential and so she was given prophylactic anti-emetics with each course.

At presentation her weight was 38.9 kg (2nd centile), her height was 148 cm (2nd centile) and her BMI was 17.8 (25th centile). See Figure 31.1 for her growth chart. Although she had a good response to chemotherapy

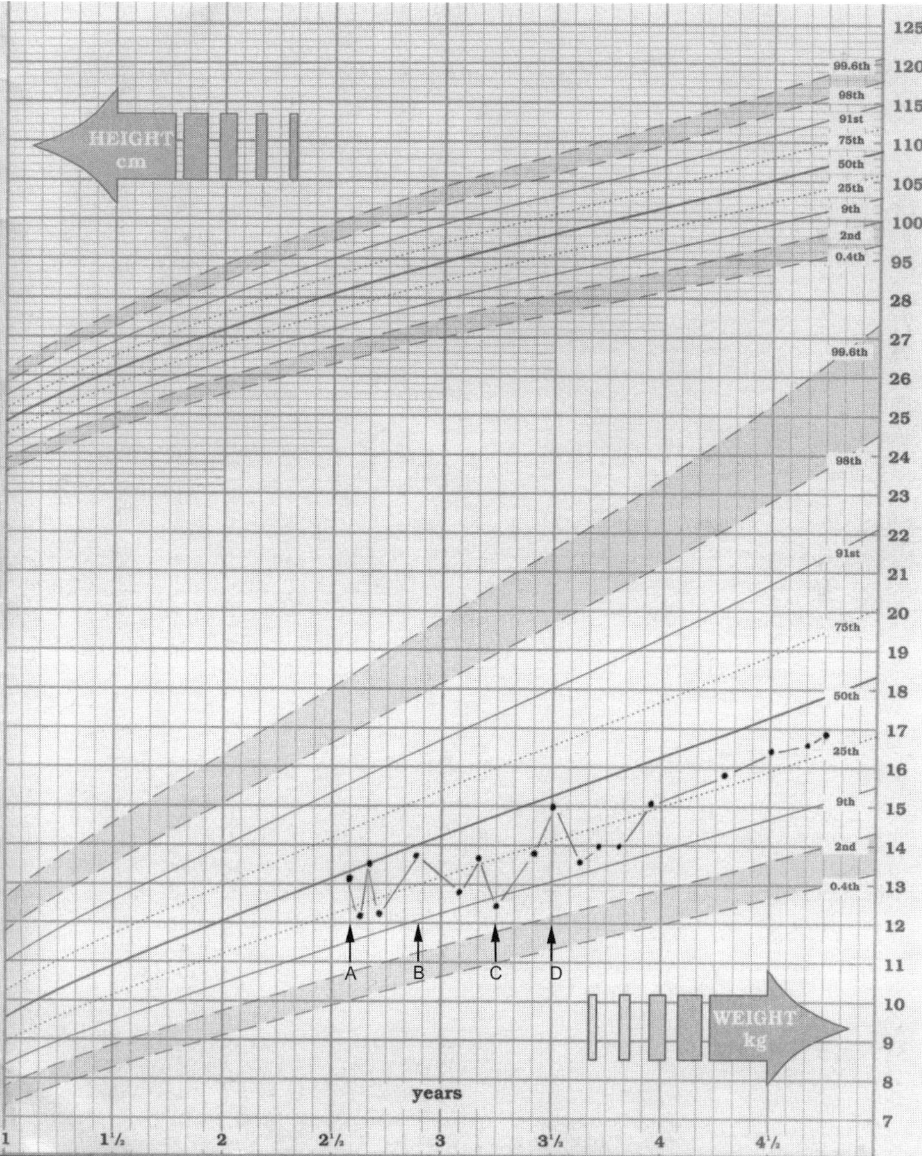

Fig. 31.1 Growth chart for Sally O. (A) Diagnosis. (B) Tumour resection. (C) Enteral nutrition. (D) Veno-occlusive disease leading to oedema.

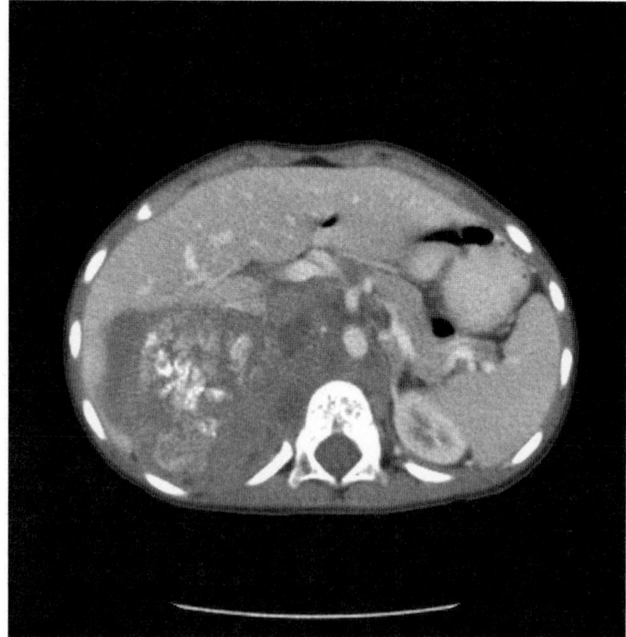

Fig. 31.2 Computed tomography of abdomen showing neuroblastoma (arrow). Note space-occupying effect within abdominal cavity, which can lead to significant problems establishing adequate enteral nutrition.

she began to loose interest in food and her weight fell to 33.9 kg. Her mood deteriorated and she became withdrawn and depressed. PN was provided during her admissions for chemotherapy and management of her neutropenia. Severe mucositis, prolonged periods of fever and malaise and the development of Clostridium difficile-positive diarrhoea all contributed to her problems. Although initially fed via a nasogastric tube, for cosmetic reasons she finally refused to continue with this route. A gastrostomy tube was inserted and a feeding programme established which ultimately lead to clinical, nutritional and mental improvement.

Case study 2

A 2-year-old girl presented with a short history of lethargy, back pain and abdominal pain. Examination suggested an abdominal mass and further imaging confirmed the presence of large mass seen to be arising from the superior pole of the left kidney and measuring 16 × 12 × 9 cm (Figure 31.2). Biopsy confirmed this to be a neuroblastoma. Chemotherapy included cisplatin, carboplatin, etoposide, cyclophosphamide, adriamycin and vincristine. Macroscopic surgical resection was undertaken after about 12 weeks. Further chemotherapy and radiotherapy to the abdomen were administered. The complete cycle of intensive treatment lasted 10 months. At presentation her weight was 13.2 kg (50th centile), her height was 84 cm (25th centile) and her BMI was 18.7 (75th centile). See Figure 31.3 for her growth chart. The provision of chemotherapy resulted in reduced nutritional intake, and PN was required. The weeks following surgery were complicated by persistent diarrhoea and, during radiotherapy, she had anorexia and vomiting. Both are recognized complications limiting the use of the enteral route for feeding. All problems had to be anticipated and addressed by active nutritional support.

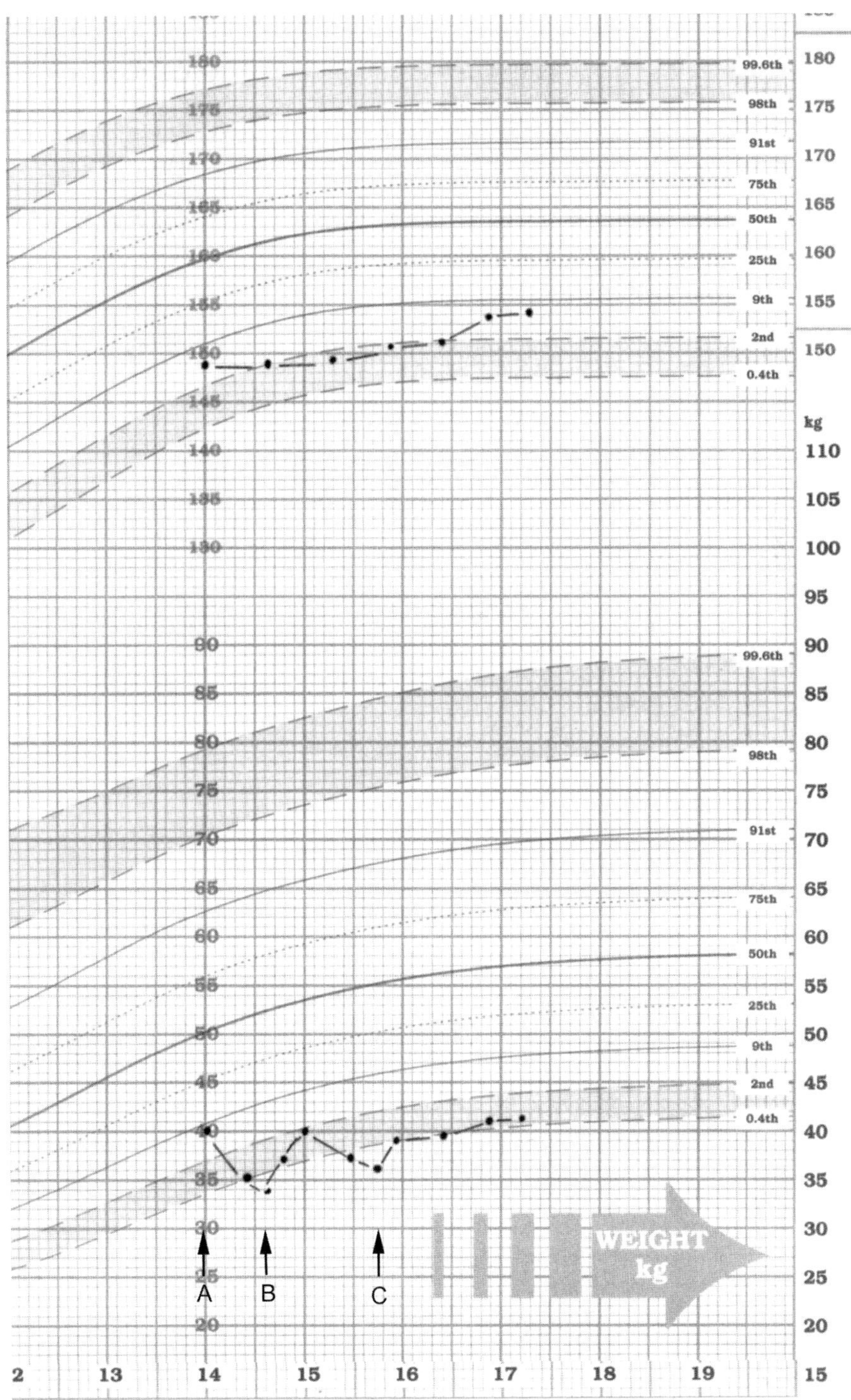

Fig. 31.3 Growth chart for Sammy H. (A) Diagnosis. (B) Parenteral nutrition. (C) Enteral nutrition.

References

1. Rogers PC, Melnick SJ, Ladas EJ, Halton J, Baillargeon J, Sacks N (2008) Children's Oncology Group (COG) Nutrition Committee. *Pediatr Blood Cancer*, **50**(Suppl 2), 447–50.
2. Ladas EJ, Sacks N, Meacham L, *et al.* (2005) A multidisciplinary review of nutrition considerations in the pediatric oncology population: a perspective from Children's Oncology Group. *Nutr Clin Pract*, **20**, 337–93.
3. Martin E, Belleton F, Lallemand Y, *et al.* (2006) Malnutrition in pediatric oncology: prevalence and screening. *Arch Pediatr*, **13**(4), 352–7 [Epub 20 Feb 2006].
4. Mauer AM, Burgess JB, Donaldson SS, *et al.* (1990) Special nutritional needs of children with malignancies: a review. *J Parenter Enteral Nutr*, **14**(3), 315–24.
5. Andrassay RJ, Chwals WJ (1998) Nutritional support of the paediatric oncology patient. *Nutrition*, **14**, 124–9.
6. Hays DM, Merritt RJ, White L, Ashley J, Siegel SE (1983) Effect of total parenteral nutrition on marrow recovery during induction therapy for acute nonlymphocytic leukemia in childhood. *Med Paediatr Oncol*, **11**, 134–40.
7. Lange BJ Gerbing RB, Feusner J, *et al.* (2005) Mortality in overweight and underweight children with acute myeloid leukemia. *J Am Med Assoc*, **293**, 203–211.
8. Ptetsch JB, Ford C (2000) Children with cancer: measurements of nutritional status at diagnosis. *Nutr Clin Pract*, **15**, 185–8.
9. Oeffinger KC, Hudson MM (2004) Long term complications following childhood and adolescent cancer: foundation for providing risk based healthcare for survivors. *CA Cancer J Clin*, **54**, 208–36.
10. Ladas EJ, Sacks N, Brophy P, *et al.* (2006) Standards of nutritional care in pediatric oncology. A Children's Oncology Group study. *Pediatr Blood Cancer*, **46**, 339–44.
11. Ladas EJ, Sacks N, Meacham LR, *et al.* (2005) A review of the nutritional practices for the pediatric oncology population: assessment, intervention, nursing, pharmacology, quality of life, and survivorship. *Nutr Clin Pract*, **20**, 377–93.
12. Huhmann MB, August DA (2008) Review of American Society for Parenteral and Enteral Nutrition (ASPEN) clinical guidelines for nutrition support in cancer patient: nutrition screening and assessment. *Nutr Clin Pract*, **23**(2), 182–8.
13. Koletzko B, Goulet O, Hunt J, Krohn K, Shamir R (2005) Guidelines on Paediatric Parenteral Nutrition of the European Society of Paediatric Gastroenterology, Hepatology and Nutrition (ESPGHAN) and the European Society for Clinical Nutrition and Metabolism (ESPEN). *J Paediat Gastroenterol Nutr*, **41**, S1–S4.
14. Loser C, Aschl G, Hebyterne X, *et al.* (2005) ESPEN guidelines on artificial enteral nutrition—percutaneous endoscopic gastrostomy (PEG). *Clin Nutr*, **24**, 848–61.
15. Stiller CA, Kroll ME, Eatock EM (2007) Incidence of childhood cancer 1991–2000. In: Stiller CA (ed.), *Childhood Cancer in Britain: Incidence, Survival, Mortality*. Oxford: Oxford University Press.
16. Sacks N, Ringwald Smith K, Hale G (2004) Nutritional support. In: Altman A (ed.), *Supportive Care of Children with Cancer*, pp. 243–61. Baltimore MD: John Hopkins University Press.
17. American Academy of Pediatrics (1999) Nutritional management of children with cancer. In: Kleinmann RE (ed.), *Pediatric Nutrition Handbook*, pp. 709–17. Elk Grove Village, IL: AAP.
18. Bessler S (1999) Nutritional assessment. In: Samour PQ, Helm KK, Lang CE (eds), *Handbook of Paediatric Nutrition*, pp. 19–47. Gaithersburg, MD: Aspen.
19. Wright CM, Booth IW, Buckler JMH, *et al.* (2002) Growth reference charts for use in the United Kingdom. *Arch Dis Childh*, **86**, 11–14.
20. Kuczmarski R, Ogden C, Grummer-Strawn L, *et al.* (2002) 2000 CDC growth charts for the United States—methods & development. National Center for Health Stats. *Vital Health Stat*, **11**(246), 1–190.
21. Van 't Hof, Hashke F, Group E-GS (2000) Euro growth references for body mass index (BMI) and weight for length (WfL). *J Pediatr Gastroenterol Nutr*, **31**(Suppl 1), S48–59.

22. Frizancho AR (1981) New norms of upper limb fat and muscle areas for assessment by nutritional status. *Am J Clin Nutr*, **34**, 2540–5.
23. Tanner JM, Whitehouse RH (1975) Revised standards for triceps and subscapular skinfolds in British Children. *Arch Dis Child*, **50**, 142–5.
24. Brennan B, Gill M, Penneалls O, Eden O, Thomas A, Clayton P (1998) Insulin like growth factor, IGF binding protein 3 & IGFBP protease activity: relation to anthropometric indices in solid tumours or leukaemia. *Arch Dis Child*, **80**, 226–30.
25. Solomon SM, Kirkby DF (1990) The re-feeding syndrome: a review. *J Parenter Enteral Nutr*, **14**, 90–7.
26. Department of Health (1991) *Report on Health and Social Subjects, No. 41. Dietary Reference Values for Food, Energy and Nutrients for the United Kingdom*. London: HMSO.
27. Food and Nutrition Board Institute of Medicine (2002) *Dietary Reference Intakes Energy, Carbohydrate, Fiber, Fat, Fatty Acids, Cholesterol, Protein and Amino Acids*. Washington, DC; National Academy Press.
28. Young VR (1977) Energy metabolism & requirements in the cancer patient. *Cancer Res*, **37**, 2336–47.
29. Peacock JL, Inculet RI, Corsey R, *et al.* (1987) Resting energy expenditure and body cell mass alterations in non-cachetic patients with sarcomas. *Surgery*, **102**, 465–72.
30. McCarthy H, McNulty H, Dixon M, Eaton-Evans MJ (2008) Screening for nutrition risk in childhood—validation of a new tool. *J Hum Nutr Diet*, **21**, 395–6.
31. Kondrup J, Allison JP, Elia M, Vellas B, Plauth M (2003) ESPEN Guidelines for nutrition screening. *Clin Nutr*, **22**, 415–21.
32. Pietsch JB, Ford C, Whitlock JA (1999) Nasogastric tube feeding in children with high risk cancer: a pilot study. *J Pediatr Hematol Oncol*, **21**, 111–14.
33. Deswarte-Wallace J, Firouzbakhsh S, Finkelstein JZ (2001) Using research to change practice: enteral feeding for pediatric oncology patients. *J Pediatr Oncol Nurs*, **18**, 217–33.
34. Den Broeder E, Lippens RJ, van 't Hof MA, *et al.* (1998) Effects of nasogastric tube feeding on the nutritional status of children with cancer. *Eur J Clin Nutr*, **52**, 494–500.
35. Langdana A, Tully N, Molloy E, Bourke B, Meara A (2001) Intensive enteral nutrition support in paediatric bone marrow tranplantation. *Bone Marrow Transpl*, **27**, 741–6.
36. Barlaug M, Kruse A, Shroeder H (2008) Percutaneous endoscopic gastrostomy in paediatric cancer patients. *Ugerskr Laeger*, **170**(23), 2027–31.
37. Han Markey T (2000) Nutritional considerations in paediatric oncology. *Semin Oncol Nurs*, **16**, 146–51.
38. Koletzko B, Goulet O, Hut J, Krohn K, Shamir R (2005) Guidelines on Paediatric Parenteral Nutrition of the Paediatric Gastroenterology, Hepatology & Nutrition ESPGHAN) and the European Society for Clinical Nutrition and Metabolism (ESPEN). *J Paediat Gastroenterol Hepatol Nutr*, **41**, S1–S4.
39. Kumpf VJ (2006) Parenteral nutrition associated liver disease in adult & paediatric patients. *Nutr Clin Pract*, **21**(3), 279–90.
40. Askins MA, Moore BD 3rd (2008) Psychosocial support of the pediatric cancer patient; lessons learned over the past 50 years. *Curr Oncol Rep*, **10**, 469–76.

Chapter 32

Nutritional care of older people

Jane Hopkinson and Christopher Bailey

Introduction

> I look at the wrinkly bits of skin and think 'I am really getting old now'.... The doctor says 'well, you are 70, you must expect it!'
>
> (Craig, age 71 years)

Craig is associating his weight loss with age. He is one of the 84 interviewees aged ≥60 years who have taken part in the Macmillan Weight and Eating Studies (MWES).[1–4] These studies have been conducted in the UK to investigate how people with advanced cancer might be helped to live with weight loss and eating difficulties: symptoms of cancer–cachexia syndrome (CCS).

In this chapter we consider whether age is an important consideration in the management of CCS. We are nurses with clinical experience in the rehabilitation of elderly people (J.H.), cancer care (J.H., C.B.) and the conduct of research with older people with cancer (J.H., C.B.). The issues we raise are relevant to the practice of all members of the multidisciplinary cancer care team.

'Age discrimination' and clinical decision-making

Older people living with cancer are cared for in the context of discourses about age and ageing. Ageism is an example. Help the Aged (based in the UK), defines ageist attitudes as:

> ... positive and negative images that are accepted and considered to represent older people. Unfortunately, the negative stereotypes tend to be more predominant and accepted. Some negative stereotypes suggest all older people are: Sick and disabled, impotent, ugly, poor, depressed, isolated, demented, unable to learn, and unproductive.[5]

Similarly, the Victoria State Government in Australia has described ageism as making assumptions that people have memory and physical impairments because of their age and are unable to change.[6] These are just two examples that demonstrate ageism crosses national boundaries. When ageism informs behaviour, it can lead to age discrimination.

Help the Aged advises the public that they are experiencing age discrimination if they feel they have been treated differently because of their age. For example, if they have 'Been told by a doctor or nurse your symptoms are just "down to getting old".'[5]

Do you think Craig was experiencing age discrimination when his doctor advised him that he should expect wrinkly skin (caused by weight loss) at his age? Perhaps he was. Alternatively, he may be describing good clinical practice in lay people's language. We will argue that age-related factors should be taken into account when making clinical decisions about the management of CCS.

Setting the scene

The proportion of older people is increasing in western populations. In the UK in 2001, the percentage of people aged ≥65 years was 18%, double what it was in 1931.[7] Those aged ≥80 years constitute the fastest-growing age group.[8] From a global perspective, data from the United Nations suggest that the percentage of the world's population aged ≥60 years will double from 11% in 2007 to 22% in 2050.[9] These trends are important because the incidence of most cancers is age dependent.[10] In the USA, data show that in the ≥75 years age group, numbers of people diagnosed with cancer are expected to rise from 389 000 in 2000 (30% of the cancer population) to nearly 1 102 000 in 2050 (42% of the cancer population).[11] Such demographic changes have clear consequences for health care worldwide. In the UK, for example, the King's Fund estimates that the projected increase in the proportion of the population aged ≥65 years from 16% in 2006 to 22% in 2031 will lead to a substantial increase in the demand for services.[12,13] Similarly, in the USA it is anticipated that the ageing of the population will lead to substantial increases in the number and age of cancer patients:[11] The number of people in need of cancer treatment, together with their age when they need it, will also rise, bringing a 'growing demand for more supportive, palliative, and general medical services.'[11]

A number of factors are reported to affect older people with cancer, including other chronic disabling conditions (comorbidities). Data from a Dutch cancer registry show that 63% of newly diagnosed patients aged 65–79 years reported serious comorbidities including previous cancer, cardiovascular disease, chronic obstructive pulmonary disease, hypertension and diabetes. For those aged ≥80 years, this rose to 67%.[14] Comorbidity is an important consideration for people with cancer because it has been shown to be an independent predictor of survival.[15] De Vries *et al.* (2007) list potential problems experienced by older people with cancer, including affective disorders such as depression, inadequate social support, functional impairments, nutritional complications, and loss of auditory or visual acuity.

Older people may experience exclusion from health care through the combined effects of professional roles and market principles.[16] In the UK, it has been argued that professional groups in the health services act as gatekeepers, controlling older people's access to health and social care. Disability and ill-health in older age can be regarded as a normal part of the ageing process and not be seen as priorities for diagnosis and treatment.

Historically questions have been raised about equity of treatment for older people with cancer. Leading clinicians have asked why cancer in the elderly is so badly treated[17] and have pointed to 'bulging files' on the undertreatment of older people.[18] More recent research has continued to identify discrepancies. In breast cancer, for example, age may have been used to decide on treatment options 'too rigidly', with elderly women denied surgery on the basis of their chronological age alone.[19] This, and other similar evidence, supports the argument that we must not allow age to remain 'an important and independent risk factor for receiving inadequate care'.[20]

Normal physiological ageing

Age does change our bodies in ways that may be relevant to nutritional care. The normal process of ageing includes loss of muscle mass, decline in appetite, and diminished taste and smell acuity.[21] This normal ageing process can contribute to the risk of poor nutritional status by making shopping, food preparation and eating difficult. There is debate around the extent to which diet and exercise can slow normal physiological ageing. What is agreed is that 'as people grow old, the probability of important losses of function increases, but the ageing process remains highly individual.'[22] The timing of structural and functional losses across the course of life is dependent on many individual and environmental factors, and losses are not inevitable.

Nutritional care of people with CCS

The pharmacological and nutritional management options for primary and secondary cachexia are described earlier in this book. Developing understanding of how social context can influence the eating habits and nutritional status of people with cancer is a new avenue of study. Interventions such as family counselling have been theorized to help patients manage weight- and eating-related problems.[23] Evidence is emerging that supportive psychosocial intervention can mitigate weight- and eating-related distress and may have beneficial effects on appetite.[24]

Nutritional care of older people with CCS

Looking to the literature for guidance on whether the nutritional care of older people with cancer should differ from those of younger age groups, there is little to inform practice.

We searched electronic data bases: CINAHL, EMBASE, BNI, Medline, PsychINFO, and Web of Knowledge from 2006 to 2008. Literature was excluded during abstract selection if it was about: (i) prevention of cancer or ageing; (ii) ageing in non-cancer/healthy subjects; (iii) age-related cancer incidence; (iv) biochemistry of ageing and/or the genetic contribution to ageing, (v) management of cancer was not considered in relation to age; (vi) methodological/methods issues. The selected sample comprised 21 from 1107 abstracts, revealing how few publications have considered age-related issues in the nutritional care of people with cancer. The findings can be summarized as follows.

- Physiological ageing should inform treatment decisions, such as dosage of chemotherapy agents and anticachexia medication, but there are no evidence-based guidelines for practice.
- Physiological ageing makes (i) complications of treatments more difficult to manage (e.g. because of reduced renal function), (ii) drug interactions more likely (e.g. because of comorbidity), and (iii) may contribute to the progression of malnutrition and CCS.
- Geriatric assessment and care pathways may facilitate optimal treatment outcomes (including optimal nutritional care) in older people with cancer.
- There may be age-specific consequences for cancer survivors that require tailored supportive (including nutritional) care.

Therefore an evidence base and/or guidelines on how physical change that can accompany age should be taken into account when making clinical decisions on the pharmacological management of CCS have yet to be developed. Physiological age, not chronological age, is argued to be important, as it is factors such as functional status and comorbidity that influence treatment outcomes not chronological age.

Little attention seems to have been paid to the question of whether nutritional interventions and counselling should be tailored to take account of physiological ageing—for example, screening for the decline in taste acuity that can accompany normal ageing and increase nutritional risk.

Age as a factor in the nutritional care of people with cancer

From the issues outlined above, it can be seen that the nutritional care of older people with cancer is complex. Considerations include the implications of physiological ageing on medication use and differences in the nutritional requirements of older versus younger people. There is, however, another layer of complexity: the way psychosocial factors, such as ageist attitudes, may lead to a requirement for age-sensitive management of nutritional issues in people with cancer.

In western society, growing old has become associated with physical and mental frailty and growing dependency on others. Perhaps the tension between the privileged cultural values of individual responsibility and independence and negative stereotypical images of ageing, lead to resistance to identifying with being aged; resistance that has implications for the delivery of nutritional care to an older person with cancer. Before we discuss these implications, we will set out some of the evidence that has led us to believe that ageism influences people's self-management of diet.

Macmillan Weight and Eating Studies (MWES)

Only a minority of the patients who were interview participants of MWES identified with being old. Just ten of them suggested age as being a contributory factor to weight loss and/or changing eating habits. These people identified with the cultural portrayal of ageing and unquestioningly accepted that with age they would lose weight, eat less and be less active (changes that do accompany normal physiological ageing):

> You have got to learn to live with (weight loss and loss of appetite) and learn to die with it. It is hard for me to explain to you, but I am an old man now.
>
> (William, age 66 years)

Attributing appetite and weight loss to age justified inaction in response to involuntary weight loss or poor appetite:

> Just can't eat quite so much 'cause I'm an old (person).
>
> (Alan, age 67 years)

However, the majority of interviewees did not identify with being old. Across the course of the MWES, 145 interviews have been conducted, exploring the experience of living with CCS for 95 people, 84 of whom were aged ≥60 years. Less than a third of these 95 people mentioned age. This seems surprising given the reminders in our everyday lives of relationships between age, ageing, diet and weight. For example, food products are marketed with claims of benefits for older people, such as calcium to counter osteoporosis. When reference was made to age, it was typical to talk of others as being old or others as having the characteristics of older people. Anna has been given dietary advice for someone with a small appetite, but discounts it, as being appropriate for other older people.

> The advice (the dietitian) gave I found was terrible .... And it was probably applied to old people.
>
> (Anna, age 64 years)

A possible explanation for the MWES participants electing to talk about others as aged, or electing not to talk about age at all, might be that they were behaving as defended subjects.[25] They may have been resisting the adoption of identity that invites negative stereotyping.

Self-management of diet to achieve optimal intake is important for achieving best outcomes from curative and possibly palliative treatments. Yet it seemed that suboptimal dietary intake could result, in part, from weight loss and small appetite either being dismissed as a normal part of ageing or discounted as a problem so as to avoid characterizing oneself as ageing. Ageist attitudes (the stereotypical images of the older person), which older people with CCS may themselves be influenced by, could lead to inappropriate nutritional intake for optimal health and well-being.

Our thesis—that ageist attitudes held by patients can lead to suboptimal eating behaviours—raises the possibility that socially constructed ideas about age may need to be taken into consideration when planning the delivery of supportive nutritional care to people living with cancer. The idea is based on information gathered from a small sample of people with advanced cancer living in a single region of the UK, so it should be generalized with caution. It is of value because of the research questions it generates and its possible implications for the nutritional care of older people with cancer.

Implications of MWES for future research

There is still much work to be done to understand the implications of age for the management of CCS. There is need for empirical work to establish if proactive provision of nutritional advice to older people with cancer can improve outcomes from active treatment and palliative care. This would seem a promising line of enquiry, as there is some evidence that intervention in response to problems can bring about change in dietary intake in older people with cancer[26,27] and that nutritional status is related to morbidity and survival. Geriatric assessment has been proposed as a useful tool for the identification of problems that place an older person with cancer at nutritional risk.[14,28,29] It is a method that could be tested for its ability to initiate timely nutritional support.

Implications of MWES for nutritional care of older people with cancer

The way in which the meaning of age informs behaviour might be as important as physiological (not chronological) age to the nutritional management of older people with cancer. There is the potential for ageist attitudes to inform not only the behaviour of healthcare professionals, but also the behaviour of patients. What is important for practice is to be alert to the possibility of ageist attitudes acting as a psychosocial obstacle to optimal self-management of weight and eating problems by patients.

Conclusion

We have drawn on a scope of literature to argue that physiological changes associated with ageing should be taken into account when deciding on the pharmacological management of CCS. Nutritional interventions, including counselling, might also be enhanced by consideration of changes in the senses, appetite and nutritional requirements that are associated with age. Our own work suggests that ageist attitudes may present a socially constructed obstacle to the achievement of optimal nutritional care of older people with cancer. The obstacle lies not solely with the attitudes of healthcare professionals, but with older people themselves. In conclusion, it is not chronological age that is an important consideration in the delivery of nutritional care, but the person's physiological status and the meanings they attribute to age. The way forward is to assess these factors in the context of cancer care, so that they can inform clinical decisions and result in better nutritional care of older people with cancer.

References

1. Hopkinson JB, Wright DNM, Corner JL (2006) The experience of weight loss in people with advanced cancer. *J Adv Nurs*, **54**(3), 304–12.
2. Hopkinson JB, Wright DNM, McDonald JW, Corner JL (2006) The prevalence of concern about weight loss and change in eating habits in people with advanced cancer. *J Pain Sympt Manag*, **32**(4), 322–31.
3. Hopkinson JB (2007) How people with advanced cancer manage change in eating habits. *J Adv Nurs*, **59**(5), 454–62.
4. Hopkinson JB, Corner JL (2006) Helping patients with advanced cancer live with concerns about eating. *J Pain Sympt Manag*, **31**(4), 293–305.
5. Help the Aged (2008) What is age discrimination? Available at: http://www.helptheaged.org.uk/en-gb/Campaigns/Campaigns_old/FightingAgeism/WhatIsAgeDiscrimination/default.htm? (accessed 13 July 2008).
6. Victoria State Government (2008) Challenging ageist attitudes. Available at: http://www.health.vic.gov.au/agedcare/publications/wellforlife/wellforlife_hs32.pdf (accessed 13 July 2008).
7. Victor CR (2005) *The Social Context of Ageing: A Textbook of Gerontology*. London: Routledge.
8. Office for National Statistics (2008) *More Pensioners than Under-16s for the First Time Ever*. Newport: ONS.

9. United Nations (2007) *World Population Ageing.* New York: UN Publications.
10. Di Maio M, Perrone F (2003) Quality of life in elderly patients with cancer. *Health Qual Life Outcomes,* **1**, 44.
11. Edwards BK, Howe HL, Ries LAG, *et al.* (2002) Annual report to the nation on the status of cancer 1973–1999, featuring implications of age and ageing on U.S. cancer burden. *Cancer,* **94**(10), 2766–92.
12. Office for National Statistics (2006) *UK Population to Rise to 65m by 2016.* Newport: ONS.
13. Rosen R, Smith A, Harrison A (2006) *Future Trends and Challenges for Cancer Services in England: A Review of Literature and Policy.* London: King's Fund.
14. de Vries M, van Weert JC, Jansen J, Lemmons VE, Maas HA (2007) Step by step development of clinical care pathways for older cancer patients: necessary or desirable? *Eur J Cancer,* **43**(15), 2170–8.
15. Lichtman SM (2003) Guidelines for the treatment of elderly cancer patients. *Cancer Control,* **10**(6), 445–53.
16. Walker A (1999) Older people and health services: the challenge of empowerment. In: Purdey M, Banks D (eds), *Health and Exclusion.* London: Routledge.
17. Fentiman IS, Tirelli U, Monfardini S, *et al.* (1990) Cancer in the elderly: why so badly treated? *Lancet,* **335**(8696), 1020–2.
18. Fentiman IS (1996) Are the elderly receiving appropriate treatment for cancer? *Ann Oncol,* **7**, 657–8.
19. Rai S, Stotter A (2005) Management of elderly patients with breast cancer: the time for surgery. *Aust NZ J Surg,* **75**, 863–5.
20. Bernardi D, Errante D, Tirelli U, Salvagno L, Bianco A, Fentiman IS (2006) Insight into the treatment of cancer in older patients: developments in the last decade. *Cancer Treat Rev,* **32**, 277–88.
21. Roberts SB, Rosenberg I (2006) Nutrition and aging: changes in the regulation of energy metabolism with aging. *Physiol Rev,* **86**, 651–67.
22. Lazarus RS (1999) *Stress and Emotion: A New Synthesis,* p. 165. London: Free Association Press.
23. McClement SE (2005) Cancer anorexia–cachexia syndrome: psychological effect on the patient and family. *J Wound Ostomy Continence Nurs,* **32**(4), 264–68.
24. Hopkinson JB, Fenlon D, Nicholls P, *et al.* (2009) *Helping People Live with Advanced Cancer: An Exploratory Cluster Randomised Trial to Investigate the Effectiveness of the Macmillan Approach to Weight Loss and Eating Difficulties (MAWE).* London: Macmillan Cancer Support.
25. Hollway W, Jefferson T (2000) *Doing Qualitative Research Differently: Free Association, Narrative and Interview Method.* London: Sage.
26. Demark-Wahnefried W, Morey MC, *et al.* (2005) Results of Project LEAD (Leading the Way in Exercise and Diet)—a trial testing an intervention of telephone-counselling and mailed materials in improving physical functioning among older breast and prostate cancer survivors. *J Clin Oncol,* **23**(16S), 8138.
27. Snyder DC, Sloane R, Haines PS, *et al.* (2007) The Diet Quality Index—Revised: a tool to promote and evaluate dietary change among older cancer survivors enrolled in a home-based intervention trial. *J Am Diet Assoc,* **107**(9), 1519–29.
28. Extermann M, Hurria A (2007) Comprehensive geriatric assessment for older patients with cancer. *J Clin Oncol,* **25**(14), 1824–31.
29. Hurria A, Lichtman SM, Gardes J, *et al.* (2007) Identifying vulnerable older adults with cancer: integrating geriatric assessment into oncology practice. *J Am Geriatr Soc,* **55**, 1604–8.

Chapter 33

Nutrition and comorbidities

Marvin Omar Delgado Guay

Introduction

The intersection of ageing and cancer implies more than simply an increase in the incidence and prevalence of the disease. Cancer may present and respond to treatment differently in older patients. Older patients are also more likely than younger patients to present with concurrent comorbid conditions and/or functional disabilities.[1–4] The presence of comorbidities complicates the screening, diagnosis, treatment, and management of cancer in older adults.[5–8] Oncology patients aged >70 years average three diagnosed comorbid conditions in addition to their cancer.[9] Comorbidity is an important prognostic indicator. Cancer patients with higher levels of comorbidity have poorer survival, functional status, and quality of life than patients with no comorbid conditions.[1,3] In this chapter we discuss the potential influences of comorbidities and their treatment on metabolism and nutrition in cancer patients.

Comorbidities

The significance of comorbidities was described more than 30 years ago by Feinstein.[10] Comorbidity is defined as the presence of one or more health conditions among people diagnosed with an index disease, such as cancer. Comorbidity has been evaluated using different assessment tools.[1,11–13] The Charlson Index is the most commonly used scale in studies of cancer patients[1,14] and provides an overall score based on a composite of values weighted by level of severity and assigned for any of 19 selected conditions. There are other measures that have undergone formal scale development with accompanying tests of reliability and validity, such as the Kaplan–Feinstein Index,[15] and the Greenfield Index which assess the effects of coexisting conditions on the level and types of treatment for cancer patients.[16] Other measures include the Cumulative Illness Rating Scale (CIRS)[17] that is used increasingly in studies of comorbidity and cancer; the National Institute of Aging (NIA) and the National Cancer Institute (NCI)[18,19] include 27 major medical categories and illness severity; and the Adult Comorbidity Evaluate (ACE-27)[20] designed to assess comorbidity among cancer patients (an adaptation of the Kaplan–Feinstein Index). The independent, prognostic significance of new measures of comorbidity should be assessed, in conjunction with other measures, such as physical function, to enhance current measures of medical assessment.[21,22] It is also important to examine the independent effects of individual comorbid conditions on the duration and quality of life in specific forms of cancer. Older cancer patients with comorbid conditions are less likely than patients without comorbid conditions to receive invasive, definitive therapy.[23]

Comorbidities and advanced cancer

Cachexia affects more than 5 million people in the USA (Table 33.1).[24] A number of disparate disease states can develop cachexia, including congestive heart failure, chronic obstructive

Table 33.1 Patients with different comorbidities affected by cachexia in the USA

Disease	Patients with comorbidity	Patients with cachexia (%)
Heart failure	4 800 000	20
AIDS	900 000	10–35
COPD	16 000 000	20
Kidney failure	375 000	40
Rheumatoid arthritis	2 100 000	10
Cancer	1 368 000	35

AIDS, acquired immune deficiency syndrome; COPD, chronic obstructive pulmonary disease.

pulmonary disease, inflammatory bowel disease, rheumatoid arthritis, human immunodeficiency virus (HIV), tuberculosis, and malaria. Patients with these conditions may also develop cancer. Individuals who are cachectic because of a pre-existing condition such as chronic obstructive pulmonary disease (COPD) are more likely to experience progression to severe cachexia after their cancer diagnosis. The specific therapies for these individual comorbid conditions could help or hinder the management of cancer cachexia. For example, beta-blocker and angiotensin-converting enzyme (ACE) inhibitor therapy used for congestive heart failure patients might have a favourable effect on resting energy expenditure and muscle wasting. Other therapies such as corticosteroids for COPD may increase appetite but will also enhance the peripheral catabolic effects on muscle and promote insulin resistance.

Patients with cancer should also be evaluated for thyroid abnormalities (thyroid-stimulating hormone), hypoadrenalism (a.m. cortisol), vitamin B_{12} deficiencies, vitamin D deficiencies (25-hydroxy cholecalciferol) and hypogonadism (bioavailable testosterone). These abnormalities are easily treated with replacement therapy which may attenuate catabolism, improve symptoms, function and quality of life.

Congestive heart failure

Congestive heart failure (CHF) is a devastating major public health problem with poor prognosis.[25,26] The prognosis worsens once cardiac cachexia has been detected. Cachexia predicts a poor prognosis independently of the stage of the heart failure. Mortality at 18 months in CHF patients with cardiac cachexia was higher (50%) compared to CHF patients without cachexia 17%.[27] Patients with CHF who develop cachexia not only lose muscle mass but also total fat mass and bone mineral density.[28] Cachexia in CHF is not associated with structural cardiac changes, left ventricular ejection fraction, severity classes according to the New York Heart Association (NYHA), or with the exercise duration.[29] Cardiac cachexia has been defined as the non-oedematous weight loss of >6% observed over a period of >6 months.[30] Patients with CHF have an increased resting metabolic rate which can be up to 70% of their daily energy expenditure.[31] The metabolism of CHF patients shows a shift towards catabolism with most of the mechanisms implicated in the wasting process being activated early in the development of CHF. These mediators include catecholamines, cortisol, natriuretic peptides, proinflammatory cytokines, and heat shock proteins.[32] Activation of the renin–angiotensin–adosterone–system tends to follow the activation of proinflammatory cytokines in the course of CHF. Elevated levels of tumour necrosis factor (TNF)-α, interleukin (IL)-1 and IL-6 are described in patients with cardiac cachexia[33] and are associated with poor long and short prognosis.[34] TNF may worsen endothelial dysfunction,[35] reduce exercise endurance, downregulate albumin synthesis in the liver and promote satiety signals in the hypothalamus.[36,37]

Endocrine dysfunction also plays a role in the nutritional abnormalities of CHF patients. Levels of GH are elevated three-fold in cachectic patients with CHF compared to non-cachectic and healthy subjects. Cachectic CHF patients also have significantly higher levels of plasma ghrelin than non-cachectic patients, suggesting a state of 'ghrelin resistance'.[38] A preliminary trial of a ghrelin infusion in NYHA class III cachectic patients for 3 weeks increased food intake and produced a non-significant increase in body weight and lean body mass.[39] CHF patients who are insulin resistant have increased severity of disease and impairment in functional capacity of skeletal muscle.[40]

Patients with CHF may also develop decreased appetite and food intake related to changes in taste and smell, dietary advice on salt and calorie intake, social isolation, and derangements in bowel perfusion. Deficiencies in both macronutrients and micronutrients may affect patients with CHF.[2] Loop diuretics increase urinary excretion of micronutrients especially thiamine and selenium. Thiamine supplementation and other micronutrients (e.g. vitamins C, E, magnesium, selenium, zinc, coenzyme Q10)[41,42] might improve left ventricular ejection fraction.[43] Finally, Rozentryt *et al.*[44] reported that patients with cardiac cachexia might benefit from enteral support of 600 kcal daily in addition to their normal diet or placebo for 6 weeks. There were significant improvements in weight, 6 min walking distance and total fat mass.

Several other factors contribute to the progressive deterioration of nutritional status in patients with CHF. CHF patients develop changes in bowel perfusion and bowel oedema, because of blood shunted from arterioles to venules at low flow rates.[45] This can lead to fat malabsorption, protein loss, and translocation of bacteria and endotoxins through the intestine wall to the circulation.[46,47] These endotoxins in the circulation may precipitate the increment of proinflammatory cytokine production and perpetuate the cachexia syndrome.

Nutrition itself still seems to be a major factor in treatment strategies, because CHF patients are at risk of multiple deficiencies of micro- and macronutrients, and the supplementation of vitamins and branched-chain amino acids may be of benefit.[48] Serum levels of calcium, bone mineral content and bone mineral density are lower in cachectic CHF patients.[49]

Pharmacological therapies such as ACE inhibitors and beta-blockers have the potential to delay or prevent the onset of cardiac cachexia.[48] ACE inhibitors are implicated in the improvement of insulin resistance[50] and reduced weight loss in patients with CHF.[51] Experimentally, administration of an ACE inhibitor to tumour-bearing mice attenuated their weight loss compared with control animals.[52]

The use of beta-blockers may decrease resting energy expenditure,[53] inhibit catecholamine-induced lipolysis[54] and mediate an increase of skeletal muscle mass in animal models and other catabolic conditions.[55,56] Patients with CHF treated with carvedilol have significant increase in weight compared to placebo-treated patients.[57]

As cardiac cachexia represents a chronic inflammatory state; interventions towards anti-inflammatory strategies have been considered. The use of neutralizing antibodies such as etarnecept and infliximab showed a lack of efficacy in CHF patients. Statins have pleiotropic effects which may prove to be useful for cachexia, including the reduction of proinflammatory cytokines in some settings.

The cachectic cancer patient with a history of CHF might therefore benefit from continued use of medications such as beta-blockers, ACE inhbitors and statins. Beta-bockers are very effective in other catabolic states such as children with burns, and along with ACE inhibitors they have been effective in preliminary trials involving cancer patients and animal models.[58] Some investigational interventions such as ghrelin and ghrelin mimetics have also shown positive results in patients with left ventricular dysfunction.

Chronic kidney disease

More than 25% of patients receiving haemodialysis are malnourished.[59] Patients with advanced chronic kidney disease (CKD) are prone to wasting because of several factors, including the dialysis procedure, comorbid conditions, chronic inflammation and insulin resistance or deficiency.[60] Patients with cachexia related to CKD have increased energy expenditure, anorexia, hypoalbuminaemia, and loss of protein stores and sarcopenia.[61] Clinical wasting is an important risk factor for mortality in CKD and is reported to have a prevalence of 30–60%.[62] This maladaptive metabolic state often coexists with inflammation[63] and increased concentrations of circulating cytokines, such as TNFα, IL-1, and IL-6, which correlate with the degree of cachexia in individuals.[64] Anorexia is caused by several factors including gastroparesis, glucose absorption from the dialysate, medications, and zinc deficiency.[65] The poor appetite seen in haemodialysis patients also appears to be associated with lower branched-chain amino acid levels but not with higher free tryptophan levels and higher free tryptophan:large neutral amino acids ratios.[66] Higher levels of ghrelin and poor appetite are observed in haemodialysis patients. Preliminary studies show that the subcutaneous administration of synthetic ghrelin stimulates food intake among dialysis patients over the intermediate term.[67]

Interventions that may be effective for this complex entity include a combination of intradialytic nutritional supplementation, anticytokine therapy, erythropoietin supplementation, and nutritional support.[68]

Diabetes mellitus

Diabetes, a serious and economically devastating illness that is reaching epidemic proportions in both industrialized and developing countries, poses a major threat to public health in the twenty-first century. Of the more than 200 000 Americans with diabetes who succumb annually to diabetes-related complications, most die of coronary heart disease or other cardiovascular disease conditions.[69] The causes of diabetes in patients with advanced disease are multifactorial[70] with an increased incidence of diabetes in older people, patients taking diabetogenic medications such as corticosteroids, obese patients, and in those with metabolic changes secondary to cancer. Patients diagnosed with cancer who have pre-existing diabetes are at increased risk for long term all-cause mortality compared to those without diabetes.[71] Childhood survivors of cancer are at increased risk of developing the metabolic syndrome[72] and diabetes is more common in survivors than the general population.[73]

Box 33.1 General management of patients with advanced cancer with diabetes with a prognosis of weeks to months

- Relax all dietary restrictions.
- Consider referral to specialist palliative care and/or the diabetes team (if available).
- Reduce blood glucose monitoring to an acceptable minimum.
- Reduce dose of oral hypoglycaemic as appetite reduces.
- Early identification and treatment of oral candida.
- Avoid use of metformin due to unpleasant side-effects.
- Reduce necessity of steroids and investigate about the symptoms of hyperglycaemia.
- Counsel patient and family members about these measures. Document your counselling.

It is important to recognize that medications commonly used in cancer, such as corticosteroids and some diuretics, are known to precipitate hyperglycaemia. Control of blood glucose levels via diet and glucose-lowering medicines (insulin and/or oral agents) and careful monitoring are essential components of glycaemic control.[70] Unfortunately the glycaemic management in the context of advanced cancer may vary and there are no specific evidence-based clinical guidelines for glycaemic control.[74] When individuals with diabetes have advanced cancer or another chronic illness, they often become anorectic[75,76] and are at increased risk of hypoglycaemic episodes. In these individuals it is important and appropriate to shift the goal of therapy from tight control of blood glucose to maintain comfort and enhance quality of life (Figure 33.1).

Patients with long term diabetes can present with a variety of complications including muscle atrophy and cachexia. An animal model for spontaneous diabetes is associated with profound skeletal muscle atrophy and a significant loss of skeletal muscle protein.[77]

Type 1 diabetes mellitus	*Type 2 diabetes mellitus*
With stable nutritional status: Maintain current therapy. Monitor BG every 3rd day: 2×/day before meals and as needed based on symptoms.	**With stable nutritional status:** Maintain current therapy. Monitor BG weekly fasting initially, taper to 1–2×/month unless symptomatic.
With weight loss/anorexia: Reduce insulin dose based on BG values. Consider change to intermediate-acting from long acting. Monitor BG twice daily. Once stable resume monitoring every 3rd day.	**With weight loss/anorexia:** Reduce oral medication dose by 50%. Monitor BG weekly fasting 3×. then 1–2× month unless symptomatic.
With nausea and vomiting: Change to short-acting insulin. Once stable, shift to intermediate-acting. Monitor BG twice daily. Once stable resume monitoring every 3rd day.	**With nausea and vomiting:** Discontinue oral agents while symptomatic. Monitor BG fasting every other day. Once stable resume weekly 3× then 1–2×/month.
BG > 250 mg/dl: Change to short-acting insulin. Once stable, shift to intermediate-acting. Monitor BG twice daily. Once stable resume monitoring every 3rd day.	**BG > 250 mg/dl:** Short acting insulin 2–4× daily. Shift to intermediate acting when stable. Monitor BG 2–4× daily before scheduled insulin dose. Taper to daily fasting when stable, then 2× week.
Actively dying (last few days to last week of life): Consider discontinue drug therapy. Discontinue monitoring if insulin is stopped.	**Actively dying (last few days to last week of life):** Discontinue oral agents. Discontinue BG monitoring.

Fig. 33.1 Management of patients with diabetes mellitus type 1 and type 2 with advanced illnesses and at the end of life. BG, blood glucose.

Several factors that play a causal role in the development of diabetes also play a causal role in the onset of cachexia. The use of insulin in patients with diabetes can inhibit proteolysis by blocking ubiquitin-mediated proteasomal activity.[78] Interestingly, although treatment with insulin stimulates weight gain in cachectic cancer patients, lean tissue mass is not affected.[79] This suggests that pathways leading to cachexia in different primary disease states do not entirely overlap.

Diabetic neuropathic cachexia is a rare complication in patients with diabetes and the most uncommon form of diabetic neuropathy.[80,81] It is characterized by a bilateral, painful neuropathy usually involving the anterior thighs, with rapid weight loss. Patients affected by this entity are usually middle-aged type 2 diabetics on oral agents, and most patients recover spontaneously, although residual deficits may persist. No specific therapy has been found useful, although proper nutrition is very important to avoid further deterioration.

Diabetes appears to share some features of cancer cachexia including insulin resistance, elevated inflammatory markers, autonomic nervous system and skeletal muscle dysfunction. Some of the therapies for diabetes such as insulin and thioglitazones have been used in trials for cancer cachexia and in animal models. On the other hand, therapies for appetite stimulation in diabetics with advanced cancer such as corticosteroids or megestrol could raise glucose levels, while anabolic agents such as testosterone may be helpful by increasing insulin sensitivity. Finally, the cancer patient's position in the disease trajectory might determine the usefulness of a particular intervention (e.g. tight glucose control with insulin) or a medication may be continued because it (e.g.metformin) demonstrates antitumour activity.[82]

Nutritional changes in patients with chronic obstructive pulmonary disease

The majority of patients diagnosed with lung cancer also have COPD. The two conditions may share inflammatory mechanisms and elevated serum proinflammatory cytokines.[83] Patients with COPD have systemic manifestations (possibly related to systemic inflammatory mediators) that are associated with impaired functional capacity, worsening dyspnoea, reduced health-related quality of life, and increased mortality.[84] COPD is often accompanied by loss of fat-free mass and by skeletal muscle weakness[85] with alterations in muscle function and structure. The skeletal muscle atrophy seen in COPD patients is specific to muscle fibre type IIA/IIx[86] and is a significant determinant of exercise capacity in patients with COPD independent of disease severity. Patients with severe COPD who experience muscle wasting develop increased risk for hospital readmission after exacerbation and increased need for mechanical support.[87]

Muscle inactivity, especially at the time of exacerbation, is an important mechanism of peripheral muscle dysfunction in patients with COPD.[88,89] Physical inactivity itself favours systemic inflammation in patients with COPD, as a consequence of a reduced function of the transcription factor peroxisome proliferator-activated-γ coactivator.[90] Since the progression of skeletal muscle dysfunction in COPD is strongly associated with enhanced oxidative stress and reactive oxygen species (ROS), COPD patients with cancer might be especially responsive to an intervention that includes immune modulation and exercise (please refer to Chapters 11 and 29 respectively).[91]

Patients with COPD have a high prevalence of osteoporosis (even in milder stages of the disease)[92] and their bone mineral density correlates with fat-free mass. Vertebral compression fractures are relatively common among these patients.[93] The mechanism proposed for these changes in bone structure are secondary to activation of osteoclasts by systemic inflammatory cytokines, including IL-6, IL-1, and TNFα.[94]

Systemic inflammatory changes in COPD also predispose these patients to insulin resistance by blocking signalling through the insulin receptor and increasing their risk of metabolic syndrome and type 2 diabetes. The use of corticosteroids for COPD also increases the risk for developing diabetes. Agents used for other diseases may prove to be useful for muscle wasting in COPD patients. The use of peroxisome proliferator-activated receptor agonists, such as fibrates (clofibrate and fenofibrate) and thiazolidinediones, may have therapeutic potential in treating systemic features of COPD, including cachexia and systemic inflammation. Preliminary results of ghrelin administration in cachectic patients with COPD showed improved body composition and functional capacity.[95] Further research is needed to determine the role of these agents in cachexia and COPD and other chronic diseases.

References

1. Satariano WA, Silliman RA (2003) Comorbidity: implications for research and practice in geriatric oncology. *Crit Rev Oncol Hematol*, **48**, 239–48.
2. Witte KKA, Clark AL (2002) Nutritional abnormalities contributing to cachexia in chronic illness. *Int J Cardiol*, **85**, 23–31.
3. Yancik R, Havlik RJ, Wesley MN, *et al.* (1996) Cancer and comorbidity in older patients: a descriptive profile. *Ann Epidemiol*, **6**, 399–412.
4. Kennedy BJ (2000) Aging and cancer. *Oncology*, **14**, 1731–33.
5. Piccirillo JF, Feinstein AR (1996) Clinical symptoms and comorbidity: significance for the prognostic classification of cancer. *Cancer*, **77**, 834–42.
6. Satariano WA (2000) Comorbidities and cancer. In: Hunter CP, Johnson KA, Muss HB, (eds), *Cancer in the Elderly*, pp. 477–99. New York: Marcel Dekker.
7. Ford ME, Havstad SL, Fields ME, *et al.* (2008) Effects of baseline comorbidities on cancer screening trial adherence among older African American men. *Cancer Epidemiol Prev*, **17**(5), 1234–39.
8. Zeber JE, Copeland LA, Hosek BJ, *et al.* (2008) Cancer rates, medical comorbidities, and treatment modalities in the oldest patients. *Crit Rev Oncol/Hematol*, **67**(3), 237–42.
9. Extermann M, Overcash J, Lyman GH, Parr J, Balducci L (1998) Comorbidity and functional status are independent in older cancer patients. *J Clin Oncol*, **16**, 1582–87.
10. Feinstein AR (1970) The pre-therapeutic classification of co-morbidity in chronic disease. *J Chron Dis*, **23**, 455–69.
11. Mandelblatt JS, Bierman AS, Gold K, *et al.* (2001) Constructs of burden of illness in older patients with breast cancer: a comparison of measurement methods. *Health Serv Res*, **36**, 1085–107.
12. Klabunde CN, Warren J, Legler JM (2002) Assessing comorbidity using claims data: an overview. *Med Care*, **40**(8 Suppl), IV-26–IV-35.
13. Gijsen R Hoeymans N, Schellevis FG, *et al.* (2001) Causes and consequences of comorbidity: a review. *J Clin Epidemiol*, **54**, 661–74.
14. Charlson ME, Pompei P, Alex KL, MacKenzie CR (1987) A new method of classifying prognostic comorbidity in longitudinal studies: development and validation. *J Chron Dis*, **40**, 373–83.
15. Kaplan MH, Feinstein AR (1974) The importance o classifying initial co-morbidity in evaluating the outcome of diabetes mellitus. *J Chron Dis*, **27**, 387–404.
16. Greenfield S, Blanco DM, Elashoff RM, Ganz PA (1987) Patterns of care related to age of breast cancer patient. *J Am Med Assoc*, **257**, 2766–70.
17. Extermann M (2000) Measuring comorbidity in older cancer patients. *Eur J Cancer*, **36**, 453–71.
18. Yancik R, Wesley MN, Ries LA, *et al.* (1998) Comorbidity and age as predictors of risk for early mortality of male and female colon carcinoma patients: a population-based study. *Cancer*, **82**, 2123–34.
19. Yancik R, Wesley MN, Ries LA, *et al.* (2001) Effect of age and comorbidity in postmenopausal breast cancer patients aged 55 years and older. *J Am Med Assoc*, **285**, 885–92.
20. Piccirillo JF, Creech C, Zequeira R, Anderson S, Johnson AS (1999) Inclusion of comorbidity into oncology data registries. *J Reg Man*, **26**, 66–70.

21. Repetto L, Ratino L, Audisio RA, *et al.* (2002) Comprehensive geriatric assessment adds information to Eastern Cooperative Oncology Group performance status in elderly cancer patients: an Italian Group for Geriatric Oncology Study. *J Clin Oncol*, **20**, 494–502.
22. Repetto L, Balducci L (2002) A case for geriatric oncology. *Lancet Oncol*, **3**, 289–97.
23. Newchaffer CJ, Penberthy L, Desch CD, Retchin SM, Whittemore M (1996) The effect of age and comorbidity in the treatment of elderly women with nonmetastatic breast cancer. *Arch Intern Med*, **156**, 85–90.
24. Morley JE, David RT, Wilson MMG (2006) Cachexia: pathophysiology and clinical relevance. *Am J Clin Nutr*, **83**, 735–43.
25. Von Haehling S, Doehner W, Anker SD (2007) Nutrition, metabolism, and the complex pathophysiology of cachexia in chronic heart failure. *Cardiovasc Res*, **73**, 298–309.
26. Stewart S, MacIntyre K, Hole DJ, Capewell S, McMurray JJ (2001) More 'malignant' than cancer? Five year survival following a first admission for heart failure. *Eur J Heart Fail*, **3**, 315–22.
27. Anker SD, Ponikowski P, Varney S, *et al.* (1997) Wasting as independent risk factor for mortality in chronic heart failure. *Lancet*, **349**, 1050–53.
28. Anker SD, Sharma R (2002) The syndrome of cardiac cachexia. *Int J Cardiol*, **85**, 51–66.
29. Florea VG, Moon J, Pennell DJ, *et al.* (2004) Wasting of the left ventricle in patients with cardiac cachexia: a cardiovascular magnetic resonance study. *Int J Cardiol* **97**, 15–20.
30. Anker SD, Negassa A, Coats AJ, *et al.* (2003) Prognostic importance of weight loss in chronic heart failure and the effect of the treatment with angiotensin-converting enzyme inhibitors: an observational study. *Lancet*, **3**, 1077–83.
31. Obiesan T, Tooth MJ, Kendall D (1996) Energy expenditure and symptom severity in men with heart failure. *Am J Cardiol*, **77**, 1250–52.
32. Genth-Zotz S, Bolger AP, Kalra PR, *et al.* (2004) Heat shock protein 70 in patients with chronic heart failure: relation to disease severity and survival. *Int J Cardiol*, **96**, 397–401.
33. Levine B, Kalman J, Majer L, Fillit HM, Packer M (1990) Elevated circulating levels of tumor necrosis factor in severe chronic heart failure. *N Engl J Med*, **323**, 236–41.
34. Von Haehling S, Genth-Zotz S, Anker SD, Volk HD (2002) Cachexia: a therapeutic approach beyond cytokine antagonism. *Int J Cardiol*, **85**, 173–83.
35. Rauchhaus M, Doehner W, Francis DP, *et al.* (2000) Plasma cytokine parameters and mortality in patients with chronic heart failure. *Circulation*, **92**, 1479–86.
36. Langhans W, Hrupka B (1999) Interleukins and tumor necrosis factor as inhibitors of food intake. *Neuropeptides*, **33**, 414–24.
37. Chojkier M (2005) Inhibition of albumin synthesis in chronic diseases: molecular mechanisms. *J Clin Gastroenterol*, **39**(Suppl 2), S143–46.
38. Nagaya N, Uematsu M, Kojima M, *et al.* (2001) Elevated circulating level of ghrelin in cachexia associated with chronic heart failure: relationships between ghrelin and anabolic/catabolic factors. *Circulation*, **104**, 2034–8.
39. Nagaya N, Moriya J, Yasumura Y, *et al.* (2004) Effects of ghrelin administration of left ventricular function, exercise capacity, and muscle wasting in patients with chronic heart failure. *Circulation*, **110**, 3674–9.
40. Swan JW, Anker SD, Walton C, *et al.* (1997) Insulin resistance in chronic heart failure: relation to severity and etiology of heart failure. *J Am Coll Cardiol*, **30**, 527–32.
41. Witte KK, Clark AL, Cleland JG (2001) Chronic heart failure and micronutrients. *J Am Coll Cardiol*, **37**, 1765–74.
42. Shimon I, Almog S, Vered Z, *et al.* (1995) Improved left ventricular function after thiamine supplementation in patients with congestive heart failure receiving long term furosemide therapy. *Am J Med*, **98**, 485–90.
43. Witte KK, Nikitin NP, Parker AC, *et al.* (2005) The effect of micronutrient supplementation on quality-of-life and left ventricular function in elderly patients with chronic heart failure. *Eur Heart J*, **26**, 2238–44.

44. Rozentryt P, Michalak A, Nowak JU, *et al.* (2005) The effects of enteral supplementation in patients with cardiac cachexia—a prospective, randomized, double-blind placebo controlled trial. 3rd Cachexia Conference, Rome, Italy. Abstract Book, p. 82.
45. King D, Smith ML, Lye M (1996) Gastro-intestinal protein loss in elderly patients with cardiac cachexia. *Age Ageing* **25**, 221–3.
46. King D, Smith ML, Chapman TJ, *et al.* (1996) Fat malabsorption in elderly patients with cardiac cachexia. *Age Ageing* **25**, 144–9.
47. Anker SD, Egerer KR, Volk HD, *et al.* (1997) Elevated soluble CD14 receptors and altered cytokines in chronic heart failure. *Am J Cardiol* **79**, 1426–30.
48. Ventadour S, Attaix D (2006) Mechanisms of skeletal muscle atrophy. *Curr Opin Rheumatol*, **18**, 631–5.
49. Anker SD, Clark AL, Teixeira MM, *et al.* (1999) Loss of bone mineral in patients with cachexia due to chronic heart failure. *Am J Cardiol*, **83**, 612–15.
50. Yusuf S, Gerstein H, Hoogwerf B, *et al.* for the HOPE Study Investigators (2001) Ramipril and the development of diabetes. *J Am Med Assoc*, **286**, 1882–5.
51. Anker SD, Negassa A, Coats AJ, *et al.* (2003) Prognostic importance of weight loss in chronic heart failure and the effect of treatment with Angiotensin-converting-enzyme inhibitors: an observational study. *Lancet*, **361**, 1077–83.
52. Sanders PM, Russel ST, Tisdale MJ (2005) Angiotensin II directly induces muscle protein catabolism through the ubiquitin–proteosome protelytic pathway and may play a role in cancer cachexia. *Br J Cancer*, **93**, 425–34.
53. Lamont LS, Brown T, Riebe D, Caldwell M (2000) The major components of human energy balance during chronic beta-adrenergic blockade. *J Cardiopulm Rehabil*, **20**, 247–50.
54. Langin D (2006) Adipose tissue lipolysis as a metabolic pathway to define pharmacological strategies against obesity and the metabolic syndrome. *Pharmacol Res*, **53**, 482–91.
55. Herndon DN, Hart DW, Wolf SE, *et al.* (2001) Reversal of catabolism by beta-blockade after severe burns. *N Engl J Med*, **345**, 1223–9.
56. von Haehling S, Lainscak M, Springer J, Anker SD (2009) Cardiac cachexia: a systematic overview. *Pharmacol Ther*, **121**(3), 227–52.
57. Anker SD, Coats AJ, Roecker EB, *et al.* (2002) Does carvedilol prevent and reverse cardiac cachexia in patients with severe heart failure? Results of the COPERNICUS study. *Eur Heart J*, **23**, 394 (abstract).
58. Nagaya N, Kojima M, Kangawa K (2006) Ghrelin, a novel growth hormone-releasing peptide, in the treatment of cardiopulmonary-associated cachexia. *Intern Med*, **45**(3), 127–34.
59. Garg AX, Blake PG, Clark WF, *et al.* (2001) Association between renal insufficiency and malnutrition in older adults: results from the NHAMES III. *Kidney Int*, **60**, 1867–74.
60. Alp Ikizler T (2007) Protein and energy intake in advanced chronic kidney disease how much is too much? *Semin Dialysis*, **20**, 5–11.
61. Raj DSC, Sun Y, Tzamaloukas AH (2008) Hypercatabolism in dialysis patients. *Curr Opin Nephrol Hypertens*, **17**, 589–94.
62. Mak RH, Cheung W, Cone RD, Mark DL (2006) Mechanisms of disease: cytokine and adipokine signaling in uremic cachexia. *Nat Clin Pract Nephrol*, **2**, 527–34.
63. Mak RH, Cheung W (2006) Energy homeostasis and cachexia in chronic kidney disease. *Pediatr Nephrol*, **21**, 1807–14.
64. Mak RH, Cheung W (2007) Cachexia in chronic kidney disease: role of inflammation and neuropeptide signaling. *Curr Opin Nephrol Hypertens*, **16**, 27–31.
65. De Schoenmakere G, Vanholder R, Rottey S, *et al.* (2001) Relationship between gastric emptying and clinical and biochemical factors in chronic hemodialysis patients. *Am J Kidney Dis*, **16**, 1850–5.
66. Bossola M, Scribano D, Colacicco L, *et al.* (2009) Anorexia and plasma levels of free tryptophan, branched chain amino acids, and ghrelin in hemodialysis patients. *J Renal Nutrition*, **19**, 248–55.

67. Ashby DR, Ford HE, Wynne KJ, *et al.* (2009) Sustained appetite improvement in malnourished dialysis patients by daily ghrelin treatment. *Kidney Int*, **76**(2), 199–206.
68. Kalantar-Zadeh K, Stenvinkel P, Bross R, *et al.* (2005) Kidney insufficiency and nutrient-based modulation of inflammation. *Curr Opin Clin Nutr Metab Care*, **8**, 388–96.
69. Winer N, Sowers JR (2004) Epidemiology of diabetes. *J Clin Pharmacol*, **44**, 397–405.
70. Quinn K, Hudson P, Dunning T (2006) Diabetes management in patients receiving palliative care. *J Pain Sympt Manag*, **32**, 275–86.
71. Barone BB, Yeh HC, Snyder CF, *et al.* (2008) Long-term all-cause mortality in cancer patients with preexisting diabetes mellitus: a systematic review and meta-analysis. *J Am Med Assoc*, **300**(23), 2754–64.
72. Talvensaari KK, Lanning M, Tapanainen P, *et al.* (1996) Long-term survivors of childhood cancer have an increased risk of manifesting the metabolic syndrome. *J Clin Endocrinol Metab*, **81**, 3051–5.
73. Stava CJ, Beck ML, Feng L, Lopez A, Busaidy N, Vassilopoulou-Sellin R (2007) The frequency of DM was higher among survivors than in the general U.S. population. *J Cancer Surviv*, **1**(2), 108–15.
74. Poulson J (1997) The management of diabetes in patients with advanced cancer. *J Pain Sympt Manag*, **13**(6), 339–46.
75. Tice MA (2006) Diabetes management at the end of life. *Home Healthcare Nurse*, **24**, 290–3.
76. McCoubrie R, Jeffrey D, Paton C, Dawes L (2005) Managing diabetes mellitus in patients with advanced cancer: a case note audit and guidelines. *Eur J Cancer Care*, **14**, 244–8.
77. Zhao Ch, Wang Z, Robertson MW, Davies JD (2008) Cachexia in the non-obese diabetic mouse is associated with CD4+ T cell lymphopenia. *Immunology*, **125**, 48–58.
78. Bennett RG, Hamel FG, Duckworth WC (2000) Insulin inhibits the ubiquitin-dependent degrading activity of the 26S proteasome. *Endocrinology*, **141**, 2508–17.
79. Lundholm K, Korner U, Gunnebo L, *et al.* (2007) Insulin treatment in cancer cachexia: effects on survival, metabolism, and physical function. *Clin Cancer Res*, **13**, 2699–706.
80. Neal, JM (2009) Diabetic neuropathic cachexia: a rare manifestation of diabetic neuropathy. *Southern Med J*, **102**, 327–9.
81. Yuen, KCJ, Day JL, Flannagan DW, Rayman G (2001) Diabetic neuropathic cachexia and acute bilateral cataract formation following rapid glycaemic control in a newly diagnosed type 1 diabetic patient. *Diabetic Med*, **18**, 854–7.
82. Jiralerspong S, Palla SL, Giordano SH, *et al.* (2009) Metformin and pathologic complete responses to neoadjuvant chemotherapy in diabetic patients with breast cancer. *J Clin Oncol*, **27**, 3297–302.
83. Barnes PJ, Celli BR (2009) Systemic manifestations and comorbidities of COPD. *Eur Respir J*, **33**, 1165–85.
84. Agusti A, Soriano JB (2008) COPD as a systemic disease. *Chron Obstruct Pulmon Dis*, **5**, 133–8.
85. Gosker HR, Kubar B, Schaart G, *et al.* (2003) Myopathological features in skeletal muscle of patients with chronic obstructive pulmonary disease. *Eur Respir J*, **22**, 280–5.
86. Swallow EB, Reyes D, Hopkinson NS, *et al.* (2007) Quadriceps strength predicts mortality in patients with moderate to severe chronic obstructive pulmonary disease. *Thorax*, **62**, 115–20.
87. Marquis K, Debigare R, Lacasse Y, *et al.* (2002) Midthigh muscle cross-sectional area is a better predictor of mortality than body mass index in patients with chronic obstructive pulmonary disease. *Am J Respir Crit Care Med*, **166**, 809–13.
88. Man WD, Soliman MG, Nikeletou D, *et al.* (2003) Non-volitional assessment of skeletal muscle strength in patients with chronic obstructive pulmonary disease. *Thorax*, **58**, 665–9.
89. Agusti A, Morla M, Sauleda J, Miralles C, *et al.* (2002) Skeletal muscle apoptosis and weight loss in chronic obstructive pulmonary disease. *Am J Respir Crit Med*, **166**, 485–9.
90. Rememls AH, Gosker HR, Schrauwen P, Langen RC, Schols AM (2008) Peroxisome proliferator-activated receptors: a therapeutic target in COPD? *Eur Respir J*, **31**, 502–8.

91. Barreiro E, de la Puente B, Minguella J, *et al.* (2005) Oxidative stress and respiratory muscle dysfunction in severe chronic obstructive pulmonary disease. *Am J Respir Crit Care Med*, **171**, 1116–24.
92. Jorgensen NR, Schwarz P (2008) Osteoporosis in chronic obstructive pulmonary disease patients. *Curr Opin Pulm Med*, **14**, 122–7.
93. Carter JD, Patel S, Sultan FL, *et al.* (2008) The recognition and treatment of vertebral fractures in males with chronic obstructive pulmonary disease. *Resp Med*, **102**, 1165–72.
94. Bolton CE, Ionescu AA, Shiels KM, *et al.* (2004) Associated loss of fat-free mass and bone mineral density in chronic obstructive pulmonary disease. *Am J Respir Crit Care Med*, **170**, 1286–93.
95. Nagaya N, Itoh T, Murakami S, *et al.* (2005) Treatment of cachexia with ghrelin in patients with COPD. *Chest*, **128**(3), 1187–93.

Chapter 34

Patients in the developing world

Richard Harding and Liz Gwyther

Introduction

Resource-poor countries can be found across Sub-Saharan Africa, Asia, Latin America, and the former Eastern/Central European states. Two related factors influence the context of providing nutritional care to the cancer patient in a developing country setting. First, the epidemiology of malignant disease. Cancer care has been overlooked in poorer countries, where generalized poverty, human immunodeficiency virus (HIV)/acquired immune deficiency sydrome (AIDS), maternal health and tuberculosis have attracted the majority of research and donor interest. However, cancer is now recognized as a public health problem in Africa, and projections indicate rising incidence. Second, the resources available at the patient/family level, and at the state health system level, are limited. Therefore, the potential and options for nutritional assessment and care may be relatively few in comparison with well-resourced health care systems and higher household incomes.

The 'best practice' and evidence-based clinical guidance presented in this volume are likely to be based on research data generated in resource-rich settings. This is a result of the fact that research activity in resource-poor settings has been described as 'moribund',[1] and is a contributory factor to health inequalities. Guidance and policy must advocate assessment and intervention strategies that are feasible, accessible and appropriate as well as effective in these settings. Therefore, when proposing nutritional care in resource-poor countries we must consider where most of the research evidence has been generated, how relevant and applicable the evidence is, what is possible in poorer settings, patient preferences and cultural meanings and choices in relation to food and nutrition, the prevalent malignancies, and differing patient needs. Recommendations and protocols can be adapted to these settings to ensure that patient needs are met in an effective, feasible and appropriate way.

In this chapter we present an overview of the evidence of the epidemiological, economic and health systems contexts, and clinical examples of current practice in the assessment and management of nutritional need in cancer patients. We present examples from African settings where practice has evolved to provide multidisciplinary cancer palliative care that is responsive and appropriate to the local situation.

Health care provision and uptake in resource-poor countries

In countries where families already live in poverty, poor health can push them from poverty to destitution. If a head of household is incapacitated then the extended family will also suffer (HIV-related mortality has often led grandparents, aunts and uncles to take on additional parenting roles). In resource-rich countries, housing, money, heating, and food may be provided under the remit of the welfare state. Where such a backdrop of support does not exist, then the responsibility of activities such as income generation and basic nutrition may become the responsibility of the health care provider. Indeed, it is common in Africa for services either to provide, or to link closely with agencies that do provide, sewing groups for women affected by HIV to generate income, gardens to produce food, micro-loans, and food parcels.

Patient contact with health care providers is sometimes rare due to socio-economic factors, lack of health care expectations, and distance to facilities. In addition, when considering who might be the professional agency to most feasibly offer nutritional advice and support, it is important to consider the preferred, or actual, source of advice and care in a particular setting. For example, traditional healers are often the first contact of choice, and there are numerous examples of 'western'-style providers (e.g. medical/nursing clinics) working closely with traditional healers to educate them in both direct provision of advice and care and how/when to refer patients to clinics. Such providers who are 'embedded' in communities have cultural acceptance and influence that is reflected in traditionally held belief and practice. These health care providers have credibility among the community, and so endorsement by traditional healers of 'western' nursing and medicine offer feasible and acceptable routes to care for patients and families.

Cultural dimensions of care are essential in considering clinical guidance for nutrition in the cancer patient. For example, it is essential to understand local belief regarding food and its impact on the body and health, local sources of credible advice in care, food preferences and availability, who within the family grouping may have a role in preparing nutrition for the patient, beliefs on the origin of diseases and whether nutrition can play a role in its management, and economic access to different nutritional sources.

Epidemiology of cancer in resource-poor countries

Across Africa, cancer rates are expected to increase by 400% over the next 50 years.[2] It has been estimated by the World Health Organization (WHO) that there are more than 0.5 million annual cancer deaths in Africa[3] and that by 2020, 70% of new cancer cases will be in the developing world.[4] The African continent is, however, characterized by resource and infrastructure challenges that render governments least able to address the disease burden, where survival rates are consequently significantly lower than those in developed countries, and where patients' expectations for disease-modifying oncological treatment are low.[5,6]

Indeed, the imperative to address the challenge posed by cancer resulted in the 'London Declaration on Cancer Control in Africa', calling upon research institutions, international organizations, the pharmaceutical industry, national governments and civil society in developed and developing countries to unite to deliver comprehensive cancer care to the continent.[7,8]

A thorough overview of cancer in Sub-Saharan Africa[9,10] has raised the hitherto lack of attention to malignant disease in Africa. The reviewers identify that the lifetime risk of a female dying of cancer is double that of developed countries. They also highlight the fact that cancer trends in Africa are generally unknown, although there are data that report, for example, the comparatively high incidence of liver cancer in Africa, and the incidence of Kaposi Sarcoma secondary to HIV infection.

Cancer is a common presentation of advanced AIDS, particularly in more advanced disease progression. Non-Hodgkin lymphoma and cervical cancer are often seen in HIV clinics. Although the advent of antiretroviral therapy (ART) has brought enormous improvements in HIV morbidity and mortality, it is still a relatively new therapeutic intervention, and as time since the introduction of ART increases, and the chronic disease phase extends correspondingly, evidence suggests that both malignant and cerebrovascular disease are emerging as causes of death in patients who have accessed ART.

Status of research

In developed countries, clinicians, researchers and policy-makers strive to ensure that patients receive evidence-based health care interventions. There is a strong moral imperative to conduct research in poorer countries, and patients in resource-poorer settings deserve no less than effective care. Indeed, it could be argued that there is a stronger need for research and audit in these settings to ensure best allocation of scarce resources.[11] However, a systematic review of the scientific and 'grey' literature on palliative care in Sub-Saharan Africa, taking a broad approach to include both descriptive and outcome data, found very little evidence despite innovative examples of palliative care delivery by skilled, trained practitioners.[12]

Several key barriers to the generation of robust data on advanced cancer patients in developing settings have been identified.[13] First, there is the lack of well-developed, validated outcome tools for this population, although this is now being remedied with the African Palliative Care Association Palliative Outcome Scale (POS) that has been developed by a multiprofessional clinical and academic group and tested in eight countries using a full protocol to test validity and reliability. The POS addresses the key areas of concern in advanced care, and has been revalidated in a number of settings around the world. It has sound psychometric properties, is brief (10 items), and has been used successfully around the world (Europe, Latin America, USA, Australia) in research and improving clinical practice through audit methods.

The lack of attention to paediatric advanced disease research globally has particular resonance for Africa, where the rates of paediatric mortality from progressive disease are much higher than in those in rich countries where research often originates.

The generation of research evidence in resource-poor settings must be appropriate to local need, culturally appropriate and relevant, use tools validated in local populations, and be generated locally in partnership with local stakeholders. Consultation with local stakeholders has, for example, informed identification of which areas of research are needed in advanced disease[14] and to ensure that tools reflect local need and opinion.[15] We have much further to go to ensure that an evidence base relevant to resource-poor settings is achieved,[16] and to ensure that allocation of resources to research activity is seen as an essential step in improving outcomes for patients and families in settings where resources are scarce.[17]

Cancer and nutrition in the developing world

Consideration of nutrition and cancer in the developing world is complicated by the impact of poverty on health. In a recent study from Malawi[18] it was found that more than half the children with cancer are severely malnourished at admission to care.

A recent UNICEF[19] report (Table 34.1) highlights many challenges for health care of mothers and children. It identifies a number of key factors contributing to maternal and child mortality. First on the list are 'poorly resourced, unresponsive culturally inappropriate health and nutrition services', and second on the list is 'food insecurity'.

Table 34.1 Key statistics for Sub-Saharan Africa[19]

Gross national income per capita for 2006	US$851
% population living on <US$1/day	35%
Life expectancy	
1970	48 years
1990	45 years
2006	40 years
% aged <5 years underweight	28%
Mortality rate for children <5 years	111/1000 live births

Health care is provided against a background of poverty and substandard living conditions, so that ensuring a clean water source and safe disposal of excreta are essential interventions for the improvement of general health care.

An Essential Nutrition Action Program in Ethiopia, Malawi and Sudan providing therapeutic or nutrition-dense foods in the community measured an 80% recovery rate from severe acute malnutrition and a reduction in mortality rate to 4% at costs of between US$12 and $132 per year of life gained.[19]

Causative and preventive nutrition

It is estimated that development of up to 50% of all cancers may be diet-related.[20] Identifying diet–cancer links is an important focus for campaigns to prevent cancer through educating communities. In South Africa, lifestyle risk factors for developing cancers include both those found in the western world and those of developing countries. These risk factors include: high body mass, low intake of fruit and vegetables, physical inactivity, unsafe sex, tobacco and alcohol use, and smoke from solid fuel fires.[21]

There has been an increase in oesophageal cancer especially in the Eastern Cape Province of South Africa linked to nutritional factors, particularly consumption of maize containing *Fusarium* ssp. which produce mycotoxins implicated in the development of oesophageal cancer. Oesophageal cancer is the second leading cancer in African males and the third leading cancer in African females in South Africa. There is also an increased risk of developing oesophageal cancer with tobacco smoking. Maize is a dietary staple in Africa but has low levels of niacin, riboflavin, vitamin C and other micronutrients. A diet of maize without additional fruit and vegetables further increases the risk of developing cancer.

Liver cancer also has links to dietary factors as well as to hepatitis B infection. Additional risk factors include alcohol consumption, and aflatoxin produced by *Aspergillus* spp. found in ground nuts and maize.

The high incidence of stomach cancer in the developing world is associated with the consumption of smoked, pickled and preserved food, a high salt intake, alcohol consumption, smoking tobacco, and low fruit and vegetable intake. The use of refrigeration has resulted in a reduction in the incidence of stomach cancer in the developed world.

Treatment and nutrition

Many patients in Africa present late to health care facilities and a high proportion of patients, many of whom have potentially curable cancer, receive inadequate or no treatment.[22] Further, a high proportion of patients choose to consult a traditional healer either as their first health consultation or as their preferred care provider. For example, 57% of Ugandans[23] do not see a health worker but seek health care from the traditional healer. There is also a requirement for patients to pay for the costs or to cost share their medical treatment and this makes cancer treatment unaffordable. Ocean Road Cancer Institute, the only cancer treatment centre in Tanzania, is able to provide services at no charge as the Tanzanian government pays for the cost of care.[22] An additional logistical challenge is the fact that patients travel long distances to the hospital and stay for the whole duration of their treatment which is at least 6 weeks of radiotherapy and 6–8 months of chemotherapy. With the shortage of health care workers in Africa, many health care facilities require family members to act as caregivers in hospitals as well as at home (see Case report 1).

Effective control of cancer requires training of health care professionals and the establishment of facilities to provide treatment and public education programmes. Priorities for public education programmes and cancer treatment need to be based on the pattern of cancer within the specific country.

The suffering of the poor with AIDS or cancer in developing countries demands not the same response as that provided to the rich but a greater response. It is essential to scale up cancer control programmes[24] that include prevention and treatment and to provide comprehensive palliative care.

Goals of nutritional support within cancer treatment are to maintain or improve nutritional status and to increase tolerance of, and the response to, cancer therapy. Most successful nutritional support involves provision of a normal healthy balanced diet. For example, in situations of poverty, there is often inadequate intake of fruit and vegetables which is exacerbated under conditions of drought. Oral supplementation to normal feeding such as fortified maize meal, consisting of precooked maize supplemented with soya to increase the protein content of the meal and added micronutrients, is an effective intervention. The fortified maize meal can be prepared to the consistency required by each patient.

Micronutrient supplementation itself has been found to improve nutritional status and well-being of both cancer and AIDS patients.[25,26]

As in the developed world, there are particular problems in nutrition for patients with head and neck tumours. Patients with oesophageal cancer often present late and surgical interventions may be required to improve feeding such as dilation or stenting of the oesophagus or the insertion of a gastrostomy feeding tube (see Case report 2). Nutrition is then provided through a soft diet or liquid formula feeds. The formula feed needs to be nutritionally balanced, lactose free, of low osmolality and contain essential micronutrients.

Parenteral nutrition is very rarely available other than in a tertiary hospital setting.

A number of nutritional problems are experienced by cancer patients as a result of therapy such as mucositis, xerostomia, dysphagia, anorexia, nausea, cramps, diarrhoea, radiation enteritis and malabsorption. These all require careful assessment and advice to patient and family members with the involvement of a dietitian, if available.

Malnourished patients have a reduced response to anticancer treatment and reduced tolerance to treatment, are more susceptible to infection, and have decreased survival.[27] Cachexia may occur in up to 80% of patients with advanced cancer.[28] This percentage may be higher in the resource-poor setting where patients on diagnosis are malnourished. The features of cancer cachexia are abnormal metabolism of fats, carbohydrates and proteins, and associated symptoms include anorexia and fatigue.

Palliative care

Nutrition and feeding are fundamental aspects of nurturing. Families caring for patients with advanced cancer are distressed by food refusal in the face of severe weight loss due to anorexia. The issues are similar to those found in resource-rich countries (e.g. see Chapter 19). Sensitive counselling is required, providing information that food requirements are less, that additional food does not improve the patient's outcomes, and advice regarding control of associated symptoms. Offering different foods and small portions can help to allay family members' anxieties around feeding and the fear that their loved one is starving to death. As with all aspects of palliative care, it is essential to individualize nutritional care.

The presentation of food can assist in nutrition support. Smaller portion sizes may be more acceptable to patients. They may prefer food at a particular temperature and it is important to allow flexibility in eating times. Cold food produces less aroma and may be more acceptable for patients experiencing nausea. Some patients develop taste abnormalities, and sweet or spicy food may help overcome these.

Meals are a social event. It may be important for the patient to be at the meal even if not eating very much or if only sipping liquids. If the patient is unable to join the family at meals, the family may join the patient after meals for social time with the patient. If patients have difficulty swallowing or if they drool while eating, they may prefer privacy at meals.

Medications available as appetite stimulants in the resource-poor setting are practically limited to steroids. The appetite stimulant effect is of short duration and side-effects of steroids need to be considered before prescribing these medications. On the whole, other appetite stimulants are not available other than illegally grown cannabis.

Children's issues

Eighty-five per cent of the world's children live in developing countries where access to adequate care is limited and children's health is already compromised through infectious diseases and malnutrition.[29]

The impact of the AIDS epidemic in Sub-Saharan Africa has adversely affected the lives of millions of children, creating orphans and aggravating poverty. It has been estimated that in South Africa in 2006, 70% of children were living in poverty.[30] Care and interventions to assist children need to take into account the fact that children need to grow and develop in addition to receiving appropriate treatment for their illness. Thus food security programmes, educational and developmental activities should be part of children's services.

There are challenges to assessing the nutritional status of children. In general, the road-to-health charts are used, measuring height for age and weight for age with malnutrition measured against expected weight for age. However, in cancer this measurement may be affected by the weight of the tumour. In children with abdominal tumours, the tumour mass may weigh more than 10% of the child's total body weight.[29] More accurate assessment methods include triceps skinfold to measure fat mass, and/or mid-arm circumference measuring lean body weight. These methods are available but not used routinely in paediatric services. Biochemical tests (plasma proteins) are of limited value in the developed world. These measurements are affected by fever and presence of infection, and laboratory tests are not available for assessment of nutritional status in the developing world setting.

The prevalence of malnutrition at diagnosis of cancer averages 50% in children with cancer in developing countries.[29] Malnutrition may be as a result of socio-economic circumstances or as a result of illness with reduced food intake, losses due to malabsorption, or increased needs due to changes in fat and carbohydrate metabolism.

Malnutrition may develop during treatment due to symptoms such as change in taste, nausea and cancer treatment effects—including mucositis and malabsorption. Malnutrition impacts on the child's tolerance of therapy and on survival, and increases the risk of comorbidities. There is evidence that dietary supplementation can reverse malnutrition and improve the tolerance of chemotherapy. However, evidence for nutritional interventions improving survival is not reported.

Case reports

Case 1. Thendai

Thendai is an 8-year-old boy whose home is in northern Tanzania. He was referred to Ocean Road Cancer Institute (ORCI) in Dar es Salaam for treatment of Burkitt lymphoma.

He has massively swollen cervical lymph nodes which have affected his ability to swallow. Before coming to ORCI he was only eating small quantities of thin maize meal porridge or soup and, on admission, was thin and easily fatigued.

He has been admitted to ORCI for 6 months of chemotherapy. ORCI is the only cancer treatment centre in Tanzania, and because of the costs of travel, patients requiring oncology treatment stay in the hospital for the duration of therapy, typically 6 weeks of radiotherapy or 6 months of chemotherapy.

Thendai's father has come with him to care for him during his treatment while his mother and siblings work the land at home. The hospital cannot afford to pay for food for both patient and family member, so his father was sharing Thendai's meals.

The circumstances of the patient and family members were identified by a local faith-based organization which raises funds for and provides meals for many patients and the family members who come to them for care. This organization recognized Thendai's special needs and has been providing nutritious semi-solid meals for Thendai which have greatly helped his response to chemotherapy, with minimal side-effects, his weight gain and his growth. Thendai has a great deal more energy and spends his days playing soccer with other children in the hospital grounds and attending classes when these are available in the hospital so that he does not fall too far behind in his schooling. His oncology team anticipates that his cancer will be cured by the treatment he is receiving.

Case 2. Mathews

Mathews presented to Groote Schuur Hospital with stage IV oesophageal cancer, complaining of dysphagia and retrosternal pain. He was initially treated with internal radiation therapy which produced a minimal improvement in his ability to swallow and had initially increased his pain levels. Mathews was referred to Helderberg Hospice in Cape Town for symptom management and nutritional support. He was severely cachetic. A syringe driver was set up with morphine sulphate 30 mg/24 h and haloperidol 5 mg/24 h. Constipation was controlled by regular use of suppository laxatives. The hospice staff started regular frequent feeds with a fortified nutritional shake mixed with milk and consulted a dietitian and the local surgeon.

The surgeon reviewed the clinical notes from Groote Schuur Hospital and indicated that he felt it would be possible to insert a percutaneous endoscopic gastrostomy (PEG) feeding tube to facilitate feeding and in the anticipation that the cancer would progress and result in complete obstruction of the oesophagus.

Mathews was counselled as to the implications of the PEG feeding tube and consented to the surgery. It became easier to provide nutrition and fluids to Mathews who started to gain weight. He became self-sufficient in mixing his food and in administering the feed through a funnel into the PEG tube. When he was not using the tube this was curled up under his shirt. His medication was also given via the PEG tube.

Mathews went home to his sister and continued to attend day hospice, gaining weight and taking an active role in the day hospice proceedings. The success of this procedure encouraged the hospice staff and the surgeon who worked two sessions per week as a consultant at the local state hospital. Three other patients with cancer of the oesophagus underwent successful PEG procedures until the hospital authorities decided that there were no longer the resources to spend on this procedure for patients with a short prognosis.

Mathews travelled back to his home in rural South Africa but returned to hospice 3 weeks later again in a severely emaciated state. He no longer had the PEG tube in place and it transpired that he had found feeding difficult as it was socially and culturally unacceptable to utilize this method of feeding in his home village, and he had pulled the tube out. There had been no counselling services to support his continued use of the PEG tube or to improve his community's understanding of the circumstances. He had tried to take his liquid morphine orally as well as liquids for nourishment but was unable to swallow successfully. It appeared that he had complete oesophageal obstruction. He was admitted to the hospice, again his medication was delivered via a syringe driver and pain control was achieved. He also received fluids via hypodermoclysis. He died 2 days later.

Conclusion

Nutritional support is an important aspect to consider in implementing cancer control programmes alongside other socio-economic interventions. There continues to be a need for research on nutritional status and nutritional interventions, especially in poorly resourced countries with high burden of disease and poor socio-economic conditions.

References

1. Volmink J, Dare L (2005) Addressing inequalities in research capacity in Africa. *Br Med J*, **331**(7519), 705–6.
2. Morris K (2003) Cancer? In Africa? *Lancet Oncol*, **4**(1), 5.
3. Sepulveda C, Habiyambere V, Amandua J, *et al.* (2003) Quality care at the end of life in Africa. *Br Med J*, **327**(7408), 209–13.
4. Ramsay S (2001) Raising the profile of palliative care for Africa. *Lancet*, **358**(9283), 734.
5. Mufunda J, Chatora R, Ndambakuwa Y, *et al.* (2006) Emerging non-communicable disease epidemic in Africa: preventive measures from the WHO Regional Office for Africa. *Ethn Dis*, **16**(2), 521–6.
6. World Health Organization (2006) *The African Regional Health Report: The Health of the People.* Geneva: WHO.
7. AfrOx. *2007 Declaration on Cancer Control in Africa.* Available at: http://www.afrox.org/declaration.html (accessed 6 January 2009).
8. Murray SA, Grant E, Mwangi-Powell F (2005) Health in Africa: time to wake up to cancer's toll. *Br Med J*, **331**(7521), 904.
9. Parkin DM, Sitas F, Chirenje M, Stein L, Abratt R, Wabinga H (2008) Part I: Cancer in Indigenous Africans—burden, distribution, and trends. *Lancet Oncol*, **9**(7), 683–92.
10. Sitas F, Parkin DM, Chirenje M, Stein L, Abratt R, Wabinga H (2008) Part II: Cancer in Indigenous Africans—causes and control. *Lancet Oncol*, **9**(8), 786–95.
11. Higginson IJ, Bruera E (2002) Do we need palliative care audit in developing countries? *Palliat Med*, **16**(6), 546–7.
12. Harding R, Higginson IJ (2005) Palliative care in sub-Saharan Africa. *Lancet*, **365**(9475), 1971–7.
13. Harding R, Powell RA, Downing J, *et al.* (2008) Generating an African palliative care evidence base: the context, need, challenges, and strategies. *J Pain Sympt Manag*, **36**(3), 304–9
14. Harding R, Stewart K, Marconi K, O'Neill JF, Higginson IJ (2003) Current HIV/AIDS end-of-life care in sub-Saharan Africa: a survey of models, services, challenges and priorities. *BMC Public Health*, **3**, 33.
15. Harding R, Dinat N, Mpanga Sebuyira L (2007) Measuring and improving palliative care in South Africa: multiprofessional clinical perspectives on development and application of appropriate outcome tools. *Prog Palliat Care*, **15**(2), 55–9.
16. Powell RA, Downing J, Radbruch L, Mwangi-Powell F, Harding R (2008) Advancing palliative care research in Sub-Suharan Africa: from Venice to Nairobi and beyond. *Palliat Med.*, **22**, 885–7.
17. Harding R (2008) Palliative care in resource-poor settings: fallacies and misapprehensions. *J Pain Sympt Manag*, **36**(5), 515–7.
18. Israels T, Chirambo C, Caron HN, Molyneux EM (2008) Nutritional status at admission of children with cancer in Malawi. *Pediatr Blood Cancer*, **51**(5), 626–8.
19. UNICEF. The state of the world's children 2008. Available at: http://www.unicef.org/sowc08/docs/sowc08.pdf (accessed 30 October 2008).
20. Simpson P (1995) Cancer and nutrition. In: Pervan P, Cohen LH, Jaftha T (eds), *Oncology for Health-Care Professional*, pp. 571–85. Lansdowne, Western Cape: Juta & Co.
21. Norman R, Mqoqi N, Sitas F (2006) Lifestyle-induced cancer in South Africa. In Steyn K, Fourie J, Temple N (eds), *Lifestyle-induced cancer in South Africa*, pp. 142–85. Cape Town: South African Medical Research Council.
22. International Network for Cancer Treatment and Research (2008) Available at: http://www.inctr.org/ (accessed 30 October 2008).
23. Jagwe J, Merriman A (2007) Uganda: delivering analgesia in rural Africa: opioid availability and nurse prescribing. *J Pain Sympt Manag*, **33**(5), 547–51.
24. Krakuaer E (2008) Just palliative care: responding responsibly to the suffering of the poor. *J Pain Sympt Manag*, **36**(5), 505–512.

25. Department of Health (2001) *South African National Guidelines on Nutrition for People Living with TB, HIV/AIDS and other Chronic Debilitating Conditions*. Available at: http://www.doh.gov.za/docs/factsheets/guidelines/tb/index.htm (accessed 6 January 2009).
26. Gwyther L, Finch L, Garanganga E, *et al.* (2006) Nutrition. In: Gwyther L, Merriman A, Mpanga Sebuyira L, Schietinger H (eds), *A Clinical Guide to Supportive and Palliative Care for HIV/AIDS in Sub-Sarahan Africa*. Alexandria, VA: National Hospice and Palliative Care Organization.
27. Bruera E, Fainsinger RL (1993) Clinical management of cachexia and anorexia. In: Doyle D, Hanks GWC, MacDonald N (eds), *Oxford Textbook of Palliative Medicine*, pp. 548–57. Oxford: Oxford University Press.
28. Del Fabbro E, Dalal S, Bruera E (2006) Symptom control in palliative care—Part II: cachexia/anorexia and fatigue. *J Palliat Med*, **9**(2), 409–21.
29. Sala A, Pencharz P, Barr RD (2004) Children, cancer, and nutrition—a dynamic triangle in review. *Cancer*, **100**(4), 677–87.
30. Marston J (2006) *Palliative Care for Children and Young People in South Africa.* Hospice Palliative Care Association, South Africa.

Chapter 35

Involuntary weight loss and altered body image in patients with cancer anorexia–cachexia syndrome

Susan E. McClement

Introduction

Patients with advanced cancer frequently experience anorexia, involuntary weight loss, muscle wasting, and profound fatigue.[1] These symptoms are manifestations of the cancer anorexia–cachexia syndrome (CACS), a complex process of metabolic abnormalities resulting in skeletal muscle catabolism and fat loss.[2] Patients can experience involuntary and unabated weight loss, despite the maintenance of adequate nutritional intake, and often look like victims of famine.[3]

Because marked weight loss and muscle wasting are poor prognostic indicators,[4] much research attention has been directed toward understanding the underlying biological mechanisms of involuntary weight loss in cancer patients, and the evaluation of anticachexia therapies.[5] However, experiencing unwanted physical changes in one's body due to illness also affects body image, and can result in social isolation, lowered self-esteem, anxiety, depression, and a decreased quality of life.[6,7] Holistic care of cachectic patients and their families requires that we attend to both the biomedical and psychosocial impacts of cancer cachexia.[8] This multidimensional understanding of cancer cachexia is foundational to the development and testing of interventions aimed at supporting patients who experience involuntary weight loss and their families.

The purpose of this chapter is to examine the experience of involuntary weight loss and altered body image from the perspectives of advanced cancer patients and their families.

Body image: conceptual issues

The construct of body image is complex. Early definitions of body image that focused exclusively on individual perception and satisfaction with one's physical appearance[9] have given way to an appreciation that body image is a multidimensional experience encompassing a person's body-related self-perceptions, self-attitudes, beliefs, feelings, and behaviours.[10] Current thinking about body image now also acknowledges the construct's inherent subjective and perceptual elements, and the ways in which it can be influenced by historical, contextual, environmental, and developmental variables.[11]

Body image has been examined from a variety of theoretical perspectives, including cognitive behavioural theory, psychodynamic theory, terror management theory, and self-discrepancy theory.[12] The application of these diverse theoretical perspectives speak to the complexity of the body image construct and have the potential to provide varied and unique insights about body image that have relevant clinical application. For example, self-discrepancy theory posits that patients with alterations in body image that are discrepant from the ideal body image to which they aspire, evaluate that alteration both from their own personal perspective, and from the perspectives they perceive others hold of them. Such evaluations generate body image emotions, and drive behaviour arising from these emotions.[13] Thus in order to intervene effectively, clinicians must explore both patients' own thoughts and emotions about their altered bodies, and the assumptions they ascribe to others.

The impact that cancer and its treatment can have on body image is well recognized in the psycho-oncology literature.[14] Despite the fact that body image has been identified as an important research outcome, it has not been clearly defined and/or been conflated with terms such as stigma, self-esteem and self-consciousness.[13]

Moreover, attempts to operationalize body image in cancer research tend to be unidimensional, thereby failing to distinguish distinct facets subsumed within the body image construct, such as 'positive versus negative', and 'secure versus insecure' body image.[15] Conceptually driven research and theoretically derived interventions are contingent upon conceptual clarity. Therefore, conceptual 'muddiness' concerning body image is inherently problematic from a research perspective. Caution must be exercised to ensure congruence between body image measures and research aims.

Salience of weight loss and body image in CACS research

Research examining unintentional and non-treatment-related weight loss in patients with advanced cancer has been conducted. This work has focused on such issues as the impact of nutritional counselling, the effects of weight loss on performance status and global quality of life scores, and the relationships between weight loss, appetite, the inflammatory response, and survival duration.[16–20] Attention has also been directed toward the development and testing of instruments aimed at assessing the subjective improvement anorectic–cachectic patients have in their mood, sense of well-being, body image, and ability to derive pleasure from eating.[21,22] However, a thorough understanding of cancer anorexia–cachexia involves more than knowledge garnered solely from biomedical research.[23] Psychosocial research examining the experiential aspects of CACS-related wasting from the perspective of patients and families is also important (Box 35.1).[23]

Box 35.1 Importance of research examining the experience of involuntary weight loss in people with cancer cachexia

- The patient and family constitute the unit of care. Thus, an 'insider's' understanding of the experience from the perspective of patients and families is needed to develop meaningful psychotherapeutic interventions.
- Clinicians must be able to support patients who experience health-stigma resulting from the reactions of others to weight loss.
- Patients need assistance in maintaining a dignified appearance while managing feelings arising because of physical changes
- Social support networks have the capacity to support or erode cachectic patients' reintegration into society.
- Altered physical appearance is associated with a fractured sense of patient dignity, loss of will to live, increased desire for death, depression, hopelessness, and anxiety.

First, the development of meaningful psychosocial interventions requires that clinicians understand the emic or lived experience of involuntary weight loss and altered body image from those affected by it; namely patients and their family members.

Second, the changes in physical appearance and bodily functioning seen in patients with CACS may provoke negative reactions and behaviours of others, making patients feel unworthy, inadequate and unwelcome. This experience, known as health-related stigma, leads to the social disqualification of individuals and populations who are identified with particular health problems.[24] The reactions of others toward one's body are felt deeply. An understanding of the nature and extent of health-related stigma experienced by patients may help clinicians develop interventions designed to support those who feel stigmatized to enhance their resilience and limit their feelings of vulnerability.

Third, Price[25] theorizes that those with life-threatening illnesses may have greater body image needs than healthy individuals, in order to sustain contact with others who might lend support. These include maintaining a comfortable and dignified physical appearance and managing verbal accounts of how one's physical body makes one feel.

The importance of supportive social networks in illness has been described in the literature,[26] and the social support network within which individuals manage life crises such as cancer has been shown to influence adaptation.[27,28] Supportive social networks are the optimal context within which body image is developed and sustained. They are also the context within which an altered body image is reintegrated into society.[29] This suggests that patient perceptions of social support should be assessed as part of the patient's psychosocial care, as they impact the body image.

Fifth, CACS-related wasting is a highly visible external sign of serious illness and is perceived as a harbinger of death, particularly for family members who often pressure patients to eat and petition health care providers to implement aggressive nutritional interventions.[30–32] Given that the patient and family constitute the unit of care, awareness of family perspectives regarding the involuntary wasting of their relative is essential.

Finally, empirical work conducted by Chochinov *et al.* examining the construct of dignity in end-of-life care suggests that changes in physical appearance can erode advanced cancer patients' sense of dignity.[33] A cross-sectional cohort study of terminally ill cancer patients with a life expectancy of less than 6 months ($n = 213$) was conducted toidentify demographic and disease-specific variables related to dignity in the terminally ill, and to discern the extent to which those near the end of life perceive that they are able to maintain a sense of dignity. Among the 16 patients in this study who experienced a fractured sense of dignity, appearance emerged as the strongest predictor of an undermined sense of dignity ($\chi^2 = 7.29$; $P = 0.007$). These patients also reported loss of will to live, increased desire for death, depression, hopelessness, and anxiety.[33]

Given the profound impacts of cachexia on body image, and the fact that to date, the physical wasting seen in CACS is largely irreversible, research describing the experience of unintentional weight loss is warranted, with an aim to inform the development of psychological interventions to help modulate CACS-related distress.

Empirical work

Though still in its infancy, research examining experiences of cancer cachexia-related weight loss and changes in body image is beginning to appear in the literature.

Guided by Paterson and Zderad's humanistic nursing theory and Wolcott's framework for qualitative data analysis, Hopkinson *et al.*[34] examined the experience of weight loss and its management from the perspective of advanced cancer patients with heterogeneous diagnoses ($n = 30$), their caregivers ($n = 23$), and nurse specialists ($n = 14$) in the south of England. Findings revealed that whereas all patients were aware that they had lost weight, not all patients expected weight loss to occur as part of their disease. Patients also varied regarding the concern that weight loss engendered for them.

Weight loss that became visible to others was distressing for some patients because it symbolized both physical disease and emotional weakness. By contrast, other patients commented upon the health benefits of weight loss such as improved mobility. Some patients in the study believed that they were personally responsible for maintaining their weight during the illness through the consumption of adequate caloric intake. Other patients felt helpless in response to a loss of control over unabated weight loss—feelings exacerbated by expressions by health care providers that nothing could be done to alleviate this symptom.

Because nurses felt they had little to offer patients losing weight, they were careful not to initiate discussion about this symptom, preferring to address weight loss only if it was raised by the patient or family. Consequently, a reactive versus proactive style of symptom management tended to ensue.

Drawing on the tenets of social theory and constructions of the self as derived from the chronic illness literature, Hinsley and Hughes[35] conducted conversational interviews with a purposive sample of palliative patients with heterogeneous cancer diagnoses living in the community in southeast England ($n = 12$). Findings of the study revealed that, in addition to weight loss, the other symptoms experienced as part of their cachexia made patients feel self-conscious; a feeling exacerbated by the reactions of other people toward their changed appearance, and one that resulted in patients limiting their social interaction with others, and/or dressing to try and avoid drawing attention to their weight loss.

Patients described their bodies with reference to images of emaciation, and reported feeling physically unattractive and sexually undesirable. Accordingly, some patients revealed the need to protect their loved ones from seeing the physical ravages of marked weight loss.

Patients also experienced feelings of fear and uncertainty regarding the meaning of weight loss as part of their illness and were frustrated that they were not able to reverse this loss. They were living a restricted life characterized by loss of autonomy and feelings of being a burden to others.

McClement *et al.* conducted a qualitative study based on the tenets of grounded theory to explore the perspectives of cachectic palliative cancer patients ($n = 15$) attending an outpatient pain and symptom management clinic, and their families ($n = 5$), regarding the experience of involuntary weight loss and wasting. Data were collected through audiotaped individual face-to-face interviews, which were transcribed verbatim and analysed using constant comparative analysis techniques.

The overarching theme to emerge was that of 'dealing with a body in shambles'; an experience encompassing the physical, emotional, and social changes and challenges arising from disease-related weight loss with which patients and family members had to contend. A brief overview of these changes and challenges and the strategies used to deal with them is provided here.

Physical changes and challenges

It was evident that in addition to experiencing involuntary weight loss, patients in this study suffered from a myriad of other symptoms including, but not limited to, overwhelming fatigue, anorexia, nausea, vomiting, diarrhoea, constipation and gastrointestinal bleeding. Accordingly, patients needed to talk about weight loss within the context of their overall illness experience. In addition to weight loss, fatigue was identified as highly problematic for patients, because of its negative impact on their quality of life. Said this patient: 'The thing that bothers me most is feeling tired all the time and having no energy. I lay on the chesterfield all day long. It is ridiculous. I have no life.' Family members were also aware of the multiple symptoms that patients experienced, frequently tracking their prevalence and severity between doctor's visits.

Participants evoked graphic images to convey the physical changes that were happening to their bodies. Statements such as, 'I look like a concentration camp survivor starving in Dakau' and, 'This bony thing shows up in the mirror every morning, and my eyes fall on this creature on the other side of the mirror' speak to the experience of emaciation, excessive depletion and carnage of the physical body that rendered it foreign and almost unrecognizable to its owner.

Emotional changes and challenges

Patient interviews were replete with references to the feelings and emotions they experienced as a result of losing weight. Because many of the patients interviewed for this study were overweight prior to their cancer diagnosis and treatment, they were startled when they realized just exactly how much weight they had lost. Paradoxically in some cases, weight loss was welcomed, because of the putative health benefits of a lower body mass index and less abdominal fat. In other instances, the ability to wear smaller-sized clothing, something not previously experienced despite efforts at dieting, were enjoyed. Said one woman, 'I always wanted to be a size 4, and now I am!'

Such joy was fleeting, however. Once it was clear that the weight loss was continuing unabated despite efforts to prevent it, both patients and family members expressed feelings of fear, anxiety, and loss of control. Moreover, such weight loss served as a frightening symbol and potent reminder of the gravity of the patient's medical condition and a foreshadowing of things to come; something captured eloquently by this study participant: 'It means you're slowly dying. You're losing your life energy, your life essence, slowly but surely. It tells you that maybe you'll loose more weight. You'll just be a pile of bones with a covering of skin. That's what it tells me.'

Relationship changes and challenges

Patients experiencing weight loss reported changes in the nature of their social interactions with others. Particularly distressing were encounters in which patients' physical bodies had changed so much that they were 'beyond recognition' to friends and acquaintances. Said this participant: 'I was 5 feet from him before he could figure out who it was. I cried, because he was a very, very good friend of mine. It seemed to confirm the fact that I was so skinny. That I had lost too much weight.'

As regards relationships, participants consistently reported that friends and family members often behaved awkwardly toward them; not knowing what to do or say. Some people would ask pointed questions, wanting to know about all aspects of the disease and treatment, while others would shy away from conversation or avoid interacting with the patient and family all together. For their part, participants in this study expressed the desire to be treated so as to feel 'normal'. One patient said: 'Just let me feel as normal as you. Be my friend, and treat me like you did before.'

Patient–family dyads reported role changes and relationship tensions that had their genesis in the patient's anorexia and weight loss. Family members often aggressively pressured patients to eat, and experienced patients as being stubborn and uncooperative when caloric intake was sub-optimal, or when 'junk food' as opposed to 'health food' was being consumed. Constantly reminding another adult to eat made this family member feel like she was parenting her husband versus being his partner; a role she neither wanted to assume nor enjoyed: she noted, 'The hardest is that I feel so much like I'm a parent. And I don't want to be that. I'm trying to keeping it out of our relationship.'

Strategies to deal with a body in shambles

Data revealed that patients used several strategies in an attempt to deal with the physical, emotional, and relationship changes engendered by 'a body in shambles'.

As regards the physical changes experienced, several patients indicated that it was important to eat as much as they could, even when they did not feel like doing so. Such efforts were seen as essential in trying to stave off additional weight loss. The deliberate conscious efforts connected with this are captured in such statements as 'forcing myself to eat', and 'I force many a meal'. Family members were often very actively involved in trying to fix something that the patient would eat, and would try 'anything and everything' in that regard.

When asked about the role of nutritional information and counselling from health care providers in helping patients and families deal with weight loss, two distinct types of experiences were described. Some participants identified that they had received little if any information about how they might approach their waning appetite and weight loss, and would have found such information helpful.

Conversely, others identified that they had been scheduled to meet with a dietician to talk about ways of enhancing their intake of protein and calories. Some patients appreciated the recommendation to take supplements like Ensure®, but found them to be unpalatable. Other patients found the recommendation to include high calorie foods in their diet counterintuitive because of the negative health effects associated with such foods. Said this patient: 'I met with the dietitian and she recommended trail mix and some other fattening foods. I've been off anything with fat in it, so now I'm trying to dose myself with these fattening types of foods. The kind we read we're not supposed to eat.' One participant who was outright dismissive of the dietary counselling she received commented, 'I am going back to fruit.'

Some patients reported that they tried to manage physical changes in their body by dressing to help conceal signs of wasting. This typically involved the use of layering, and wearing baggy clothes. Said this participant: 'I want my arms and legs covered, because they're scrawny. I want loose clothing like pajamas and loose tops so you wouldn't see it'. Through use of this strategy, patients hoped to minimize the negative reaction of others encountered in social settings. By contrast, family members often thought that well-tailored bright-coloured clothing drew less appearance to a gaunt frame.

A strategy patients used to minimize their feelings of social isolation involved reaching out to friends and acquaintances. While some patients were content to take the lead in initiating social contact, others resented the fact that they were saddled with this task. Said one patient of his friends: 'I have to hound them. I have to reach out to them and I have to help them, and not look to them to help me. "I am the one going through this and I'm the one having to help you", and it just doesn't seem right.'

Implications for practice and research

While limited, research examining the psychosocial domain of weight loss and changes in body image secondary to cancer cachexia is instructive (Box 35.2).

First, it underscores the importance of creating a space in the clinical encounter where health care providers can dialogue proactively with patients and families about the questions and concerns they have about weight loss. To render such discussions taboo, waiting for patients to raise issues and concerns because health professionals feel helpless to know what to do is ethically indefensible. As suggested by the work of Hopkinson *et al.*,[34] research evaluating the effect of educational initiatives for nurses regarding ways of communicating with patients and families about weight loss is indicated. Such work could include outcome measures of nurses' feelings of

Box 35.2 Implications for practice and research

- Anticipate that patients and families have concerns about weight loss, and explore this with them.
- Attend to the social aspects of the patient's illness, and interact with patients in ways that support independence and choice.
- Affirm to patients that they are valued for the person they are, irrespective of any physical changes.
- Explore desire for nutritional counselling. Anticipate that instructions to consume high caloric foods may be discrepant with patient notions of a 'healthy diet'.
- Ensure meticulous management of symptoms that have the potential to affect oral intake.
- Explore family members' feelings regarding the patients' health status, and consider referral for formalized psychosocial support.
- Meanings of illness are culturally mediated, thus consider the ways in which culture may be influencing patient and family responses to cachexia.

role-efficacy, and patient/family feelings of anxiety, helplessness, symptom distress, adaptation to illness; and satisfaction with communication.

Second, extant work speaks to the marked changes in social interaction that many cancer patients experience when living with weight loss. Health care providers must attend to the social aspects of the patient's illness, and interact with patients in ways that support independence and choice, and affirm to them that they are valued for the person as they are, irrespective of any physical changes that have occurred as a result of their illness. This has such implications for practice as communicating with the patient about those aspects of his/his life not affected by the disease; learning about the patient's biography, attending to those aspects of life that are valued most; and identifying and facilitating patient participation in those activities that are most meaningful, given a limited life expectancy.[36]

Third, nutritional information and counselling is viewed as important by some patients and families in managing weight loss. Therefore, the desire for such services needs to be determined and opportunities to access them provided in a timely manner, as part of the patient's plan of care. Those providing such counselling need to be aware that messages to consume high caloric foods may run counter to patient and family perceptions of a healthy diet, and rather than consume protein dense foods, some patients may opt to maximize fruit and vegetable intake. This type of low energy density dietary pattern among cancer patients identified previously in the literature and is problematic because it places patients at great risk of malnutrition.[37]

Fourth, research reveals that some patients are deliberately forcing themselves to eat in the face of anorexia. This behaviour, identified in a grounded theory study by Schragge *et al.*,[38] is known as 'shifting to conscious control'; a process used by cancer patients to manage the social and emotional consequences of declining intake. Clinicians can support patients in the use of this strategy through meticulous control of symptoms negatively impacting oral intake.

Fifth, declining intake and weight loss causes tension between many patients and families who may hold disparate views about the most appropriate approach to dealing with these symptoms.[23–25,39,40] The anxiety, helplessness, and role changes experienced in families in response to the patient's illness suggests the need for psychosocial interventions aimed at ameliorating this distress and optimizing family functioning. Such intervention may take the form of a therapeutic family support group session wherein the feelings and concerns of members' could be safely vetted, strategies for ameliorating them devised, and their efficacy in helping family members to cope evaluated.

Finally, the majority of research examining experiences of weight loss, conducted in the USA, the UK and Canada, has produced relatively consistent findings.[23] An even greater global understanding of the experience of weight loss would be realized were research to be conducted with diverse cultural samples. The meanings ascribed to illness symptoms are culturally mediated.[8,41] Research accessing the experiences of different cultural groups will help to optimize our understanding about weight loss and changes in body image in patients with CACS and their families, and provide the basis for developing culturally appropriate interventions.

Conclusion

Cancer cachexia is a pervasive clinical problem that profoundly affects cancer patients and their families, yet little is known about the psychosocial issues spawned by the experience of weight loss and changes in body image.

The work conducted to date, however, suggests that psychosocial interventions may mitigate the distress that patients and families experience. Systematic cross-disciplinary research aimed at both characterizing the nature and prevalence of psychological distress occurring because of involuntary weight loss, and developing psychotherapeutic interventions in response to them, is urgently needed. Without it, clinicians will be bereft of empirically based interventions to offer advanced cancer patients and their families.

References

1. Tsai JS, Wu CH, Chiu TY, Hy WY, Chen CY (2006) Symptom patterns of advanced cancer patients in a palliative care unit. *Palliat Med*, **20**, 617–22.
2. Billingsley KG, Alexander HR (1996) The pathophysiology of cachexia in advanced cancer and AIDS. In: Bruera E, Higginson I (eds), *Cachexia–Anorexia in Cancer Patients*, pp. 1–22. Oxford: Oxford University Press.
3. MacDonald N, Easson AM, Mazurak VC, Dunn GP, Baracos VE (2003) Understanding and managing cancer cachexia. *J Am Coll Surg*, **197**, 143–61.
4. DeWys WD, Begg C, Lavin PT, *et al.* (1980) Prognostic effect of weight loss prior to chemotherapy in cancer patients. Eastern Cooperative Oncology Group. *Am J Med*, **80**, 491–497.
5. Baracos VE (2006) Cancer-associated cachexia and underlying biological mechanisms. *Annu Rev Nutr*, **26**, 435–61.
6. Bessell A, Moss TP (2007) Evaluating the effectiveness of psychosocial interventions for individuals with visible differences: a systematic review of the empirical literature. *Body Image*, **4**, 227–38.
7. Grogan S (2006) Body image and health: contemporary perspectives. *J Health Psychol*, **11**, 523–30.
8. McClement SE, Woodgate RL (1997) Care of the terminally ill cachectic cancer patient: interface between nursing and psychological anthropology. *Eur J Cancer Care*, **6**, 295–303.
9. Pruzinsky T (2004) Enhancing quality of life in medical populations: a vision for body image assessment and rehabilitation as standards of care. *Body Image*, **1**, 71–81.
10. Herbozo S, Thompson JK (2006) Development and validation of the verbal commentary on physical appearance scale: considering both positive and negative commentary. *Body Image*, **3**, 335–44.
11. Rudiger JA, Cash TF, Roehrig M, Thompson JK (2007) Day-to-day body-image states: prospective predictors of intra-individual level and variability. *Body Image*, **4**, 1–9.
12. Cash TF, Pruzinsky T (eds) (2002) *Body Image: A Handbook of Theory, Research and Clinical Practice*. New York: Guilford Press.

13. White CA (2000) Body image dimensions and cancer: a heuristic cognitive behavioral model. *Psychooncology*, **9**, 183–92.
14. Hopwood P (1993) The assessment of body image in cancer patients. *Eur J Cancer*, **29A**, 276–81.
15. Fisher S (1990) The evolution of psychological concepts about the body. In: Cash TF, Pruzinsky T (eds), *Body Images: Development Deviance and Change*, pp. 3–20. New York: Guilford Press.
16. Halfdanarson TR, Thordardottir EO, West CP, Jatoi A (2008) Does dietary counseling improve quality of life in cancer patients? A systematic review and meta-analysis. *J Support Oncol*, **6**, 234–7.
17. Melnyk SE, Cash TF, Janda LH (2004) Body image ups and downs: prediction of intra-individual level and variability of women's daily body image experiences. *Body Image*, **1**, 225–35.
18. O'Gorman P, McMillan DC, McAndle CS (1998) Impact of weight loss, appetite, and the inflammatory response on quality of life in gastrointestinal cancer patients. *Nutr Cancer*, **32**, 76–80.
19. Sarna L, Lindsey AM, Dean H, Brecht ML, McCorkle R (1993) Nutritional intake, weight change, symptom distress, and functional status over time in adults with lung cancer. *Oncol Nurs Forum*, **20**, 481–9.
20. Davidson W, Ash S, Capra S, Bauer J (2004) Cancer Cachexia Study Group. Weight stabilisation is associated with improved survival duration and quality of life in unresectable pancreatic cancer. *Clin Nutr*, **23**, 239–47.
21. Cella DF, VonRoenn J, Lloyd S, Browder HP (1995) The Bristol–Myers Anorexia/Cachexia Recovery Instrument (BACRI): a brief assessment of patients' subjective response to treatment for anorexia/cachexia. *Qual Life Res*, **4**, 221–31.
22. Ribaudo JM, Cella D, Hahn EA, *et al.* (2000) Re-validation and shortening of the Functional Assessment of Anorexia/Cachexia Therapy (FAACT) questionnaire. *Qual Life Res*, **9**, 1137–46.
23. Poole K, Frogatt K (2002) Loss of weight and loss of appetite in advanced cancer: a problem for the patient, the carer, or the health professional? *Palliat Med*, **16**, 499–506.
24. Weiss MG, Ramakrishna J, Somma D (2006) Health-related stigma: rethinking concepts and interventions. *Psychol Health Med*, **11**, 277–87.
25 Price B (2000) Altered body image: managing social encounters. *Int J Palliat Nurs*, **6**, 179–85.
26. Wortman C (1984) Social support and the cancer patient: conceptual and methodologic issues. *Cancer*, **15**(10 Suppl), 2339–62.
27. Lepore SJ, Glaser DB, Roberts KJ (2008) On the positive relation between received social support and negative affect: a test of the triage and self-esteem threat models in women with breast cancer. *Psychooncology* [Epub Jul 9].
28. Bloom JR (2008) Improving the health and well-being of cancer survivors: past as prologue. *Psychooncology*, **17**, 525–32.
29. Price B (2000) Altered body image: managing social encounters. *Int J Palliat Nurs*, **6**, 179–85.
30 McClement SE (2005) Cancer anorexia–cachexia-syndrome [CACS]: psychological impact on the patient and family. *J Wound Ostomy Continence Nurs*, **32**, 264–8.
31. McClement SE, Degner LF, Harlos MS (2004) Family responses to declining intake in a terminally ill relative: Part I: "Fighting Back". *J Palliat Care*, **20**, 93–100.
32. McClement SE, Degner LF, Harlos MS (2003) Family beliefs regarding the nutritional care of a terminally ill relative. *J Palliat Med*, **6**, 737–48.
33. Chochinov HM, Hack T, Hassard T, Kristjanson LJ, McClement S, Harlos M (2002) Dignity in the terminally ill: a cross-sectional, cohort study. *Lancet*, **360**, 2026–30.
34 Hopkinson J, Wright D, Corner J (2006) Exploring the experience of weight loss in people with advanced cancer. *J Adv Nurs*, **54**, 304–12.
35. Hinsley R, Hughes R (2007) The reflections you get: an exploration of body image and cachexia. *Int J Palliat Nurs*, **13**, 84–9.
36. McClement SE, Chochinov HM, Hack TF, Kristjanson LJ, Harlos M (2004) Dignity-conserving care: application of research findings to practice. *Int J Palliat Nurs*, **10**, 173–9.

37. Hutton JL, Martin L, Field CJ, *et al.* (2006) Dietary patterns in patients with advanced cancer: implications for anorexia–cachexia therapy. *Am J Clin Nutr*, **84**, 1163–70.
38. Shragge JE, Wismer WV, Olson KL, Baracos VE (2007) Shifting to conscious control: psychosocial and dietary management of anorexia by patients with advanced cancer. *Palliat Med*, **21**, 227–33.
39. Strasser F, Binswanger J, Cerny T, Kesselring A (2007) Fighting a losing battle: eating-related distress of men with advanced cancer and their female partners. A mixed-methods study. *Palliat Med*, **21**, 129–37.
40. McClement SE, Harlos M (2008) When advanced cancer patients won't eat: family member responses. *Int J Palliat Nurs*, **14**, 185–91.
41. Justice C (1995) The natural death while not eating: a type of palliative care in Banares, India. *J Palliat Care*, **11**, 38–42.

Index